MEDICAL OFFICE
Administration

A Worktext

MEDICAL OFFICE Administration

A Worktext

THIRD EDITION

BRENDA A. POTTER, BS, CPC-I, CPC

Medical Administrative Program Director

Minnesota State Community & Technical College

Moorhead, Minnesota

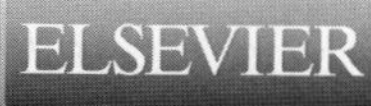

ELSEVIER
SAUNDERS

3251 Riverport Lane
St. Louis, Missouri 63043

MEDICAL OFFICE ADMINISTRATION: A WORKTEXT ISBN: 978-1-4377-2739-5

ISBN: 978-1-4377-2739-5

Executive Content Strategist: Jennifer Janson
Associate Content Development Specialist: Elizabeth Bawden
Content Coordinator: Laurel Berkel
Publishing Services Manager: Julie Eddy
Senior Project Manager: Marquita Parker
Design Manager: Teresa McBryan

Printed in the United States of America

Last digit is the print number: 9 8 7 6 5 4 3 2

All our dreams can come true, if we have the courage to pursue them.

—Walt Disney

To my husband—your boundless love and support enabled the pursuit of this and many other dreams.

To my children and grandchildren—you are the most precious gift I have ever received. May you realize your dreams.

To my parents and family—thank you for your constant encouragement and support.

To my students and students everywhere—as you have inspired me, so may I inspire you.

I am truly blessed and forever grateful for your presence in my life.

Editorial Review Board

Preface

The best interest of the patient
is the only interest to be considered.
- Dr. William J. Mayo, 1910

No better words than these can describe the focus of and purpose for the third edition of *Medical Office Administration*. The patient is, indeed, the very purpose of anyone's work in health care. Whether employed in the business aspect of a medical office or in direct patient care, each patient is the very reason for our presence in the office. The health care industry is very patient focused and customer-sensitive (as it should be), and we must recognize that the patient is indeed our customer.

Changes in the industry continue at an accelerated pace, and new electronic technologies continue to alter the face of health care. Health records are becoming increasingly computerized, allowing a patient's health information to be accessed almost instantly, wherever and whenever needed. Some individuals in health care office careers now work from home. Computers have made their way into the examination room, the operating room, and nearly every department of a health care organization. The face of medical transcription and medical coding is changing at a rapid pace.

Medical Office Administration, Third Edition, explores the career of a medical administrative assistant, beginning with an examination of the profession and the health care industry, and continuing on to the daily responsibilities of a medical administrative assistant. The text is organized into five units and 16 chapters which are designed to prepare the student for employment as a medical administrative assistant.

Medical Office Administration, Third Edition, is intended to meet the medical administrative competencies developed by the Commission on Accreditation of Allied Health Education Programs (CAAHEP) Competencies and the Accrediting Bureau of Health Education Schools (ABHES) Competencies. Procedure checklists included in this text provide a detailed outline to help students to meet administrative competencies and instructors to evaluate those competencies. The text can be used by anyone who desires to understand the day-to-day business activities of a medical office.

In updating this third edition of *Medical Office Administration,* my basic focus included enhancing the exercises, activities, and discussion points that encourage students to problem-solve and think critically. Although memorization of some facts may be necessary, it is my belief that students must be able to apply their factual knowledge to the myriad of situations that may arise in a medical office. The text encourages this skill through features that present the complexities of the medical office environment:

- The text includes enhanced reading content, as well as questions, activities, and discussion.
- Medisoft Version 18 medical management software is available with the text as a package or separate option. Several chapters include computer activities that encompass a variety of realistic work situations, from appointment scheduling and registration, to billing and insurance claims. It is highly recommended that students use the Medisoft software component to ensure their readiness for the work world.

Procedure

- Procedure boxes offer step-by-step instructions for performing specific administrative tasks.

HIPAA Hint

- The HIPAA Hint feature emphasizes important HIPAA points that apply to everyday events in a medical office.

Checkpoint

- Checkpoint features in each chapter give students the opportunity to apply knowledge gained in the chapter to a situation that requires critical thinking.

You Are the Medical Administrative Assistant

- You Are the Medical Administrative Assistant is a feature that allows the reader to apply knowledge learned in the chapter to realistic medical office scenarios.
- Competency assessment checklists (found in Appendix 2) detail the individual steps required to complete a full range of administrative procedures and allow the instructor or student to evaluate performance.

Throughout my various career experiences in both health care and the business world, I have lived and breathed what students will experience in the workplace. In my role as a medical administrative program director at Minnesota State Community and Technical College in Moorhead, Minnesota, I have assisted hundreds of students in gaining employment in health care organizations. Exceptional patient service is essential to the success of a health care organization and is a common thread woven throughout this text. How we interact and treat others is crucial to the success of any organization. It is my sincere hope that every day we make a positive difference in the lives of those we meet, and that this text enables students to make that positive difference for patients.

Brenda A. Potter, BS, CPC-I, CPC

Acknowledgments

My heartfelt thanks to everyone involved in this project, especially:

- To Elizabeth Bawden, Associate Content Development Specialist, whose thoughtfulness, dedication, and attention to detail made this work a reality;
- To Jennifer Janson, Content Strategist, whose guidance made this project possible;
- To Teresa McBryan, Manager, Art & Design, whose skills made this project look terrific;
- To the McKesson Corporation, for graciously providing the Medisoft software and related support for this work;
- To the reviewers whose commentary helped refine this edition;
- To my colleagues at Minnesota State Community & Technical College, who have continued to provide feedback and encouragement that has enabled this work to evolve;
- To my students, past and present, who inspired and who are the reason for this work.
- And in fond memory of Susan Cole, Executive Editor, whose vision and support contributed to the overall success of this work.

Your presence and encouragement made this text possible. I could not have done this without you. I am eternally grateful to all of you.

Contents

CHAPTER 1 The Career of a Medical Administrative Assistant

LEARNING OUTCOMES

On successful completion of this chapter, the student will be able to

1. Identify various titles for office positions usually filled by a medical administrative assistant and list the places where an assistant might find related employment.
2. Describe the typical job duties of a medical administrative assistant.
3. Explain the desired personal qualities of a medical administrative assistant.
4. Demonstrate appropriate professional appearance for a medical administrative assistant.
5. Identify professional skills needed by a medical administrative assistant.
6. Describe the importance of a student portfolio and begin a portfolio.
7. Identify employment information (e.g., earnings, employment trends, and forecasts related to the medical administrative assistant profession).
8. Name professional organizations and related certifications for medical administrative assistants.

COMMISSION ON ACCREDITATION OF ALLIED HEALTH EDUCATION PROGRAMS (CAAHEP) CORE CURRICULUM FOR MEDICAL ASSISTANTS

- Use Internet to access information related to the medical office.
- Discuss legal scope of practice for medical assistants.
- Perform within scope of practice.

ACCREDITING BUREAU OF HEALTH EDUCATION SCHOOLS (ABHES) PROGRAMMATIC EVALUATION STANDARDS FOR MEDICAL ASSISTING

Graduates

- Comprehend the current employment outlook for the medical assistant.
- Have knowledge of the general responsibilities of the medical assistant.
- Demonstrate professionalism by:
  - Exhibiting dependability, punctuality, and a positive work ethic.
  - Exhibiting a positive attitude and a sense of responsibility.
  - Exhibiting initiative.
  - Expressing a responsible attitude.
  - Being courteous and diplomatic.
  - Conducting work within scope of education, training, and ability.

VOCABULARY

certified administrative professional (CAP)
certified coding specialist (CCS)
certified coding specialist–physician based (CCS-P)
certified healthcare documentation specialist (CHDS)
certified medical administrative specialist (CMAS)
certified medical assistant (CMA)
certified professional coder (CPC)
certified professional coder–hospital (CPC-H)
certified professional coder–payer (CPC-P)
compassion
confidentiality
empathy
medical administrative assistant
medical assistant
medical transcriptionist
registered healthcare documentation specialist (RHDS)
registered medical assistant (RMA)
student portfolio

Wanted: Enthusiastic, caring, empathetic individual with an interest in health care to work in a large or small office with few or many coworkers. Must be able to handle the stress of a heavy workload and be able to multitask on a daily basis.

This is quite an interesting job description, isn't it? Although such an advertisement probably would never appear in a newspaper, it is very descriptive of what many employers expect of a medical administrative assistant.

You selected this career for your own reasons. You may have an interest in health care, you may enjoy working with people, or maybe you were looking for a career where you could make a difference.

Students who elect to pursue a career in the medical office may or may not already have an idea of what a medical administrative assistant does. Working in a medical office is exciting, rewarding, and challenging. It seems that every day there is something new to learn about the health care field.

Just what will be expected of you on the job? Quite a bit, actually! Let's begin to take a look at all that is involved in the career of a medical administrative assistant.

Career Description

When you are seeking employment as an administrative assistant in health care, one of the first things to note is the many different titles that are used for this type of administrative position.

In this text, the title **medical administrative assistant** has been carefully chosen to identify an individual who serves patient and organizational needs by performing a huge variety of office support or business functions within a health care organization. This position is identified by a variety of titles in the marketplace, a few of which are listed in Box 1-1. The title *medical administrative assistant* is used because *administrative assistant* is a commonly used and accepted term for an individual who performs office support functions, and *medical administrative assistant* identifies an individual who performs these activities in a health care setting (Fig. 1-1).

BOX 1-1

Possible Titles for a Medical Administrative Assistant

- Medical Office Assistant
- Medical Office Associate
- Medical Office Specialist
- Medical Receptionist
- Medical Secretary/Transcriptionist
- Patient Registration Specialist
- Patient Services Coordinator
- Patient Services Representative
- Patient Services Specialist
- Patient Services Assistant

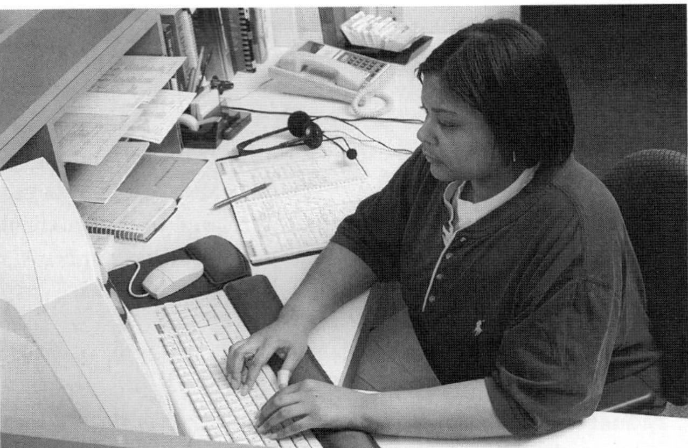

Figure 1-1 A medical administrative assistant uses a computer to perform many of a medical office's administrative support functions.

Job Duties

Although a variety of job titles exist for the position of medical administrative assistant, the essential duties remain the same. What might those duties include?

Job responsibilities for a medical administrative assistant can vary widely, depending on the specific duties of the position in a particular organization. Each organization has its own, unique needs that are dependent on the nature and structure of the organization. For example, an assistant's responsibilities may be very different whether employed by a one-physician private practice, an orthopedic practice, or a multispecialty group practice of 100 physicians or more. Common administrative responsibilities of an assistant are listed in Box 1-2, but an assistant's job responsibilities may include *any* or possibly *all* of the duties listed in Box 1-2 and, depending on the employer, the job description may even include additional duties.

BOX 1-2

Duties of a Medical Administrative Assistant

- Schedule appointments.
- Screen and make telephone calls.
- Obtain and verify patient registration information.
- Transcribe medical dictation.
- Maintain medical records.
- Prepare correspondence.
- Code procedures and diagnoses for physician services.
- Perform billing and collection procedures.
- Prepare insurance claims.
- Perform financial and bookkeeping procedures.
- Arrange outside appointments and admissions.
- Manage office activities.

It is a medical administrative assistant's job to provide office support for the efficient operation of the entire medical office. Administrative responsibilities are also part of another multiskilled position known as **medical assistant.** The term *medical assistant* is used to describe an individual who is qualified to perform both *administrative* and *clinical* duties in a medical office. The clinical responsibilities of a medical assistant also will vary with the needs of the office and can include some or all of the clinical duties listed in Box 1-3. Clinical responsibilities can vary from state to state as a state defines the scope of clinical practice for a medical assistant.

It is important for a student in a medical office–related program to clearly understand the differences between the job responsibilities of a medical administrative assistant and those of a medical assistant. A medical administrative assistant performs administrative duties, and a medical assistant may perform administrative duties, clinical duties, or both, depending on the needs of the health care organization in

BOX 1-3

Clinical Duties of a Medical Assistant

- Use precautions necessary in a health care environment.
- Obtain patient's medical history.
- Obtain patient's vital signs.
- Collect specimens for testing.
- Perform routine laboratory and diagnostic tests.
- Prepare patient for examination.
- Prepare the office for patient examinations and treatments.
- Assist with examinations and procedures.
- Prepare and administer medications.
- Apply sterilization procedures.
- Provide patient education.
- Maintain patient immunization records.

which he or she works. The terms *medical administrative assistant* and *assistant* are used interchangeably within this text to represent the same position, but the terms *medical administrative assistant* and *medical assistant* cannot be used interchangeably because of the scope of their responsibilities. Both the medical administrative assistant and the medical assistant perform the administrative skills of the office, and those administrative skills are presented within this text.

A Typical Day at the Office

What is it really like to work in a medical office? Typical job descriptions highlight the major job responsibilities, but many other things happen as part of everyday activities. From one day to the next, each day can be quite different from another, which makes the job quite surprising and challenging. No matter what a day brings, a medical administrative assistant has the opportunity to make a difference in someone's life by providing the best possible service to patients each and every day.

As mentioned previously, the responsibilities of an assistant will be influenced greatly by the type of organization in which he or she works. In a large organization, an assistant sometimes specializes in a specific area of responsibility or in a combination of specific areas, such as billing, insurance, registration, appointments, transcription, or medical records. In a small organization, an assistant often has a variety of different responsibilities and may even be responsible for all of the administrative responsibilities identified in Box 1-2. No matter what type of organization, an assistant is expected to have impeccable communication skills—both the written and spoken word—because an assistant is a vital communication link between a patient and a health care provider. Telephone procedures are an important, critical function performed by a medical administrative assistant in the daily operations of any medical office.

In addition to those administrative duties previously mentioned, an assistant may be asked to assume other office responsibilities, such as arming and disarming alarm systems used for office security; maintaining supply records; managing the administrative staff; or devising, reorganizing, and implementing procedures to improve patient services. In addition, each and every day an assistant must be ready for any possible medical emergency that could present itself in the office. Some days can go by in the blink of an eye, and other days will give an assistant the opportunity to catch up on office tasks that were postponed because of a heavy patient load. An assistant must be prepared for all possible circumstances while at work in a medical office and will have to be able to adjust to an unpredictable workload.

Personal Qualities

If the ability to perform the office duties were all that a medical administrative assistant had to bring to the position, it might be easy for many individuals to simply learn the steps of a procedure and repeat them on the job. But there are other attributes that are important for a medical administrative assistant to possess. Granted, a medical administrative assistant's ability to perform the tasks necessary for the position is important, but equally important are the personal qualities and characteristics that a medical administrative assistant possesses and refines while receiving training in the profession.

As you begin your education for this position, you should always keep in mind the qualities and characteristics that are necessary to provide patients with the best possible service. Exceptional service for patients is extremely important. Patients are the reason for the work of medical professionals, and health care is a very serious business that affects people's lives every day. Patients deserve your very best.

What are some of the personal qualities and characteristics that employers look for in potential employees?

Empathy

Empathy is probably one of the most highly desired qualities of a medical administrative assistant and of many other health care professionals. **Empathy** means that an individual has an understanding of what another individual is experiencing. In other words, a health care professional can identify with a patient. For example, the parents of a child who is ill may be waiting for the results of some diagnostic tests. A medical administrative assistant might offer a quiet place for the parents to sit with their child. An assistant, knowing the parents may be experiencing some stress, would try to make their office visit as comfortable as possible. An empathetic assistant responds to a situation with an understanding of what a patient and the patient's family might be experiencing.

Compassion

Working in a medical office can, at times, be hectic, but it is also very rewarding. Every day, a medical administrative assistant has an opportunity to make a difference in people's lives by providing assistance to patients with varying medical concerns. Compassionate individuals display genuine caring and concern for people. They are kind and considerate and often put another's feelings ahead of their own. Assistants are usually very friendly individuals who enjoy working with people.

Sometimes a patient's experience or that of a family with an ill family member can be very difficult emotionally. An assistant, while interacting with a patient, should not become so personally and emotionally involved with the situation that he or she cannot perform assigned job duties. However, an assistant will be personally touched by such experiences, and some situations, indeed, will be very trying, but an assistant will have to remember the boundaries of professional behavior.

Dependability

A physician expects the front office staff to provide office support when and where needed and to manage the activities of the office with as little intervention as possible from the physician. Staff members must be punctual in reporting to work on time, taking only the specified amount of time for coffee and lunch breaks, and covering the front desk at all times. If a staff member is ill, he or she may have to secure a replacement or notify the supervisor early enough that a substitute can be found for the day.

Teamwork

To provide the best possible patient service, all office staff members must work as a team, and staff members must be able to depend on one another to accomplish the work of the office. Teamwork means that all staff members, regardless of their position, work for the common good of patients. Remember the quote from the founders of the Mayo Clinic that was mentioned in the preface of this text: "The best interest of the patient is the only interest to be considered." Working as a team means putting aside personal differences and doing everything possible to achieve the best outcome for the patient.

Confidentiality

All health care personnel are expected to hold confidential all that they hear, see, or do with regard to patients and their care. A patient's medical history and treatment often are very sensitive issues, and all health care personnel must take the utmost care in ensuring that such issues remain secret. **Confidentiality** is a legal expectation in the medical office that is required under the Health Insurance Portability and Accountability Act (HIPAA), a federal law, and confidentiality is a professional ethical expectation as well.

Attention to Details

A medical administrative assistant must be well organized and thorough in performing the daily activities of the office. Because of the serious nature of many patients' health care needs, an assistant must be precise and accurate when performing office duties.

Positive Work Ethic

The personal qualities that have been discussed here are all important components of a positive work ethic. An assistant who possesses a positive, or strong, work ethic is a positive individual who takes the initiative to make sure things that need to get done in the office get done. Such an individual is proactive and anticipates needs before the need is even apparent. An individual with this type of attitude is not afraid of hard work and sees that a task is carried through to completion; these qualities are highly desirable and valued in the workplace.

Other Desirable Personality Traits

When interviewing new employees, employers look for a variety of personal attributes. Employees of a medical office should be friendly and compassionate individuals who are respectful of others and good listeners and enjoy working with people. An assistant who, in addition to the traits mentioned, is honest, courteous, sincere, conscientious, and professional will have a greater chance of being hired.

Professional Appearance

Another highly desired personal quality is a professional appearance. The type of clothing worn and other things a person does regarding his or her outward appearance and interactions with others create a lasting impression. This impression must be a good one. The medical administrative assistant is often the first person a patient sees when entering a medical office, and it is extremely important for a medical administrative assistant to possess a professional appearance and be well groomed. A professional appearance will positively influence a patient's confidence in the medical staff.

A very important thing to remember when choosing clothing and preparing for work in a medical office is that **health care is very conservative.** Outrageous fads, outlandish clothing, and the like have no place in a health care setting. An extreme or peculiar appearance could destroy patient confidence in the office staff. Conservative clothing does not mean that clothing must be fancy, lavish, or expensive—it means that clothing should be modest or traditional. Even some casual clothing can be conservative and yet professional—for example, a pair of khaki pants and a coordinating collared shirt would be tasteful and very appropriate for some offices.

Dress Codes

The type of business clothing worn by assistants is largely dependent on the facility in which they work. A variety of apparel may be chosen for individuals in this position. The type of clothing worn in a medical office ranges all the way from casual dress and uniforms to business attire. Most health care organizations have dress codes that define appropriate appearance for the employees in the organization. A dress code is a necessary reference when you are determining what is suitable to wear to work. Some medical employers may prefer to select a uniform or variations of a basic uniform for their employees, to ensure that all staff members are

BOX 1-4

Sample Dress Code Policy

Happy Valley Medical Group is dedicated to providing quality care to patients, and employees are expected to dress in a professional manner.

Employees are expected to follow the dress code as specified below.

1. Identification must be worn at all times. Badges should be attached to clothing near the collar level and must be visible to patients. Badges should not be defaced with stickers or pins.
2. Clothing should be neat and pressed without tears, frayed edges, or stains. No jeans, capri pants, shorts, sweatpants, or leggings may be worn. Clothing should not be too tight or too loose.
3. Hair should be neat and controlled and should not interfere with patient care. Beards and mustaches should be neat and trimmed.
4. Jewelry may be worn but should be kept to a minimum. Items should not dangle or make excessive noise and cannot be a potential hazard to a patient. Body piercing other than ears is not allowed.
5. Shoes and hosiery must be worn at all times. Shoes must be closed-toed. Open-toed or backless shoes, flip flops, or slippers are not allowed.
6. Fingernail polish may be worn but in a subdued color and must be kept neat and free of chips. Artificial nails are not allowed. Fingernails should be kept clean and short.
7. Fragrance-free hygiene products should be used. Strong perfumes and aftershaves should not be worn.
8. Employees with tattoos must place a bandage over the tattoo or must keep the tattoo covered with clothing.

dressed appropriately for the environment and present a unified appearance. A sample dress code for a health care facility is listed in Box 1-4.

Uniforms

Uniforms are popular in some medical offices (Fig. 1-2). A uniform may be casual in style or may have a business look. Casual uniforms, often referred to as scrubs, consist of a comfortable pair of pants (available in many colors), a colorful smock-type top that allows the wearer to wear a shirt of some kind underneath, and a pair of clean white tennis shoes or white nurse's shoes. This type of uniform is extremely comfortable and wears well. Comfortable shoes are an added bonus with the uniform in that assistants can expect to spend long hours on their feet, and comfortable shoes help to minimize the chance that foot problems may result from this type of work. A disadvantage of wearing a casual uniform is that if the front desk staff and nursing or other staff members wear the same type of uniform, patients may confuse the front desk staff with others in the office.

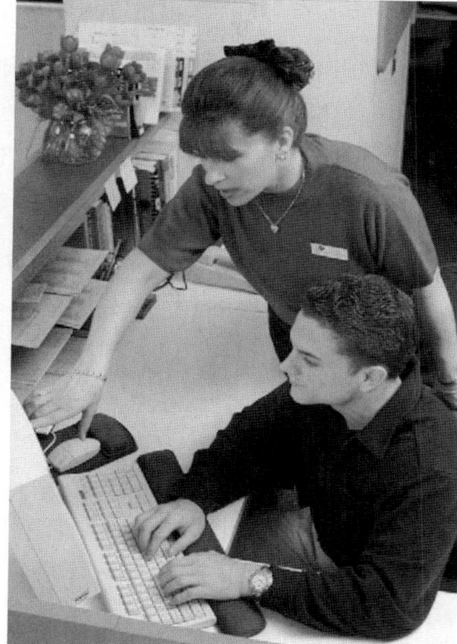

Figure 1-2 A variety of attire is suitable for the medical office. What type of office attire is each employee wearing in this setting? (From Bonewit-West K: *Today's Medical Assistant,* ed 2, St Louis, Saunders, 2013.)

A business uniform consists of a collection of business apparel in a few color choices. The basic pieces of the uniform are available for purchase in colors that coordinate with one another. For example, the uniform pieces might be available in navy, khaki, and burgundy. Employees could then choose from uniform components in one or more of the selected colors. The basic pieces of the uniform would include blazers, pants, and skirts for women and jackets and pants for men. An assistant then may be allowed to wear any shirt or accessory that fits within the color scheme. Business uniforms may be provided by the employer, or the cost may be the responsibility of the employee. As personnel come and go from the facility, the uniform must be available in open stock to ensure that all assistants have a coordinated appearance.

Other Office Apparel

For those facilities that do not require uniforms for their office staff, some type of business dress will be expected to be worn to work (Fig. 1-3). The office may allow business casual dress or may require the staff to wear more formal business clothing. An employee's attire must reflect good taste. Clothing should be clean, wrinkle-free, and should fit properly. Clothing that is torn, stained, frayed, or revealing should not be worn. Denim, capri pants, sweatpants, sweatshirts, and midriff tops would be inappropriate for a medical office.

If you are not sure what to wear to work, observe what *most* of the rest of the staff members are wearing. Particularly, note what your supervisor is wearing. She or he will likely be setting an example for appropriate office attire. If there is still uncertainty, ask your supervisor whether a particular type of clothing is acceptable.

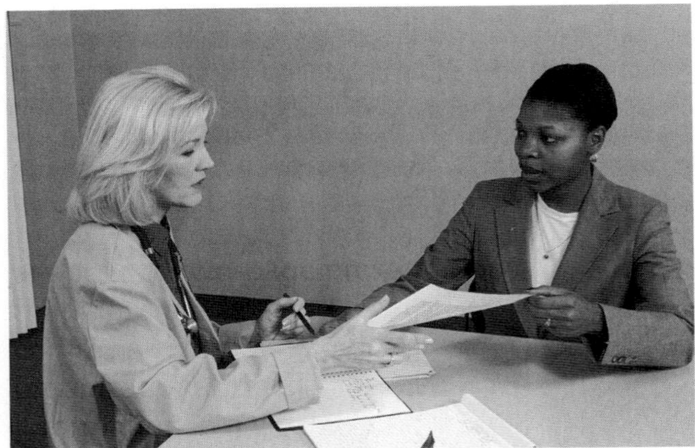

Figure 1-3 Business attire creates a professional appearance for this medical administrative assistant. (From Young A: *Kinn's The Administrative Medical Assistant,* ed 7, St Louis, Saunders, 2011.)

Personal Appearance

Medical administrative assistants should have impeccable grooming habits. Your appearance says a lot about your professionalism and integrity, and attention must be paid to every detail of your appearance.

Identification. When on duty, employees are expected to wear name badges at all times. Badges should be clean and visible to patients and should not be defaced in any way. If an employee loses a name badge, replacements are usually quickly available, but there may be a small cost to the employee.

Fingernails. Fingernails should be kept clean and trimmed because hands are often in view while an assistant is helping patients. Women who choose to wear nail polish should wear subdued colors and avoid shockingly bright or neon colors. Polished nails should be maintained and should not be allowed to chip. Because of infection concerns, assistants with direct patient contact and those who may handle patient supplies normally are not allowed to wear artificial nail coverings such as acrylic nails.

Hair. In addition to being neat and well kept, it is often wise to choose a hairstyle that is easy to maintain. Hair must be controlled and cannot interfere with job responsibilities. High-maintenance hairstyles will not hold up in a busy office. Unusual, distracting hair styles and colors are not recommended and often are not allowed.

Scents. Use of perfumes, aftershaves, and other fragrances is best avoided when you are working in a medical office. If scents are used to excess, they can wreak havoc for patients and coworkers, who may be allergic to fragrances. Make sure that a fragrance is not overpowering. Ill patients can become nauseous and are often highly sensitive to smells. Some health care organizations may require employees to use only fragrance-free hygiene products.

Jewelry and Piercing. Try to limit jewelry to three or four pieces. There is no need to decorate every appendage of the body with a piece of jewelry.

Earrings are acceptable jewelry, but posts or small hoops should be worn. If ears are pierced, avoid several earrings on one ear. Some dress codes can even limit the number of earrings in an ear and can restrict the location of piercings.

Dangling jewelry is a potential hazard for both the patient and the employee and is, therefore, a safety consideration in the workplace. Dangling earrings, bracelets, or necklaces could become caught on a patient and could be ripped from an employee. In addition, foreign, contaminated material may become trapped in jewelry, and this material could be transferred to another individual.

Piercing of other body parts, such as the tongue, nose, or eyebrow, is not allowed. Employees who have these body parts pierced are usually expected to remove the jewelry from these areas while on duty.

Tattoos. Even though tattoos are becoming more commonplace, health care organizations often do not allow them to be visible in the workplace. Depending on the nature of a tattoo, some employers may require that the tattoo be covered by a bandage or clothing when the employee is on duty. Some employers may even go so far as to send the employee home for a change of clothes if the tattoo is visible.

Footwear. Employees are expected to wear socks or some type of hosiery at all times. Shoes should be closed-toed and of low or moderate heel with nonskid bottoms that make minimal noise when walking on a hard surface. Sandals, beach flip-flops, and slipper-type shoes are not appropriate.

Dress codes are expected to be followed for the safety and comfort of patients. Remember, health care is a very serious business, and its environment is very conservative. Professional dress contributes positively to the overall atmosphere of an office. Employers simply are not happy with an unprofessional appearance.

Professional Skills

Career preparation for medical administrative assistants is available at many public and private educational institutions throughout the United States. The curriculum for this profession provides training for necessary job skills and usually consists of courses in the following areas.

Medical Terminology, Anatomy and Physiology, and Disease Processes

Medical terminology training provides an understanding of medical terms and abbreviations. Training in anatomy, physiology, and disease conditions covers the structure and function of the human body, as well as diseases and disorders that affect humans. An understanding of these subjects is essential for serving patients and conducting the business of health care. The medical administrative assistant must be able to communicate with the entire medical staff and is a vital communications link among the patient, the physician, and the rest of the office staff. Whether transcribing medical reports, processing a patient's bill, taking a message, or scheduling an appointment, an assistant must possess an exceptional command of medical language to serve as that communications link.

Medical Office Procedures and Practices

Telephone reception, appointment scheduling, medical record preparation and maintenance, and other office activities are part of the everyday activities of a medical administrative assistant. Knowledge of what, why, when, and how things are done in the medical office is expected of graduates entering the workforce.

Medical Transcription

The documentation of a patient's encounter with the health care provider is an important part of the activities of the medical office. A physician must keep accurate, complete, and legible documentation of each patient's visit. Medical transcription involves the production of medical reports that provide a legal record of a patient's visit with a health care provider. Medical reports are legal documents and are essential to continuity of patient care and a vital component of the medical record. Medical records are used to provide documentation of patient care, to supply information for billing purposes and statistical purposes, and to furnish medical information in a legal case.

Medical Coding, Billing, and Insurance

Preparing monthly statements and insurance claims for patients is an important function performed by a medical administrative assistant. Coding, billing, and submitting insurance claims are interconnected, and an understanding of each of these processes is essential for a well-trained assistant in the medical office. Proper billing practices help to ensure that the medical office stays financially stable.

Communication Skills

A medical administrative assistant must possess proper oral and written communication skills. Throughout the day, an assistant communicates with patients and coworkers, and the ability to communicate in a professional manner is a public and employer expectation.

Computer Technology

Today, almost all medical offices conduct many patient-related activities by means of a computer system. Computers are used for scheduling appointments, retaining patient registration information, billing patients, processing insurance claims, and transcribing medical reports and correspondence. The National Center for Health Statistics indicated that, in 2011, 54% of physicians' offices used an electronic medical record system for their patients' files. Offices today need medical administrative assistants with strong computer skills and keyboarding ability to maintain information in a computer system.

Internship

Many educational programs provide the opportunity for students to experience the activities of a medical office through an internship or through practical experience. During an internship, a student works in a medical office and performs many office activities under the supervision of an employee of that office. This experience is generally a nonpaid experience and allows the student to practice skills learned in school, while gaining on-the-job experience.

Student Portfolio

After enrolling in a medical office program, students should begin to collect samples of projects and course work that they complete while enrolled in the program. Students should also keep track of accomplishments and special activities in which they participated. This information is gathered to create a **student portfolio** that can later be presented to a prospective employer. Examples of information that might be kept in this portfolio include—but are not limited to—an appointment project from a medical office procedures course; a bookkeeping project from a medical billing course; samples of medical transcription, letters, and other medical office documents produced by the student; and even certificates of achievement for participation in school activities. The portfolio helps a student keep track of important items from the student's educational experience and serves as documentation to an employer of the student's capabilities.

Places of Employment

Medical administrative assistants work in a variety of organizations. A private practice, a clinic, and a hospital are probably the first locations that come to mind, but there are many other employment possibilities if a student has other interests. Assistants may find employment in such places as nursing homes, home health agencies, pharmaceutical businesses, dental offices, independent laboratory and radiologic facilities, insurance companies, and even legal firms that handle medically related cases.

CHECKPOINT

Why would education as a medical administrative assistant be beneficial for employment in a dental office?

Earnings

Information on the earnings of a medical administrative assistant can be obtained through state government agencies that provide employment services. Information is also available from the U.S. Bureau of Labor Statistics; however, this information represents a national average.

Several factors may affect potential earnings. Supply and demand for medical administrative assistants affect regional earnings. Earnings also vary regionally according to economic conditions, with salaries usually being higher in metropolitan areas. In addition, employees who obtain certification that is applicable to their field may expect to earn more than employees who do not have certification.

Employment Trends and Forecasts

Although individuals find employment in a medical office under an assortment of job titles, the employment statistics kept by the federal government usually are tracked under the occupation title of *medical secretary* or *medical assistant*. The future of employment in these areas looks promising. The U.S. Bureau of Labor Statistics forecasts that medical assisting jobs will grow much faster than average or by more than 20% between 2008 and 2018. This increase in jobs is largely due to increasing demand for health care services because of the aging of the population and longer life expectancies. As health care needs continue to grow, this increase will require health care organizations to hire additional office support staff. Because of this anticipated growth, medical administrative assistants should expect to find many opportunities when seeking employment.

Professional Organizations

Membership in a professional organization is a very practical way to keep current with changes in the profession. Membership is not required but provides many advantages to an assistant. Organizations hold conferences and conventions to communicate the latest news about a profession and to give members a chance to network with others in the field. Several organizations have professional publications that contain articles related to the profession. Many employers encourage membership in a professional organization by paying a portion or all of membership costs and sometimes by paying expenses for attending conferences or conventions. Many organizations have state and local chapters that provide excellent opportunities for professional development activities for medical administrative professionals.

Professional organizations offer one or more certification examinations that a student may be eligible to take, depending on the qualifications required to take the examination. Specific information regarding these organizations and the certifications they sponsor, as well as available professional publications and other details, is available by using the information in Table 1-1 to contact the organization desired.

American Association of Medical Assistants

Formed in 1955, the American Association of Medical Assistants (AAMA) is a professional organization that promotes and serves members of the medical assisting profession. The AAMA has identified competencies necessary for medical assistants and conducts a certification examination that assesses an applicant's knowledge of those competencies. The examination covers both administrative and clinical competencies required for employment in the profession. An individual who passes the certification examination is known as a **Certified Medical Assistant (CMA)**. In 2003, the AAMA updated the AAMA Role Delineation Study, which analyzes the professional responsibilities of medical assistants and identifies the administrative and clinical procedures performed by an entry level medical assistant. The Commission on Accreditation of Allied Health Education Programs has established Standards and Guidelines for educational programs in medical assisting. Related competencies included in those guidelines are listed at the beginning of each chapter of this text.

Members of the AAMA, in upholding the standards of their profession, have established a code of ethics to guide medical assistants in performing the ethical behaviors expected of a medical assistant. The AAMA Code of Ethics should serve as a guide for all medical administrative staff when they are performing the responsibilities of their position. To ensure that assistants stay current with changes in health care, the AAMA requires that CMAs receive the

TABLE 1-1

Professional Organizations of Interest to Medical Administrative Assistants

Organization Name	Address	Telephone No.	Internet Address and E-mail Contact
American Academy of Professional Coders (AAPC)	2480 South 3850 West, Suite B Salt Lake City, UT 84120	800-626-CODE (2633)	www.aapc.com E-mail: info@aapc.com
American Association of Medical Assistants (AAMA)	20 North Wacker Drive, Suite 1575 Chicago, IL 60606-2903	312-899-1500	www.aama-ntl.org
American Medical Technologists (AMT)	10700 West Higgins Road, Suite 150 Rosemont, IL 60018	847-823-5169 or 800-275-1268	www.amt1.com E-mail: mail@americanmedtech.org
Association for Healthcare Documentation Integrity (AHDI)	4230 Kiernan Avenue, Suite 130 Modesto, CA 95356	800-982-2182	www.ahdionline.org E-mail: ahdi@ahdionline.org
International Association of Administrative Professionals (IAAP)	10502 NW Ambassador Drive PO Box 20404 Kansas City, MO 64195-0404	816-891-6600	www.iaap-hq.org E-mail: service@iaap-hq.org
American Health Information Management Association	233 North Michigan Avenue, 21st Floor Chicago, IL 60601-5809	312-233-1100 or 800-335-5535	www.ahima.org E-mail: info@ahima.org

equivalent of 60 continuing education units (CEUs) every 5 years to retain certification.

American Medical Technologists

The American Medical Technologists (AMT) is a national group for medical assistants that conducts a certification examination different from the one conducted by the AAMA. The AMT sponsors two different certification examinations related to medical assisting: the **Registered Medical Assistant (RMA)** and the **Certified Medical Administrative Specialist (CMAS)** examinations. The AMT has established a group of administrative and clinical competencies that are assessed on each examination.

Depending on the requirements of the state in which he or she wishes to practice, a medical assisting student could take a medical assisting certification examination that is most commonly recognized by the state in which the student wishes to work. However, if a medical assisting student does not wish to work in a clinical area, a certification exam is not necessary.

American Academy of Professional Coders

Billing and insurance processing represent an integral part of today's medical office. Numerous government regulations and requirements of insurance companies make working in this area of health care an exciting challenge. The need for highly skilled individuals in this field will likely continue to increase.

The American Academy of Professional Coders (AAPC), was established in 1988, and in early 2013, there were more than 120,000 members. The AAPC certifies coders who work in physician offices, outpatient facilities, and other related facilities and is the largest certifying organization for medical coders. The organization offers six core certification examinations and 20 specialty coding certifications. Some of the more common certifications are in the following areas:

- **Certified Professional Coder (CPC)** is a professional who performs diagnosis and procedure coding in a physician-based setting.
- **Certified Professional Coder–Hospital (CPC-H)** is a professional who performs diagnosis and procedure coding for facility- or hospital-based services.
- **Certified Professional Coder–Payer (CPC-P)** certifies individuals with expertise in insurance claims processing.

Examination candidates for each of the above certifications must have 2 years of work experience or 1 year of work experience and coding-related education to be eligible to complete the exam. Candidates with less than those qualifications are allowed to take the examination, and if they pass the examination, they are awarded an apprentice status (CPC-A, CPC-H-A, CPC-P-A) with the earned credential until the work experience or work/education experience is completed.

The AAPC holds a national conference each year and has many local chapters that are available to provide educational and networking opportunities for members. The organization's publication *Coding Edge* provides many relevant articles to help members keep up with the many regulations required by the coding profession.

These types of coding certifications help individuals to maintain professional standards in the field of medical coding, an important component that is vital for billing and for handling insurance procedures in the medical office.

International Association of Administrative Professionals

The International Association of Administrative Professionals (IAAP) is an organization dedicated to advancing the profession of administrative support professionals. The organization was formed in 1942 and currently includes more than 40,000 members throughout the world.

For its members, the organization provides the following:

- Education in the form of workshops, seminars, and conferences
- Networking opportunities
- A publication, *The OfficePro*, which provides current information related to the administrative support field
- Certification examination known as the **Certified Administrative Professional (CAP)** for members and nonmembers who wish to demonstrate excellence in their field through the certification process

The national IAAP organization sponsors a conference each year in a different area of the United States. Many areas in the United States also have local chapters that sponsor continuing education events related to the administrative support profession.

Association for Healthcare Documentation Integrity

The Association for Healthcare Documentation Integrity (AHDI), formerly the American Association for Medical Transcription, is a professional group that was organized to support the members of the medical transcription profession. Each year, the AHDI holds a national meeting somewhere in the United States, and several states have their own chapters that hold regional meetings. The AHDI organization has several publications related to health care documentation, technology, and other aspects of the medical transcription profession. Transcriptionists will find sources such as these invaluable in keeping up with their profession.

The AHDI has established guidelines for the **Certified Healthcare Documentation Specialist (CHDS)** examination. This examination is given to transcriptionists who have two or more years' experience in an acute care health care setting. Such a setting would have exposed a transcriptionist to a wide variety of medical reports and many dictators, including ESL (English-as-a-second language) dictators. The AHDI also has established guidelines for the **Registered Healthcare Documentation Specialist (RHDS)** examination. This examination is intended for the transcriptionist who is not eligible to complete the CHDS examination. Recent graduates of medical transcription programs are eligible to complete the RHDS.

To obtain employment as a **medical transcriptionist**, it is not required that a transcriptionist obtain a certification or registration credential. Attainment of a credential, however, demonstrates the level of proficiency that a transcriptionist has achieved. A credential can make a difference to an employer who is interested in hiring a transcriptionist.

American Health Information Management Association

The American Health Information Management Association (AHIMA) is a nationally recognized organization whose members are chiefly responsible for the management of personal health information in a health care facility. This includes ensuring the quality of medical records, managing health care statistics, and implementing medical coding systems.

This organization also sponsors two coding certification examinations that may be of interest to medical administrative assistants: **Certified Coding Specialist (CCS)** and the **Certified Coding Specialist–Physician-Based (CCS-P)** examinations.

Additional Certifications

Many other professional organizations sponsor their own certification examinations. Even worldwide companies—Microsoft, for example—sponsor certification examinations that assess an individual's ability to use their product. Although some examinations are not as widely known as others, they still may be highly regarded by a health care employer. When considering a certification examination, an individual may wish to consult employers in the area about their preference for hiring certified individuals. It is also important to research certifying organizations and only consider certifications from reputable groups.

Continuing Education

Once assistants finish their formal education, take any certification examinations desired, and secure employment in their field, their education is still far from over. Health care is a dynamic field that is changing constantly. Workshops, seminars, and college courses designed to keep medical administrative assistants informed of the latest changes and the newest technologies are often available. Professional organizations sponsor conferences, or independent study options may allow members and nonmembers to attend and upgrade their skills and knowledge about their field. A genuine interest in learning new things is a very desirable trait in an employee, and employers often encourage staff members to attend these conferences to keep current with health industry advances.

SUMMARY

The health care field offers numerous employment opportunities for medical administrative assistants. Employers look for individuals with the right training and qualities, who will provide exceptional service to their patients. An individual who wishes to be hired as a medical administrative assistant will have to receive appropriate educational preparation to perform many duties in the medical office. Even after an assistant is employed, he or she must keep current in the field. Professional organizations related to medical office responsibilities provide a wealth of information and support to enhance the career of the medical administrative assistant.

YOU ARE THE MEDICAL ADMINISTRATIVE ASSISTANT

Picture yourself as a medical administrative assistant in a medical practice. What would you do in the following situations?

1. The parents of a 2-year-old child with cancer are bringing him to the office because he has taken a turn for the worse. The parents come in carrying the child, who obviously is very weak and has lost all of his hair. As the assistant, what could you do to make their visit more comfortable?
2. The clinic manager wants to hire an additional staff person to help cover the front desk in the office. The labor market is tight, and the manager thinks that a person with no office experience or medical background would be all right for the position. Do you agree? Why?
3. On a coffee break, a coworker mentions that she would like to get a tattoo on her ankle. How would you reply?

Suggested Readings

The 7 Habits of Highly Successful People by Stephen Covey explores the basic principles that individuals can use to approach personal and professional situations. It is highly regarded in the business world and is a must read for business professionals.

Many *Chicken Soup for the Soul* books are on the market today. These books provide wonderful stories that eloquently portray empathy, compassion, kindness, and other desirable human virtues.

Who Moved My Cheese? by Spencer Johnson is a motivational book designed to help individuals deal with change in their lives.

REVIEW EXERCISES

Exercise 1-1 True or False

Read the following statements and determine whether the statement is true or false. Record the answer in the blank provided. T = true; F = false.

_____ 1. It is common in large health care organizations for a medical administrative assistant to specialize in a specific administrative area of the organization.

_____ 2. CCS means "certified corporate secretary."

_____ 3. *Patient services specialist, medical office specialist, medical secretary*, and *medical administrative assistant* are job titles that could be used to describe the same position.

_____ 4. Composing a letter to a patient may be part of an assistant's responsibility.

_____ 5. Continuing education is necessary for an assistant to remain a valued employee.

_____ 6. Handling telephone calls is part of a medical administrative assistant's responsibility.

_____ 7. Wearing the latest styles is important for the medical administrative assistant who wishes to present a professional appearance.

_____ 8. Casual clothing is acceptable attire in some medical offices.

_____ 9. A medical administrative assistant's appearance may influence a patient's perception of that assistant.

_____ 10. Uniforms are the only type of clothing appropriate for a medical administrative assistant on the job.

_____ 11. If the office staff and the nursing staff wear the same uniform, a patient may confuse the office staff and the nursing staff.

_____ 12. To become a medical transcriptionist, an assistant must be certified.

_____ 13. To transcribe medical reports, one must have knowledge of medical terminology.

_____ 14. The study of human anatomy and physiology covers the structure and function of the human body.

_____ 15. Because most patient contact occurs in person in the medical office, it is not necessary for a medical administrative assistant to have proper written communication skills.

_____ 16. Computer skills are not widely used in the medical office today.

_____ 17. Membership in a professional organization is mandatory for all medical administrative assistants.

Exercise 1-2 Administrative and Clinical Duties in the Medical Office

Identify whether the following duties in the medical office are administrative or clinical. Record the answer in the blank provided. A = administrative; C = clinical.

_____ 1. Prepare insurance claim.

_____ 2. Take and record patient's blood pressure.

_____ 3. Sterilize instruments.

_____ 4. File medical records.

_____ 5. Provide assistance to physician during a procedure.

_____ 6. Obtain patient's medical history.

_____ 7. Perform routine laboratory test.

_____ 8. Prepare treatment room for patient.

_____ 9. Schedule appointments.

_____ 10. Record patient's payment on account.

_____ 11. Prepare statement of patient's account.

_____ 12. Remove patient's bandage.

_____ 13. Take and record patient's temperature.

_____ 14. Make daily bank deposit.

_____ 15. Record patient's change of address.

Exercise 1-3 Desirable Personality Traits of a Medical Administrative Assistant

Desirable personality traits of a medical administrative assistant are listed here. Match the characteristics on the left with their meanings on the right. Record the answer in the blank provided. Each answer is used only once.

a. Keeps information secret
b. Thorough
c. Envisions things from the patient's perspective
d. Appropriately dressed
e. Caring
f. Works well in a group
g. Friendly
h. Reliable
i. Truthful
j. Arrives on time

______ 1. Compassionate
______ 2. Dependable
______ 3. Conscientious
______ 4. Honest
______ 5. Confidential
______ 6. Personable
______ 7. Team player
______ 8. Punctual
______ 9. Empathetic
______ 10. Well groomed

Exercise 1-4 Professional Organizations

Match each statement below with its associated organization. Choose the best answer. Some answers may be used more than once. Record the answer in the blank provided.

a. American Association of Medical Assistants
b. American Medical Technologists
c. International Association of Administrative Professionals
d. Association for Healthcare Documentation Integrity
e. American Health Information Management Association
f. American Academy of Professional Coders

______ 1. Conducts the CMA certification examination
______ 2. Professional organization for health information personnel
______ 3. Conducts the CPC, CPC-H, and CPC-P and several specialty coding certification examinations
______ 4. Professional group for medical transcriptionists
______ 5. Conducts the CAP examination
______ 6. Conducts the RMA examination
______ 7. Conducts the CCS and CCS-P coding certification examinations
______ 8. Publishes *The OfficePRO*
______ 9. Conducts the CHDS and RHDS examinations
______ 10. Largest certification organization for medical coders
______ 11. Conducts a certification examination that certifies individuals with expertise in insurance claims processing

Exercise 1-5 Professional Appearance

Read each statement regarding personal appearance, and determine whether or not the appearance is professional. Record the answer in the blank provided. Y = Yes, this is professional; N = No, this is not professional.

______ 1. Bright red nail polish
______ 2. Navy blazer and pants
______ 3. Pierced tongue
______ 4. Jogging suit
______ 5. Conservative hairstyle
______ 6. Green-tinted hair
______ 7. Khaki pants and coordinating shirt
______ 8. Denim skirt
______ 9. Tennis shoes with white uniform
______ 10. Lightly worn cologne
______ 11. Visible tattoo
______ 12. Two or three pieces of jewelry

ACTIVITIES

ACTIVITY 1-1 MEDISOFT INSTALLATION AND BACKUP

Install the Medisoft Version 18 software that accompanied your book or was purchased separately. Be sure to follow the instructions exactly. See Appendix III which includes additional information pertaining to installation. If problems occur during installation, contact Elsevier Technical Support listed on the Evolve site for this text. The practice that will be used for exercises within this text is the Medisoft Tutorial practice entitled "Happy Valley Medical Clinic." The words "Medical Group (Tutorial Data)" will appear on the Medisoft title bar when the Happy Valley Medical Clinic practice is open. Be sure to consult Evolve for tips and updates on using Medisoft.

To verify that the correct data has installed, perform the following:

1. Open Medisoft using one of the following options:
   a. On the computer desktop, double-click the icon labeled **Medisoft Advanced Demo** or
   b. Click **Programs>Medisoft>Medisoft Advanced Demo.**
2. Verify that the practice entitled **Medical Group (Tutorial Data)** is open. The practice name appears after Medisoft Advanced at the top of the Medisoft window. If no practice name appears, click **File>Open Practice>Medical Group**, then click **OK.** (If the tutorial is not on the list, click **Add tutorial** on the right side of the practice window and after the tutorial has installed, open the practice as previously instructed.
3. Click **Lists>Patients/Guarantors and Cases.**
4. Click the **Radio** button for **Patient** on the right side of the **Field** box. In the **Field** box, click the drop-down arrow and click **Last name, First name.** The patient list should sort alphabetically. The first patient on the list should be Dwight Again and the last patient should be Anthony Zimmerman.
5. To close the patient list, click the "X" in the upper right corner of the patient list window. (Be careful not to click the "X" to close the program.)

To set backup options, perform the following:

6. Click **File>Program Options.** Under the **General** tab, place a check before **Remind to Back Up on Program Exit.** Click **Save.**
7. To close Medisoft, click the "X" in the upper right corner of the Medisoft window. When prompted for backup, click **Backup Data Now** if you wish to back up your data you have entered. A backup is not needed after this short activity, but information should be backed up when a significant amount of data has been entered. A backup can restore data should information be lost from the program. The backup message states "A backup of your data should be made on a different disk or tape. A backup is a copy of your data files that can be used if your working data files are lost or damaged."
8. If backup data has been selected, a message may appear stating that users of the software will need to exit. This *does not* apply to student users if software is normally accessed by a student on an individual computer, not a networked computer. Click **OK.**
9. It is recommended that a backup be placed on a USB or external storage device in case the user's computer should crash, but the C: drive of a personal computer could be used. In the **Destination File Path and Name** box, click **Find** and insert the location where the backup will be located.
10. Click **Start Backup.** Click **OK** when the Backup complete message appears. Click **Close.** (It is NOT necessary to restore data when starting the program. Previously input data will be available when the program is reopened. Data **should only be restored** in case of a loss of data due to a computer malfunction. Data can be restored by selecting **File>Restore>Restore Data>OK.** The location of the backup file will need to be specified in order to restore the information.)

ACTIVITY 1-2 MEDISOFT HELP FEATURE

1. Open Medisoft using one of the following options:
   a. On the computer desktop, double-click the icon labeled **Medisoft Advanced Demo** or
   b. Click **Programs>Medisoft>Medisoft Advanced Demo.** Verify that the practice entitled **Medical Group (Tutorial Data)** is open.
2. Click **Help>Medisoft Help.**
3. When the **Help** window opens, click the **Contents** tab. Click the + sign before **Scheduling Appointments.** Click **Appointments>New Appointment Entry.** Note that information pertaining to **New Appointment Entry** will appear on the right-hand side of the window.
4. Click the **Index** tab. Enter the word **patient** in the **keyword** box. Locate **Patient entry – Name, Address Tab.** Information pertaining to the **Name, Address Tab** will appear on the right-hand side of the window.
5. Click the **Search** tab. Enter the word **co-payment** in the **keyword** box. Topics in which the word **co-payment** appears will display below the **keyword** box. Locate **Patient entry.** Information pertaining to the **co-payment within patient entry** will appear on the right-hand side of the window.
6. Topics can be printed by clicking the **Print** icon on the top left side of the **Help** window. Print one of the topics listed in this activity and hand it in to your instructor.

ACTIVITY 1-3 EMPLOYMENT OPPORTUNITIES

Research employment opportunities using the Internet, newspapers, or any other source. Find at least three openings for which a medical administrative assistant or medical assistant would be qualified. Find at least one opening outside your state. Take note of the titles of the positions advertised. On each of the listings, highlight the information that identifies educational requirements, personal qualities, and other information regarding medical administrative assistants that is discussed in Chapter 1.

ACTIVITY 1-4 PROFESSIONAL ORGANIZATIONS

Research the professional organizations identified in this chapter. You might be interested in the following:

a. Does the organization have a local chapter in your area?
b. Is the organization sponsoring any workshops in your area in the near future?
c. Where and when is the next annual convention or national meeting?
d. How much are dues?

ACTIVITY 1-5 MEDICAL ADMINISTRATIVE ASSISTANT INTERVIEW

Interview a person who is currently working as a medical administrative assistant. Prepare a list of interview questions to be approved by your instructor.

ACTIVITY 1-6 PROFESSIONAL APPEARANCE

Chapter 1 gives examples of professional and unprofessional appearance for the medical office. Using magazines, newspapers, the Internet, or any other sources available, find two pictures of professional business dress appropriate for the medical office, one picture of an appropriate uniform for the medical office, and two pictures of unprofessional appearance.

Locate an example of a dress code for a health care organization in your local area. Using the dress code as a guide, identify whether your examples would comply with the dress code, and explain the reasons for your answer.

ACTIVITY 1-7 PROFESSIONAL APPEARANCE

Professional appearance is so important in a health care facility. Patients' confidence in the health care staff will be influenced by the staff's appearance. Review the chapter information presented on professional dress and any class discussions on the subject, and then dress professionally for class on a date specified by the instructor.

ACTIVITY 1-8 STUDENT PORTFOLIO

Start a portfolio that will be used to gather samples of your work while you are in school. An accordion-style paper folder can be used to hold many items. Discuss with your instructor what items should be included in the portfolio. Periodically review your portfolio, placing like items together.

ACTIVITY 1-9 MEDICAL OFFICE CERTIFICATIONS

Research certifications and their associated examinations from the organizations mentioned in this chapter. Find answers to such questions as the following:

a. What types of certifications are available?
b. What are the requirements to take a certification examination?
c. How much does a certification examination cost?
d. Locate a list of the topics covered in the exam and sample test questions.

ACTIVITY 1-10 SOFTWARE CERTIFICATIONS

Research computer software certifications such as the MOS certification from Microsoft. Find answers to the questions listed in Activity 1-9 for those organizations.

ACTIVITY 1-11 PERSONAL QUALITIES

Review the personal qualities of an assistant as presented in this chapter and in class discussions. Identify some of your strongest qualities, and explain why you believe they are your strongest qualities.

ACTIVITY 1-12 AMERICAN ASSOCIATION OF MEDICAL ASSISTANTS

Using the AAMA's website, locate the following:

- Medical Assistant Code of Ethics
- Medical Assistant Creed
- Educational Competencies for the Medical Assistant
- AAMA Role Delineation Study

ACTIVITY 1-13 MEDICAL OFFICE SCENARIOS

Consider the following role-playing situations. What are the appropriate responses to the situations given?

a. A coworker named Nancy, on a whim, wants something new for her hair. She decides a really "funky" thing to do would be to color her hair (temporarily) green. She tells you about this idea during your lunch break. What do you say?
b. Another coworker, David, and a few of his buddies have decided that it would be fun to pierce their lips and noses. David reports to work one day with a silver stud through his lower lip and another through his nose. He asks what you think about his new jewelry. What do you say?
c. You would like to join a professional organization. You are willing to pay the membership fee, but how would you approach your supervisor to ask to attend a 2-day conference next month? You would like your employer to give you the time to attend, so you will not have to use your vacation days.

DISCUSSION

The following topics can be used for class discussion or for individual student essay.

DISCUSSION 1-1

What is the importance of the statement, "Patients are the reason for the work of medical professionals"?

DISCUSSION 1-2

Discuss the application of the Medical Assistant Code of Ethics to the position of medical administrative assistant.

DISCUSSION 1-3

Several employees want to wear jeans to work. Are jeans appropriate for the medical office? Why or why not?

DISCUSSION 1-4

You want to work in a medical office and have decided to become a medical administrative assistant. Why do you want to work in health care?

Bibliography

American Academy of Professional Coders. Website. www.aapc.com. Accessed April 7, 2013.

American Association of Medical Assistants: *AAMA Role Delineation Study*. www.aama-ntl.org. Accessed November 24, 2010.

American Health Information Management Association. Website. www.ahima.org. Accessed November 28, 2010.

American Medical Technologists. Website. www.amt1.com. Accessed November 24, 2010.

Association for Healthcare Documentation Integrity. Website. http://www.ahdionline.org. Accessed November 28, 2010.

National Center for Health Statistics, Centers for Disease Control and Prevention: *NCHS Data Brief No. 98 July 1012, Physician Adoptions of Electronic Health Record Systems: United States*. www.cdc.gov. Accessed April 7, 2013.

International Association of Administrative Professionals. Website. www.iaap-hq.org. Accessed December 1, 2010.

Johns Hopkins Health System. Website. www.hopkinsmedicine.org. Accessed December 1, 2010.

MayoClinic. Website. www.mayoclinic.org. Accessed November 28, 2010.

St. Joseph Mercy Health System/University of Michigan. Website. www.sjmercyhealth.org. Accessed December 16, 2006.

UCLA Medical Center. Website. www.uclahealth.org/workfiles/documents/volunteering/dresscode.pdf. Accessed November 29, 2010.

UCLA Medical Center: *Employee News*, April 2008. http://townhall.mednet.ucla.edu/restored/hs_news/0804p04.html. Accessed November 28, 2010.

U.S. Department of Labor, Bureau of Labor Statistics: *Occupational Outlook Handbook, 2010* 11th ed. www.bls.gov/oco. Accessed December 1, 2010.

CHAPTER 2 The Health Care Team

LEARNING OUTCOMES

On successful completion of this chapter, the student will be able to

1. Identify the different members of the health care team and explain the roles of health care team members within a health care organization.
2. Identify various medical specialties.
3. Describe common settings for the delivery of health care.
4. Use medical practice management software to enter practice and employee information.

COMMISSION ON ACCREDITATION OF ALLIED HEALTH EDUCATION PROGRAMS (CAAHEP) CORE CURRICULUM FOR MEDICAL ASSISTANTS

- Use the Internet to access information related to the medical office.
- Discuss licensure and certification as it applies to health care providers.

ACCREDITING BUREAU OF HEALTH EDUCATION SCHOOLS (ABHES) PROGRAMMATIC EVALUATION STANDARDS FOR MEDICAL ASSISTING

Graduates

- Compare and contrast the allied health professions and understand their relation to medical assisting.
- Understand medical assistant credentialing requirements and the process to obtain the credential.
- Comprehend the importance of credentialing.

VOCABULARY

ambulatory
assisted living facility
board certified
clinic
day surgery
emergency department or emergency room (ED, ER)
home health
hospice care
hospital
inpatient
managed care
mid-level provider
nonphysician practitioner (NPP)
nursing home
outpatient
outpatient surgery center
physician extender
primary care
private practice
provider
public health agency
reciprocity
residency
residents
rotation
triage
urgent care center

Who are the significant players on the health care team? What do they do for the patient? What is required of these professionals?

It is important that a medical administrative assistant know the answers to these questions so that the assistant understands (1) how these professionals interact with patients and one another and (2) each professional's role in the health care setting. Medical administrative assistants provide many support functions for these professionals, and knowledge and understanding of each professional's role enable an assistant to perform those functions to the highest degree possible.

In addition, this chapter examines the common types of facilities in which health care is provided to supply a frame of reference for the places in which a medical administrative assistant may work. Although a medical administrative assistant may work in a variety of locations, the most common location is a clinic, whether a private practice or group practice, which is the focus of the chapters in this text.

Many different employment opportunities are available for people who have an interest in health care. No matter where a health care professional may work, however, anyone who enters a health care profession should do so with one focus in mind: patient service. Patients are the reason that a health care facility and its staff members provide health care services, and excellent service can be provided only with continuous and heartfelt consideration for all patients. More simply put: Patients are the reason for our work.

Health Care Providers

The term **provider** or **providers** is used in health care to describe the individuals who are chiefly responsible for coordinating and delivering health care services. Providers examine patients, order laboratory or radiologic testing, and may prescribe medications, treatments, or therapies for illness or injury. They also provide preventive health care. Physicians, nurse practitioners, and physician assistants, to name a few, are examples of providers. A provider relies on many other health care professionals to supply many of the necessary services related to a patient's visit to a health care facility.

Physician

A physician's practice of medicine involves providing preventive care or coordinating treatment for patients' illnesses or injuries. As mentioned previously, a physician also relies on other health care professionals to provide additional services for patients. For example, a physician who is treating a patient with a suspected fracture will order a radiograph, but a radiology technologist will actually take the radiograph. Then a radiologist (another physician) will interpret the radiograph and will report the findings to the treating physician. Although physicians may not actually conduct all treatments or therapies, they are chiefly responsible for developing and overseeing the treatment plans for their patients.

A physician (Fig. 2-1) is usually the leading health care professional in most of today's medical offices. Although many offices do employ other providers—such as physician assistants, nurse practitioners, and certified nurse midwives—a physician or a group of physicians must supervise the activities of those health professionals and is ultimately responsible for their actions.

Physician Education

The road to becoming a physician is long, difficult, and very costly. A student who wishes to become a physician usually completes a 4-year bachelor's degree program in a science, such as biology or chemistry, or completes a program designated as "pre-med." Such a program provides the student with the base of knowledge necessary to continue in medical school.

After the student has completed 4 years of college and is accepted into medical school, he or she spends the next 4 years in the medical school program. The first 2 years of medical school are spent learning the foundations of medical practice: anatomy and physiology, pharmacology, chemistry, microbiology, medical law and ethics, and treatment and examination of patients. During the third and fourth years of medical school and under the supervision of a physician, the medical student works with actual patients to gain first-hand knowledge of patient treatment. This experience is known as a **rotation** because the student rotates through various departments in a medical facility such as internal medicine, psychiatry, surgery, pediatrics, and so forth. This medical rotation allows a medical student to experience all types of specialties to determine in which specialty he or she would like to study and eventually establish a practice.

On graduation from medical school, a student is awarded the degree of doctor of medicine (MD) or doctor of osteopathy (DO). Of 154 medical schools in the United States, 129 prepare MDs and 25 prepare DOs, with a total of more than 16,000 medical students graduating each year.

Both MDs and DOs are physicians who are required to be licensed to practice medicine. Each type of physician is trained to treat illness and injury and to provide preventive health care. Both MDs and DOs perform surgery and prescribe medication. One of the key differences between these two types of physicians is that the osteopath's (DO's) education focuses on the body as a whole, rather than on a particular organ system or body area. Osteopathic medical treatment incorporates musculoskeletal manipulations of the body with an emphasis on the importance of a healthy musculoskeletal system for good health. Training for MDs focuses on the particular specialty in which the physician chooses to specialize.

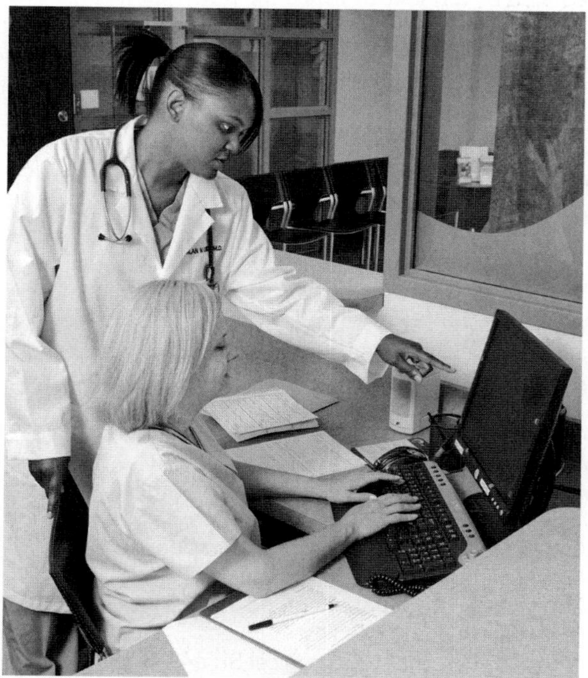

Figure 2-1 A physician may receive medical training as an MD or DO and is chiefly responsible for developing and overseeing the treatment plans for her patients. (From Young A: *Kinn's The Administrative Medical Assistant,* ed 7, St. Louis, Saunders, 2011.)

Physician Licensure

Before a medical school graduate is allowed to practice medicine, the graduate must be licensed by the state in which he or she wishes to work. All states, the District of Columbia, and all U.S. territories have their own medical licensing board that oversees the practice of medicine within their region. These boards are known by different names in different states, such as Board of Medical Examiners, Board of Medicine, and State Medical Board, to name a few. Each board is responsible for defining and regulating the practice of medicine within its jurisdiction. Many boards also maintain public access to a physician database that assists consumers in obtaining information regarding physicians licensed to practice within that jurisdiction and in identifying physicians who have had disciplinary action taken against them.

Application for licensure requires that a doctor must be a graduate of an accredited medical school, and that he or she must have passed a licensing examination that is acceptable to the Board to which the graduate has applied. In the United States, physicians who are MDs must pass the U.S. Medical Licensing Examination (USMLE) and osteopathic physicians must pass the Comprehensive Osteopathic Medical Licensing Examination (COMLEX). Applicants for licensure must disclose their medical history and any record of arrests or convictions. Each state establishes its own requirements for licensure; however, many states allow a physician who is licensed in another state to obtain a license in that state through an agreement called **reciprocity.** Reciprocity allows the physician who has met the requirements in one state to obtain a license in another state without retaking licensing examinations.

Once licensed, the physician must renew his or her license as required by the state in which the physician works. Renewal takes place on a regular basis. For example, a physician may be required to renew his or her license every 2 years. States normally require that the physician take part in a specified amount of continuing education as part of renewing a license to practice.

Residency

After graduating from medical school and obtaining licensure from the state in which he or she works, the physician may apply to complete a residency in a specialty of his or her choice. These graduates are known as **residents,** and this period of education is known as a **residency.** Residents are physicians who are licensed to practice medicine, but they are also students who are continuing their education in a chosen specialty. Residency training programs for medical specialties vary in length from 3 to 7 years, depending on the specialty.

Because the body of medical knowledge is so extensive, many doctors choose to specialize or further concentrate their medical study in a specific area of medicine. Thus, most medical school graduates continue on in some type of residency program.

Board Certification

Once he or she has completed a residency in a specialty area, the resident may choose to take an examination related to his or her specialty to become **board certified.** The resident also may practice for a few years before taking the board certification examination. Both MDs and DOs may choose to become certified by a medical board after completing their residency training and any other requirements necessary for board certification.

The 24 member boards of the American Board of Medical Specialties set certification standards for MDs (Box 2-1). Each board listed in Box 2-1 sets the standards for its specialty. Within some specialties, subspecialties allow a physician to further specialize his or her practice of medicine. For example, a physician who specializes in surgery may wish to further specialize in pediatric surgery, or an obstetrician may wish to further specialize in reproductive endocrinology. Overall, the American Board of Medical Specialties consists of more than 145 specialties and subspecialties for MDs.

If the physician successfully completes the board certification examination, the physician is then known as a diplomate and is said to be board certified. Achievement of the designation board certified indicates that the physician is recognized as an expert in his or her chosen field.

Table 2-1 describes the scope of practice or focus of care of many of the more common medical specialties.

BOX 2-1

American Board of Medical Specialties Member Boards

American Board of Allergy and Immunology
American Board of Anesthesiology
American Board of Colon and Rectal Surgery
American Board of Dermatology
American Board of Emergency Medicine
American Board of Family Medicine
American Board of Internal Medicine
American Board of Medical Genetics
American Board of Neurological Surgery
American Board of Nuclear Medicine
American Board of Obstetrics and Gynecology
American Board of Ophthalmology
American Board of Orthopedic Surgery
American Board of Otolaryngology
American Board of Pathology
American Board of Pediatrics
American Board of Physical Medicine and Rehabilitation
American Board of Plastic Surgery
American Board of Preventative Medicine
American Board of Psychiatry and Neurology
American Board of Radiology
American Board of Surgery
American Board of Thoracic Surgery
American Board of Urology

TABLE 2-1

Common Specialties in Health Care Facilities

Specialty	Scope of Practice
Allergy and immunology	Specialists in allergy and immunology treat patients with immune system disorders ranging from asthma and hypersensitivity to substances to treatment of HIV and AIDS.
Anesthesiology	Anesthesiologists provide care for surgical patients. Anesthesiologists are responsible for constantly monitoring patients' vital signs during surgery. In addition, anesthesiologists provide treatment for patients who suffer from acute and chronic pain conditions.
Cardiology	Cardiologists specialize in treating disorders of the heart and vascular system. Interventional cardiologists specialize in using diagnostic testing to measure the function of the heart and blood vessels.
Dermatology	Dermatologists treat disorders of the skin, including management of skin cancer. They have training in surgical techniques used to treat integumentary disorders. In addition, they are trained to recognize manifestations of systemic diseases in the integumentary system.
Emergency medicine	An emergency physician practices both in a prehospital setting and in the emergency room. They treat all ages of patients—from young to old—and are chiefly responsible for saving patients from death or severe impairment after a serious injury or illness.
Endocrinology	An endocrinologist treats patients with disorders of the endocrine system, including diabetes, menstrual problems, and dysfunction of adrenal, thyroid, and pituitary gland(s).
Family medicine	Family medicine practitioners provide health care for patients of all ages, infant to elderly. Family medicine physicians treat patients with a wide range of health care disorders and refer patients who have more serious disorders to specialists. Family medicine professionals are primary care specialists and often referred to as family practice physicians.
Gastroenterology	A gastroenterologist treats patients with disorders of digestive tract organs, including the esophagus, stomach, liver, gallbladder, pancreas, and small and large intestines.
Hematology	A hematologist treats disorders of the lymphatic system, blood, and spleen.
Infectious disease	An infectious disease specialist treats a multitude of different diseases that affect almost any body system. Patients with a bodily disease that requires careful treatment with medication may need an infectious disease specialist.
Internal medicine	Specialists treat disorders and injuries of internal organs and are referred to as internists. They provide care for adults with a myriad of health problems.
Nephrology	A nephrologist's primary focus is disorders of the kidneys and related organs.
Neurology	Physicians in this specialty treat disorders of the brain, spinal cord, and the rest of the nervous system.
Neurosurgery	These surgeons provide treatment for patients who may need surgery on the brain, the spinal cord, or another part of the nervous system. Neurosurgeons also perform surgery on the spine itself because of the close proximity of the spine to the spinal cord.
Obstetrics and Gynecology (OB-GYN)	OB-GYN physicians serve female patients by providing care for reproductive system disorders and prenatal and postnatal care.
Oncology	Most people equate oncology with cancer or malignant tumors, but oncologists also treat patients who may have benign tumors.
Ophthalmology	Ophthalmologists treat eye disorders and are trained to recognize manifestations of systemic diseases in the eye.
Orthopedic surgery	Orthopedic surgeons examine patients with musculoskeletal disorders and operate on patients who require surgery for correction of a musculoskeletal problem.
Otolaryngology	These physicians treat patients with allergic disorders and patients with disorders of the ear, nose, and throat. They also perform surgery on patients who need surgical treatment of a condition of the ears, nose, and throat.
Pathology	Pathologists are responsible for examination of surgical specimens, autopsies, and testing of bodily substances in the laboratory.
Pediatrics	Pediatricians provide primary care to children up to age 18. Pediatricians also may choose to subspecialize.
Physical medicine and rehabilitation	Known as a physiatrist, a physician in this specialty is responsible for restoring body function for patients with disabilities resulting from illness or injury. They may treat patients who suffer from neck or back pain, or who have had a debilitating bodily injury from trauma or a disease process.

Continued

TABLE 2-1

Common Specialties in Health Care Facilities—cont'd

Specialty	Scope of Practice
Plastic surgery	These surgeons provide surgery to patients requiring reconstruction of skin or underlying structures.
Psychiatry	Psychiatrists provide psychotherapy and medication to patients with psychological disorders. Psychotherapy involves helping patients regain good mental health through discussions and counseling.
Pulmonology	Pulmonologists treat patients with disorders of the respiratory system.
Radiology	Radiologists are responsible for the radiology department of a health care facility. They interpret diagnostic radiologic tests that have been done by a radiologic technologist, and they are involved in the radiologic treatment of some patients.
Rheumatology	Rheumatologists treat disorders of the musculoskeletal system, including diseases and injuries.
Sports medicine	Sports medicine physicians seek to promote health and fitness in patients and treat musculoskeletal injuries resulting from sports activities.
Surgery	A general surgeon provides surgical services to patients with many common conditions. A surgeon may choose to further specialize in areas such as vascular surgery, pediatric surgery, and hand surgery, to name a few.
Urology	A urologist treats disorders of the entire urinary system and the adrenal glands.

BOX 2-2

American Osteopathic Boards

American Osteopathic Board of Anesthesiology
American Osteopathic Board of Dermatology
American Osteopathic Board of Emergency Medicine
American Osteopathic Board of Family Physicians
American Osteopathic Board of Internal Medicine
American Osteopathic Board of Neurology and Psychiatry
American Osteopathic Board of Neuromusculoskeletal Medicine
American Osteopathic Board of Nuclear Medicine
American Osteopathic Board of Obstetrics and Gynecology
American Osteopathic Board of Ophthalmology and Otolaryngology
American Osteopathic Board of Orthopedic Surgery
American Osteopathic Board of Pathology
American Osteopathic Board of Pediatrics
American Osteopathic Board of Physical Medicine and Rehabilitation
American Osteopathic Board of Preventative Medicine
American Osteopathic Board of Proctology
American Osteopathic Board of Radiology
American Osteopathic Board of Surgery

The American Osteopathic Association (AOA) provides 18 board examinations for specialization of osteopathic physicians (Box 2-2).

Board certification is not required for physicians but is highly desirable. Board certification indicates that a physician has achieved a certain level of expertise in his or her chosen field. Whether or not a physician chooses to take a board examination, he or she may choose to practice in a particular medical specialty. Both MDs and DOs may choose a specialty.

Primary Care Specialties

Primary care specialties include the greatest number of physicians because a primary care specialty involves treating patients with numerous and various ailments. Primary care physicians are physicians who treat disorders of all parts of the body. They provide care for patients' routine health needs on a regular basis and when necessary, they refer patients to other physicians for more specialized care.

According to the American Medical Association (AMA), primary care specialties include family practice and general practice, internal medicine, obstetrics and gynecology (OB-GYN), and pediatrics. *The Occupational Outlook Handbook* (Bureau of Labor Statistics, 2010–2011) reports that 47% of MDs are in a primary care specialty and the American Osteopathic Association reports that approximately 60% of DOs are primary care providers.

Current Trends

Many years ago, it was common for a physician to practice independently in a small office located either within his or her own home or, perhaps, in a small storefront on the main street in town. Physicians were on call almost every day of the week and received little support from fellow physicians, owing to the geographic distances between them. Since the 1950s, increasing specialization in medicine has led many physicians to group together in multispecialty clinics.

In today's health care environment, physicians are much more likely than they were in years past to work as part of a group practice. A group practice offers some relief for physicians in providing emergency coverage for patients. A group practice allows physicians to communicate more readily with one another and gives physicians within the group access to one another's expertise. This arrangement also allows the practice to pool resources to buy more state-of-the art equipment to diagnose and treat patients and to provide additional health care services.

Another change that has been seen in the delivery of health care over the past 40 years is the increase in the number of female physicians. In 1970, medical practices consisted of mostly male physicians as more than 92% of physicians at that time were male. In 2006, that number was reduced to 72%, with female physicians making up nearly 28% of all physicians.

Currently, the health care industry is undergoing a shift in the types of physicians that will be needed to fill jobs in the future. The growing number of **managed care** insurance plans today means that even more primary care physicians will be needed to serve the U.S. population.

Managed care plans normally require that a patient see a primary care physician, who acts as a "gatekeeper," when seeking help with a medical problem or for preventive care. The gatekeeper role means that the primary care physician always sees the patient first (except in emergency cases) and refers the patient to a specialist only when necessary. The use of primary care physicians results in an overall reduction in health care costs for the consumer. More information on managed care is provided in Chapter 12.

Another trend in recent years is the addition of health care providers who are not physicians. **Mid-level providers** are nonphysician health care providers who provide direct patient care. Also known as **physician extenders** or **nonphysician practitioners (NPPs)**, they are able to treat and diagnose patients. Examples of such providers are physician assistants, nurse practitioners, nurse midwives, and nurse anesthetists. The addition of these health care providers increases patient access to health care. This is particularly important in rural areas where health care providers can be scarce. The *Occupational Outlook Handbook 2010–2011* reports that in 2007, the American Medical Association reported that 75% of physicians worked in metropolitan areas and only 25% worked in rural areas. The National Rural Health Association reports that number to be lower with only 10% of physicians practicing in rural areas, even though 25% of the population lives in what can be defined as a rural area. The addition of mid-level providers to a medical practice serves the public well because these providers increase the availability of health care across the United States.

CHECKPOINT

Explain why a group practice may want to employ more primary care physicians than specialists.

Physician Assistant

Physician assistants (PAs) provide routine health care under the supervision of a physician. They examine patients and may order and interpret laboratory tests, make diagnoses, and provide treatment. They can treat injuries that require sutures, splints, or casts and often assist a physician in surgery. In most states, PAs may prescribe medications. Depending on the requirements of the state, the extent of the PA's duties may be decided by the state regulating agency or by the supervising physician.

Admittance into many PA training programs requires a minimum of 2 years of undergraduate education and some work experience in health care. PA programs last about 2 years. The PA curriculum consists of health-related courses and clinical experiences in areas such as OB-GYN, emergency medicine, pediatrics, and surgery.

Almost all states and the District of Columbia require that PAs pass the Physician Assistants' National Certifying Examination before they can practice in their state. Once a PA has passed the examination, he or she is allowed to use the credential PA-C (physician assistant-certified). PAs must complete 100 continuing education hours every 2 years to keep their certification. In addition, PAs must complete a recertification examination every 6 years or complete an alternative program for recertification. PAs often work in primary care or may specialize in an area of medicine such as general surgery, orthopedics, emergency medicine, or geriatrics. PAs who work in a surgery-related specialty may assist during surgical procedures.

Nurse Practitioner

A nurse practitioner is an advanced practice registered nurse who diagnoses and treats patients with acute or chronic problems, illness, or injury, or who may provide well care to patients. Nurse practitioners can specialize in one of many specialties, including but not limited to family medicine, pediatrics, women's health, oncology, gerontology, or psychiatry.

Nurse practitioners are allowed to prescribe medications in most states, but the types of medications that they are allowed to prescribe may vary among states. Similar to PAs, nurse practitioners usually work under the supervision of a physician. The extent of the supervision required is determined by the state in which they work.

As mentioned previously, a nurse practitioner is an advanced practice nurse who has met additional educational and clinical requirements beyond those needed to obtain a master's degree in nursing. A nurse practitioner course of study usually lasts 2 years.

Similar to other health care providers, as mentioned previously, certification and licensure requirements for nurse practitioners vary from state to state. Some states require that nurse practitioners pass a certification examination before they are eligible for licensure. A nurse who has passed the certification examination is known as a Certified Nurse Practitioner (CNP). Continuing education will be required to maintain licensure.

Certified Nurse Midwife

Somewhat similar in practice to a nurse practitioner, a certified nurse midwife (CNM) is an advanced practice registered nurse who provides primary health care services for women. A CNM conducts routine yearly physical examinations for women, delivers babies, prescribes medications, and provides prenatal and postnatal care for routine (i.e., without serious complications) obstetrics patients. CNMs are licensed in all states and the District of Columbia. Both certified nurse midwives and certified midwives (CMs) provide primary health care services to women, but the CNM has training in both nursing and midwifery and the CM has training in just midwifery.

Podiatrist

A doctor of podiatric medicine (DPM), also known as a podiatrist, treats disorders of the foot and lower leg. Podiatrists treat a variety of foot disorders, from corns, calluses, and bunions to foot disorders caused by diabetes. Podiatrists are allowed to prescribe drugs, perform surgery, treat fractures, and order tests to diagnose foot problems. They make customized inserts, known as orthotics, to correct foot abnormalities and even custom design shoes.

Most applicants to a college of podiatric medicine have a bachelor's degree before they seek admission. Podiatric colleges offer a 4-year curriculum that includes courses in a variety of sciences, as well as clinical rotations in clinics and hospitals. A graduate of a college of podiatric medicine is known as a DPM. After becoming a DPM, podiatrists usually complete a residency training of 1 to 3 years. Residents receive advanced education in anesthesiology, surgery, and related areas.

To practice podiatric medicine, podiatrists must be licensed by the state in which they work. All states have outlined the requirements for licensure to practice in their state. Many states have reciprocity agreements that allow podiatrists to easily obtain licensure in more than one state.

Psychologist

Many different types of psychologists are available, but the most common type of psychologist is the clinical psychologist, who is employed in a hospital, clinic, or counseling center. A clinical psychologist attains a doctor of psychology (PsyD) degree and treats patients with mental health disorders and assists them in adjusting to their life circumstances. Depending on the focus of their training, other psychologists may earn a doctor of philosophy (PhD) degree.

A psychologist differs from a psychiatrist in that a psychiatrist is trained as a medical doctor and a psychologist is not. A psychiatrist can prescribe medications for patients. Psychologists often advise a patient's medical doctor regarding the patient's progress, which, in turn, may indicate the need to medicate the patient. A psychologist generally cannot prescribe medication; however, a couple of states do allow psychologists to prescribe some medications. If a patient needs medication for a psychiatric illness, such medication can be prescribed by a psychiatrist or by a primary care physician.

In addition to a doctoral degree, a psychologist must meet state requirements for certification or licensure to counsel patients. Such requirements normally include passing a certification examination and completing a specified amount of continuing education for certificate or license renewal.

Chiropractor

A Doctor of Chiropractic (DC), also known as a chiropractor, treats patients with disorders associated with the musculoskeletal or nervous system. Chiropractors believe that musculoskeletal problems can cause problems throughout the body and may obstruct the body's ability to fight disease.

Chiropractors do not prescribe drugs or perform surgery; instead, they treat patients, when appropriate, by manipulating or adjusting the spine. They also may treat patients via ultrasound, massage, or heat therapy.

A bachelor's degree usually is required for admission to a chiropractic college. Chiropractic programs consist of 4 years of study, with the student taking science courses during the first 2 years and completing clinical experiences and related courses during the last 2 years. There are also chiropractic specialty boards that further focus a chiropractor's education.

Chiropractors, similar to other health care providers, must be licensed by the state in which they work. All states and the District of Columbia regulate the practice of chiropractic within their boundaries. Some states have reciprocity agreements that allow chiropractors with a license in another state to easily apply for a license to practice in their state.

Optometrist

Optometrists (also known as doctors of optometry [ODs]) perform eye examinations and prescribe corrective lenses to correct vision problems. Optometrists provide a large portion of the primary eye care in the United States.

Both optometrists and ophthalmologists perform eye examinations and can prescribe corrective lenses for patients. The difference between the two is that the ophthalmologist is an MD who performs eye surgery, prescribes medications, and treats all types of eye diseases. Optometrists are allowed to diagnose vision problems, prescribe corrective lenses, or provide vision therapy, and they are permitted to prescribe certain medications to treat some eye diseases.

Most optometry students have a bachelor's degree on entrance to an optometry school. The optometry curriculum consists of courses in health and visual sciences and usually takes 4 years to complete.

All states and the District of Columbia require licensure of optometrists who wish to practice within their boundaries. Optometrists are required to be graduates of an accredited college of optometry and must pass a licensure examination. Continuing education credits are required for license renewal.

Nurse Anesthetist

Nurse anesthetists are advanced practice registered nurses who work under the supervision of an anesthesiologist. They administer all types of surgical anesthesia and monitor a patient's vital signs intraoperatively and postoperatively, and they provide approximately 65% of all anesthesia administered in all types of health care facilities.

The Council on Certification of Nurse Anesthetists is responsible for conducting the certification examination and for certifying nurse anesthetists. Continuing education and current licensure as a nurse are required for recertification every 2 years.

CHECKPOINT

What advantage(s) would result if a health care facility chose to hire health care providers other than physicians to provide health care services for patients?

Nursing Professionals

Registered Nurse

Registered nurses (RNs) constitute the largest health care occupation in the United States. RNs work in many different settings, from clinics and hospitals to nursing homes, home health, public health, and health-related administrative positions.

The chief focus of the nursing profession is the caring process. Nurses help patients recover from or live with illness or injury, observe patient progress, administer medications, and assist physicians. Nurses are also essential in providing health education to patients.

Depending on the location in which they work, job conditions can vary greatly. Nurses in administration may spend many hours behind a desk and/or computer. Nurses who are involved in direct patient care may spend long hours on their feet. Some nursing positions require work at all hours of the day or night every day of the week; work hours for other positions may extend from 8 AM to 5 PM, Monday through Friday.

Educational opportunities for an RN vary. An associate's degree in nursing (2 years) provides education for an entry-level position as an RN. The Bachelor of Science degree in nursing (BSN) (4 years) provides further training should a nurse wish to pursue a position in management or education. BSNs have many more career opportunities because of their advanced educational preparation.

All RNs must take a national certification examination. Successful completion of the certification examination is a standard requirement for licensure. Each state establishes specific requirements for licensure as an RN.

Licensed Practical Nurse

Licensed practical nurses (LPNs) or licensed vocational nurses (LVNs in Texas and California) (Fig. 2-2) provide basic patient care, such as taking vital signs, performing laboratory tests, providing patients with hygiene care, and reporting patient progress. In some states, they are allowed to start intravenous lines and administer prescribed medications. LPNs usually work under the supervision of a physician or an RN. As RNs have moved into more supervisory positions, LPNs have become more directly involved in patient care, with LPNs performing many of the nursing duties in a medical office.

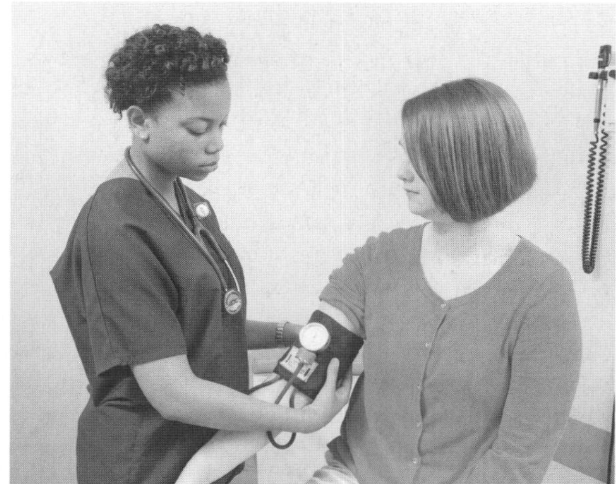

Figure 2-2 Licensed practical nurses perform many of the basic patient care duties in a medical office, such as taking vital signs and documenting patient progress. (From Young A: *Kinn's The Administrative Medical Assistant,* ed 7, St. Louis, Saunders, 2011.)

Educational requirements for LPNs vary from state to state. Most programs are 1 year in length; a few programs are 2 years in length. Education includes health-related classroom courses, as well as clinical experience. To work as an LPN or LVN, all states require that LPNs and LVNs must be graduates of an approved program who have passed an examination for licensure.

Certified Nursing Assistant

Certified nursing assistants (CNAs) provide personal care for patients in hospitals and nursing homes. CNAs assist patients with eating and personal hygiene. The nature of CNA work is physically demanding, with CNAs often having to lift and transfer patients. Nursing assistants must be careful to avoid injury while at work. All nursing professionals, including RNs, LPNs, and CNAs, are particularly vulnerable to injury because of the nature of their work.

To work as a CNA, an individual usually takes a short course (approximately 3 weeks in length) that involves classroom study and clinical experience and then is usually required to take a state certification examination.

Allied Health Professionals

Medical Administrative Assistant

As detailed in Chapter 1, a medical administrative assistant provides administrative support for many of the business functions of a medical office (see Box 1-2). Depending on the make-up of the health care organization, a medical administrative assistant's responsibilities may be quite diverse or may be specialized. Many other titles may describe this position such as administrative medical assistant, medical office specialist, medical secretary, or others, as found in Box 1-1.

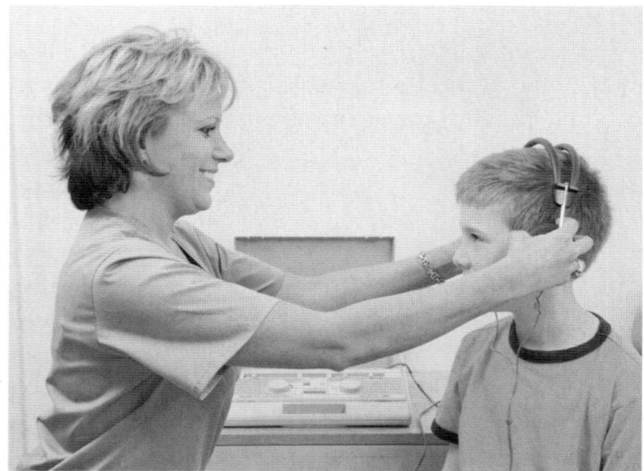

Figure 2-3 A certified medical assistant is qualified to perform clinical, as well as administrative, duties in the medical office. (From Young A: *Kinn's The Administrative Medical Assistant*, ed 7, St. Louis, Saunders, 2011.)

Medical Assistant

As mentioned in Chapter 1, medical assistants (Fig. 2-3) are qualified to perform administrative and clinical duties in the medical office. In smaller offices, medical assistants may actually perform both clinical and administrative duties, but in a larger office, the medical assistant may specialize in either administrative or clinical duties. Practices with a larger patient volume are often more "departmentalized" than are practices with a smaller patient volume, and a medical assistant is likely to be assigned specific duties.

In some states, medical assistants who will be performing certain clinical duties are required to pass the national certification examination. Two national organizations, the American Association of Medical Assistants (AAMA) and American Medical Technologists (AMT), provide certification for medical assistants, depending on the requirements of the state in which the assistant wishes to work. The assistant also may be required to be a graduate of an accredited medical assistant program before becoming certified or registered. Chapter 1 provides additional information about these organizations (see Table 1-1). Examination is not required for assistants who perform office duties only.

Medical Transcriptionist

A medical transcriptionist's chief responsibility is to transcribe physician dictation. An accurate recording of a patient's encounters with health care providers is a critical component of any medical record.

Medical transcriptionists must possess an extensive knowledge of anatomy and physiology, medical terminology, and disease processes, and they must have a great deal of computer ability and keyboarding skill. These are all necessary for creating medical reports, office chart notes, letters, and other essential components of the medical record.

Although it is not necessary for employment, the credential certified medical transcriptionist (CMT) is awarded by the Association for Healthcare Documentation Integrity to individuals who pass both written and practical portions of the medical transcription certification examination. A medical assistant or medical administrative assistant also may perform the duties of a transcriptionist in the medical office.

Medical Coder

Billing and insurance processing are vital to the financial health of a medical office. Medical coders assign procedure and diagnosis codes based on the information contained in a patient's medical record to receive payment for those services from health insurance plans.

There are general coding certifications as well as many types of specialty coding certifications available from the largest coding certification organization, the American Academy of Professional Coders (AAPC). The AAPC provides two basic certifications—the Certified Professional Coder (CPC) and the Certified Professional Coder–Hospital (CPC-H)—and has 23 other certifications for individuals wishing to further demonstrate their expertise in coding.

Health Information Professionals

Three types of professionals work with health information: registered health information technicians (RHITs), registered health information administrators (RHIAs), and cancer registrars. Individuals who work in the health information profession are primarily responsible for reviewing the health information (medical records) of patients treated in health care facilities. Review of health information is done to ensure that records are organized appropriately and are complete and accurate.

This health care profession is unusual in that persons who work in this profession have little to no contact with patients. They work primarily behind the scenes, maintaining medical records and supplying information for patient billing and insurance claims.

Registered Health Information Technician

Health information technicians are graduates of a 2-year health information program. After graduating from an accredited program, the graduate may choose to take a credentialing examination to become an RHIT. The examination is offered by the American Health Information Management Association, a professional organization for health information professionals. Health information technicians are responsible for day-to-day maintenance and management of the medical record and may be involved in diagnostic and procedural coding of health care services for billing purposes.

Registered Health Information Administrator

An RHIA is an individual who has successfully completed a bachelor's degree program in health information and has passed a national certification examination.

RHIAs usually are employed as directors of health information (medical records) departments in health care facilities. They are chiefly responsible for coordinating health information department activities, such as medical transcription,

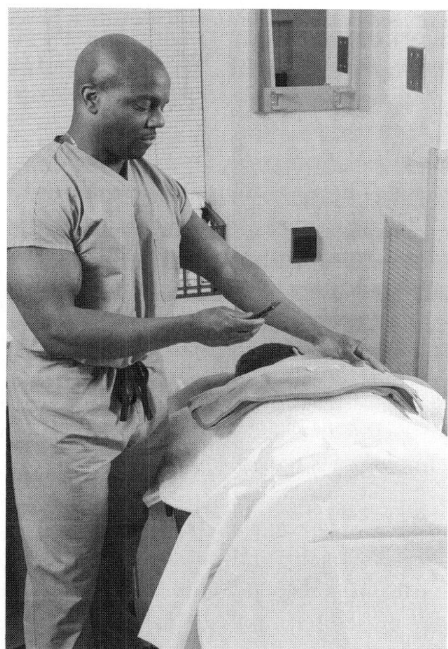

Figure 2-4 A physical therapist provides treatments to help improve or restore a patient's mobility.

records review, coding, and even tumor registry. RHIAs supervise the health information staff and ensure that a facility's health information practices conform to national accreditation standards.

Cancer Registrar

Information related to history, diagnosis, and treatment of patients with cancer is compiled by a cancer registrar. Codes are used to identify type of cancer, tumor location and extent, and treatments provided to the patient. In addition, the cancer registrar performs valuable follow-up with patients and physicians to gather information on patient progress. This information then is sent to state cancer registries and is available for physicians and public health officials for detection, prevention, and treatment of cancer and for cancer research. Certified tumor registrar (CTR) certification is available through the National Cancer Registrars Association.

Physical Therapist

A physical therapist (PT) (Fig. 2-4) provides treatment to improve or restore a patient's ability to move when the patient is affected by disease or injury. Therapists develop treatment plans that may involve exercise, ultrasound, or application of heat or cold to alleviate a patient's pain. PTs often consult with the patient's provider to plan an appropriate mode of treatment. If a PT is not able to bring about full restoration of a patient's mobility, the therapist works to limit the effects of the disability on the patient's overall health.

To become licensed as a PT, an individual first must be a graduate of an accredited physical therapy program, either a master's or doctoral degree program with almost all programs at the doctorate level. On graduation, a therapist must pass a licensing examination to be able to practice.

Physical Therapy Assistant

A physical therapy assistant (PTA) provides physical therapy treatments as assigned by a supervising PT. Such treatments include exercise, ultrasound, massage, application of heat or cold packs, and possibly traction. The job of a physical therapy assistant is often physically demanding, requiring lifting of patients and administration of various therapies as directed by a PT.

PTA programs generally last 2 years. Most states require that PTAs have at least an associate's degree, and some states require licensing of PTAs.

Occupational Therapist

Whereas a PT works with patients to help restore or improve the function of the body, an occupational therapist (OT) works with patients to restore skills needed for daily living. These range from personal skills (e.g., dressing, eating, grooming) to everyday living skills (e.g., homemaking, budgeting, using transportation). Sometimes, a patient is not able to be restored to a former level of functioning and must adapt to his or her impairment and learn ways to compensate for the loss of function. The OT's objective is to bring the patient to the maximum level of functioning possible.

All states regulate this profession. OTs must graduate from an accredited program with a minimum of a bachelor's degree and must pass a certification examination.

Occupational Therapy Assistant

Just as PTAs provide treatments as planned by PTs, occupational therapy assistants (OTAs) provide treatments as planned by OTs. OTAs can help patients learn how to perform tasks of daily living after they have suffered an illness or injury. They may teach patients how to transfer to a wheelchair properly or cook a meal, or they may even plan recreational activities with patients.

Most states regulate OTAs and require them to be graduates of accredited 2-year programs and to have passed a certification examination. Once the assistant has passed the certification examination, he or she is known as a certified occupational therapy assistant (COTA).

Respiratory Therapist

Respiratory therapists are concerned with the treatment and care of patients with respiratory dysfunction. They evaluate the patient's ability to breathe and deliver treatments ordered by the patient's provider. Training for a respiratory therapist generally lasts 2 years; some programs are 4 years in length. Most states (48) require respiratory therapists to become licensed. To be licensed, graduates of accredited programs take the examination from the National Board of Respiratory Care to become a certified respiratory therapist (CRT). If a CRT has completed sufficient education and experience, he or she may take an examination to become a registered respiratory therapist (RRT). The RRT credential is usually required of persons in a supervisory role.

Radiology Technologist

The field of radiology provides many different services within the health care industry. Radiology involves not only the use of x-rays in radiography but also the use of ultrasound, computed tomography (CT), and magnetic resonance imaging (MRI).

Radiology technologists or radiographers (Fig. 2-5) are responsible for taking x-ray images of parts of the body. They may administer contrast material (or dye) to the patient to allow better visualization of the body's internal structures. Radiologic technologists can specialize in many fields, such as ultrasound, CT scanning, MRI, nuclear medicine, or mammography.

Ultrasound technologists use ultrasound to create images of a patient's body for interpretation by the physician. Ultrasound technologists are known as sonographers and may even specialize in taking ultrasound images of specific parts of the body.

Programs that train radiologic technologists last from 1 to 4 years, with 2 years being the most common program length. Sometimes, health care professionals from other fields will cross-train in a 1-year radiology program.

About two thirds of U.S. states require licensure of radiologic technologists. Licensure requires successful completion of a certification examination offered by the American Registry of Radiologic Technologists (ARRT). A registered radiologic technologist (RT) renews his or her certification by providing evidence regarding continuing education and compliance with ARRT Standards of Ethics. Many employers prefer to hire registered RTs, but in some states, it is not necessary to be certified to perform this occupation. In 2007, 40 states required licensure of radiologic technologists.

Clinical Laboratory Technologist and Technician

Laboratory testing of a patient's bodily substances is often an integral part of the process of arriving at an accurate diagnosis of the patient's condition. Clinical laboratory personnel analyze urine, blood, and other body substances and tissues to establish whether bacteria or foreign substances are present or to determine the level of certain components in the body. Laboratory personnel identify cell characteristics and determine the quantities of cells present within the body.

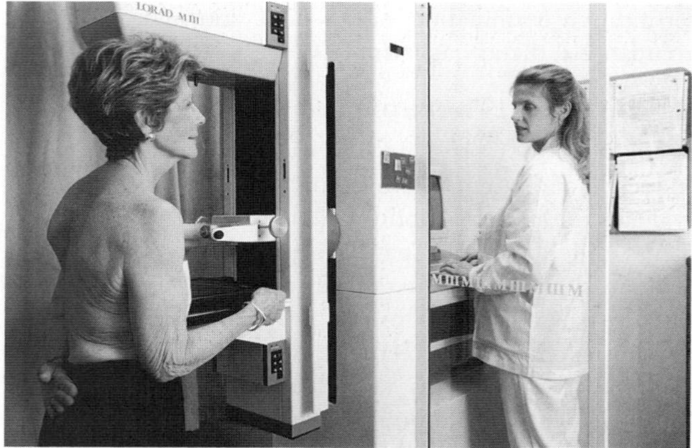

Figure 2-5 The field of radiology involves radiographs, ultrasound, CT scans, and MRI for diagnosing patient illness, as well as the use of radiology to treat patients. (From Young A: *Kinn's The Administrative Medical Assistant*, ed 7, St. Louis, Saunders, 2011.)

The difference between the training of clinical laboratory technologists and that of technicians is that technologists usually have a bachelor's degree and technicians may have an associate's degree or a vocational diploma or certificate. Technologists generally are responsible for conducting more sophisticated tests and may be found in supervisory roles. Technicians usually perform more routine or less complicated tests within the medical laboratory. Licensure to work as a medical technologist is required in some but not all states.

Pharmacist

The pharmacist is an integral part of the health care team. It is the pharmacist's responsibility to dispense medications to patients as prescribed by their physician. The pharmacist also counsels patients about the proper use of medications that they are taking. Pharmacists may work in clinics or hospitals, or they may work in retail pharmacies. Regardless of where a pharmacist is located, he or she can be in close contact with the physician when necessary for the well-being of the patient.

Students are required to complete a doctor of pharmacy (PharmD) degree program. After graduation, the graduate is eligible to take the state licensing examination. All states require pharmacists to be licensed to practice.

Social Worker

Sometimes employed in hospital or clinic settings, as well as in private practices, social workers help people deal with difficult life circumstances such as unemployment, serious or chronic illness, family or social problems, and other circumstances that may impair a person's ability to handle everyday life. A master's degree in social work usually is required for an individual to work in a health care setting; in addition, some type of certification, licensure, or registration is required for such social workers in the United States.

Licensure, Certification, and Registration

As mentioned previously, most health care professionals must be licensed before they can treat patients. Each state establishes the requirements for licensure in a particular health care field. Requirements usually include graduation from an accredited educational institution and completion of a specified professional examination. Such examinations usually are given by the national organization associated with a particular profession.

Not all professions require licensure. Some health professions have a certification or registration process. Certification or registration is not always required for an employee to work in certain fields. Certification is awarded by the national organization associated with a particular profession. An individual who desires certification must meet the organization's requirements for certification, which typically include taking a credentialing examination. On successful completion of an examination, the individual may use the "certified" designation. Some professions may offer more than one certification examination.

The registration process for a profession involves meeting specific requirements. Those requirements may involve special educational requirements or possibly an examination, or they simply may consist of payment of a registration fee.

Licensure, certification, and registration in a medical field usually must be renewed every few years. To be eligible for renewal of a license, certificate, or registration, most states or organizations require that a health professional have a minimum number of continuing education units (CEUs) in his or her field. Continuing education activity may include attending conventions, seminars, or workshops; taking college courses; and even reviewing independent study materials. The purpose of requiring CEUs is to ensure that individuals in the profession keep current with changes that are occurring in their profession. Individuals must constantly be aware of industry changes if they are to perform their jobs properly. Ultimately, such strict guidelines for licensure, certification, or registration protect the health, safety, and welfare of the public.

Professional Organizations

Nearly every health profession has a professional organization that plays a large part in establishing and maintaining high standards for the profession. As mentioned previously, these organizations often are involved in the development and administration of licensure and certification examinations. Many organizations offer continuing education programs for their membership and serve as a valuable resource for health information that helps members meet certification and/or licensure requirements; they also provide opportunities for members to network with others in their profession.

Health Care Facilities

The public can receive health care treatment in many different types of facilities. The facilities described here are some of the most common places where health care is provided.

Clinic

In a **clinic** or medical office, a physician or group of physicians and possibly other providers (e.g., nurse practitioners, physician assistants, nurse midwives) provide care to patients. This care is referred to as **ambulatory** or **outpatient** care because the patient comes and goes within a 24-hour period and is usually treated within a span of a few hours. A clinic is a chief location for primary care or routine outpatient care delivery. Patients who receive outpatient care usually have routine health concerns and do not have a condition severe enough to warrant an overnight stay in the hospital. Occasionally, ambulatory care patients do arrive at a clinic with a serious medical condition that necessitates admission to a hospital.

Some very large group practices include at least one physician who can provide care in each of the major specialty areas. Large group practices are prevalent throughout the United States, with physicians from varying specialties practicing together at a single clinic location.

One of the largest and probably most famous multispecialty groups in the United States is the Mayo Clinic, located in Rochester, Minnesota. This clinic, which is a prime example of health care availability at its finest, draws patients from around the globe. In 2009, the Mayo Clinic employed nearly 3,700 physicians and scientists; 3,200 residents, fellows, and students; and an allied health staff of more than 49,000 employees at its three main clinic sites in Rochester, Minnesota, Scottsdale, Arizona, and Jacksonville, Florida. In that year, their three sites served over 500,000 patients. In addition to providing top-quality patient care, the Mayo Clinic is a teaching facility at which physicians and other health care professionals are educated. The Mayo Clinic has greatly influenced the trend toward specialized medicine and group practice. In his speech to the graduating class of Rush Medical College in 1910, Dr. William J. Mayo stated, "The sum total of medical knowledge is now so great and wide-spreading that it would be futile for any one man...to assume that he has even a working knowledge of any part of the whole." Dr. Mayo recognized, even 100 years ago, that specialization in medicine was not only inevitable but necessary.

It is quite common today for large clinics to also provide specialized health care at satellite offices or branch clinics. Some branch clinics are located in rural areas to allow greater access to health care for rural residents, and some branch clinics are located in suburban areas of a large city. Branch clinics usually provide primary care on a regular basis and occasionally have specialists who work at the clinic on an intermittent basis. An example of this type of arrangement would be a dermatologist who has office hours at a branch clinic every Tuesday. Rotation of specialists allows access to specialized health care for individuals who might not otherwise have access to that specialized care without traveling a great distance. Branch clinics also are a considerable source of referrals to specialists at a larger clinic.

Physicians who practice in group practices enjoy several advantages. First, physicians in a group practice can consult with one another quickly when faced with a difficult diagnosis. Second, physicians who work in a clinic setting usually have reduced responsibility for being available during hours when the clinic is closed because on-call responsibility is shared with other group physicians. In addition, overhead costs, such as costs of staff, equipment, and buildings, are shared among the entire clinical practice. A large group practice usually is run by a board of directors that makes decisions on facility operation and management, thereby relieving the group's physicians of having to oversee all aspects of a medical office. A group practice arrangement is supportive for physicians within the practice.

Private Practice

In a **private practice,** a physician provides outpatient medical care from an office in which the physician may be the only provider, or the physician may be part of a group practice that operates independently of any university or insurance company affiliation. Some physicians prefer to have their own private practices because they may want the freedom to make decisions about how the practice is run. Physicians who operate a private practice usually maintain an affiliation with at least one hospital so that they may have the right to admit patients when necessary for hospital care. Physicians in private practice may have increased on-call duty and also often shoulder the responsibility of running the medical office.

Hospital

Hospitals vary greatly in the types of services they provide. In general, a **hospital** provides **inpatient** health care—that is, health care that requires the patient to stay overnight (longer than a 24-hour period) and have the constant attention of nursing staff at the hospital. Hospitals are designed to provide care for patients with acute conditions; therefore, usually all of the services and equipment (lab, radiography, surgery) needed to serve patients are located within the hospital. Hospitals also may offer outpatient services for patients. They can be operated for profit or as nonprofit organizations.

Hospitals often differ in the types of services they provide. Some hospitals are designated trauma centers, meaning that they are appropriately equipped and staffed to handle certain types of emergency cases, such as critically injured adult or pediatric patients. Such trauma centers may even have helicopter service to bring critical patients to the hospital. The American College of Surgeons has defined national standards for trauma care and has identified four levels of trauma care ranging from Level I to Level IV, with Level I providing the highest level of care.

Some hospitals specialize in the type of care they provide. For example, a children's hospital may provide inpatient care for persons younger than 18 years. A rehabilitation hospital may accept patients who need rehabilitative services because of illness or injury. A psychiatric hospital may provide inpatient or outpatient mental health care.

Emergency Room

Most people are familiar with the emergency department in a hospital. The **emergency department (ED)** or **emergency room (ER)** is the place within a hospital that receives patients who are acutely, seriously, or critically ill or injured. Emergency departments are open 24 hours a day, every day. Sometimes patients with health concerns such as abdominal pain, severe headache, and musculoskeletal injuries go to the ER because their regular health care provider is unavailable or because the office is closed. Of course, accident victims and patients with critical illnesses such as stroke or heart attack also end up in the ER. The ER provides care to all types of patients with acute conditions, and, if a patient's condition warrants hospitalization, an attending physician will admit the patient.

Urgent Care Center

An urgent care center might bring to mind thoughts of an emergency room; however, an urgent care center and an emergency room are not the same thing.

Urgent care centers can be found in various locations. Some urgent care centers are located within an ER. Even though ERs are open 24 hours a day, urgent care centers located in an ER may or may not be open 24 hours a day (patients may not even be able to tell where the ER starts and where the urgent care center ends).

In a combination urgent care center/ER, patients are received at a central desk area, where a medical administrative assistant takes registration data. The assistant then communicates the patient's arrival to a nurse, who interviews the patient, takes vital signs, and assesses the level of care that the patient may need. This assessment is known as **triage**. At this point, depending on the type of care needed, the decision usually is made by the nurse about whether the patient will be seen in urgent care or as an emergency patient.

One big difference for the patient is the amount of money that will be charged for the visit. The cost of urgent care treatment is ordinarily much less than the cost of treatment provided in an ER. If at any time the patient requires care greater than that provided in urgent care, the patient will be transferred to the ER.

Urgent care centers are convenient because they provide care for patients who require the attention of a physician but do not have an appointment. These centers sometimes are referred to as walk-in clinics because patients can walk in without an appointment and are seen by a health care provider. Patients usually are seen in the order in which they arrive, but acutely ill or injured patients may be given priority over other patients. In addition to hospital settings, urgent care centers may be found in clinic settings. Urgent care centers within a clinic may follow a clinic's regularly scheduled hours or may be open for extended hours.

The tremendous advantage of urgent care centers is that urgent care provides patients with immediate access to health care. No appointment is necessary. The centers provide care for patients' illnesses and injuries ranging from very routine cases such as ear infections, sore throats, and urinary tract infections to more serious cases such as fracture, appendicitis, and severe infection.

A recent development in provision of urgent care services is the establishment of quick health care access in shopping malls and other business establishments. Such places may advertise that patients are seen within 15 minutes, and health care is provided by a nurse practitioner or PA for routine ailments such as sore throats, ear infections, and other problems that need immediate attention. These facilities may consist of only one examination room and often are staffed only by the health care provider.

Outpatient (Ambulatory) Surgery Center

As mentioned previously, delivery of health care services has changed drastically since the 1980s. During those years, there was a tremendous shift to outpatient delivery of surgical services. Many surgical procedures that used to require one or more nights in the hospital are now available to patients on an outpatient basis. At an **outpatient**, or **ambulatory, surgery center** (sometimes called **day surgery**), patients receive instructions to prepare for surgery (e.g., no food or water after midnight) and arrive at the center an hour or two before their scheduled surgery.

Patients then are passed through a series of preoperative steps to ready them for surgery. They sign necessary forms, have vital signs taken, and put on surgical garments. In many instances, patients even walk to the surgical suite (accompanied by a health professional) for their surgery.

After surgery, patients are taken to a recovery area to wait for the effects of any anesthesia or intraoperative medications to dissipate. In the recovery area, family members often are allowed to visit the patient until the patient is ready to be discharged. At the time of discharge, patients are given postoperative instructions to be followed after they are discharged.

Many different types of surgeries can be performed on an outpatient basis. All patients are not alike, however; in some instances, because of other preexisting medical conditions, a patient may be a surgical risk and may require inpatient hospitalization. Also, problems may arise during a surgical procedure, and a patient may require hospitalization as a result of complications during surgery.

On the whole, outpatient surgery has made an impact in keeping costs down for patients and insurance plans by allowing patients to recuperate at home instead of in the hospital.

Home Health

Home health care has become big business. Home health care refers, of course, to care given to a patient in his or her own home. With the rising costs of health care, insurance companies, physicians, and patients have been looking for ways to access health care while sparing some expense. Most insurance companies are willing to pay for home health care services because this often is less costly than having a patient hospitalized.

Home health care agencies make it possible for patients to receive health care in their own home instead of traveling to a health care facility. Of course, not all health care can be delivered at home, but health care such as physical therapy, occupational therapy, respiratory therapy, speech therapy, and intravenous treatment often is delivered in the patient's home.

Hospice Care

Hospice care provides medical, psychological, and spiritual care for terminally ill persons who have a life expectancy of less than 6 months. In addition, support is provided for family members. Care can be provided in a person's home, or hospice care may be provided in a health care facility. Hospice care places a great emphasis on quality of life at the end of life and provides palliative medical care that eases pain and suffering. Physician and nursing services, counseling, social services, and physical and speech therapies are just some of the many services offered through hospice care.

Nursing Home, Assisted Living

Nursing homes and assisted living facilities provide continual care to patients (usually called residents). The residents live within the facility and receive the level of health care that they need.

Nursing homes provide round-the-clock care for their residents. Residents may be elderly and feeble with multiple health problems, or they may be young individuals who have a serious or life-threatening health problem that does not justify inpatient hospitalization but who are too ill to be cared for at home. RNs, LPNs, and CNAs provide round-the-clock care to residents, with physicians visiting the nursing home when necessary to see patients.

Assisted living facilities may be located with, or separate from, a nursing home. These facilities provide residents with the level of health care required for their particular health situation. Residents live in an apartment-type setting and may require services such as assistance with medication. Meals may be eaten in a central dining area or within the resident's apartment. An assisted living facility can give patients the security of having others around to help when needed but can leave the resident with a great deal of autonomy.

CHECKPOINT

Nursing homes are required to have a certain number of RNs on duty at all times. A clinic may choose to hire LPNs to work with patients and may or may not have an RN present in the facility. Given what you know about the makeup of those facilities, explain why a clinic may not be required to hire RNs.

Public Health

Public health agencies provide an assortment of health care services. The chief focus of most public health agency activities is on keeping the community healthy. Public health programs provide education about healthful living habits, and they work to involve community members in promoting a healthful way of life. Public health agencies also work to prevent or control epidemics and are responsible for tracking and reporting infectious and communicable diseases to their respective state health departments. They also provide health care services at little or no cost to low-income individuals.

SUMMARY

After reading this chapter, the medical administrative assistant should recognize the various duties of the health care professionals who work in a medical office. No one individual can do everything for a patient, and each member of the health care team is needed if comprehensive patient services are to be provided. Whether working at a clinic, hospital, urgent care center, or other health care facility, all members of the health care team contribute to the patient's care experience.

YOU ARE THE MEDICAL ADMINISTRATIVE ASSISTANT

Picture yourself as a medical administrative assistant in a medical practice. What would you do in the following situations?

1. You are working in a group practice with five primary care physicians, one pediatric nurse practitioner, and a physician's assistant. Give a response to the following:
   a. A mother calls about her 3-year-old child who has a possible ear infection. Explain to the mother the role of a nurse practitioner.
   b. A 20-year-old man walks into the clinic with a finger laceration that requires simple closure with approximately four sutures. Is it appropriate to offer the services of another health care provider in addition to those of a physician?

REVIEW EXERCISES

Exercise 2-1 True or False

Read the following statements and determine whether each statement is true or false. Record the answer in the blank provided. T = true; F = false.

_______ 1. A physician's assistant performs the same duties as a medical assistant.

_______ 2. An MD is responsible for coordinating the treatment of a patient's condition.

_______ 3. Wellness education has decreased in recent years.

_______ 4. The most common type of physician in practice in the United States is a doctor of osteopathy.

_______ 5. A person who is entering medical school must have a license to practice medicine to be enrolled.

_______ 6. The state board of physician practices regulates the practice of medicine in each state.

_______ 7. A license to practice medicine is granted for life.

_______ 8. Primary care physicians provide care for a wide variety of disorders and diseases.

_______ 9. An OD is a medical doctor.

_______ 10. Some nurse practitioners are allowed to prescribe medication.

_______ 11. Persons who live in a nursing home are known as residents.

_______ 12. A psychologist is a medical doctor.

_______ 13. Professional organizations typically provide continuing education opportunities for their members.

_______ 14. Anyone who wishes to work as a medical transcriptionist is required to obtain CMT certification.

_______ 15. Clinics typically provide outpatient care.

_______ 16. A physician who works in a clinic setting can expect more on-call duty than an MD in private practice.

_______ 17. All hospitals are designated trauma centers.

_______ 18. The terms "urgent care center" and "emergency room" are synonymous.

_______ 19. The terms "urgent care center" and "walk-in clinic" are synonymous.

_______ 20. The terms "urgent care center" and "outpatient surgery center" are synonymous.

_______ 21. Home health services often save money for patients and insurance companies.

_______ 22. A physician's residency is typically 1 year in length.

_______ 23. A group practice can help alleviate after-hours responsibility for physicians.

_______ 24. Prescription privileges for some health care providers can vary from state to state.

_______ 25. Hospice services are always administered in a patient's home.

_______ 26. Physicians are known as mid-level providers.

_______ 27. The terms "mid-level provider" and "physician extender" are synonymous.

Exercise 2-2 Medical Specialties

Identify the medical specialists or subspecialists who would treat patients with the following conditions. Some cases are repeated to demonstrate the fact that more than one specialty may serve the patient. Refer to Table 2-1 for descriptions of specialties. You may need to consult a medical dictionary or other medical reference for definitions of medical terms that are unfamiliar. Choose the specialty that best fits the patient's condition as listed. Record your answer in the space provided.

_______ 1. Patient has Graves disease.
(a) Neurology
(b) Endocrinology
(c) Ophthalmology
(d) Gastroenterology

_______ 2. Patient has recurrent tonsillitis.
(a) Plastic surgery
(b) Thoracic surgery
(c) Otolaryngology
(d) Dermatology

______ 3. Patient is 10 years old; needs a routine checkup.
(a) Pediatric surgery
(b) Allergy and immunology
(c) Ophthalmology
(d) Pediatrics

______ 4. Male patient is 10 years old; needs a routine checkup.
(a) Physical medicine and rehabilitation
(b) Internal medicine
(c) Family practice
(d) Urology

______ 5. Patient has a seizure disorder.
(a) Neurology
(b) Radiology
(c) Dermatology
(d) Cardiology

______ 6. Patient is given the diagnosis of manic depression.
(a) Cardiology
(b) Gastroenterology
(c) Anesthesiology
(d) Psychiatry

______ 7. Patient breaks out in hives repeatedly after eating certain foods.
(a) Urology
(b) Allergy and immunology
(c) Gastroenterology
(d) Orthopedics

______ 8. Patient is pregnant.
(a) Geriatric medicine
(b) OB-GYN
(c) Hematology
(d) Rheumatology

______ 9. Patient has chondromalacia patella.
(a) Orthopedics
(b) Dermatology
(c) Radiology
(d) Endocrinology

______ 10. Patient has Parkinson disease.
(a) Otolaryngology
(b) Pathology
(c) Neurology
(d) OB-GYN

______ 11. Patient is 35 years old; has influenza.
(a) Family practice
(b) Cardiology
(c) Nephrology
(d) Ophthalmology

______ 12. Patient has paronychia.
(a) Dermatology
(b) Thoracic surgery
(c) Plastic surgery
(d) Allergy and immunology

______ 13. Patient has congestive heart failure.
(a) Allergy and immunology
(b) Hematology
(c) Nephrology
(d) Cardiology

______ 14. Patient is being referred for a CT scan.
(a) Pediatrics
(b) Colon and rectal surgery
(c) Pathology
(d) Radiology

______ 15. Patient has brain lesion that requires surgery.
(a) Psychiatry
(b) Neurologic surgery
(c) Plastic surgery
(d) Nuclear medicine

______ 16. Patient has a corneal abrasion.
(a) Ophthalmology
(b) Hematology
(c) Gastroenterology
(d) Otolaryngology

______ 17. Patient has persistent diarrhea.
(a) Cardiology
(b) Neurology
(c) Gastroenterology
(d) Nuclear medicine

______ 18. Patient has a breast lump.
(a) Urology
(b) Neurologic surgery
(c) OB-GYN
(d) Rheumatology

______ 19. Patient has diabetes mellitus.
(a) Urology
(b) Endocrinology
(c) Gastroenterology
(d) Cardiology

______ 20. Patient has recurrent anxiety attacks.
(a) Psychiatry
(b) Neurology
(c) Dermatology
(d) Radiology

______ 21. Patient has a blood disorder.
(a) Neurology
(b) Endocrinology
(c) Pathology
(d) Hematology

______ 22. Patient has tuberculosis.
(a) Cardiology
(b) Infectious disease
(c) Oncology
(d) Rheumatology

______ 23. Patient has pain from a chronic back injury.
(a) Surgery
(b) Physical medicine and rehabilitation
(c) Pulmonology
(d) Neurology

Exercise 2-3 The Health Care Team

In each group, identify the professional acronym or abbreviation given with the **best** description of the profession. Use each answer only once. Record your answer in the blank provided.

(a) PharmD
(b) RN
(c) MD
(d) DPM
(e) CNP

______ 1. Observes patient progress, administers medications, and provides health education to patients; this nurse may be found in a supervisory role

______ 2. Dispenses medication and counsels patients on usage of the medication

______ 3. Advanced practice nurse; provides health care under the supervision of a physician; may specialize in family medicine, pediatrics, or women's health

______ 4. Physician

______ 5. Doctor who specializes in disorders of the foot

(a) OD
(b) DO
(c) CNM
(d) PA
(e) LPN, LVN

______ 6. Provides routine health care under the supervision of a physician

______ 7. Physician whose training is based on the fundamental belief that a healthy musculoskeletal system is essential to good health

______ 8. Nurse who works under the supervision of a physician or an RN; may be responsible for charting patient progress, taking vital signs, and administering intravenous lines

______ 9. Advanced practice nurse who provides routine yearly physical examinations for women and provides prenatal and postnatal care

______ 10. Doctor who conducts visual examinations

(a) DC
(b) CMA
(c) OT
(d) RHIT
(e) RHIA

______ 11. Individual trained in clinical and administrative tasks in the medical office

______ 12. Treats patients by manipulating or adjusting the spine

______ 13. Generally found as an administrator of a medical records department; supervises activities such as transcription, records review, and coding

______ 14. Provides therapy to help patients regain daily living skills

______ 15. Technician responsible for maintenance of the medical record

(a) PT
(b) CMT
(c) CRT
(d) RT
(e) CPC

______ 16. Takes radiographs, CT scans, or MRI

______ 17. Provides therapy to patients with respiratory dysfunction

______ 18. Transcribes medical reports

_____ 19. Assigns procedure and diagnosis codes to process a patient's charges for health care services

_____ 20. Provides therapy to help patients regain bodily function; may use exercise, massage, or ultrasound

Exercise 2-4 Health Care Facilities

Identify the type of health care facility that provides the health care service(s) listed. Choose the answer that most often fits the identified health care service(s). Record your answer in the space provided.

_____ 1. Chief function is to provide ambulatory care; appointments are usually required.
(a) Hospital
(b) Urgent care center
(c) Assisted living facility
(d) Nursing home
(e) Clinic

_____ 2. Provides operative services that do not require inpatient hospitalization.
(a) Assisted living facility
(b) Outpatient surgery center
(c) Home health
(d) Urgent care center
(e) Trauma center

_____ 3. Provides inpatient care for patients with acute conditions.
(a) Home health
(b) Urgent care center
(c) Public health
(d) Hospital
(e) Clinic

_____ 4. Takes patients on a walk-in basis.
(a) Urgent care center
(b) Public health
(c) Hospital
(d) Group clinic practice
(e) Private practice

_____ 5. Provides health education services and immunizations and reports occurrences of infectious disease.
(a) Private practice
(b) Public health
(c) Clinic
(d) Home health
(e) Assisted living

_____ 6. Residents live in an apartment-type setting and may receive assistance when taking medication.
(a) Public health
(b) Private practice
(c) Assisted living
(d) Group clinic practice
(e) Trauma center

_____ 7. Provides care for patients in their residence.
(a) Home health
(b) Public health
(c) Nursing home
(d) Assisted living
(e) Private practice

_____ 8. Physician provides medical care from an office in which he or she is the only provider.
(a) Group clinic practice
(b) Home health
(c) Urgent care
(d) Hospital
(e) Private practice

_____ 9. Place that would receive a patient who is critically injured.
(a) Clinic
(b) Emergency room
(c) Public health
(d) Home health
(e) Group clinic practice

_____ 10. Provides care for a patient who may be too ill to be at home but whose health condition does not warrant hospitalization.
(a) Public health
(b) Home health
(c) Private practice
(d) Nursing home
(e) Trauma center

_____ 11. Provides palliative care for terminally ill patients and support for family members.
(a) Public health
(b) Nursing home
(c) Ambulatory surgery center
(d) Hospice
(e) Home health

Exercise 2-5 Vocabulary

Read each definition and choose the vocabulary term that best matches the definition. Record your answer in the space provided.

______ 1. Period of physician training in a specialty.
(a) Reciprocity
(b) Ambulatory care
(c) Managed care
(d) Residency

______ 2. Individual who is chiefly responsible for coordinating and delivering health care services to the patient.
(a) Provider
(b) Managed care
(c) Inpatient care
(d) Resident

______ 3. Managed care patient must see this type of physician before seeing a specialist.
(a) Primary care physician
(b) Board-certified physician
(c) Ambulatory care
(d) Inpatient

______ 4. Physician licensed in one state is allowed to obtain a license in another state.
(a) Board-certified physician
(b) Reciprocity
(c) Residency
(d) Group practice

______ 5. Patient admitted to the hospital.
(a) Inpatient
(b) Ambulatory
(c) Outpatient
(d) Residency

______ 6. Physician who has passed an examination in a chosen specialty.
(a) Private practice
(b) Managed care
(c) Board-certified physician
(d) Primary care

______ 7. Requires a patient to see a primary care physician/provider before seeing a specialist.
(a) Primary care
(b) Managed care
(c) Ambulatory care
(d) Public health agency

______ 8. Assessment of patient to determine services needed.
(a) Rotation
(b) Triage
(c) Reciprocity
(d) Ambulatory

ACTIVITIES

ACTIVITY 2-1 UPDATE PRACTICE INFORMATION IN MEDISOFT

1. Using the instructions below and information listed under step No. 3, update practice information for the Happy Valley Medical Clinic.
2. Open Medisoft and the **Medical Group Tutorial** as previously instructed in Chapter 1.
3. Click **File>Practice Information.**
4. In the **Practice Information** window, update the following information as needed under the **Practice** tab:
Practice Name: Happy Valley Medical Clinic
Street: 5222 E. Baseline Rd.
City: Gilbert
State: AZ
ZIP: 85234
Phone: 800-333-4747
Fax: 012-555-0001
Type: Medical
Tax ID: 005623516
Practice type: Group
Entity type: Nonperson
Leave remaining blanks empty. (In future exercises, if no instructions are given, leave blanks empty.)
Click **Save.**

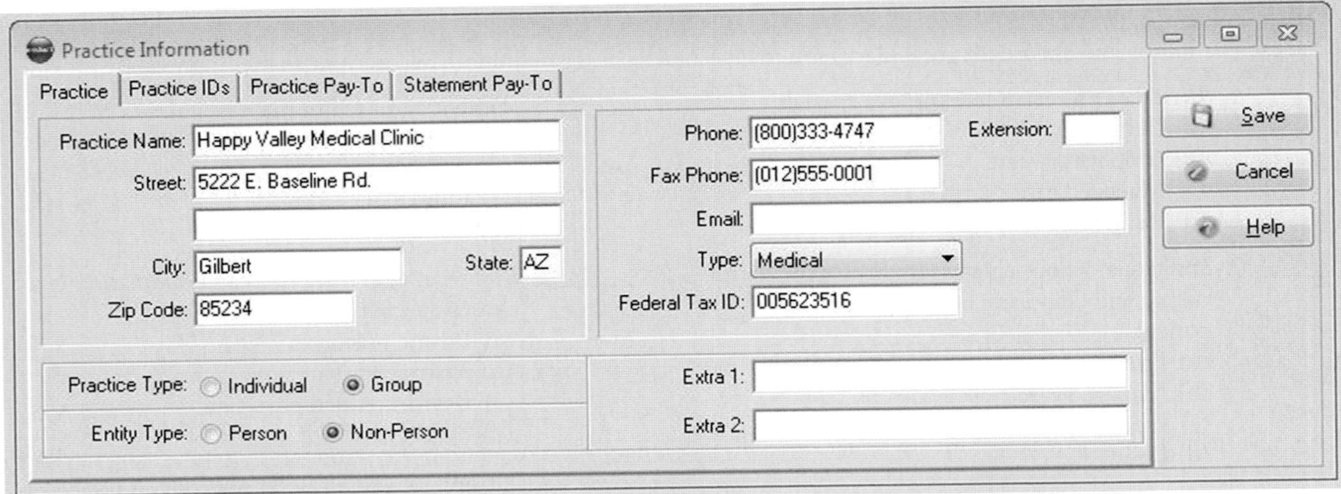

ACTIVITY 2-2 ADDING PROVIDER INFORMATION IN MEDISOFT

Using the instructions and information provided in the table below, update provider information and create files for new providers who work at Happy Valley Medical Group.

With Medisoft open, click **List>Provider>Providers.** Click **New.**

1. In the **Address** tab, fill in the information for each provider from the first table below. Place a check mark to select **Signature on File** and **Medicare Participating.** Leave the **Code**, **Email** and **Home Phone** blanks empty. Leave blanks empty where no information is provided.
2. As the information for each new provider is complete, click **Save.** Repeat the above instructions for each new provider.

Last Name	First Name	MI	Credential	Street	City	State	Zip Code
Marks	Timothy	I	PA	1234 Main Ave.	Farmington	AZ	85000
Martinez	Jana	J	DO	1234 Main Ave.	Farmington	AZ	85000
O'Brian	Emily	P	CNP	1234 Main Ave.	Farmington	AZ	85000

Last Name	Office	Fax	Cell	Signature on File	SOF Date	Medicare Part	License No.
Marks	(012)555-0000	(012)555-0001	(012)555-8828	TRUE (YES)	1/2/2013	TRUE (YES)	551193
Martinez	(012)555-0000	(012)555-0001	(012)555-3777	TRUE (YES)	1/2/2013	TRUE (YES)	235663
O'Brian	(012)555-0000	(012)555-0001	(012)555-4832	TRUE (YES)	1/2/2013	TRUE (YES)	388338

3. Use the information in the table below to update the information for the existing providers who are associated with Happy Valley Medical Group. Click **List>Provider>Providers.** Highlight the provider's name and click **Edit** to update the provider's information.
4. As the information for each existing provider is updated, click **Save.** Repeat No. 3 and No. 4 instructions for each provider.
5. When completed, click **Close**.

Last Name	First Name	MI	Credentials	Street 1	City	State	ZIP	Office	Fax	Cell	Signature on File	SOF Date	Medicare Part	License Number
Queayeman	Dean	F	M.D.	5222 E. Baseline Rd	Gilbert	AZ	85234	(800)333-4747	(000)333-4748	(000)333-6257	TRUE	2/4/2009	TRUE	710495
O'Brian	Emily	P	CNP	1234 Main Ave	Farmington	AZ	85000	(012)555-0000	(012)555-0001	(012)555-4832	TRUE	1/2/2013	TRUE	388338
Martinez	Jana	J	DO	1234 Main Ave	Farmington	AZ	85000	(012)555-0000	(012)555-0001	(012)555-3777	TRUE	1/2/2013	TRUE	235663
Mallard	Julia	D	M.D.	5222 E. Baseline Rd.	Gilbert	AZ	85234	(800)333-4747	(000)333-4748	(000)331-2367	TRUE	5/1/2008	TRUE	49872
Morris	Melvin	O	D.C.	5222 E. Baseline Rd.	Gilbert	AZ	85234	(800)333-4747	(000)333-4748	(000)313-6720	TRUE	12/2/2009	TRUE	234589

Last Name	First Name	MI	Creden-tials	Street 1	City	State	ZIP	Office	Fax	Cell	Signature on File	SOF Date	Medicare Part	License Number
Lee	Robert	E	M.D.	5222 E. Baseline Rd.	Gilbert	AZ	85234	(800)333-4747	(000)333-4748	(000)333-2341	TRUE	2/3/2010	TRUE	234598
Winks	Shelly	L	D.O.	5222 E. Baseline Rd.	Gilbert	AZ	85234	(800)333-4747	(000)333-4748	(000)313-3847	TRUE	4/8/2011	TRUE	234522
Marks	Timothy	I	PA	1234 Main Ave.	Farmington	AZ	85000	(012)555-0000	(012)555-0001	(012)555-8828	TRUE	1/2/2013	TRUE	551193
Hinckle	Wallace		M.D.	5222 E. Baseline Rd.	Gilbert	AZ	85234	(800)333-4747	(000)333-4748	(000)331-3311	TRUE	4/8/2011	TRUE	234523

ACTIVITY 2-3 MEDICAL ASSISTANT SCOPE OF PRACTICE

Research the scope of practice and identify the requirements for licensure for a medical assistant in your state.

ACTIVITY 2-4 HEALTH CARE PROFESSIONS

Conduct further research on a health care profession. Choose a profession and identify the chief responsibilities, education, required training, potential earnings, and future expectations for that career. Research can be done with written sources, personal interviews, and Internet resources. Present your findings to the class.

ACTIVITY 2-5 PROFESSIONAL ORGANIZATIONS

Identify professional organizations for some of the professions mentioned in this chapter. Obtain answers to the following items or questions:

- Name of organization
- Location of organization's headquarters
- Does the organization provide educational materials or links on its website?
- Does the organization have an annual convention or conference? If so, where is the next one held?

ACTIVITY 2-6 PSYCHIATRIST OR PSYCHOLOGIST?

Both a psychiatrist and a psychologist are involved in helping patients restore good mental health or live with mental disorders. They are both trained in assessing psychiatric disorders and can be involved in counseling and diagnosing patients. Research the types of assessments and therapies used by these professionals by using the Internet or other reference materials or by interviewing health professionals.

ACTIVITY 2-7 MEDICAL SPECIALTIES

Research the various member boards of the American Board of Medical Specialties or the American Osteopathic Boards. Identify specialties and subspecialties of each member board.

ACTIVITY 2-8 MEDICINE IN THE MOVIES

Many movies have been made about the health care profession. Watch a movie that takes place in a health care setting. Some suggestions are *Patch Adams* and *The Doctor*. Be prepared to discuss the accuracies and inaccuracies of the film.

ACTIVITY 2-9 REFLECTION ON DR. MAYO QUOTE

Write a short paragraph relating the quotation by Dr. William Mayo regarding the sum total of medical knowledge to the variety of professionals who are part of the health care team. Why is this quotation fitting for this chapter?

ACTIVITY 2-10 LOCAL HEALTH CARE FACILITIES

Examine health care facilities in your local area. Can you find examples of the following types of facilities in your area?

- Clinic
- Hospital
- Hospice
- Nursing home
- Public health agency
- Home health agency
- Urgent care center
- Assisted living facility

ACTIVITY 2-11 STATE BOARDS FOR MEDICAL PRACTICE

Research the state board that regulates the practice of medicine in your state. Check for information on the following:

- Official name of the state board
- Licensing and renewal requirements
- Medical practice guidelines
- Disciplinary actions
- Physician database

DISCUSSION

DISCUSSION 2-1

Discuss health care delivery and needs in rural areas of the United States.

Bibliography

American Academy of Nurse Practitioners: *FAQs about Nurse Practitioners*. www.aanp.org. Accessed December 22, 2010.

American Academy of Professional Coders: *Certification*. www.aapc.com. Accessed December 27, 2012.

American Association of Colleges of Podiatric Medicine: *FAQs*. www.aacpm.org. Accessed December 22, 2010.

American Association of Nurse Anesthetists: *Becoming a CRNA*. www.aana.com. Accessed December 22, 2010.

American Board of Specialties: *Specialties and Subspecialties*. www.abms.org. Accessed December 19, 2010.

American College of Nurse Midwives: *FAQ* www.acnm.org. Accessed December 22, 2010.

American Hospice Foundation: *What Is Your Hospice IQ?* www.americanhospice.org. Accessed December 22, 2010.

American Medical Association: *Statistics History*. www.aama-assn.org. Accessed December 20, 2010.

American Osteopathic Association: *What Is a DO?* www.osteopathic.org. Accessed December 19, 2010.

American Osteopathic Association: *About Osteopathic Medicine*. www.osteopathic.org. Accessed December 19, 2010.

American Osteopathic Association: *AOA Specialty Certifying Boards*. www.osteopathic.org. Accessed December 20, 2010.

Association of American Medical Colleges: *Medical Education*. www.aamc.org. Accessed December 20, 2010.

Bureau of Labor Statistics, U.S. Department of Labor: *Occupational Outlook Handbook, 2010–2011*. www.bls.gov/oco/. Accessed December 19, 2010.

Federation of State Medical Boards: *Directory of State Medical and Osteopathic Boards*. www.fsmb.org. Accessed December 19, 2010.

Mayo Clinic: *Mayo Clinic Facts–2009*. www.mayoclinic.org. Accessed December 20, 2010.

Mayo Clinic: *Mayo Clinic Model of Care*. www.mayoclinic.org. Accessed December 22, 2010.

National Rural Health Association: *What's Different About Rural Health Care?* www.ruralhealthweb.org. Accessed December 20, 2010.

United States Medical Licensing Examination: *FAQ*. www.usmle.org. Accessed December 22, 2010.

Wikipedia: *Trauma center*. en.wikipedia.org. Accessed December 22, 2010.

CHAPTER 3 Medical Law

LEARNING OUTCOMES

On successful completion of this chapter, the student will be able to

1. Describe different types of law and their origins.
2. Define and apply legal terminology and concepts.
3. Explain the essential components of a contract and how contract law applies to the physician–patient relationship.
4. Describe medical malpractice and negligence.
5. Explain legal proceedings in a typical medical malpractice suit.
6. Explain confidentiality and the protection of confidentiality.
7. Identify requirements for reporting injury, disease, and medical incidents.
8. Explain advance directives.
9. Describe the purpose of the Uniform Anatomical Gift Act.
10. Describe the purpose of the Controlled Substances Act of 1970.
11. Describe the purpose of Good Samaritan statutes.
12. Identify components of the Health Insurance Portability and Accountability Act (HIPAA) of 1996.
13. Explain the concept of risk management.

COMMISSION ON ACCREDITATION OF ALLIED HEALTH EDUCATION PROGRAMS (CAAHEP) CORE CURRICULUM FOR MEDICAL ASSISTANTS

- Use Internet to access information related to the medical office.
- Discuss legal scope of practice for medical assistants.
- Explore issue of confidentiality as it applies to the medical assistant.
- Describe the implications of HIPAA for the medical assistant in various medical settings.
- Discuss licensure and certification as it applies to health care providers.
- Compare and contrast physician and medical assistant roles in terms of standard of care.
- Compare criminal and civil law as it applies to the practicing medical assistant.
- Explain how the following impact the medical administrative assistant's practice and give examples:
  a. Negligence.
  b. Malpractice.
  c. Statute of Limitations.
  d. Good Samaritan Act(s).
  e. Uniform Anatomical Gift Act.
  f. Living will/Advanced directives.
  g. Medical durable power of attorney.
- Respond to issues of confidentiality.
- Discuss all levels of government legislation and regulation as they apply to medical assisting practice, including U.S. Food and Drug Administration (FDA) and Drug Enforcement Agency (DEA) regulations.

ACCREDITING BUREAU OF HEALTH EDUCATION SCHOOLS (ABHES) COMPETENCIES FOR MEDICAL ASSISTING

Graduates

- Demonstrate professionalism by maintaining confidentiality at all times.
- Conduct work within scope of education, training, and ability.
- Comply with federal, state, and local health laws and regulations.
- Follow established policy in initiating or terminating medical treatment.
- Monitor legislation related to current health care issues and practices.
- Perform risk management procedures.

VOCABULARY

abandonment
administrative law
advance directive
case law
civil law
common law
compensatory damages
confidentiality
consent
consideration
contract
criminal law
damages
defendant

VOCABULARY—cont'd

deposition
durable power of attorney for health care
emancipated minor
executive branch
expressed consent
implied consent
informed consent
interrogatories
judicial branch
law
legal capacity
legislative branch
litigation
living will
malpractice
mature minor
offer and acceptance
plaintiff
punitive or exemplary damages
respondeat superior
res ipsa loquitur
risk management
standards of care
statute of limitations
statutes
statutory adult
statutory law
subpoena
subpoena duces tecum

A medical administrative assistant must have a broad overview of medical law and how it affects the individuals who work in a health care organization. Legal issues regarding medical practice can affect an assistant directly or indirectly. Knowledge of the law and its concepts as it applies to health care helps a medical administrative assistant understand the complexities of health care delivery, demonstrates how legal and ethical issues affect members of the health care team, and provides an assistant with an understanding of the legal forces that are at work every day in the health care environment. Such knowledge is invaluable to a medical office as it lessens the possibility of litigation against the office.

Legal Concepts and Terms

What Is Law?

Laws are written rules established by a society's government. Laws indicate what is and what is not acceptable behavior. All citizens who belong to a society are obligated to follow that society's laws.

Because change seems to be a constant in today's world, laws are continually updated to reflect society's changes. For example, in the early 1900s, automobiles were owned by an elite few. Now, automobile ownership is commonplace. Because of the proliferation of automobiles today, laws have been developed to govern how they are used. All people who drive automobiles are obligated to follow these laws. If they do not, they are subject to fines or arrest, or both. Technological changes often cause laws to be changed. Likewise, as changes occur elsewhere in society, laws are enacted or are changed to reflect those changes.

Origin of Law

Laws can originate at the federal, state, or local level. The fundamental law at the federal level is the U.S. Constitution. Each state, as well, has its own constitution.

The structure of the government is identified in a constitution: at the federal level, the U.S. Constitution; at the state level, each individual state's constitution. At the state level and at the federal level, the structure of the government consists of three parts—legislative, judicial, and executive branches—each with its own authority.

The **legislative branch,** which consists of senators and representatives elected by the people, is responsible for establishing laws. Within state and federal jurisdictions, these enactments are known as **statutes** or **statutory law.** Statutory law is also referred to as legislative law.

The chief function of the judicial system is interpretation of laws. The **judicial branch,** or the court system, establishes **common law,** also known as **case law,** by deciding cases brought before the court. These cases, once decided, establish a precedent, and the court's decision serves as a model for future cases of a similar nature that come before the court. An extensive court system exists at both state and federal levels.

The **executive branch** at both the state level and the federal level is responsible for ensuring that the laws within its jurisdiction are observed. The president of the United States and the governors of each state serve as the executive power within their respective jurisdictions.

Even at the local level, cities and towns operate with much the same government structure. County and municipal courts (judicial) handle local violations; commissioners or other locally elected representatives (legislative) are involved, as well as a leader of the municipality—a mayor (executive).

To avoid substantial conflict between federal, state, and even local governments, the U.S. Constitution has established that the Constitution is the primary law of the land and that no state may take away rights that are ensured by the Constitution. State law cannot contradict or supersede federal law. No state can take away rights that are guaranteed by federal law.

Administrative Law

Because establishing laws to govern the many facets of society would be overwhelming for elected officials of the legislative branch of government, legislatures give authority to government agencies (either state or federal agencies) to establish regulations and enforce those regulations, or **administrative laws,** within their jurisdiction. There are many government agencies; for example, the DEA establishes guidelines for the manufacture and dispensing of potentially addictive prescription drugs. The Environmental Protection Agency (EPA) establishes regulations that safeguard the environment. The Centers for Medicare and Medicaid Services (CMS) oversees the administration of Medicare and Medicaid benefits. The FDA ensures the safety of drugs, food, and other biological products that we use. These federal agencies then are charged with carrying out enforcement of administrative law within their authority.

Civil and Criminal Law

Legal cases pertaining to health care can be either civil or criminal in nature. **Civil law** involves the relationship between individuals or groups. Civil cases are brought with the contention that one party did something that adversely affected or injured another party. An individual who alleges that a health care worker was negligent in providing care is making a civil claim. Civil cases usually involve the injured party asking for a sum of money to compensate for damages that he or she has incurred.

Criminal law, on the other hand, involves the relationship between an individual and the government. By enacting laws, legislatures determine what constitutes criminal behavior and what punishment is suitable for a crime. If an individual breaks a law, the government has the responsibility to uphold the law to protect the rest of society. For example, a health care worker who assists a patient in obtaining prescription drugs illegally would face criminal charges because the worker violated the law. The penalty for violating criminal law can include fine or incarceration, or both.

Standards of Care

In the health care field, health care professionals are required to perform in a manner that is consistent with expectations of their profession. This concept is known as **standards of care.**

In other words, a health care professional is expected to carry out his or her duties as other reasonable health care professionals in the profession would carry out their duties. For example, in a particular situation, a physician is expected to perform as other reasonable and prudent physicians would perform. In turn, a nurse is expected to perform as other reasonable and prudent nurses would perform. Physicians and other health care professionals are held to standards of care for their particular profession and are expected to perform as others in their profession would perform. If they fail to perform up to standards for their profession, they risk being accused of malpractice. Health care workers are each held to their own particular standard of care.

Respondeat Superior

Is the employer responsible for the wrongdoings of an employee? Most often, yes. The Latin phrase ***respondeat superior*** means "let the master answer." Essentially, this establishes liability on the part of the employer for the actions of an employee. This means that when an employee performs job duties, the employer (e.g., physician, clinic, hospital) may be held responsible for any negligence or wrongdoing of the employee.

Respondeat superior is an important concept of the law because it pertains to many of the activities that take place in the medical office. To protect a health care facility, a physician, and themselves, it is vital for assistants and everyone else who works in a medical office to understand the meaning of this term.

Because it would be virtually impossible for physicians to conduct all the business of a practice, physicians hire an office staff to help perform many of the administrative (business) and clinical functions necessary to run a medical office. All employees are deemed to act at the direction of or on behalf of the physician or the practice, and the physician and the practice are responsible for the actions of employees.

If an employee of the medical practice performs an act that harms a patient, the physician and the medical practice can be held liable because the employee represents the physician and the medical practice. A patient may elect to sue the physician, the medical practice, and even the employee. Generally, claimants will sue the party or parties that have the most to lose—typically, the physician and the medical practice—although it is also possible that an employee may be sued if he or she has some responsibility for the situation in question. An assistant should be very careful to perform only those job duties that have been assigned and should be careful to never say or do anything that is beyond the scope of their position. Nothing should ever be done that might be construed as giving medical advice.

Consider the following inappropriate comments by someone without proper training:

Patient calling the office: "I'd like to make an appointment to see Dr. Anderson. My big toe is red and swollen and is oozing pus around the toenail."

Untrained assistant: "You probably have an ingrown toenail. Have you tried soaking the nail? If not, I can make an appointment for you this afternoon."

Such a comment could be interpreted as practicing medicine without a license. If a patient calls with a question about how to treat a condition or asks what to do about a certain medical situation, the assistant must let the staff members who are specifically trained to respond to such situations do so. It is inappropriate for an assistant to suggest a diagnosis or treatment. That is not an assistant's job responsibility.

Res Ipsa Loquitur

A Latin phrase meaning "the thing speaks for itself," ***res ipsa loquitur*** (pronounced reez IP-sah LOH-kwe-tur) refers to the idea that evidence speaks for itself. If a patient has an infection caused by a surgical sponge left in a surgical site, it is likely that the sponge was the cause of the patient's infection, and that the patient would not have experienced such an infection if all sponges had been removed. To put it simply, sponges should not be left in patients. An obvious mistake on the part of a health care provider is usually negligence, and it provides enough evidence for a legal action.

CHECKPOINT

Identify whether the following situations could be malpractice on the part of a health care professional:

1. A nurse gives the wrong dosage of a drug, and that dosage causes harm to the patient.
2. A patient calls the clinic with chest pain, and the nurse fails to inform the physician of the phone call. Later in the day, the patient suffers a massive heart attack while at home and dies.
3. A physician fails to notify a patient of normal laboratory results.
4. A physician fails to inform the patient of suspicious Pap smear results. The patient is not informed of the need for follow-up care, and 1 year later she is given the diagnosis of cervical cancer.

Contract Law

The basis for many civil suits, or civil **litigation,** involving medical practice is founded in **contract** law. Litigation refers to a lawsuit, and a contract is a legal agreement between two parties that creates an obligation. Establishment of a contract creates a duty for one party to do something because another party has agreed to do something in return.

Essentials of a Contract

Many times, when someone hears the word *contract*, what comes to mind is something that is written and then signed by both parties. However, a contract may be written or verbal. The physician–patient relationship is based on a contractual agreement. Most physician–patient relationships are established through an oral contract.

A contractual agreement is said to exist if each of the following four criteria have been met.

Offer and Acceptance. This is the initial step in establishing a contract. **Offer** means that the first party has offered to provide something, such as goods or a service. **Acceptance** means that the second party has accepted the first party's offer. Therefore, when a physician offers service to a patient and the patient accepts the service, the beginning steps of a contract have commenced.

Legal Subject Matter. The topic or subject matter of a contract must be a legal act or object. A contract would not exist if the subject matter was an illegal item, nor would a contract exist if the action to be performed was illegal (e.g., prescribing illegal drugs to treat a condition).

Legal Capacity. **Legal capacity** refers to a party's ability to enter into a contract. Generally, an individual must be 18 years of age or older to enter into a contract. Minors (individuals younger than age 18) usually cannot enter into a contract. However, there are certain exceptions to this requirement. One exception is an individual who has been declared by the court to be an **emancipated minor,** meaning that the individual is younger than age 18 but is capable of making adult decisions despite not having reached adulthood. Generally, an emancipated minor meets one of the following conditions:

- The minor is married, separated, divorced, or widowed
- The minor is a parent
- The minor is in the armed forces
- The minor resides away from home and supports himself or herself

Some states recognize that minors are **statutory adults** who may consent to medical treatment at 14 years of age. Statutory adults also have the right to confidentiality in relation to their medical records, even though parents may be obligated to pay for a minor's medical care.

Other states recognize some minors as **mature minors** who are capable of making medical decisions without parental consent. Mature minors generally are unable to give consent for medical treatment except in cases involving pregnancy, requests for contraception, treatment for sexually transmitted diseases, substance abuse, and psychiatric care. Usually, if a minor is 14 years of age or older and seeks treatment for the aforementioned conditions, information regarding treatment must be kept confidential and cannot be released to the minor's parents without the minor's consent. Not all states recognize mature minors, statutory adults, or emancipated minors, and states vary greatly in providing medical treatment to minors.

Another component of legal capacity is that an individual who enters into a contract must be of sound mind and must be capable of making decisions that are in his or her best interest. If a patient is younger than the age of 18, a parent or guardian usually is needed to give consent for medical care. If the patient is not of sound mind (mentally incompetent) or is incapable of making his or her own decisions, a guardian or someone with legal authority will make the decision for the patient. A patient with a known psychiatric disorder, low IQ, or a medical condition that affects his or her thinking may not have the legal capacity to consent to treatment. Persons who are under the effects of some medications temporarily may not be able to enter into a contract.

Consideration. In completing a contractual agreement, something of value is exchanged between the two parties. This is known as **consideration**. If a physician examines a patient and determines a diagnosis, the professional opinion or advice of the physician is something of value. The patient, after receiving the physician's treatment and diagnosis, will then pay the physician for the services provided. The physician's professional advice and the patient's money are the items of value that are exchanged.

CHECKPOINT

Could a patient with Alzheimer disease enter into a contract?

The Physician–Patient Relationship

A physician–patient relationship is present if the four criteria of a contract are met. If a patient alleges wrongdoing on the part of a physician, it will be important to establish the existence of a relationship or contract between the physician and the patient. If a relationship does not exist, the physician could possibly not be held liable.

Physicians are free to choose whom they will accept as patients. Some physicians with a large patient load may have to stop accepting new patients because they have an obligation to provide care for their existing patients. For example, obstetrics and gynecology physicians may have to restrict the number of obstetrics patients they accept so as to avoid overloading their practice. If confronted with an emergency situation, however, a physician must provide care for the patient until care can be transferred to another physician or facility.

Once a physician–patient relationship has been established, it is important for the physician to provide services to the patient as needed. Establishment of the physician–patient relationship creates an obligation on the part of the physician to provide ongoing treatment to the patient if needed.

Terminating a Contract

If a physician can no longer provide services for a patient, the physician must notify the patient that he or she is no longer able to provide care for the patient.

A physician who finds it necessary to discharge a patient from care should consult an attorney as to the appropriate steps to take to terminate care. Usually, the physician is advised to complete the following:

1. Send a letter via certified mail with a return receipt notifying the patient of the termination. The return receipt is necessary to verify delivery of the letter to the patient.
2. Specify in the letter the reason for dismissing the patient. Reasons for dismissal may include the patient's noncompliance with treatment, the patient's failure to keep scheduled appointments, threats from the patient, the physician's retirement or relocation to another location, or even termination of an insurance contract with the physician's health care organization.
3. Give the patient names of other physicians who may be available to provide care.
4. Offer to provide care for a reasonable period (typically 30 days) until the patient can make other arrangements for medical care. It is widespread practice that the physician is obligated to provide care for a reasonable period and may even be obligated for a longer period for emergency care.
5. Offer to provide the patient's records to another physician on receipt of a signed release of information from the patient.

Sometimes, a patient decides to terminate the relationship with a physician. If a patient is currently being treated for a medical condition, it is important that the physician confirm the patient's wishes. This termination should be confirmed by writing a letter to the patient to verify his or her intent to sever the relationship.

In all cases of termination of the physician–patient relationship before patient care is finished, the termination should be well documented by the physician in the patient's chart. No matter who initiated the termination, medical record documentation is vital to protect the physician and the practice should litigation arise from any treatment situation. According to the American Medical Association's Council on Ethical and Judicial Affairs, "A physician may not discontinue treatment of a patient as long as further treatment is medically indicated, without giving the patient reasonable notice and sufficient opportunity to make alternative arrangements for care."

Abandonment. If a physician does not properly meet his or her obligation to treat the patient, the physician could be held responsible for abandoning the patient.

Abandonment might be alleged if a patient is admitted to the hospital and the physician does not see the patient in the hospital and makes no arrangements for another physician to take his or her place. A physician who suddenly closes the practice doors one day without notifying patients and making arrangements for subsequent treatment might also be found guilty of abandonment, as might a physician who is constantly unavailable for follow-up treatment of chronically ill patients. Even a physician who performs a surgical procedure and does not provide the necessary follow-up care could be found guilty of abandonment. A physician who does not provide follow-up care because a patient has a large outstanding balance on an account could also be found guilty of abandonment. Once a person has been accepted as a physician's patient, the physician has an obligation to treat the patient unless the relationship has been terminated appropriately.

Legal Action Against a Medical Practice

Occasionally in medical practice, a patient alleges that something has gone wrong in the physician–patient relationship. Because of an adverse outcome, a patient may assert that he or she has been injured through the negligent actions of the physician or one of the physician's employees. If a patient decides to pursue litigation, or legal action, the patient (who initiated the suit) is known as the **plaintiff** and the physician or allied health employee, or the practice (party or parties accused of wrongdoing), or both, is known as the **defendant.**

Statute of Limitations

Cases regarding medical malpractice must be brought forward within a reasonable time. This period, known as the **statute of limitations,** varies from state to state. If the state statute of limitations is 2 years for a medical malpractice suit, a patient may bring suit within 2 years of the alleged injury, or when the patient becomes aware of the injury.

In the case of injury to a minor, the statute of limitations may be figured from the time the patient reaches the age of majority. For example, if a child is injured at 5 years of age and the statute of limitations is 2 years in the state where the child resides, the child may have a right to sue even at age 19 because the statute of limitations may not begin to run until the child reaches 18 years.

In some states, a plaintiff who alleges medical malpractice is required to obtain expert opinion from another physician to support allegations made against a physician. If this is not done in a timely manner, the suit may be dismissed. Some states allow only 3 months for expert opinions to be obtained.

Medical Malpractice and Negligence

According to the *Miller-Keane Encyclopedia and Dictionary of Medicine, Nursing, and Allied Health*, **malpractice** is "any professional misconduct, unreasonable lack of skill or fidelity in professional duties, or illegal or immoral conduct." A widely held view of malpractice is of a physician failing to do something that a reasonable and prudent person would do, or of a physician doing something that a reasonable and prudent person would not do.

Because of their advanced training, physicians are held to their profession's standards of care when they administer medical care. Physicians may be liable if they act or if they do not act. They can be found guilty of malpractice if they make a mistake while administering medical treatment, or if they fail to recognize treatment that should be given in a particular situation. The actions of a physician will be compared with those of other physicians in the determination of whether the physician acted as other physicians would have acted.

Malpractice is a type of negligence. To prove negligence in a court of law, an individual must be able to demonstrate all of the following:

1. Duty—an obligation or duty existed on the part of the physician to provide services for a patient. What is important here is the determination of whether a physician–patient relationship existed and the physician was obligated to provide some type of care for the patient. The physician–patient relationship was described earlier in this chapter.
2. Breach of duty—the physician did not meet his or her obligation to the patient and failed to provide proper care for the patient. It must be demonstrated that the physician either failed to act (omission) or acted in an improper manner (commission).
3. Causation—the physician's failure caused the patient's injury. It must be proved that however the physician acted, the physician's action was the direct cause of the patient's injury.
4. Damages or injury—the patient suffered damage or injury. Once the first three points have been met and damage or injury to the patient has been proved, the patient may be awarded some type of compensation for injury or suffering.

Any allied health professional can be found negligent when working with or caring for patients. Professionals in the health care setting perform their job in accordance with standards of care for that position. If the standards of care have not been met because the professional failed to do something or did something incorrectly, allegations of negligence may be a very real possibility. It is up to all health care professionals to minimize the possibility that these types of allegations will ever occur.

Effects of Medical Malpractice Suits

A medical malpractice case can be devastating to a physician, staff, and health care facility. Litigation places a physician's and a facility's reputation at stake. Information about a case may appear on television or radio or in a newspaper. Even if a physician is found not guilty and wins, or if a suit is dismissed or settled without admission of guilt, his or her reputation may be damaged by the publicity of the suit. Also, involvement in a suit can cause financial strain and can be emotionally draining.

Physicians sometimes may elect to settle a suit before it even reaches the trial stage. If the plaintiff will settle for a nominal amount, a physician may choose to settle instead of going to trial. Frequently, settlements do not admit wrongdoing but are made because they may be cheaper than defending a lawsuit. A physician's malpractice insurer may decide to settle with a plaintiff and may even do so without the approval of the physician. Insurers will weigh the chances of successful outcomes of the trial, along with the potential cost of going to trial, and will determine whether it is prudent to settle a suit before trial.

In a U.S. Department of Justice 2000–2004 study of medical malpractice insurance claims in seven states (Florida, Illinois, Maine, Massachusetts, Missouri, Nevada, and Texas), 95% of medical malpractice suits were settled before trial. The study additionally noted that most malpractice claims are closed without any payout to claimants (plaintiffs). In Maine, Missouri, and Nevada, only one third of cases resulted in a malpractice insurance payout to a claimant. In Illinois, only 12% of cases resulted in an insurance payout. Even though the likelihood of a successful suit on the part of a plaintiff is low, health care professionals must be diligent in reducing even the possibility of medical malpractice claims within their medical facilities.

Legal Proceedings

Once a patient has decided to pursue litigation against a physician or health care facility, an assistant should be prepared to receive legal requests for information. The pretrial phase of a lawsuit involves much information gathering on the part of both parties. Information regarding any malpractice case should not be given without consultation with the attorney who is representing the physician or clinic. If the opposing party's attorney asks questions of any medical office employees, all employees must refrain from giving any information whatsoever to the attorney. The slightest comment could be potentially damaging.

A chart explaining the process of a typical medical malpractice case is shown in Figure 3-1. At any time during the process illustrated in this figure, the parties may agree to a settlement. An alternative to settlement or trial is the arbitration process. Parties who agree to have a case decided by arbitration do so knowing that the decision of the arbitrator will be final.

Interrogatories

Before a trial begins, a set of written questions may be asked of the opposing party by either the plaintiff or the defendant. These questions are known as **interrogatories.** The purpose of interrogatories is to obtain basic factual information such

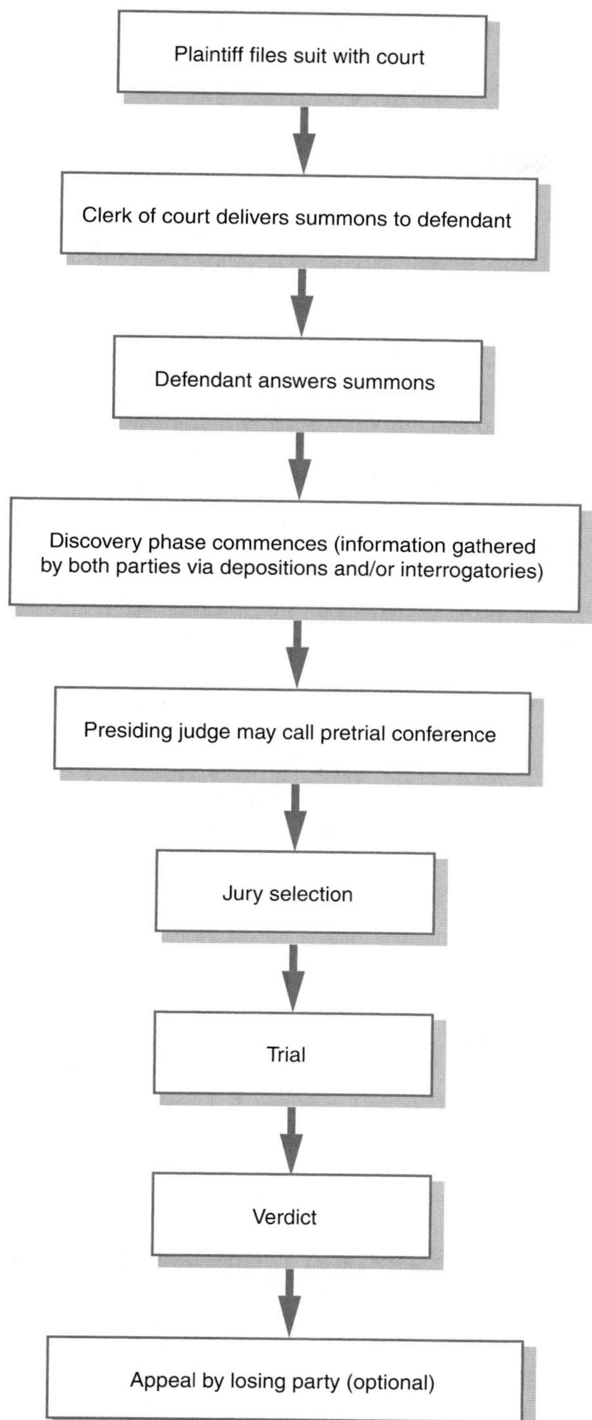
Plaintiff files suit with court
Clerk of court delivers summons to defendant
Defendant answers summons
Discovery phase commences (information gathered by both parties via depositions and/or interrogatories)
Presiding judge may call pretrial conference
Jury selection
Trial
Verdict
Appeal by losing party (optional)

Figure 3-1 Flow chart of the possible sequence of a medical malpractice case.

as dates of employment, details of education, and other pertinent professional qualification information. These questions are answered in writing under oath and should be answered in consultation with an attorney.

Depositions

Sometimes, a physician must be an expert witness (having treated the patient) and must give testimony regarding the patient's claim of injury against a third party. It is not always necessary for witnesses to testify in court. Witnesses or experts can give testimony outside the courtroom in a process known as a **deposition.** A deposition may be held in a medical facility or at an attorney's office, with the latter being more common. Generally, it is preferred that depositions be held away from a medical office to avoid drawing attention to a group of attorneys who visit the physician at the office.

Usually taken before trial, a deposition is a written record of the sworn testimony of a witness. This testimony, given in question/answer format, similar to courtroom proceedings, is taken by a court reporter that has been retained by one of the parties to record the proceedings of the deposition. Before the deposition begins, the witness is sworn in, just as if he or she were in a courtroom. Attorneys who represent each party to the suit take part in the deposition and ask questions of the witness—the same as in a courtroom. Attorney may arrange depositions of expert witnesses who support their client's case. Also attorneys may arrange to depose persons who are witnesses for the opponent's side of the case in order to obtain more information about the circumstances of the case. Physicians often give depositions for patients who may have been injured in an accident, such as an automobile accident, work accident, etc.

In the deposition of a physician, opening questions usually relate to the physician's professional qualifications (e.g., where he or she attended medical school, whether he or she has board certification, where he or she practices). Once this foundation has been laid, questions center around the patient's visits with the physician and the physician's professional opinion of the patient's injuries (Box 3-1).

After the deposition has concluded, the court reporter prepares an original and copies of the deposition in written form. The court reporter sends a rough draft of the deposition for review to the person who gave the testimony. Any necessary corrections (changes in testimony are not allowed, but errors may be corrected) are made by the witness and returned to the court reporter.

BOX 3-1

Portion of a Sample Deposition

Q When did you first see Jennifer Singer as a patient?
A June 16, 1998.
Q And what was her chief complaint at that visit?
A Pain and swelling of the right knee.
Q What was the condition of her right knee at that time?
A She had significant infrapatellar swelling and erythema. Her range of motion was restricted.
Q What did she say caused her injury?
A She reported that she was in a motor vehicle accident and her knee struck the dashboard.
Q Were her injuries consistent with a motor vehicle collision?

Q = questions by an attorney; A = answers by a physician.

Corrections then are made to the deposition, and the original of the deposition is filed with the court. Copies of the deposition may be ordered by the attorneys if they wish. The court reporter charges the attorney who arranged for the deposition for the original. If the physician is an expert witness in the case, the physician charges the attorney who arranged for the deposition for the testimony. Any additional copies ordered are charged to the ordering party. A physician who is a defendant in a case is not allowed to charge for testimony.

Subpoena

If a case goes to trial, it may be necessary to order an individual to appear in court. This order is known as a **subpoena** (pronounced sub-PE-nah). A subpoena instructs an individual to appear in court at a certain time and place. If an individual fails to do so, that individual is subject to a penalty imposed by the court.

Physicians may appear in court for a variety of reasons. They may be called in a civil or criminal trial. Most commonly, they are called as expert witnesses to give their professional opinion about a party's injury. Remember, as an expert witness, a physician normally charges a fee for giving testimony because they are rendering their professional opinion.

Subpoena Duces Tecum

In cases involving a patient from a physician's practice, it will become necessary for the patient's medical record to be submitted into evidence at a trial. An order to produce a patient's medical record for use at a trial is known as a subpoena duces tecum (pronounced sub-PE-nah DU-kes TE-kum). If a record is subpoenaed, the assistant or another employee of the clinic who is responsible for the medical record may be called on to identify the record. A photocopy of the record is usually acceptable to submit into evidence, and the patient's original record remains in the clinic. In a legal case, it is acceptable to charge the patient's attorney a reasonable fee for photocopying the patient's record.

The medical administrative assistant who has received a subpoena duces tecum will be expected to bring a copy of the patient's record to the court at the time and place specified. It is the physician's responsibility to give meaning to the record; it is the medical administrative assistant's responsibility to verify that the record belongs to a certain individual and that the content is original and has not been altered or falsified.

The Assistant as a Witness

When served with a subpoena or subpoena duces tecum, a medical administrative assistant should consult the legal counsel retained by the clinic or the physician. An attorney will instruct the assistant about the proper procedures to follow in obeying the subpoena.

When appearing in court as a witness, a medical administrative assistant should do the following:

- Answer only the question asked by the questioning attorney. Do not offer additional information.
- Answer each question truthfully.
- Be sure that the question asked is understood. If not, state, "I don't understand the question."
- If an answer to a question is unknown, do not be afraid to say, "I don't know."
- Explain the facts in easy to understand terms.
- Never cover up any discrepancies in the record.
- Dress appropriately. Professional appearance adds to witness credibility.

Damages

When a case is initially filed with the court, damage amounts requested by the plaintiff are specified. **Damages** are monetary amounts requested by a plaintiff in consideration for injuries that the plaintiff alleges to have received.

If the defense of a malpractice case is unsuccessful and a physician or practice loses the case, damages to be awarded to the plaintiff will be specified by the jury. Common damages sought in actions against a medical practice or a physician (or both) include compensatory and punitive damages.

Compensatory damages are awarded to compensate the plaintiff for injuries or losses suffered as a result of the wrongdoing of the defendant. These awards are meant to compensate for damages such as physical injury, loss of wages due to inability to work, emotional suffering, or loss of companionship.

Punitive, or **exemplary, damages** are usually the most severe. Multimillion dollar awards that one hears about in the media usually consist of substantial punitive damage amounts. Punitive damages are awarded to do exactly what the word punitive means: to punish. This damage award is given to punish a defendant for something that was very wrong. If a defendant acted recklessly when treating a patient, this likely will be taken into account when damages are considered.

Large punitive damage amounts are intended to deter others from similar conduct and are intended to make an "example" of the case. Because punitive damages can be so high, some states have set limits as to the punitive damage amounts that can be awarded. Punitive damages may be awarded along with compensatory damages.

Legal Topics Related to the Medical Office

The Practice of Medicine

To legally practice medicine, a physician must be licensed to practice in each state in which he or she practices medicine. The state board of medical examiners in each state is responsible for the physician licensure process.

What constitutes the practice of medicine in each state is established by the state's medical practice act. The purpose of each medical practice act is to regulate the practice of medicine to protect the public. A definition of practicing medicine usually includes some or all of the following:

- A person is engaged in the practice of diagnosing and treating disease.
- A person provides or prescribes treatment for the physical or mental ailments of persons in order to receive compensation.

- A person uses the title "medical doctor" or "doctor of osteopathy" or any other similar abbreviation with his or her name.

In most states, health care providers other than physicians—physician assistants, nurse practitioners, and so forth, as well as alternative health care providers such as massage therapists, hypnotists, and acupuncturists—are allowed to practice their profession, provided that they practice within the scope of practice as defined by the state's medical practice act.

It is extremely important for an assistant to never say or do anything that could be construed as giving medical advice and/or treatment to a patient without the physician's approval. An assistant should be careful to never say such things as, "You probably have strep throat" or "You should put ice on a sprained ankle." Through such statements, an assistant is giving medical advice or a diagnosis and very likely could be accused of practicing medicine without a license. In addition, a patient could suffer an injury from taking such an action. It is not unusual for a physician to instruct the front desk staff that they should never give out a bandage at the front desk because that simple act could be construed as giving medical treatment.

It is possible, however, for physicians to establish protocol that is to be used within a health care facility in certain situations. For example, if a patient with a possible leg fracture enters the clinic, the assistant may have been given previous instructions to transport the patient in a wheelchair. This action is not only practical but is necessary to avoid possible further injury to the patient. Additionally, established protocol may authorize that radiographs of the patient's injury should be taken before the physician actually sees the patient.

Consent

To treat patients, a physician must obtain **consent** for medical treatment from the patient. Consent is either expressed or implied by the patient. To give consent for medical treatment is to give approval for medical treatment.

Expressed consent is a statement from the patient that the physician should provide medical treatment for the patient. Expressed consent may be given by the patient either verbally or in writing. The nature of the proposed medical treatment will determine whether the consent should be written. Consent for routine care, such as examinations and basic diagnostic tests, is usually given verbally. If medical treatment is invasive, or if it requires administration of a medication, written consent is usually given. Written consent is used for such procedures as surgery, administration of immunizations, and removal of lesions and for certain laboratory or radiologic examinations, such as testing for the human immunodeficiency virus and computed tomographic scans that require the use of contrast medium.

Implied consent is given very often in a medical office. Patients may not even realize when they are giving implied consent. Implied consent is evidenced by a patient's actions. If a physician asks a patient to open his mouth and say, "Ah," and the patient does it, the patient is giving consent to the physician to examine his throat. Even the very act of arriving for an appointment with a physician is implied consent—implying that the patient wants to be treated.

In a life-or-death situation, consent is not required to treat a patient. It is implied, or assumed, that a patient would want his or her life saved. Even if a patient cannot communicate, the medical staff will commence and continue treatment until the patient is out of danger. The consent of a patient or relative is not necessary for initiation of life-saving treatment.

To give consent, patients must have full knowledge of their medical condition and the proposed treatment for the condition. Whenever consent is given by patients, it must be an **informed consent.** Informed consent means that patients have been given information about their medical condition, the treatment alternatives for their condition, and why treatment is recommended. They must be told of the potential benefits and risks of each treatment and likely outcomes related to each treatment. They also must be informed of what may happen if they choose not to treat the condition, and they must receive this information in language that they understand. Informed consent may not be a one-time event but could occur over time. A patient who is receiving treatment for a chronic condition over several encounters with a physician will accumulate information over the course of those visits and will use that information to make an informed decision regarding the next steps of treatment.

Consider the following examples of informed consent:

- A patient has been given the diagnosis of high blood pressure. The physician gives in detail the treatment options (e.g., various medications, dietary changes) and the risks associated with each option. The physician also must inform the patient of what may happen if the patient does not treat the condition (the patient may be at risk for serious health complications, such as a stroke).
- A patient sees a surgeon for a suspicious mole. The physician may recommend excision of the mole but must inform the patient of possible scarring, infection, and other consequences. The physician also may inform the patient that if he or she chooses to wait to remove the lesion and it is malignant, serious complications could occur.
- A patient sees his physician for knee pain. The physician prescribes medication for the pain. The patient does not improve and is referred by the physician to an orthopedic specialist. The specialist examines the patient and orders physical therapy. The patient fails to improve, and the physician recommends diagnostic arthroscopy based on the patient's failure to improve and the persistent pain.

Confidentiality

The concept of health care **confidentiality** means that communication between a patient and a health care professional must be kept secret. Federal legislation known as HIPPA provided the groundwork for the first comprehensive federal protection of the confidentiality of health care information for all individuals. In addition, an individual state may provide greater protection of a patient's medical privacy.

BOX 3-2

Summary of the HIPAA Privacy Rule

The Office of Civil Rights of the United States Department of Health and Human Services has created a document entitled *Summary of the HIPAA Privacy Rule.*

This document is available in PDF format on the Department of Health and Human Services website at www.hhs.gov. The document contains concise information on application of HIPAA and covers information regarding the following:

- What Organizations are Subject to HIPAA Rules
- What Information is Protected
- Permitted Uses and Disclosures of Information
- Authorized Uses and Disclosures of Information
- Limiting Uses and Disclosures to the Minimum Necessary
- Notice and Other Individual Rights
- Administrative Requirements of Health Care Organizations
- Personal Representatives and Minors
- Enforcement and Penalties for Noncompliance

Confidentiality is important to a patient's health care because an assurance of confidentiality encourages a patient to disclose sensitive information to health care professionals because the patient knows that it will not be openly or freely shared with others. Without a guarantee of confidentiality, a patient may be reluctant to divulge important information that may have an impact on his or her health. For instance, if a physician asks about a patient's social habits and the patient answers no to questions of illegal drug use when the patient has actually used illegal drugs, this could have a serious impact on the patient's treatment for his or her condition.

All information regarding a patient's medical treatment is considered confidential information. Confidentiality in the medical office setting means that patient information is to be kept secret or private, and that this information is to be kept among those who provide care for the patient and may not be divulged to anyone else without the patient's permission. Assistants must keep everything confidential that they see, hear, and do in the office.

The first overall federal protection of the confidentiality of medical information took effect in April 2003 with the Health Insurance Portability and Accountability Act (HIPAA) (Box 3-2). Even though it is legally mandated, it is also absolutely ethically expected that all health care providers should continually protect the confidentiality of health care information. Additional information on HIPAA protected information is given in Chapter 9, Health Information Management.

Release of Confidential Information

From time to time it becomes necessary to release to a third party, information regarding a patient's medical care. In most cases, a patient's medical information should be released only with the patient's written consent. It is inappropriate to release any information regarding a patient's health care treatment or services without that consent. There are a few exceptions to this rule, as mentioned below, but it is generally held that each patient owns the right to decide who may have access to his or her medical record. Release of information documentation is discussed in greater detail in Chapter 9, Health Information Management (see Fig. 9-28).

Required Release of Medical Information

In some instances, a health care provider is required to release confidential information about the patient, whether or not the patient has authorized its release. Generally, a provider or other health care professional is expected to keep all health information confidential unless a written authorization to release information is obtained from the patient. However, confidential information about a patient may have to be released in the following instances:

- Injuries that occur as the result of a crime are required to be reported. The law requires that this information be reported to law enforcement authorities. Providers cannot hide information that health care treatment was provided for a patient who was injured in connection with a crime.
- Public health laws may require release of information. If a patient has certain communicable or infectious diseases, he or she may be a threat to public safety, and information regarding the patient's illness is usually sent to the public health department.
- If the patient is a serious threat to someone (including themselves) or to society (e.g., the patient threatens to harm someone [Box 3-3], authorities or individuals may be notified of the concern.
- If a provider is subpoenaed as part of a legal action, information may have to be given as testimony in a court of law.

In the absence of a specific legal requirement for disclosure, it is wise for the assistant to leave it up to the provider to determine whether information should be disclosed without signed authorization to do so. Once confidential information is disclosed, it has been revealed and cannot be truly confidential again.

Under no circumstances should any health care professional *ever* discuss a patient's medical treatment or diagnosis with anyone (the patient's family or anyone else), unless it is necessary as part of providing continuing care to the patient. This includes all health care professionals in the medical office. Adult family members are not entitled to information about other adult family members unless the patient gives permission.

Details regarding any patient's visit can be discussed with other health care personnel but *only* if the details are needed for personnel to provide continued care or service to the patient. Situations in which this would apply may include (1) giving information to billing personnel within the office as they complete the billing process, (2) asking the nurse to verify a patient's medications because the physician's dictation is inaudible, or (3) verifying laboratory tests that were ordered for a patient. More information on legal issues as they pertain specifically to a patient's health information can be found in Chapter 9.

BOX 3-3

Tarasoff v. Regents of University of California; Morgan V. Fairfield

Following are examples of why confidentiality may have to be breached by a physician or other health care providers. These are real cases.

Tarasoff v. Regents of University of California (1976)

Prosenjit Poddar, an adult male, became obsessed with a student named Tatiana Tarasoff. A friend encouraged Poddar to get professional help. Poddar saw a psychiatrist, was given medication, and was scheduled for weekly appointments with a psychologist. During the appointments, Poddar confessed to having fantasies about harming, maybe killing, Tarasoff. A friend told the psychologist that Poddar planned to buy a gun. Poddar stopped therapy, and the psychologist asked campus police to question Poddar. When questioned, Poddar denied any plan to harm Tarasoff.

Two months later, Poddar stabbed Tarasoff to death. Poddar was convicted of murder, but because of a technicality, the conviction was overturned. Poddar then left the country.

Tarasoff's family filed a civil suit against the university, psychiatrist, psychologist, and campus police for negligence. The court found for the plaintiff and concluded that the therapists had a duty to warn Tarasoff of possible impending danger.

Morgan v. Fairfield

In a more recent case, Morgan v. Fairfield (1997), the Ohio Supreme Court ruled against Dr. Brown, a psychiatrist/consultant, and the Fairfield Family Counseling Center. A psychiatric patient, Matt Morgan, had made threats against his father and was subsequently hospitalized and given the diagnosis of a schizophreniform disorder. After being released from the hospital, he received follow-up care from Dr. Brown, who later discontinued Matt's medication. Matt's mother repeatedly reported to the doctor that her son's condition was deteriorating. The parents made repeated attempts to have Matt involuntarily committed but were unsuccessful. On July 25, 1991, Matt Morgan shot and killed his parents and seriously injured his sister. The plaintiffs alleged that the doctor did not obtain an adequate medical history, improperly discontinued the patient's medication, and failed to monitor the patient's condition. The case reached the Ohio Supreme Court, where the Court ruled in favor of the plaintiffs.

These cases illustrate the point that confidentiality should not be protected if society or an individual is in danger. In instances such as these, the need for society or an individual to know of the threat is greater than the need to protect the patient's confidentiality.

From *Tarasoff v. Regents of University of California*, 17 Cal. 3d 425, 551 P. 2d 334, 131 Cal. Rptr. 14 (1976); American Association of Community Psychiatrists. AACP Newsletter, Vol. 11, No. 3, Summer 1997.

As mentioned previously, in certain instances, minors may receive treatment without parental consent. Such instances include treatment for pregnancy, contraceptive prescription, sexually transmitted diseases, drug and other substance abuse, and psychiatric problems. Information regarding those treatments cannot be released to the parent without the approval of the minor. Because these conditions are so serious and fundamental to the well-being of the minor, this information is kept confidential; it is even kept from the patient's parents.

Imagine how many minors with concerns related to these conditions would seek treatment if they knew their parents would know everything. Treatment of minors is often a "sticky" situation, and a physician in conjunction with legal counsel should establish guidelines consistent with legal requirements to protect disclosure of confidential information.

Mandated Reportable Injury, Disease, and Occurrences

To protect the public from outbreaks of disease, the government requires that certain medical occurrences must be reported to the state health department.

Public health laws in every state require physicians to report certain occurrences of disease, injury, and other medical events. Requirements for reporting vary from state to state. These occurrences include such items as the following:

- Births and deaths
- Suspected abuse (child, adult, or elderly)
- Treatment of patients with injuries from a violent act, such as stabbing, shooting, or poisoning
- Communicable or infectious diseases (Box 3-4)

Information received by state health departments is then compiled on a national scale by the Centers for Disease Control and Prevention (CDC) in Atlanta, Georgia. Each week, the CDC publishes the *Morbidity and Mortality Weekly Report,* which reports instances of certain diseases and death statistics from every state. Collected information is used in planning health initiatives and is vital in protecting the public from communicable or infectious diseases.

Confidentiality Agreements

Every health care professional should be required to sign a confidentiality agreement (Fig. 3-2). These agreements are signed by employees at the beginning of employment and should be signed at every employment anniversary. Even those who volunteer at a health care facility should be required to sign a confidentiality agreement. When signed, such an agreement acknowledges the assistant's understanding of the facility's policy regarding confidentiality of health information. After it has been signed, the agreement should be placed in the employee's file in the human resources office.

The importance of protecting patient confidentiality cannot be stressed enough. In the course of business in a medical

BOX 3-4

Conditions Reportable to State Department of Health

AIDS
Anthrax*
Arboviral infection
Botulism*
Brucellosis*
Campylobacteriosis*
Cancer (invasive and in situ carcinomas)
Carbepenem-resistant *Enterobacteriaceae*
CD4 test results
Chickenpox (varicella)
Chlamydial infection
Cholera*
Clostridium perfringens intoxication
Coccidiomycosis
Creutzfeldt-Jakob disease
Cryptosporidiosis
Diphtheria*
Enterococcus, vancomycin resistant (VRE)*
Escherichia coli (*Shiga*-toxin producing strains)*
Foodborne or waterborne outbreaks
Giardiasis
Glanders
Gonorrhea
Haemophilus influenzae infection*
Hantavirus*
Hemolytic-uremic syndrome
Hepatitis A, B, C
Human immunodeficiency virus (HIV) infection
Influenza
Klebsiella pneumonia Carbapenemase (KPC)–producers
Laboratory incidences with possible release of category A agents or novel influenza virus
Lead blood level greater than or equal to 10 µg/dL
Legionellosis
Listeriosis*
Lyme disease
Malaria*
Measles (rubeola)*
Melioidosis
Meningitis, bacterial*
Meningococcal disease (invasive)
Mumps
Nipah virus infections
Nosocomial outbreaks in institutions
Pertussis*
Plague*
Poliomyelitis*
Pregnancy in person infected with perinatally transmissible disease
Psittacosis
Q fever*
Rabies (animal or human*)
Rocky Mountain spotted fever
Rubella*
Salmonellosis*
Scabies outbreaks in institutions
Severe acute respiratory syndrome (SARS)
Shigellosis
Smallpox
Staphylococcus aureus, methicillin resistant (MRSA)*
Staphylococcus aureus, vancomycin resistant (VRSA)*
Staphylococcus enterotoxin B intoxication
Streptococcal infections–invasive
Syphilis
Tetanus
Tickborne encephalitis viruses and fevers
Toxic shock syndrome*
Trichinosis
Tuberculosis*
Tularemia*
Tumors of the central nervous system
Typhoid fever*
Unexplained critical illness/death in otherwise healthy person
Unusual disease clusters
Vibriosis
Viral hemorrhagic fevers
Weapons of mass destruction suspected event
Yellow fever

From North Dakota State Department of Health, 2013.
**Requires submission of sample to public health laboratory.*

office, an assistant and all other employees frequently are required to deal with sensitive, personal information about a patient's health care treatment. A patient's right to complete confidentiality must be protected. Any health care employee who does not respect confidentiality of medical information is not only acting illegally and may be subject to civil and criminal penalties but also will likely become unemployed. Some unfortunate cases of confidentiality breaches have made national headlines. In 2008, Britney Spears (the singer/songwriter) was hospitalized, and during her hospitalization, her medical records were inappropriately accessed by health care workers who were NOT providing care for her. As a result of these breaches, several individuals were terminated from their employment. There have been other cases of famous individuals who have been the victims of confidentiality breaches. Every patient deserves protection of their confidentiality and every individual in a medical office has a responsibility to ensure that each patient's confidentiality is protected.

Protecting Patient Confidentiality

In a medical office, an assistant must be aware of several possible locations in which health care confidentiality may be breached. Several precautions can and must be taken to guard

Happy Valley Medical Group
Confidentiality Agreement

I understand that all information regarding patients and their health care is considered confidential. Information may be written, verbal, or in computerized format. Any information regarding patients that is acquired during the course employment at Happy Valley Medical Group shall be considered confidential.

I understand that confidential information must never be disclosed for nonemployment related purposes. Disclosure of confidential information outside of my assigned duties will constitute unauthorized release of confidential information and can be considered reason for termination of employment.

By signing this document, I acknowledge that I understand this statement and agree to abide by all policies and procedures pertaining to confidentiality of patient information.

________________________ ____________
Employee Signature Date

________________________ ____________
Witness Signature Date

Figure 3-2 Sample of a confidentiality agreement.

against the possibility of a confidentiality breach in a typical medical office setting.

Photocopiers/Printers. Various types of documents are copied in the medical office, including a patient's medical record for release, an insurance claim form, or an appointment schedule, to name a few. Sometimes, after a copy is made, originals may be inadvertently left in the copier (Fig. 3-3). When making copies, an assistant should double-check the area around the copier to ensure that no items are left. If copies are made in error, they should be disposed of properly by shredding or other secure disposal.

It is also important to remember that with today's copier and printer technology, it is possible to send and store electronic copies of documents within a device's memory. Documents can be scanned and stored or can be sent electronically to the device for printing. It is imperative to ensure that any such documents are kept confidential.

With the increased use of electronic health records, copies of patients' health records are usually printed from a computer. One must be careful that only those records that are needed are printed. If extra pages are printed, they should be properly disposed of as described in the following section entitled Information Disposal.

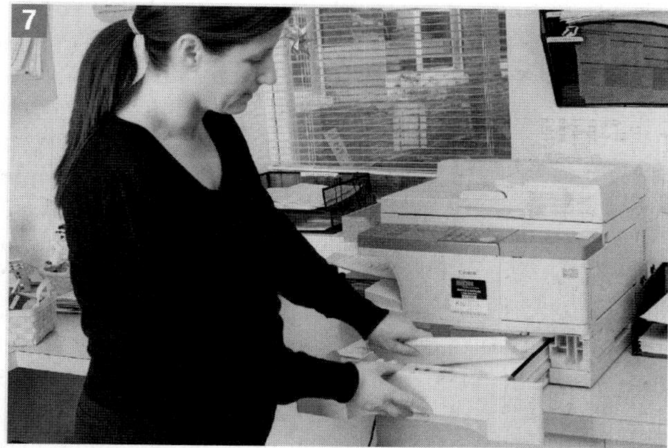

Figure 3-3 An assistant must be careful to remove all medical documents from a copier after photocopies have been made. (From Chester GA: *Modern Medical Assisting*. Philadelphia, WB Saunders; 1999.)

Information Disposal. Failure to protect anything that contains a patient's name, chart number, or any other identifying piece of information could bring about a breach in confidentiality. Copies of laboratory slips, copies of the appointment schedule, photocopies made in error, and anything else with identifying information on it could identify a patient, the procedure that he or she has undergone, or the patient's diagnosis. A patient's name on a slip of paper may seem harmless, but imagine the personal implications for the patient if the slip of paper contained orders for testing for sexually transmitted diseases.

Anything with information that identifies a patient (e.g., name, chart number, phone number, address) must be destroyed. It is not sufficient to throw away the information—the information must be destroyed so that it cannot be read. Using a shredder is an easy way to ensure that information is destroyed before it leaves the clinic. Some offices may hire a professional disposal service that agrees to pick up confidential trash and destroy it. If an office decides to use such an outside company, a confidentiality agreement should be signed, stipulating that the hired company agrees to protect the confidentiality of information it has been entrusted to destroy.

If a shredder is used, it should be placed in an area of the office where it is not seen by patients. A patient who sees an assistant who is shredding documents may get the wrong idea about the use of the shredder and may believe that vital information is being shredded. The shredder is used solely for the purpose of destroying sensitive medical documents that are no longer needed.

Computer Equipment. Technology has brought some new concerns about safeguarding information stored in a computer system. Several problems may arise when a computer is used in a medical office.

If a computer system includes all of the basic office tasks, such as billing, appointment scheduling, registration, and maintenance of medical records, access to different areas of the system usually is restricted. Employees should be given access only to those parts of the system that they will need to accomplish their job duties.

For example, in a large clinic with several different departments, an assistant who works in the billing and insurance area may need access to the appointment scheduling portion of the system in order to verify dates of service for medical charges. An assistant who works in patient registration may have access to the registration and appointments section of the system but would probably not need to have access to the billing portion. Physicians may have access to everything within the system or may have limited access also. Computer systems also can be set to allow some individuals to have read-only access to some areas, while others may have full access and the ability to change information. Access rights would be determined by each individual organization.

Every computer system should be password protected. Each employee should be required to log on with a unique, employee identification and should use a password that only he or she knows. Using the employee identification, a computerized system then tracks all of the areas the employee visits and what is accessed. If a confidentiality breach occurs, a system log helps identify where the breach might have occurred. In a password-protected system, each user should change his or her password frequently to help avoid any security breaches. At no time should an assistant allow his or her identification and password to be used by anyone else.

Most health care facilities have networked computer systems that must be protected from outside computer hackers. Hackers intentionally try to break the security of computer systems in order to obtain sensitive information or to destroy information contained in the system. It is the responsibility of every medical office to protect the integrity of its information system and to eliminate the possibility of any security breaches.

An assistant can take several steps to protect computer information. Computer screens should be pointed away from areas where the public can view the screen, and screen savers should be used to cover the screen if the computer is inactive. Screen savers should be activated shortly after the computer becomes idle. Systems may have an auto log-off feature that will log a user off when the computer has been idle for a specified length of time.

Printers are used to produce appointment schedules, patient statements, insurance forms, and other office documents. They should be located in a secure area that is consistently monitored by the office staff. Print jobs should be stopped while the assistant is away from the printer area.

Telephones. Everyone in the medical office should be aware of telephone conversations near public areas. Staff members at the nurses' station or the front desk might be within earshot of the public and should be careful to protect confidentiality when speaking on the phone in these areas. Confidential information should never be given when it may be overheard by the public. Additional information regarding telephone and fax machine confidentiality is provided in Chapter 6, Interpersonal Communications.

Elevators and Hallways. Sometimes, staff members become "too comfortable" with patient information and may discuss a patient's treatment while in a public area of the clinic. A patient's medical information should never be discussed in such settings. Staff members should be very careful not to use patients' names or discuss sensitive medical information in public areas. Another person in the elevator or hallway may know the patient. A breach of confidentiality such as this would likely result in dismissal of the staff member who divulged the information.

Advance Directives

No individual can ever be certain that he or she will always be capable of making all of his or her health care decisions. At one time or another, everyone probably will know someone who is no longer able to communicate wishes for medical treatment. This may happen as the result of an accident or serious illness at any time in someone's life.

What happens when patients are so ill or incapacitated that they cannot make health care decisions for themselves? **Advance directives** are legal documents that establish a patient's wishes for medical care when he or she is no longer able to make those decisions. Almost all states recognize advance directives.

In the absence of written instructions for health care decisions, physicians consult with the patient's relatives to obtain consent for medical treatment. A patient's relatives may not be aware of the patient's wishes for medical treatment. An advance directive will inform family members of a patient's wishes if the patient has failed to do so.

The Joint Commission, an organization that reviews practices and procedures of hospitals and other health care facilities, requires hospitals to ask every patient when admitted whether he or she has an advance directive. If the patient has prepared an advance directive, a copy must be placed in the patient's chart.

One type of advance directive, a **living will,** specifies the type of treatment the patient would or would not like if in a terminal, irreversible condition. A living will communicates the patient's wishes with regard to use of life-sustaining treatment. A living will identifies whether the patient desires tube feeding, cardiopulmonary resuscitation (CPR), or other extraordinary measures to save his or her life. Once the patient is attached to a life-sustaining or life-prolonging device, it is often very difficult to have that device removed. A living will that has been prepared by the patient may spare the patient and family an undesirable, unpleasant medical situation.

A **durable power of attorney for health care**, another type of advance directive, is a document that is broader in nature and covers more possible types of medical situations. A durable power of attorney for health care is a legal document that gives authority to an individual who will make health care decisions for a person if that person is no longer able to make those decisions. If the patient is comatose or is mentally incapacitated and cannot make decisions for himself or herself, the individual designated as the durable power of attorney for health care will make the patient's decisions.

A living will is different from a durable power of attorney in that the living will communicates the patient's wishes if the patient should have an irreversible or terminal illness. Many medical situations can arise that may impede an individual's ability to decide, but not all of those situations are necessarily irreversible or terminal.

Advance directives are legal documents that must be witnessed by individuals who do not stand to benefit from the patient's medical condition. Hospital or health facility employees, blood relatives, and anyone named in a patient's will can not be witness to that patient's advance directive. Health facility employees may benefit if a patient is kept on life support and large bills result. Relatives or persons named in wills may benefit from a patient's demise. That is why a witness to an advance directive must be free from those connections to a patient and must not possibly benefit from the patient's condition. Although a relative may not be a witness, a relative can be named to make decisions as a power of attorney.

A specialized type of advance directive, a mental health directive, may or may not be available in your state. A mental health directive identifies someone who will act on an individual's behalf, should that individual be unable to make treatment decisions regarding mental health care. In such a document, an individual can specify his or her wishes regarding administration of certain medications or other treatments such as electroshock therapy. A mental health directive typically would become active only if an individual is considered incompetent to make decisions regarding personal health care.

A do-not-resuscitate order is a specific advance directive in which a patient specifies that he or she does not wish to be revived or receive CPR if his or her heart should stop. Such orders usually are noted in the charts of patients who are hospitalized.

Patients who have or desire advance directives should be sure to communicate their wishes to the health care provider. Copies of these directives should be placed in the patient's medical record, and the record should be clearly marked that the patient has an advance directive. Patients should clearly communicate their wishes to appointed decision makers and should select decision makers who will carry out their wishes. In addition, patients should inform family members about the existence of their advance directive should the patient's condition at any time warrant its enforcement.

Uniform Anatomical Gift Act

The Uniform Anatomical Gift Act, which was passed in 1968, governs the donation of body parts. Common parts of the body that are donated include heart, lungs, kidneys, liver, and corneas. An individual who wishes to donate body parts on his or her death may specify that all body parts may be donated or may identify specific parts to be donated.

Because of the advancement of medical technology and the ability to transplant body parts from one individual to another, it became necessary to control the transplantation and donation process. This is often the case with law pertaining to medicine; technological advances in medicine make it necessary to enact laws to protect society.

The basic principles of the Uniform Anatomical Gift Act include the following:

1. An individual 18 years of age and of sound mind may donate any or all parts of his or her body on his or her death.
2. If an individual has not specified donation, a relative of a deceased individual may donate any or all body parts. The relative who makes the decision usually is selected according to the following order: spouse, adult children, parents, adult brothers and sisters.
3. Gift recipients (recipients of the donation) are restricted to certain medical-related facilities (e.g., hospitals, medical schools) or to a specific individual in need.
4. An individual may revoke his or her donation at any time.
5. The facility or person designated to receive the donation has a right to reject the donation.

Just about all persons of any age are eligible to be organ or tissue donors. Age is not a factor, but an individual must be free from an active cancer, HIV, or bodily infection at the time of death. Organs (kidney, heart, lungs, liver, pancreas, and intestines), body tissues (heart valves, skin, ligaments, tendons, and corneas), and stem cells (including bone marrow) can be donated; however, organs must be used right away. Tissues and stem cells can be stored for later use. The condition of the organ or tissue is more important than its age.

Donations can be made by living individuals or by deceased individuals, but individuals younger than 18 years need the permission of a parent to make a donation. Of all transplants performed in 2004, approximately one fourth were provided through living donor donations.

Controlled Substances Act of 1970

The Controlled Substances Act (CSA) is part of the Comprehensive Drug Abuse Prevention and Control Act of 1970. The purpose of this legislation is to control the manufacture and distribution of narcotics, stimulants, depressants, hallucinogens, anabolic steroids, and chemicals used to produce a controlled substance.

All individuals involved in the handling of controlled substances are required to be registered with the DEA. Physicians and other health professionals who are authorized to dispense, prescribe, or administer drugs identified under the CSA must identify their DEA number on a patient's prescription when one of these drugs is prescribed. Manufacturers, distributors, hospitals, clinics, pharmacies, and other handlers of controlled substances are required to have a DEA number. All individuals and companies that are authorized to handle these drugs are also required to maintain a complete, accurate inventory and records of the substances and their related transactions, as well as proper security measures for storing the substances.

Drugs that are regulated by the CSA are placed on one of five schedules. Table 3-1 details each Schedule from I through V, along with examples of drugs included in each schedule. When considering placement on the schedule, the DEA considers several factors:

- Potential for abuse
- Pharmacologic effects of the drug
- Scientific knowledge of the drug
- History of abuse
- Scope, duration, and significance of abuse
- Risk to public health
- Possibility of physical addiction or psychological dependence on the drug
- Immediate precursor to a drug that is already controlled

Patients given prescriptions for Schedule II drugs must receive a written and signed prescription from the health care provider; such prescriptions may not be called in and may not be refilled without the patient seeing the provider again to obtain another prescription. Schedule III and IV drugs may be written or phoned in to a pharmacy and may be refilled with some restrictions.

Good Samaritan Statutes

Good Samaritan statutes are designed to protect health professionals who stop to render aid at the scene of an accident. Good Samaritan statutes are present to some degree in all 50 states. The intention of the statutes is to protect trained medical personnel from liability if they stop at the scene of an accident to render aid (Fig. 3-4). As is the case with many accidents, if a trained passerby arrives on the scene before an emergency response team does, treatment without delay can mean the difference between life or death.

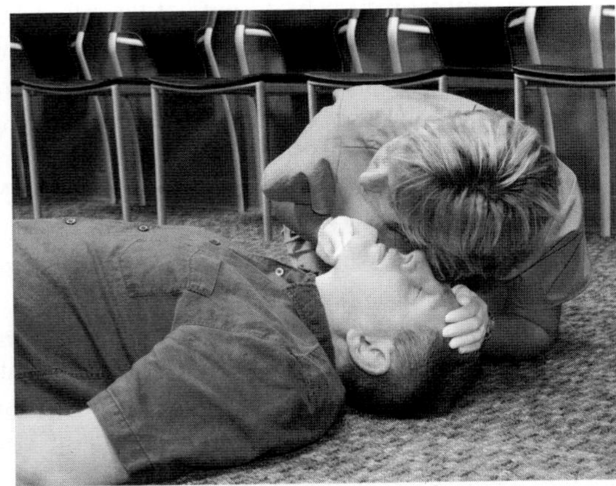

Figure 3-4 Good Samaritans who stop at the scene of an accident may be able to administer lifesaving care to a patient. Trained medical personnel generally are protected from liability when providing emergency care at the scene of an accident. This is important because seconds can count before emergency personnel arrive.

TABLE 3-1

Drug Enforcement Administration Determines Usage Requirements for Scheduled Drugs and Substances

Schedule Number	Potential for Abuse	Medical Use	Safety or Dependence Liability	Examples of Drugs or Substances
I	High	No currently accepted medical use in the United States	Lack of accepted safety for use of the drug	Heroin, LSD
II	High	Current accepted medical use in the United States with possible restrictions on use	Abuse of drug can lead to severe psychological or physical dependence	Morphine, PCP, cocaine, methadone, marijuana, methamphetamine
III	Less potential for abuse than drugs or substances in Schedule I or II	Current accepted medical use in the United States	Abuse of drug can lead to moderate or low physical dependence or high psychological dependence	Anabolic steroid, codeine, hydrocodone with aspirin or Tylenol
IV	Low potential for abuse relative to drugs in Schedule III	Current accepted medical use in the United States	Abuse of drug may lead to limited physical dependence or psychological dependence relative to drugs in Schedule III	Darvon, Talwin, Equanil, Valium, Xanax
V	Low potential for abuse relative to drugs in Schedule IV	Current accepted medical use in the United States	Abuse of drug may lead to limited physical dependence or psychological dependence relative to drugs in Schedule IV	Cough medicine with codeine

Good Samaritan statutes do not protect health care professionals from negligent, reckless behavior. A Good Samaritan usually is not held liable for injury to the patient unless the health care professional's behavior was not within standards of care and contributed to further injury of the patient. The Good Samaritan Act also does not apply to emergency cases within a medical facility.

Health Insurance Portability and Accountability Act of 1996

The Department of Health and Human Services established regulations for the first federal protection of the privacy of medical information, effective April 14, 2003. The mandate for this protection was included in the Health Insurance Portability and Accountability Act of 1996, otherwise known as HIPAA (pronounced HIP-pah). The HIPAA regulations apply to all personal health care information, including oral, paper, and electronic information.

HIPAA regulations include the following basic components.

Consumer Control

Health care consumers have new rights with regard to control of their health information. These rights include a patient's right to obtain a copy of his or her medical record and the right to request changes if an error in the record is identified. A health care entity must provide access to patient records within 30 days and may charge a fee for the cost of copying and sending records.

Boundaries

For the most part, disclosure of health information is limited to a patient's treatment or payment for health care treatment. Health care entities may not disclose personal medical information to marketers, insurers, banks, or other businesses without the permission of the patient. Employers are not given access to health care information that could be used for hiring and firing or to determine promotions, unless the individual authorizes such access. Health care facilities may use personal health care information for patient treatment, educational purposes (teaching and conducting research), and quality assurance. To provide the best possible medical care, physicians and other health care providers still have access to a patient's entire health record when providing treatment for a patient.

Accountability

For violations of a patient's right to privacy, civil and criminal penalties may be imposed. Criminal penalties are imposed when violators knowingly disclose health care information improperly, or when health care information is obtained through deceptive practices. Depending on the nature of the offense, civil penalties may cost up to $100 per violation, and criminal penalties for wrongful disclosure of information may include up to a $250,000 fine and up to 10 years in prison.

Public Responsibility

Standards are established that allow access to information for public health purposes such as public health protection, medical research, health care improvement, law enforcement activities, and health care fraud and abuse. Examples include access to health care information for emergency circumstances, identification of a deceased person, use of health care facility patient directories, and national security and defense activities.

Security

Health care organizations have a responsibility to protect the privacy of health care information. Organizations must establish clear written procedures for protection of privacy, and within the organization, a privacy officer must be designated to monitor privacy issues.

If state and federal laws conflict with regard to privacy issues, the privacy standard that is greater would apply. Some states have more stringent laws related to health care records such as HIV/AIDS information and mental health records.

Emergency Medical Treatment and Labor Act of 1986

The Emergency Medical Treatment and Labor Act of 1986 (EMTALA) was passed by Congress and helped ensure that patients with emergency medical conditions could not be turned away for medical treatment. The statute essentially stipulates that hospitals who receive Medicare funding must screen patients with medical emergencies regardless if they can pay for their medical treatment. Hospitals are obligated to stabilize patients and to transfer patients should they request it.

Risk Management

To serve patients in an appropriate manner, a medical administrative assistant must be aware of the legal and ethical responsibilities that affect the medical office and its staff. This knowledge will help to minimize the risk that any possible legal cases against the practice may be pursued. The concept of **risk management** means minimizing the potential for legal action taken against the practice.

Keep the following in mind to minimize the chances of litigation involving the office:

- Always remember that the patient is the reason that everyone in the medical office is employed.
- Remember the quote of Mayo Clinic founder, Dr. William J. Mayo, "The best interest of the patient is the only interest to be considered…". Always keep the patient's best interests at the forefront of your actions.
- When assisting a patient, keep in mind how a simple action or statement may be viewed by the patient. Every action of the assistant is assumed to be done at the direction of the physician. Be careful what you say and do.
- Health care employees who have a good rapport with patients reduce the risk of lawsuits against the practice.
- Take immediate steps to resolve any patient conflict; notify the physician if necessary.
- Keep all medical information confidential. When in doubt, don't give it out!
- Be aware of the physical environment of the facility. Things such as wet floors, loose carpeting, malfunctioning doors,

and dangling electrical cords have the potential to cause physical injury to the public.

- Report any incidents or injuries to the physician, and complete any necessary paperwork to report those events. An incident report should always be completed to document any incidents or injuries that occur in the office.

The main concept of risk management is that all employees in the medical office should be aware that the treatment or service provided for a patient should never give the patient a reason to sue. In the day-to-day operations of a medical office, tasks may become familiar, and it is sometimes easy to forget that patients in the office could potentially sue the office in the future. So, the moral of the story is *never, ever give a patient cause to even consider legal action against the office.*

SUMMARY

The law has many applications in the practice of medicine. Laws governing medicine are created by legislators, case law precedent, and federal agencies designated to supervise the medical practice. If a situation should ever arise in the medical office that could have legal implications, it is extremely important for an assistant to notify the physician if there is any question of potential liability on the part of the medical office or staff.

Knowledge of the laws that govern medicine and awareness of potentially troublesome legal areas within the clinic will help the medical administrative assistant improve service to patients while avoiding the possibility of litigation against the medical office. All employees of the medical office can be sued and can play a role in preventing legal action. Positive patient relations and good customer service go a long way toward reducing the possibility of litigation.

YOU ARE THE MEDICAL ADMINISTRATIVE ASSISTANT

Picture yourself as a medical administrative assistant in a medical practice. What would you do in the following situations?

1. A patient calls the office and states he has slipped on the ice. He would like to know the best thing to do for a possible sprained ankle. How do you reply?
2. Your physician–employer has given you a handwritten letter and asked you to type a letter discharging a patient from his care. What steps do you need to take?

REVIEW EXERCIES

Exercise 3-1 Legal Concepts and Terms

Read each statement and choose the answer that best completes the statement. Record your answer in the blank provided.

_____ 1. Type of law that governs the relationships of individuals
(a) Criminal law
(b) Administrative law
(c) Statutory law
(d) Civil law

_____ 2. Laws established by the legislative branch of government
(a) Common law
(b) Case law
(c) Statutory law
(d) Administrative law

_____ 3. Laws established by the court
(a) Common law
(b) Administrative law
(c) Statutory law
(d) Criminal law

_____ 4. Legal concept establishing that evidence speaks for itself
(a) Advance directive
(b) *Res ipsa loquitur*
(c) Standards of care
(d) *Respondeat superior*
(e) Expressed consent

_____ 5. A physician who fails to properly terminate a physician–patient relationship may be liable for _____.
(a) Consideration
(b) Abandonment
(c) *Res ipsa loquitur*
(d) *Respondeat superior*

_____ 6. Name of party who initiates a legal action against another
(a) Plaintiff
(b) Defendant
(c) Statute
(d) Mature minor

_____ 7. Federal agencies are responsible for establishing and enforcing _____ .
(a) Administrative law
(b) Common law
(c) Case law
(d) Criminal law

_____ 8. Health care professionals are required to perform in a manner that is consistent with the expectations of their profession. This is a legal concept known as _____.
(a) Abandonment
(b) Standards of care
(c) Malpractice
(d) Litigation

_____ 9. The Latin phrase *respondeat superior* means
(a) An assistant may be held liable for the actions of another staff member of the medical office.
(b) An assistant is required to keep medical information confidential.
(c) A physician may be liable for the actions of his or her employees in the medical office.
(d) The evidence speaks for itself.

_____ 10. If a physician terminates care of a patient, which of the following is incorrect?
(a) A certified letter with return receipt should be sent to the patient informing the patient of the termination of care.
(b) The physician must provide care for a reasonable period of time.
(c) The patient is not required to pay his or her outstanding bill.
(d) Termination should be documented in the patient's medical chart.

_____ 11. Which of the following is **not** required to prove a physician's negligence?
(a) Physician failed to provide proper care for the patient's medical condition.
(b) Patient suffered damage or injury.
(c) Physician's failure caused patient's injury.
(d) Patient paid physician for medical treatment.
(e) Physician had an obligation to provide service to the patient.

_____ 12. Legal agreement between two people that creates an obligation
(a) Contract
(b) Deposition
(c) Subpoena
(d) Statute

_______ 13. Establishes a time period during which legal action must commence
(a) Litigation
(b) Statute of limitations
(c) Deposition
(d) Interrogatories

_______ 14. What type of health information should **not** be released by a physician?
(a) Information legally required to be released
(b) Reporting an infectious disease to a state health department
(c) Parent requesting information about treatment of a minor for a sexually transmitted disease
(d) Reporting a patient who threatens to physically harm someone

_______ 15. If an assistant is called to court as a witness, the assistant should _______ .
(a) Offer additional information without being asked
(b) Cover up discrepancies in the record to protect the physician
(c) State "I don't know" if an answer to a question is not known
(d) Pretend to know everything
(e) Dress in jeans or other comfortable clothing because a day in court can be long

_______ 16. Which of the following is **not** part of informed consent?
(a) Patient is given information about his medical condition
(b) Patient is informed of alternative treatments for his medical condition
(c) Patient is told of potential benefits and risks of different treatment options
(d) Physician communicates in language that patient understands
(e) Patient is informed of costs of treatment

_______ 17. Which of the following is **not** good risk management practice?
(a) Develop a good rapport with patients.
(b) Ignore upset patients and give them a chance to cool down.
(c) Keep information confidential.
(d) Be alert to the physical environment of the office.
(e) Document incidents or injuries immediately.

_______ 18. Which of the following is **false** about a license to practice medicine?
(a) Each state sets its own requirements for licensure.
(b) A currently licensed physician may be eligible for a license in another state through a process called reciprocity.
(c) CEUs usually are required for renewal of a license.
(d) A physician involved in a malpractice suit is not allowed to practice.
(e) The USMLE is a licensing examination for medical doctors.

_______ 19. All of the following are reasons that a physician may stop treating a patient except _______ .
(a) The patient has failed to follow any treatment recommended by the physician.
(b) The physician is retiring from practice.
(c) The patient has failed to keep appointments with the physician.
(d) All of the above are reasons for termination.
(e) Only a and c are reasons that a physician would stop treating a patient.

Exercise 3-2 Legal Terms

In each group of statements, match each term above with the definition below that best matches the term. Record your answer in the blank provided. Each answer is used only once.

(a) Subpoena
(b) *Subpoena duces tecum*
(c) Deposition
(d) Living will
(e) Durable power of attorney for health care

_______ 1. Testimony given outside a courtroom

_______ 2. An advance directive specifying a patient's desired treatment if in a terminal irreversible condition

_______ 3. An order for an individual to appear in court

_______ 4. An advance directive giving authority to an individual to make medical decisions for an incapacitated patient

_______ 5. An order to produce medical records for trial use.

(a) Offer and acceptance
(b) Legal subject matter
(c) Legal capacity
(d) Consideration

_______ 6. The act or service to be performed is lawful.

_______ 7. Individual is an adult of sound mind.

_______ 8. One party agrees to do something, and another party also agrees.

_______ 9. Something of value is exchanged.

(a) Implied consent
(b) Expressed consent
(c) Consent
(d) Informed consent

_______ 10. To give approval for medical treatment

_______ 11. Patient is given full information about medical condition, alternative treatments, and associated risks, as well as potential benefits of each treatment.

_______ 12. This consent is evidenced by the patient's actions, that is, a patient opens her mouth when the physician asks her to do so.

_______ 13. The patient either verbally or in writing communicates the desire to have medical treatment.

Exercise 3-3 True or False

Read the following statements and determine whether each statement is true or false. Record the answer in the blank provided. T = true; F = false.

_______ 1. Risk management means reducing the possibility that a patient will sue the practice.

_______ 2. Establishing a good relationship with patients helps to reduce the chance of litigation in the future.

_______ 3. Everything an assistant says or does is believed to have been done at the direction of the physician.

_______ 4. If a patient is upset about services received in the office, it is best to point out to the patient why the patient is wrong.

_______ 5. If a patient is injured in the office, this should be reported to the physician immediately.

_______ 6. If a patient is injured in the office, a report should be completed to document the incident.

_______ 7. An assistant has little effect on whether a patient could potentially sue a medical practice.

_______ 8. Any employee of a medical office can be sued.

_______ 9. Keeping all medical information confidential is an important risk management practice of the medical office.

_______ 10. A patient who is suing a physician for malpractice may be required to obtain the testimony of an expert physician who will support the plaintiff's allegations.

_______ 11. A malpractice suit against a physician may be brought at any time during the patient's life.

_______ 12. The Uniform Anatomical Gift Act regulates gifts that a physician is allowed to receive from health industry corporations.

_______ 13. A physician may be sued for malpractice if he or she fails to act.

_______ 14. Punitive damages are awarded to compensate for lost wages.

_______ 15. Some states may set limits on the amount of punitive damages that may be awarded.

_______ 16. Both compensatory damages and exemplary damages may be awarded in a legal case.

_______ 17. Information that a patient uses to make an informed decision about a health care treatment can be given to the patient by the physician over a period of time and is not necessarily a one-time event.

_______ 18. A wife can be a witness to her husband's advance directive.

_______ 19. A physician could be sued for doing nothing.

_______ 20. A do-not-resuscitate order is a type of advance directive.

______ 21. According to the study presented in this chapter, most malpractice cases settle before going to trial, but most result in payments to plaintiffs.

______ 22. Failing to act is known as omission, and acting poorly or negligently is known as commission.

______ 23. The purpose of a state's medical practice act is to protect the public.

______ 24. All scheduled drugs require a written prescription from the physician.

______ 25. A paper shredder should be placed in a visible area so that patients can see that medical information is destroyed before it is thrown away.

______ 26. Health care employees usually are required to sign a confidentiality agreement with their employer.

______ 27. Volunteers at a health care facility should be required to sign a confidentiality agreement with the facility.

______ 28. A computer system in a medical office can track which parts of the system have been accessed by each user.

______ 29. To protect confidential information on a computer system, access can be restricted for users.

______ 30. There are no state laws protecting the confidentiality of patient's medical information.

______ 31. Oral consent of the patient is usually sufficient for release of his or her medical information.

Exercise 3-4 Legislation and Advance Directives

Read the following statements regarding the following legal topics and determine whether the statements below each topic are true or false. Record the answer in the blank provided. T = true; F = false.

Uniform Anatomical Gift Act of 1968

______ 1. This act governs the donation of body parts.

______ 2. An individual must donate all body parts to be an organ donor.

______ 3. Relatives of a deceased individual may donate any or all of the body parts of the deceased.

______ 4. Once an individual has made the decision to be an organ donor, the decision is permanent and may not be revoked.

______ 5. A medical school, a hospital, or a specific individual in need may be the recipient of an organ donation.

______ 6. Persons of all ages can be donors, but those younger than age 18 need parental permission.

______ 7. When donation of body parts is considered, the age of a person is not important; the condition of the patient's organs or the presence of disease may affect the ability to donate.

______ 8. Body tissues such as ligaments, corneas, or stem cells may be donated and stored.

______ 9. Donations can be made by living or deceased patients.

Controlled Substances Act (CSA) of 1970

______ 10. This act governs the manufacture and distribution of potentially addictive substances.

______ 11. Narcotics are regulated by the Controlled Substances Act.

______ 12. Controlled substances under this act are classified on a scale of 1 to 10, with 10 being the most addictive.

______ 13. Physicians must include their DEA number on a prescription when prescribing a controlled substance.

______ 14. The possibility that someone could be addicted to a drug is a factor that may cause a drug to be a scheduled drug.

Good Samaritan Statutes

______ 15. Less than half of the 50 states have Good Samaritan statutes.

______ 16. Good Samaritans are free from all liability if they stop at the scene of an accident.

______ 17. Good Samaritan statutes protect all health care professionals who work in an emergency room.

______ 18. The purpose of Good Samaritan statutes is to protect health care professionals from liability when they stop at an accident scene to render aid.

Advance Directives

_______ 19. A living will covers more possible health care situations than does a durable power of attorney for health care.

_______ 20. More or less, advance directives communicate a patient's wishes for health care treatment before a serious medical situation may arise.

_______ 21. Advance directives help inform a patient's family members of the patient's desire for medical treatment.

_______ 22. Every patient in a medical office must have an advance directive.

_______ 23. A living will communicates a patient's wishes for life-sustaining treatment such as tube feeding or ventilator use.

_______ 24. Once a patient is comatose, a living will is null and void.

_______ 25. Copies of a patient's living will or durable power of attorney for health care should be placed in the patient's chart.

_______ 26. A patient's relative can be a witness to the patient's advance directive.

Health Insurance Portability and Accountability Act (HIPAA) of 1996

_______ 27. HIPAA allows physicians to have complete control over the release of a patient's medical information.

_______ 28. Knowingly releasing private medical information in an improper manner is a criminal offense.

_______ 29. A patient may obtain a copy of his or her medical record.

_______ 30. When hiring an individual, an employer may access the individual's entire medical record.

_______ 31. Civil and criminal penalties may be given to persons who violate HIPAA regulations.

Emergency Medical Treatment and Labor Act (EMTALA) of 1986

_______ 32. EMTALA requires that hospitals receiving Medicare funding are required to provide a medical screening examination for emergency patients.

_______ 33. Emergency medical screening examinations must be performed regardless of a patient's ability to pay.

ACTIVITIES

ACTIVITY 3-1 SECURITY OPTIONS IN MEDISOFT

Using the following instructions, update security settings in Medisoft.

1. With Medisoft open, click **File>Program Options> HIPAA.**
2. Check the **Auto Log Off** box and enter 15 minutes in the blank provided. An auto log-off option will automatically cause the program to close to prevent unauthorized users from accessing the program should a computer be left unattended.
3. Click **Save.** A message will appear that the auto log-off will not take effect until security options are in place for the practice. At this time, the security options will not be set.
4. When completed, click **Close.**

ACTIVITY 3-2 LEGAL CASES INVOLVING MEDICAL MALPRACTICE

1. Research cases involving medical malpractice in your state. Many state sites have links to the state's judicial system. Find at least four cases involving medical malpractice, and briefly summarize each case and identify the decision of the court.
2. Research the circumstances and outcomes of the following cases involving medical practice.
   - *Fox v. Health Net of California*
   - *Albany Urology Clinic, P.C. et al. v. Cleveland, et al.*

ACTIVITY 3-3 ADVANCE DIRECTIVES

Find examples of a living will and a Durable Power of Attorney for Health Care for your state. The National Hospice and Palliative Care Organization (www.caringinfo.org) has sample forms available for every state. The American Association of Retired Persons, the American Bar Association Commission on Legal Problems of the Elderly, and the American Academy of Family Physicians have additional information on advance directives.

ACTIVITY 3-4 MANDATED REPORTABLE DISEASES AND MEDICAL OCCURRENCES

Investigate the state health department of your state. What diseases or medical occurrences are reportable in your state?

ACTIVITY 3-5 MEDICAL MALPRACTICE INFORMATION

Research medical malpractice on the Internet. Can you find answers to the following questions?

1. What is the statute of limitations for bringing a suit for malpractice in your state?
2. Is there a limit on damages in your state?
3. Which professions have the greatest incidence of malpractice involvement?
4. What places a particular specialty at greater risk for malpractice litigation?
5. How many physicians are sued for malpractice each year?
6. What are a physician's chances of being accused of malpractice at some point during his or her career?

ACTIVITY 3-6 LEGAL PROCEEDINGS

Visit a courtroom, and observe a trial in progress.

ACTIVITY 3-7 STATE MEDICAL PRACTICE ACT

Research the medical practice act and the state board governing medical practice in your state.

ACTIVITY 3-8 TREATMENT OF MINORS

Research the treatment of minors. The Guttmacher Institute (www.guttmacher.org) provides information for treatment of minors across the United States.

DISCUSSION

The following topics can be used for class discussion or for individual student essay.

DISCUSSION 3-1

Explain why a health care provider cannot guarantee medical treatment.

DISCUSSION 3-2

Explain how a medical administrative assistant can help reduce the chances of litigation involving the medical office.

DISCUSSION 3-3

Discuss the following statement from this chapter: "Technological advances in medicine make it necessary to enact laws to protect society."

DISCUSSION 3-4

Discuss the importance to the patient of each of the basic components of the Health Insurance Portability and Accountability Act of 1996. For additional information, consult the U.S. Department of Health and Human Services website.

DISCUSSION 3-5

Why should an employee be required to sign a confidentiality agreement? Are the legal requirements to keep information confidential sufficient?

Bibliography

American Academy of Family Physicians: *Respecting end-of-life treatment preferences. Sample advance directive form.* www.aafp.org. Accessed January 21, 2011.

American Medical Association: *Ending the patient-physician relationship; informed consent; patient confidentiality.* www.ama-assn.org. Accessed January 21, 2011.

Ballweg R, Stoleberg S, Sullivan E: *Physician Assistant, Guide to Clinical Practice*, Philadelphia, WB Saunders, 2003.

Brent NJ: *Nurses and the Law, A Guide to Principles and Applications*, Philadelphia, WB Saunders, 1997.

Cohen TA, Hughes KA: *U.S. Department of Justice. Bureau of Justice Statistics special report, medical malpractice insurance claims in seven states: 2000-2004.* www.ojp.usdoj.gov/bjs/pub/pdf/mmicss04.pdf. Accessed January 21, 2011.

Flight M: *Law, Liability, and Ethics for Medical Office Professionals*, ed 3, Albany, Delmar, 1998.

Group Health Research Institute: *Writing an advance directive.* www.ghc.org. Accessed January 21, 2011.

Guttmacher Institute: *Overview of abortion in the United States; Overview of minors' consent law.* www.guttmacher.org. Accessed January 21, 2011.

Huffman EK: *Health Information Management*, Berwyn, IL, Physician's Record Company, 1994.

Judson K, Blesie S: *Law and Ethics for Health Occupations*, ed 2, New York, Glencoe McGraw-Hill, 1999.

Lewis MA, Tamparo CD: *Medical Law, Ethics and Bioethics for Ambulatory Care*, Philadelphia, FA Davis, 1998.

McClinton RS: *JCAHO: Requirements for advance directives.* www.ehow.com. Accessed January 21, 2011.

Mental Health America: *Position Statement 23: Psychiatric advance directives.* www.mentalhealthamerica.net. Accessed January 21, 2011.

Minnesota Office of the Revisor of Statutes: *Minnesota statutes.* www.revisor.mn.gov. Accessed January 21, 2011.

Mid Minnesota Legal Assistance: *Minnesota advance psychiatric directive.* www.mylegalaid.org. Accessed January 21, 2011.

MSNBC: *UCLA fires workers for snooping in Spears files (as reported by the Associated Press).* http://today.msnbc.msn.com. Accessed April 12, 2011.

National Hospice and Palliative Care Organization: *Advance directives.* www.caringinfo.org. Accessed January 21, 2011.

North Dakota Board of Medical Examiners: *Medical Practice Act.* www.ndbomex. Accessed April 7, 2013.

Organ Procurement and Transplantation Network: *Data.* www.optn.org. Accessed January 21, 2011.

Texas Medical Board, Occupations Code: *Chapter 159 Physician-patient communication, Title 3. Health professions, subtitle B. Physicians.* www.tmb.state.tx.us. Accessed January 21, 2011.

United Network of Organ Sharing: *Living donation: What you need to know.* www.unos.org. Accessed January 21, 2011.

U.S. Department of Health and Human Services: *Overview of Emergency Medical Treatment and Labor Act.* www.cms.gov. Accessed January 21, 2011.

U.S. Department of Health and Human Services: *Protecting the privacy of patients' health information.* www.hhs.gov. Accessed January 21, 2011.

U.S. Department of Health and Human Services: *Health Resources and Services Administration. Organ Donation and Transplantation.* www.organdonor.gov. Accessed January 21, 2011.

U.S. Department of Health and Human Services, Office for Civil Rights: *Summary of HIPAA Privacy Rule.* www.hhs.gov/ocr/hipaa. Accessed January 21, 2011.

U.S. Drug Enforcement Agency Administration: *The Controlled Substances Act.* www.usdoj.gov. Accessed January 21, 2011.

U.S. Food and Drug Administration: *About FDA* www.fda.gov. Accessed January 21, 2011.

CHAPTER 4 Medical Ethics

LEARNING OUTCOMES

On successful completion of this chapter the student will be able to

1. Describe ethics and differentiate law and ethics.
2. Discuss the purpose of the Hippocratic Oath and other medical oaths.
3. Explain the ethical behavior of physicians.
4. Explain the ethical behavior of medical administrative assistants.
5. Discuss common ethical issues in health care and their impact on patients.
6. Describe an assistant's appropriate responses to ethical dilemmas in health care.

COMMISSION ON ACCREDITATION OF ALLIED HEALTH EDUCATION PROGRAMS (CAAHEP) CORE CURRICULUM FOR MEDICAL ASSISTANTS

- Use Internet to access information related to the medical office.
- Respond to issues of confidentiality.
- Apply HIPAA rules in regard to privacy/release of information.
- Recognize the importance of local, state and federal legislation and regulations in the practice setting.

ACCREDITING BUREAU OF HEALTH EDUCATION SCHOOLS (ABHES) COMPETENCIES FOR MEDICAL ASSISTING

Graduates

- Demonstrate professionalism by:
  - Maintaining confidentiality at all times.
  - Being cognizant of ethical boundaries.
  - Conducting work within scope of education, training, and ability.

VOCABULARY

abortion
ethics
euthanasia
medical ethics

Patients and health care providers often are faced with ethical dilemmas. Difficult medical situations create heart-wrenching decisions for patients and their health care providers. An understanding of the ethical matters that patients and their providers face helps a medical administrative assistant have empathy for patients and enables an assistant to provide thoughtful and considerate services for those patients.

Definition of Ethics

What exactly is **ethics**? According to the *Miller-Keane Encyclopedia & Dictionary of Medicine, Nursing, & Allied Health,* ethics is "systematic rules or principles which govern right conduct," and **medical ethics** refers to "the values and guidelines governing decisions in medical practice."

However, because this definition includes the word *right,* it is difficult to definitively define behavior as right or wrong, ethical or unethical. What is deemed to be right or wrong can vary among different groups in society and right or wrong does not mean the same thing to two people within the same group. Even within the medical field, each patient and treatment situation is unique; therefore, what may be "right" in one situation may not be "right" in another.

Law Versus Ethics

In Chapter 3, we learned that laws are societal rules or principles established by various branches of government. Ethics also consist of rules or principles, but they are rules or principles that define right conduct. Again, because people have different perceptions of what is right and wrong, it is sometimes very difficult to determine what ethical behavior is. Although laws and ethics are both rules, laws establish a minimum expectation of behavior. Typically, if someone violates the law, a fine or incarceration, or both, may result. Ethics, on the other hand, often are inspired by law but establish a much higher standard of behavior. Professional organizations wishing to promote high-quality behavioral standards among their members typically have a code of ethics for their members. Groups may have certain ethical expectations of their members and those members who deviate from the ethical standards established by an organization usually will find themselves with restricted membership rights and may even lose their membership rights.

History of Ethics

The topic of medical ethics is not a new one. Some early discussions of medical ethics occurred as long ago as 400 BC, when Hippocrates, the father of medicine, wrote the Hippocratic Oath (Fig. 4-1), to which today's physicians still pledge. Hippocrates was a Greek philosopher who had tremendous insight (even at that early time) into the practice of medicine. He did much to influence the practice of medicine and his influence is still seen in the practice of medicine today. On examination of the Hippocratic Oath, the following influences on modern-day medicine are seen:

- Physicians will share their knowledge of the medical profession with others.
- Physicians will not provide advice or drugs to any patient that may cause that patient's death.
- Physicians will not provide a device that accomplishes an abortion.
- When appropriate, physicians will refer patients to a specialist.
- Physicians will practice for the good of their patients.
- Patients' medical information that comes to physicians in the practice of medicine will be held confidential.

The Hippocratic Oath is an ethical code of conduct that serves as a guide for physicians in determining what constitutes "correct" professional behavior. Although the Oath is not law, it greatly influences the behavior of physicians.

CHECKPOINT

Physicians often provide treatment at no cost to their fellow physicians and their families. Is this in keeping with the Hippocratic Oath?

Ethical Behavior for Physicians

The American Medical Association (AMA), founded in 1847, is a professional organization for physicians who are dedicated to excellence in the practice of medicine. The AMA and its membership continually work to promote high-quality standards in health care delivery and to significantly influence the development of health care law in the United States. They establish policies that influence and further the practice of medicine in the United States.

The AMA has developed general principles regarding medical ethics. The AMA Principles of Medical Ethics were developed with the patient as the primary focus in the patient–physician relationship. These Principles are not laws

HIPPOCRATIC OATH

I swear by Apollo the physician, by Aesculapius, Hygeia, and Panacea, and I take to witness all the gods, all the goddesses, to keep according to my ability and my judgment the following oath:

To consider dear to me as my parents him who taught me this art; to live in common with him and if necessary to share my goods with him; to look upon his children as my own brothers, to teach them this art if they so desire without fee or written promise; to impart to my sons and the sons of the master who taught me and the disciples who have enrolled themselves and have agreed to the rules of the profession, by to these alone, the precepts and the instruction.

I will prescribe regimen for the good of my patients according to my ability and my judgment and never do harm to anyone. To please no one will I prescribe a deadly drug, nor give advice which may cause his death. Nor will I give a woman a pessary to procure abortion.

But I will preserve the purity of my life and my art. I will not cut for stone, even for patients in whom the disease is manifest; I will leave this operation to be performed by practitioners (specialists in this art). In every house where I come I will enter only for the good of my patients, keeping myself far from all intentional ill-doing and all seduction, and especially from the pleasures of love with women or with men, be they free or slaves.

All that may come to my knowledge in the exercise of my profession or outside of my profession or in daily commerce with men, which ought not to be spread abroad, I will keep secret and will never reveal.

If I keep this oath faithfully, may I enjoy my life and practice my art, respected by all men and in all times; but if I swerve from it or violate it, may the reverse be my lot.

Figure 4-1 Hippocrates, often known as the Father of Medicine, penned the Hippocratic Oath in 400 BC.

but are general statements of ethical conduct expected of AMA members. If a physician deviates from these ethical standards, he or she may not have violated the law but may likely become involved in civil litigation initiated by a dissatisfied patient, and the physician may risk loss of membership rights with the AMA as well.

AMA Council on Ethical and Judicial Affairs

The AMA's Council on Ethical and Judicial Affairs (CEJA) develops positions on ethical matters involving physicians and comments on judicial matters that involve or influence the practice of medicine. The Council continually updates the organization's position on ethical behavior of physicians in a document known as the AMA Code of Ethics. The Council is responsible for developing positions on ethical matters involving physicians and comments on judicial matters that involve or influence the practice of medicine.

A multitude of ethical issues are related to medical care. The AMA Principles of Medical Ethics establish a broad foundation for ethical behavior, but the AMA provides more specific guidance in the Current Opinions, which are introduced in the following section.

Current Opinions of the CEJA

A comprehensive listing of the Council's opinions of ethical matters, the Code of Ethics includes the Principles of Medical Ethics and opinions on topics such as social policy, interprofessional relations, hospital relations, confidentiality and media relations, fees and charges, physician records, practice matters, professional responsibilities, and the physician–patient relationship. These positions, known as Current Opinions, are reviewed and updated periodically to reflect changes in the patient–physician relationship and the delivery of health care; they are meant to serve as a guide for appropriate physician conduct.

The Current Opinions of the AMA's CEJA describe in great detail what is appropriate behavior for a physician. Even though the Current Opinions are quite detailed, they still cannot individually address every potential ethical situation that may arise in the practice of medicine. We must remember that each treatment experience with a patient is unique, and no two situations are exactly the same. Therefore, the Current Opinions are meant to serve as a guide for all physicians in the practice of medicine. A general explanation of some of the Council's Current Opinions is listed in Box 4-1, and a complete listing can be found in the ethics section of the AMA website.

Failure to Abide by Ethical Standards

Because the AMA is an organization of discretionary membership, it may choose who may be a member of the organization and who may not. Members who may have violated ethical standards almost certainly will be subject to review by the AMA. After due notice and a hearing, members in violation of the AMA's standards may be acquitted, warned, censured, suspended, or expelled from the organization's membership. The AMA does not have the power to revoke a physician's license; licensing is the responsibility of each state.

Physicians who are involved as defendants in legal proceedings also may find themselves in a disciplinary hearing with the AMA upon conclusion of the proceedings. A physician may even be acquitted in a civil or criminal proceeding, yet he or she still may face discipline by the AMA. Even though a physician has been acquitted in a legal proceeding, that physician still may lose membership rights in the AMA.

CHECKPOINT

Examine the following examples of conduct, decide whether the conduct is in keeping with the information given about the AMA Principles of Medical Ethics, and state the reason for your answer.

1. Dr. Gonzalez is an obstetrician who is practicing in a large metropolitan area. Dr. Gonzalez has decided that she will not accept any new obstetrics patients in her practice.
2. Dr. Smith is an internist who is practicing in a state that has a law against physician-assisted suicide. Dr. Smith believes that patients should have the right to choose physician-assisted suicide if they are terminally ill, so he helps a patient commit suicide.
3. Dr. Anderson is aware of a physician in her health care facility who often bills Medicare for services that have not been performed. She does not report the physician's activity to the board of directors or to Medicare officials.
4. Dr. Kowalski has developed a new technique for suturing operative wounds. He demonstrates this new technique to colleagues at the AMA's national convention.

Ethical Behavior for Medical Administrative Assistants

The American Association of Medical Assistants (AAMA) Code of Ethics serves as a guide for moral and ethical conduct for individuals employed in the medical assisting profession. These ethical standards have been developed to help medical assistants determine appropriate professional behavior in the health care workplace. Although a widely accepted ethics code is not available specifically for medical administrative assistants, the AAMA's code of ethics can serve as a guide for ethical behavior. The current version of the AAMA Code of Ethics is available on the AAMA website.

The American Academy of Professional Coders (AAPC) has created a Code of Ethics that defines ethical behavior for its members. The Code is available online and all AAPC members are expected to uphold the ethical standards within the code. If an assistant is a member of the AAPC, failure to abide by the Code of Ethics may cause the member to lose credentials from and membership in the AAPC.

BOX 4-1

Summary of Several Current Opinions of the AMA Council on Ethical and Judicial Affairs

- A physician's first concern should be the quality of care for the patient.
- A physician is allowed to participate in legal abortions.
- A physician should report instances of child, spousal, or elder abuse.
- A physician may not participate in a legally authorized execution.
- A physician may participate in research, provided the study has met acceptable standards of scientific research.
- A physician should not disclose genetic testing results to insurance companies. Such information may prevent a patient from obtaining insurance (if the patient is identified as being predisposed to a certain disease) and should be kept apart from the patient's medical record so it could not be accidentally included in a release of medical information.
- In the organ donation process, members of the health care team of the deceased or the donor cannot participate as members of the transplant team. These team members must be free from conflict of interest.
- In the treatment of patients who are terminally ill or seriously debilitated, the best interest of the patient is of utmost importance, not the burden of the patient's condition on family members or society.
- A physician is dedicated to preserving life and easing patients' suffering. When these two are not compatible, the wishes of the patient are of primary importance. Participation in euthanasia conflicts with the position of the physician to "never do harm to anyone" [as identified in the Hippocratic Oath, see Fig. 4-1].
- A physician may advertise his or her medical practice, but such an advertisement should not be deceptive or misleading.
- A physician may not talk to the media about a patient without the consent of the patient. The physician may release only authorized information. Questions about violent acts should be referred to law enforcement authorities.
- A physician shall keep patient information confidential. It may be necessary for the physician to disclose confidential information if in the best interest of society. If a patient threatens to harm himself or herself or another individual or is a threat to society, the physician has a duty to warn the individual who is threatened and the appropriate authorities.
- A physician may treat a minor patient without parental consent unless the law forbids it. The physician should encourage the minor to discuss the nature of medical care with parents.
- A physician may not collect a fee for referring patients to another physician. A physician also may not collect any type of fee or compensation from health care suppliers for prescribing their products.
- A physician should never place his or her own financial interest above a patient's best interest. Financial interest in a company should not influence a physician's decision making.
- A physician should send a patient for consultation when medically necessary or when the patient requests it.
- A physician has a right to choose whether or not to accept an individual as a patient except in cases of emergency. A physician may not refuse to accept patients because of their race, national origin, or religion.
- A physician should not engage in a romantic or sexual relationship with a patient.
- A physician should not practice medicine while under the influence of a substance that could impair the physician's medical judgment.
- A physician should not treat himself or herself or family members except in an emergency situation.
- A physician has a duty to report colleagues who are incompetent or impaired in the practice of medicine or who engage in unethical behavior.
- A physician should report incidents in which he or she believes the use of a drug or device may have been harmful.
- A physician has a duty to provide necessary health care for the poor and unfortunate.
- A physician should share his or her knowledge to advance the practice of medicine. Physicians are allowed to patent medical devices that they develop, but they are not allowed to patent medical procedures.
- A physician with an infectious disease should not put his or her patient at risk of transmission of the disease.

Adapted from American Medical Association. Current Opinions of the Council on Ethical and Judicial Affairs.

Whether or not a code of ethics exists for a particular group of employees, any employee of a health care facility is expected to perform his or her duties in a professional manner and, above all, should always exhibit ethical behavior and must always protect the confidentiality of patient information. Principles of human dignity, confidentiality of medical information, and commitment to continuing education are tantamount for anyone working as a medical administrative assistant.

CHECKPOINT

A medical administrative assistant is confronted daily with situations to which she or he must decide how to respond. The AAMA's Code of Medical Ethics provides a framework for the assistant to use in determining appropriate behavior. Consider the following instances, and determine whether the assistant's behavior is in keeping with the code of ethics.

1. An assistant volunteers to work at a local nonprofit health care organization.
2. An assistant receives additional training to upgrade job skills.
3. An assistant unnecessarily discusses a patient's medical condition with a fellow employee.
4. An assistant discusses an adult patient's medical condition with a family member.

Ethical Issues in Health Care

Ethical dilemmas regarding health care treatment, procedures, and related scientific research are often in the news. One can hardly pick up a newspaper or turn on the television without seeing an item involving medical ethics. Because health care is a multibillion dollar business that touches so many lives, hardly a day goes by without the media informing us of the results of a medical study or of a new medical breakthrough (Fig. 4-2). Technological advances in medicine often provoke society's discussion of proposed limits or boundaries for medical science. Technology has enabled such advances as the ability to further sustain life (e.g., organ transplants, synthetic body components) and create life (e.g., in vitro fertilization, artificial insemination). Such advances serve as the basis of many ethical dilemmas in the health care field because as technology advances, the legal and ethical boundaries that define the practice of medicine must catch up to address those technological changes.

The Study of Ethical Issues in Health Care

When studying medical ethics and when encountering ethical issues in medicine, it is important to remember that no two persons have exactly the same views on what is ethical, or "right," behavior. Although many people would agree that basic behaviors such as cheating, lying, and stealing are wrong, individuals differ in their definitions of the terms.

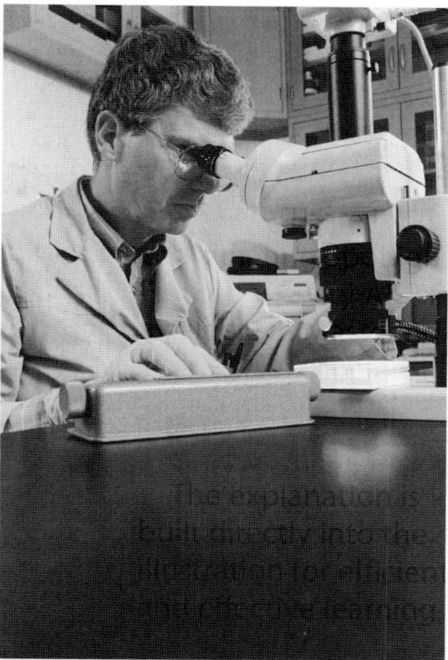

Figure 4-2 Technological advances in health care frequently push the ethical boundaries of medicine.

Consider the following example:

A patient calls the office and asks to speak to the doctor. The doctor has instructed the assistant to take messages for all calls unless the call is a potential emergency. If the assistant replies that the doctor is with a patient, and the doctor is not with a patient, is that a lie? Some people may believe so and reply instead, "I'll need to take your name and number. The doctor or nurse will call you back after your health record has been reviewed." Some people may have no problem saying "The doctor is with a patient," regardless of whether the physician is with a patient. What is considered ethical behavior for one person may not be ethical behavior for another.

A medical administrative assistant is confronted daily with patients who are coping with ethical issues. It is important for an assistant to recognize and understand the ethical issues that patients face and to respect each patient's decision without judging the patient. An assistant must have this understanding in order to continue to provide excellent customer service for patients and to treat all patients with the dignity and respect they deserve. Many issues that patients face are very difficult as well as life changing. Health care situations can be complex and very difficult for patients to face. Patients with serious health problems may have multiple options for treatment that can cause confusion, bewilderment, anger, and frustration. It is not the medical administrative assistant's position to ever counsel the patient; however, an understanding of the many different aspects of complex health care issues can help assistants have empathy for the patients they serve.

What follows is a glimpse into some of the ethical issues in health care today.

Abortion

Abortion is defined in the *Miller-Keane Encyclopedia & Dictionary of Medicine, Nursing, & Allied Health* as the "termination of pregnancy before the fetus is viable." Viable means able to sustain life. Oftentimes, people equate the term abortion with the image of a willful procedure to remove a fetus from the womb. That procedure is known as an induced abortion. However, in a health care setting, the term abortion is used to identify a miscarriage or the natural loss of a fetus, which is known as spontaneous abortion.

The ethical dilemma lies with induced abortion. The U.S. Supreme Court provided for the intentional termination of pregnancy with the 1973 landmark decision in the case of *Roe v. Wade.* In this case, the Supreme Court's ruling essentially declared that many state laws regarding abortion were unconstitutional. The Supreme Court defined the parameters for abortion as follows:

- During the first trimester, the abortion decision is between the mother and her physician.
- During the second trimester, the state may regulate abortion if the regulation is in the interest of the mother's health.
- Once the fetus is viable, the state may regulate or prohibit abortion except when abortion is necessary to protect the mother's health or life.

Although the judicial system provided women with the right to seek an abortion, executive orders issued from the Reagan administration to current day have either placed restrictions on the use of federal funding for abortion counseling or places that provide abortions or have lifted restrictions on the use of such funds. This is a highly politicized issue and will no doubt continue to be in the future.

Abortion is not merely a legal or political problem. Technological advances enable a fetus to survive outside the womb at 26 weeks' gestation or at a weight of just three fourths of a pound. Such a fetus delivered 30 years ago had no chance of survival, but medical miracles are now providing chances for life in such situations. This creates an ethical dilemma because the ability to sustain life has been greatly improved.

The major crux of the ethical dilemma with regard to abortion is the status of the fetus developing in the womb. Pro-life groups argue that a developing fetus has the rights of a person and should be regarded as such from the moment of conception. Pro-choice groups say that a woman has the right to choose what to do with her body. Another part of public opinion lies in the area between pro-life and pro-choice: the belief that the right to abortion should be determined according to the circumstances of the pregnancy, that is, abortion should be allowed in cases of pregnancy due to rape or incest but otherwise should not be allowed.

Although there are legal provisions for abortions, physicians and their employees cannot be forced to participate in abortions if they do not wish to participate.

Many people may think that the abortion issue has come to the forefront because advances in medical technology have made abortion possible. In actuality, the history of abortion reveals that abortion was a means of birth control in ancient times. Even in the early 1800s, there were no laws against abortion in the United States. In 1821, Connecticut passed the first law against abortion. By 1900, almost every state had laws against abortion. From the first part of the 1900s until the *Roe v. Wade* decision in 1973, women obtained illegal abortions. Thus, whether or not abortion was legal, women continued to have abortions.

The issue of abortion therefore is not new but is certainly controversial. It is important for medical administrative assistants to remember that it is not the assistant's place to judge. Instead, it is the assistant's place (1) to understand the law as it applies to abortion, (2) to understand the ethical viewpoints that may influence a patient's decision to seek or not seek abortion, and (3) to understand that the choice of abortion is the patient's decision to make.

CHECKPOINT

Consider the following case, and determine the appropriate action that you as a medical administrative assistant should take:

Sue Adams, an unmarried pregnant patient of the office, cannot decide whether she should have an abortion. Sue asks Dr. Johnson what she thinks should be done. How would Dr. Johnson reply?

Reproductive Rights

Reproductive capabilities have been greatly influenced by advances in medical technology. Such topics as artificial insemination, in vitro fertilization, amniocentesis, and surrogacy often spark debate as to what lengths women and men should be allowed to go to have a child.

Artificial Insemination

Artificial insemination involves injecting either the husband's sperm or donated sperm into a woman's vagina, cervical canal, or uterus in the hope that this process will result in a pregnancy that otherwise would not be possible.

Many questions arise with this reproductive issue. Should any woman be allowed to have a child using artificial insemination? Some people may argue that the possibility of pregnancy should be left to a higher being and disagree with any interference from medicine. Others may want to put "conditions" on the procedure. They may want only women who are married to be eligible to receive insemination.

How well are donors screened and their identity protected? Donors may expect to have a health screening including laboratory testing to determine if they have any medical conditions that may exclude them from being a donor. Donors can expect that their identity will not be shared with any offspring; however, a few clinics are in operation that actually discloses the identity of the sperm donor to the recipient. Should a sperm clinic set a maximum number of successful pregnancies with each donor? Many clinics do set a maximum number of times a donor is used for successful pregnancies. Imagine the problems that could occur if unlimited donation were allowed. One male donor might technically father hundreds of children within a small geographic area.

Amniocentesis

Amniocentesis is a surgical procedure in which a needle is inserted into the amniotic sac and a sample of amniotic fluid is withdrawn. Tests can be conducted on that fluid to determine whether the developing fetus has certain abnormalities, such as Down syndrome. This type of testing is routinely performed in pregnant women 35 years and older. Amniocentesis can also reveal the sex of the fetus. Should amniocentesis be required of all pregnant women 35 years and older? Do the benefits of this procedure outweigh the risks associated with it? If a woman undergoes amniocentesis or any other type of testing during pregnancy and the testing reveals what doctors believe to be a serious abnormality, should the woman be forced to abort or deliver the fetus prematurely? So far, courts generally have held that a woman of sound mind cannot be forced to undergo medical treatment against her will.

In Vitro Fertilization

In vitro fertilization involves fertilizing an ovum in a test tube or Petri dish. The fertilized embryo then is implanted in the woman's uterus in the hope that the process will result in a full-term pregnancy.

It has been many years since the first test tube pregnancy occurred (Box 4-2), and in vitro fertilization is now commonplace in treating infertility. Yet ethical issues related to this method still arise. Should a woman be implanted with more than one embryo at a time to ensure a successful pregnancy? What if five embryos are implanted and all are successful? Should selective abortion (one or more embryos are removed) be used to eliminate some of the successful embryos to give the others a better chance at survival? What happens to frozen embryos that are no longer wanted or needed?

BOX 4-2

The First Test Tube Baby?

In vitro experimentation began in the 1930s but with no success. In the early 1970s, a physician at Columbia-Presbyterian Medical Center, Dr. Landrum Shettles, was beginning to get close to the key to successful in vitro fertilization. In 1973, a Florida couple, John and Doris Del-Zio, agreed to take part in a clandestine experiment that Dr. Shettles was conducting. An egg was removed from Mrs. Del-Zio at a New York hospital; it was placed in a test tube and was carried by her husband to Columbia-Presbyterian. Once at Columbia, the egg was fertilized with John Del-Zio's sperm and was placed in a test tube in a lab incubator. An administrator, Dr. Raymond Vande Wiele, learned of the experiment and angrily seized the test tube and opened the sealed tube, thereby destroying the embryo. The Del-Zios brought suit against Columbia Presbyterian for $1.5 million. Ironically, in 1978, the Del-Zios won their suit for $50,000 shortly after the world's first test tube baby, Louise Brown, was born in England.

(For further information, see the video *American Experience: Test Tube Babies*, produced and directed by Chana Gazit and Hilary Klotz Steinman, WGBH Educational Foundation, 2006. This video was based in part on a book called *Pandora's Baby* by Robin Marantz Henig.)

Surrogate Motherhood

Many couples around the world today are infertile. Some of these couples for one reason or another choose not to adopt a child. With the advent of in vitro fertilization came the possibility that one woman could carry another woman's child. Such a possibility is called surrogacy. A woman can serve as a surrogate mother in one of two ways.

1. A husband and wife unable to have children because of the wife's infertility may ask another woman (a surrogate) to be artificially inseminated with the husband's sperm. The child then is half biologically related to the couple. On delivery of the infant, the surrogate gives the infant to the couple.
2. A woman who is unable to conceive or carry a child to term because of a uterine abnormality first may have her egg fertilized with her husband's sperm by means of the process of in vitro fertilization and then may have the fertilized embryo implanted in a surrogate. The fetus is in no way biologically related to the surrogate in this case. On delivery of the infant, the infant is given to the biologic parents.

Although no one can buy or sell another human being in the United States, a fee usually is given to the surrogate in exchange for expenses and for providing a service. Should a woman be allowed to "rent" her uterus for a pregnancy? How are surrogate mothers screened? What happens if the surrogate decides she cannot give up the baby once it is delivered? The courts have seen many cases related to the question of custody of a surrogate child.

It is plain to see that many questions arise regarding reproductive issues in medicine. Many patients will go to great lengths to conceive a child or to become parents. When serving patients in the medical office, assistants should be mindful of the emotional struggles that patients endure with regard to reproductive issues. Many questions frequently weigh heavily on the minds of both patients and their providers as they face these ethical dilemmas. In most instances, there is no "right" answer to many of these questions.

Issues Near the End of Life

Just as the question "When does life begin?" can create an ethical dilemma, so can the question "When does life end?" Does life end when the brain function ceases, or does it end when the heart stops beating?

The Patient Self-Determination Act of 1992 made it necessary for every patient to be asked on admission to a hospital or nursing facility whether he or she has an advance directive and, if not, whether he or she wants to have one. As mentioned in Chapter 3, an advance directive is a legal document that allows a patient's wishes for medical treatment to be known in the event that the patient cannot speak for himself or herself.

In a way, an advance directive allows a patient to communicate what he or she feels is a "quality of life." For example, when a patient states that he does not wish to have tube feeding, he is communicating that if he should be ill and would require tube feeding in order to survive, then—*for him*—it would not be worth surviving.

Sometimes, when faced with the end of life, a patient's choice may be to end his or her life. This choice, known as **euthanasia**, may be either passive or active. Active euthanasia involves actually taking an action that will cause someone's death. According to *Miller-Keane Encyclopedia & Dictionary of Medicine, Nursing & Allied Health,* 6th edition, passive euthanasia now is more commonly defined as foregoing life-sustaining treatment.

Assisted suicide is different from active euthanasia in that assisted suicide involves one individual helping another individual to commit suicide. The first individual does not actually inject a lethal dose or place a mask over the other's face but gives instructions to the individual on how to accomplish the intended task. In the late 20th century, many cases of assisted suicide made headlines in the United States. Generally, courts have held that it is unlawful to assist an individual in committing suicide, although two states—Washington and Oregon—have given legislative support for assisted suicide.

CHECKPOINT

Is the act of euthanasia consistent with the Hippocratic Oath? Why?

AIDS, HIV

One of the leading health care headlines in the last part of the 20th century involved the proliferation of the human immunodeficiency virus (HIV), which can lead to acquired immunodeficiency syndrome (AIDS).

Because an HIV infection has such serious social implications for those infected, health care facilities must take special precautions to safeguard the privacy of patients with HIV. When an HIV blood test is done, a patient should be asked to sign a specific HIV testing consent form to indicate that he or she is giving informed consent to have the test. Patients should be counseled as to the implications of negative and positive results of the test and must be made aware of the mandatory requirement to report a positive result.

The social stigma faced by patients with HIV and AIDS is significant. Some individuals choose to label HIV-positive patients and may think that how the patient contracted the disease is important. There is not a "good" or "bad" way to contract the disease, just as there are no "good" or "bad" patients with HIV. How a patient contracted the disease is irrelevant and does not change the fact that he or she has the disease. A positive diagnosis of HIV is devastating to a patient. Patients fear the loss of their jobs, their loved ones, and their life.

Ethical standards in health care demand that we treat all patients with compassion and that we do not discriminate because of a patient's circumstances. Serving a patient with HIV is no different from serving any other patient.

SUMMARY

During a typical workday, a medical administrative assistant deals with office situations that may involve a medical ethical issue. All members of the health care staff must exhibit ethical conduct at all times. Such conduct is expected in all situations and with all issues that may arise in a health care setting.

When faced with a medical decision, patients bring with them their own unique set of experiences and circumstances that have an impact on the decisions they make. Whatever a patient may decide with regard to his or her health care treatment, it is of the utmost importance for every health care professional to remember that, ultimately, the patient must decide for himself or herself what the treatment will be. After all, it is the patient who must live (or possibly die) with the decision.

YOU ARE THE MEDICAL ADMINISTRATIVE ASSISTANT

Picture yourself as a medical administrative assistant in a medical practice. What would you do in the following situations?

1. Julie Smith, a 16-year-old patient, has been a regular patient for years at your clinic. Her family members are regular patients of your clinic, as well. Julie is very tearful today and approaches you at the reception desk. She confides in you that she is pregnant and does not know what to do. She asks you for the name and number of the local abortion clinic in your city. (You know the name and number of the abortion clinic.) What do you do?
2. You just finished filing laboratory reports in patients' records. Among the reports was a pregnancy test for your best friend who has long hoped for a child. The results are positive. The nurse has notified your best friend of the results. You are having dinner with your friend this evening. What do you say?

REVIEW EXERCISES

Exercise 4-1 True or False

Read the following statements and determine whether the statements are true or false. Record the answer in the blank provided. T = true; F = false.

_______1. The Hippocratic Oath is a legal doctrine that must be adhered to by all physicians.

_______2. When a professional organization has a code of ethics, it is easy to determine whether a particular behavior is ethical or unethical.

_______3. The Hippocratic Oath still influences medicine today.

_______4. The Hippocratic Oath supports physician-assisted suicide.

_______5. The Hippocratic Oath supports abortion.

_______6. In the United States, abortion had not been legal until 1973.

_______7. A miscarriage is also known as an induced abortion.

_______8. An organization's code of ethics serves as a guideline for professional behavior.

_______9. The AMA establishes law that governs the practice of medicine.

_______10. The AMA may conduct a disciplinary hearing regarding a member's conduct even if the member is acquitted in a legal proceeding.

_______11. An understanding of medical ethical issues can help a medical administrative assistant have empathy for patients.

_______12. Abortion is defined as "termination of a viable pregnancy".

_______13. Executive orders can affect abortion counseling.

_______14. A physician must perform an abortion if a patient requests it.

_______15. Active euthanasia can be defined as "doing something that will cause a person's death".

Exercise 4-2 Ethical Conduct of Medical Administrative Assistants

Read each of the following examples involving medical administrative assistant conduct. Using the AAMA code of ethics (located at the AAMA's website) as a guide for ethical conduct, determine whether the conduct is ethical or unethical. Record the answer in the blank provided. E = ethical; U = unethical.

_______1. Shredding copies of a patient's insurance form that are not needed

_______2. Postponing handling records requests for patients who have not paid their bill until all other requests have been handled

_______3. Volunteering at a blood drive in the community

_______4. After seeing test results, informing a friend of another friend's serious illness

_______5. Sending medical records to a patient's employer without the patient's consent

_______6. Conversing with a patient regarding his medical condition within earshot of a lobby full of patients

_______7. Attending a regional conference for medical office personnel

Exercise 4-3 Ethical Conduct of Physicians

After completing Activity 4-1, read each of the following examples involving physician conduct. Using the information given in the AMA Principles of Medical Ethics and the Current Opinions of the CEJA (located at the AMA's website) as a guide for ethical conduct, determine whether the physician conduct listed below is ethical or unethical. Record the answer in the blank provided. E = ethical; U = unethical.

_______1. Physician grows and smokes marijuana for medicinal purposes.

_______2. Physician bills for services not rendered.

_______3. Physician refers a patient to a specialist when needed.

_______4. Physician refuses to speak to the press about a famous patient because the patient has not authorized release of information.

_______5. Physician donates services to a local homeless shelter.

_______6. A physician who specializes in obstetrics and gynecology decides to stop taking obstetrics patients so that she can concentrate her practice in gynecologic pathology.

_______7. Physician has a personal problem with alcohol abuse.

_______8. Physician fails to report suspected abuse to law enforcement authorities.

_______9. Physician works with legislators to encourage new laws governing patients' rights.

_______10. Physician suggests a pharmacy to a patient by name because the physician has part ownership of the pharmacy.

_______11. Physician accepts educational medical literature and a scale anatomic model (of nominal value) from a pharmaceutical company for use with patients in the clinic.

_______12. Physician advertises her family practice clinic in a local newspaper. Information about location and hours is provided in the advertisement.

_______13. Physician performs a legal abortion.

_______14. Physician refuses care for an emergency patient.

_______15. Physician sends a report to the Department of Transportation regarding an elderly patient who is physically unfit to drive.

_______16. Physicians may charge for a missed appointment if the patient has previously been notified that such a charge may be made.

_______17. A physician has a duty to provide critical health care to patient who cannot afford it.

_______18. A physician has a duty to notify a patient if the patient is HIV-positive.

_______19. Medical records of a retiring physician should be destroyed to protect patient confidentiality.

_______ 20. Physicians may work with chiropractors and optometrists as long as those professionals are appropriately qualified.

ACTIVITIES

ACTIVITY 4-1 CURRENT OPINIONS OF THE COUNCIL ON ETHICAL AND JUDICIAL AFFAIRS

Review and discuss the information found in sections 2 through 9 of the AMA's Current Opinions of the CEJA. The Current Opinions can be found on the AMA's website at www.ama-assn.org. Use this information to complete Exercise 4-3.

ACTIVITY 4-2 ETHICAL ISSUES

Research a medical ethical issue and identify why the issue is an ethical one by identifying the various viewpoints pertaining to the topic. Report the findings in a paper or presentation.

ACTIVITY 4-3 ETHICAL CODES

Several other ethical codes for medicine have been written throughout history. Research a medical ethical code that is not presented in this chapter, and write an essay comparing the code with the traditional Hippocratic Oath.

- Hippocratic Oath, Modern Version— written by Louis Lasagna in 1964.
- Declaration of Geneva
- Declaration of Helsinki
- Oath and Prayer of Maimonides
- Nuremberg Code

ACTIVITY 4-4 ABORTION HISTORY AND LAWS

Research the history of abortion and abortion laws in the United States.

ACTIVITY 4-5 MEDICINE IN THE MOVIES

Several films have been made regarding ethical issues in medicine. View one or more of the following films and write your reaction regarding the movie's portrayal of the ethical issue. The paper should be one to two pages long and should contain a short summary of the medical ethical issue and your reaction to the portrayal.

- *Philadelphia* (Tom Hanks)
- *One Flew Over the Cuckoo's Nest* (Jack Nicholson)
- *One True Thing* (Meryl Streep, William Hurt, Renee Zellweger)

ACTIVITY 4-6 MEDICAL OFFICE SCENARIOS

Role-play the following situations. What is the appropriate response to the situation given?

1. You are working in the medical records room at a medical office. A patient who was in today had a pregnancy test result that was positive. A nurse returns the patient's chart and comments, "The last thing she needs is another baby." How do you respond?
2. An acquaintance of one of your coworkers is pregnant and is a patient at the clinic. Your coworker knows that the acquaintance was in for an ultrasound scan because of the possibility of a twin pregnancy. Your coworker talks about going to get the scan results because she is so excited for the patient and can "hardly wait to find out the results." How do you respond?

DISCUSSION

The following topic can be used for class discussion or for individual student essay.

DISCUSSION 4-1

Why is it important for a medical administrative assistant to have an understanding of medical ethical issues? What might be different if an assistant did not study these issues?

Bibliography

American Experience: Test Tube Babies, produced and directed by Chana Gazit and Hilary Klotz Steinman, WGBH Educational Foundation, 2006.

Brent NJ: *Nurses and the Law: A Guide to Principles and Applications*, Philadelphia, 1997, WB Saunders.

Huffman EK: *Health Information Management*, Berwyn, IL, 1994, Physician's Record.

Lewis MA, Tamparo CD: *Medical Law, Ethics and Bioethics for Ambulatory Care*, Philadelphia, 1998, FA Davis.

O'Toole M: *Miller-Keane Encyclopedia & Dictionary of Medicine, Nursing, & Allied Health*, ed 6, Philadelphia, 1997, WB Saunders.

Purtillo R: *Ethical Dimensions in the Health Professions*, Philadelphia, 2005, Elsevier.

Stein R, Shear M: "Funding Restored to Groups that Perform Abortions, Other Care." *The Washington Post*, January 24, 2009.

CHAPTER 5 The Diverse Community of Patients

LEARNING OUTCOMES

On successful completion of this chapter, the student will be able to

1. Identify cultural considerations when interacting with patients.
2. Reduce language barriers.
3. Describe appropriate interactions with various types of patients.
4. Add special information about a patient to a patient's record in a medical practice management system.

COMMISSION ON ACCREDITATION OF ALLIED HEALTH EDUCATION PROGRAMS (CAAHEP) CORE CURRICULUM FOR MEDICAL ASSISTANTS

- Recognize communication barriers.
- Identify techniques for overcoming communication barriers.
- Discuss the roles of cultural, social, and ethnic diversity in ethical performance of medical assisting practice.
- Identify resources and adaptation that are required based on individual needs (e.g., culture and environment, developmental life stage, language, and physical threats to communication).

ACCREDITING BUREAU OF HEALTH EDUCATION SCHOOLS (ABHES) COMPETENCIES FOR MEDICAL ASSISTING

Graduates

- Are attentive, listen, and learn.
- Are impartial and show empathy when dealing with patients.
- Serve as liaison between physician and others.
- Use pertinent medical terminology.
- Adapt to individualized needs.

VOCABULARY

caring response
culture
culture care diversity and universality
five stages of loss

With an increasingly mobile society, many cultural differences are present throughout the United States today. A medical administrative assistant must recognize cultural differences and should have the utmost respect for all types of patients treated in the medical office and should be prepared to handle all sorts of situations. An assistant must respect each patient who comes to the practice, regardless of religion, sex, ethnic background, and other differences related to a person's lifestyle or beliefs.

This chapter focuses on those differences and how those differences affect interaction with employees of the medical office. The intention of this chapter is to expose you to some of these common cultural differences before you are introduced to the basics of communication in the next chapter. An understanding of these behavioral influences will help you communicate better with patients.

People believe and value various things. It is expected that we will not discriminate against persons who are different from us. Not only is discrimination unjust—in many instances, such as in granting credit, it is unlawful to discriminate against another individual. Human rights issues have been debated throughout history and will continue to be debated, but the staff of a medical office—regardless of what laws might be in place—should provide patients with care and service free of bias or prejudice.

Influence of Culture

What is **culture**? It is those beliefs, behaviors, and attitudes that are shared by a particular group of people and passed from one generation to the next. Culture is learned from various events and from the social environment that a patient experiences.

A patient's nationality will greatly influence his or her cultural beliefs. For example, there is varying opinion around the world today about the status of women in society. Some nationalities believe that women should be treated as equal to men. Other nationalities believe that women should not have as many rights as men do or believe that they should have very few rights at all. Women's rights are often outlined within a country's legal system. A legal system sometimes is influenced by a nation's predominant religious beliefs. In some countries, women have the same legal rights as a man, and in other countries, women may not be allowed to own property or may not be allowed to vote.

The extent of a patient's religious upbringing will also affect the patient's beliefs and attitudes regarding health care. Some religions have strong convictions about procedures such as abortion or blood transfusion. Depending on the depth of a patient's religious convictions, those beliefs can have a significant effect on his or her utilization of health care services.

Interactions With Patients of Different Cultures

Madeline M. Leininger conceived a nursing theory known as **culture care diversity and universality**. Its basic philosophy is that a patient's culture should be considered when one provides nursing services to a patient. The reasoning behind the theory is that the care a nurse provides should be consistent with a patient's cultural beliefs.

This theory is important for other staff members in the office as well. In order to provide the best service to patients, assistants who work in the medical office should be well aware that patients hold a number of different beliefs regarding what is appropriate medical care. This knowledge will help an assistant to be aware of the needs and desires of patients and will help prevent the assistant from making mistakes when communicating with patients. Awareness of differing cultural beliefs is necessary to avoid insulting or offending patients. Saying or doing the wrong thing could adversely affect a patient's relationship with the clinic staff.

A fundamental part of this discussion is that an assistant must understand that no culture is the "correct" culture and must recognize and respect cultures that are different from his or her own. To avoid the tendency to stereotype people belonging to a particular culture, this chapter does not attempt to categorize people by identifying a particular behavior with a culture but merely points out different beliefs regarding health care treatment. Some behaviors often may be associated with a particular group, but that does not mean that all people within the group will exhibit that behavior.

When a medical administrative assistant serves a patient, the assistant should begin the encounter without a predetermined set of cultural expectations of patient behavior. This may be difficult because each of us has our own perceptions and beliefs of what the health care experience should be. To provide the best possible health care experience for the patient, we should, first and foremost, serve each patient with the same respect and dignity. Failure to do so is likely to result in a poor health care experience for the patient.

Imagine the following situation: A female patient comes in with a male relative. Often persons from that patient's particular country require that a male accompany a female for a health care visit. However, the assistant should not assume that because of this cultural influence, the patient will behave in this particular manner. All individuals of one culture do not behave uniformly, although some beliefs are commonly shared by many individuals within a cultural group. Although some behaviors are widespread throughout a culture, persons of that culture do not hold a uniform set of values or beliefs. For the most part, the assistant should be aware that the behavior of a patient is likely a result of his or her own cultural influences.

A person's culture influences beliefs about the use of health care services and medicine in general. Following is a list of common patient beliefs and behaviors associated with health care treatment:

- Reluctance to have surgery or other medical procedures
- Refusal to have blood drawn or transfused
- Strong belief in use of home or natural remedies
- Aversion to taking medication
- Elders as decision makers of the family
- Support for use of alternative treatments such as herbs or acupuncture
- Refusal to allow any touching by a stranger
- Frequent use of touch in interactions
- Considering eye contact to be disrespectful
- Considering eye contact to be respectful
- Men given preferential treatment
- Condition of a terminal illness not shared with the patient
- Certain types of food not eaten
- Sexual inequality as the norm
- Use of alcohol or tobacco strongly discouraged

As you can see from this list, there is a wide range of beliefs regarding health care treatment. You must be ready for any and all of the situations that could arise when you are interacting with patients.

Expectations When Serving Patients

In dealing with patients in general, it is important to remember that many of the patients who come through the clinic doors do so because they are sick. Most of the time, illness can cause patients to behave differently than they normally would. Regardless of whether they have special cultural considerations or other concerns, sick patients may not respond to questions or instructions as otherwise healthy individuals would.

Often, patients experience physical discomfort or emotional distress because of illness. Illness often is accompanied by pain, altered bodily function, varied patterns of sleeping/eating, and general anxiety about the prospect of recovery. The stress of illness can cause patients to be quick to react or respond in a negative way. They may be short and unfriendly in their responses, and an assistant should remember not to take it personally.

Because of illness, a patient may not be able to remember directions to an appointment in a particular department or may forget instructions. It may be necessary for an assistant to repeat something several times, write it down, or escort the patient to a different location in the clinic.

An assistant may never know what problems a patient may be dealing with, but it is important to be caring and compassionate even in the most difficult situations. Even the caregivers of patients, such as adults who care for elderly parents or parents of ill children, may behave differently because of the stress related to a patient's illness.

Perhaps one of the most helpful things that you, as an assistant, should remember to do when dealing with people is to consider how you would like to be treated if you were in the patient's situation. If the patient is a loved one, how would you expect that patient to be treated?

In the text *Ethical Dimensions in the Health Professions*, the author mentions the importance of developing a **caring response**. An essential component of the caring response is the realization that the focus of all patient care is the patient. Because we have an obligation to provide high-quality services to each and every patient, it is absolutely imperative that we treat each and every patient with the same kindness, respect, and compassion. As we learned in Chapters 3 and 4, many health care situations can become problematic, but when services provided are patient focused and respectful, those services will be appropriate. Remember the words of the Mayo Clinic founders: "The best interest of the patient is the only interest to be considered." This statement should lay the groundwork for everything we do in a medical office.

Language Barriers

Our country is becoming more and more diverse every day. This diversity usually brings language differences with it. A language barrier exists if two people (e.g., a patient and an assistant) cannot communicate effectively by using a common language.

In a health care environment, language barriers create an interesting challenge. In 2001, 20% (over 55 million) of the U.S. population (all persons 5 years or older) spoke a language other than English in their home. Of those people, many can speak English, but approximately one-fourth of that 20% (or 5% of the total U.S. population) speak English poorly or cannot speak English at all (Fig. 5-1).

Language barriers can mean legal difficulties for health care providers. Because hospitals receive federal funding, they are required to make sure that patients are not discriminated against with respect to race, color, or national origin.

In 1980, a landmark case involving language barrier unfolded in Florida. An 18-year-old teenager, Willie Ramirez, went to an emergency department with a complaint of dizziness and severe headache. He and his family stated that he was *intoxicado,* which in Spanish means "nausea" or "dizziness." Medical personnel listed his initial diagnosis as a drug overdose. The patient's headache was instead related to a brain hemorrhage, and Mr. Ramirez became a quadriplegic due to the hemorrhage. A $71 million award was given to the patient for his injuries.

The Ramirez case is a tragic one, and one that possibly could have been prevented had the hospital had an interpreter available. If a patient presents with a language barrier, it will take extra effort on the part of the entire medical staff to ensure that the patient's needs are met.

English as a Second Language

According to the U.S. Census Bureau data identified in Figure 5-1, some individuals may speak another language at home, but they may also speak English well or very well. If a patient's English is difficult to understand, an attempt should be made to obtain an interpreter.

Characteristic	Total people	English-speaking ability			
		Very well	Well	Not well	Not at all
NUMBER	**280,950,438**	**(X)**	**(X)**	**(X)**	**(X)**
Population 5 years and older	225,505,953	(X)	(X)	(X)	(X)
Spoke only English at home	55,444,485	30,975,474	10,962,722	9,011,298	4,494,991
Spoke a language other than English at home					
Spoke a language other than English at home	**55,444,485**	**30,975,474**	**10,962,722**	**9,011,298**	**4,494,991**
Spanish or Spanish Creole	34,547,077	18,179,530	6,322,170	6,344,110	3,701,267
Other Indo-European languages	10,320,730	6,936,808	2,018,148	1,072,025	293,749
Asian and Pacific Island languages	8,316,426	4,274,794	2,176,180	1,412,264	453,188
Other languages	2,260,252	1,584,342	446,224	182,899	46,787
PERCENT	**100.0**	**(X)**	**(X)**	**(X)**	**(X)**
Population 5 years and older	80.3	(X)	(X)	(X)	(X)
Spoke only English at home	19.7	55.9	19.8	16.3	8.1
Spoke a language other than English at home					
Spoke a language other than English at home	**100.0**	**55.9**	**19.8**	**16.3**	**8.1**
Spanish or Spanish Creole	62.3	52.6	18.3	18.4	10.7
Other Indo-European languages	18.6	67.2	19.6	10.4	2.8
Asian and Pacific Island languages	15.0	51.4	26.2	17.0	5.4
Other languages	4.1	70.1	19.7	8.1	2.1

(X) Not applicable.

Note: Margins of error for all estimates can be found in Appendix Table 1 at <www.census.gov/population/www/socdemo/language/appendix.html>. For more information on the ACS, see <www.census.gov/acs/www/>.

Figure 5-1 Twenty percent of the U.S. population spoke a language other than English in their home. (From U.S. Census Bureau, 2007 American Community Survey.)

Sometimes a family member may serve as an interpreter for a patient who has limited English skills. There are problems that can occur with family members as interpreters. The family member may downplay the patient's complaints. The family member may not relay the patient's response exactly as given to the medical staff. Professional medical interpreters are preferred because they are trained to interpret without bias. Interpreters are employed by large medical facilities such as the Mayo Clinic in Rochester, Minnesota, which draws patients from all over the world. If a professional medical interpreter is not available at a facility, a general interpreter may be able to translate. A drawback to using a general interpreter is that the interpreter may have limited knowledge of medical terminology or procedures.

In geographic areas in which many English as a second language (ESL) patients are served, medical offices may employ bilingual health care workers to reduce the language barriers between patients and medical office staff. Figure 5-2 illustrates the concentrations of ESL populations across the United States.

Speech Difficulty

On some occasions, a patient may know English but may have difficulty speaking. An accident or a disease, such as stroke or cancer, could impair or destroy a patient's ability to speak. In this case, the patient may be able to write his or her requests. Paper and pen may be all that is needed for the patient to communicate his or her needs.

If the patient is unable to write, he or she may be able to respond to yes or no questions. If the medical administrative assistant asks a question that could be answered yes or no, the patient may be able to nod or shake the head appropriately. For instance, instead of, "When would you like your next appointment?" try saying, "Would Monday work for your recheck appointment?" and "Would you be able to come in the afternoon?"

Medical Terminology

Not everyone speaks the language of the medical office fluently. An assistant should expect that most patients in the office do not have a command of medical terminology. A medical administrative assistant should avoid creating a language barrier with a patient by using medical terminology inappropriately. An assistant should not use technical medical terms in a conversation unless the patient has used them first. For example, a patient may understand *bladder infection* but not *urinary tract infection* or understand *sore throat* but not *pharyngitis*. An assistant should take conversational cues from

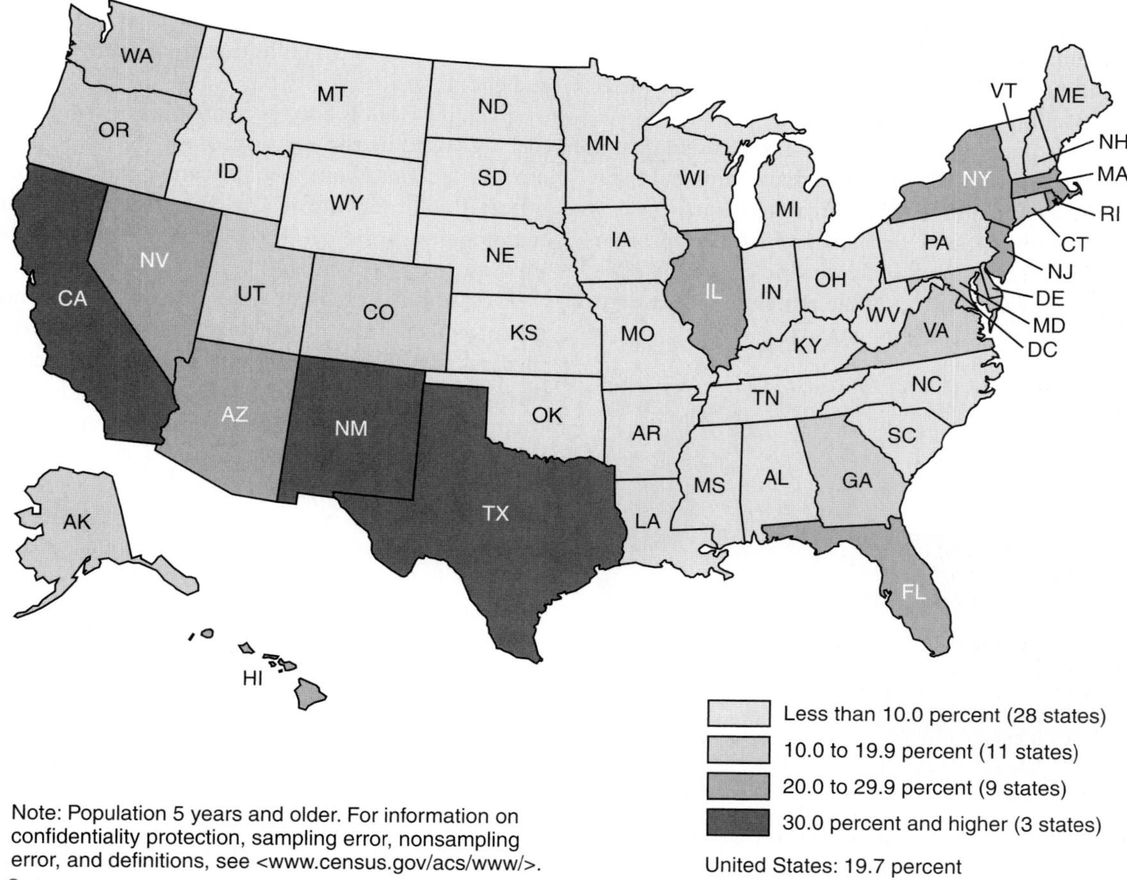

Figure 5-2 Concentrations of ESL populations across the United States. (From U.S. Census Bureau, 2007 American Community Survey.)

patients and interact with patients to their level of understanding. If a patient uses particular technical terms, it is likely that the patient has a good understanding of those terms. Obviously, if the patient is a physician or other health care professional, then it is perfectly appropriate to use medical terminology within your conversations with this patient. Otherwise, keep the conversation uncomplicated until the patient demonstrates comfort with more complex medical terms.

Specific Patient Groups

Elderly Patients

Elderly patients are frequent users of health care services and have special concerns that must be considered. These patients are served in almost every medical specialty, and an assistant must be alert to the needs of patients in this group.

The definition of a frail elderly patient, as given by the *Miller-Keane Encyclopedia & Dictionary of Medicine, Nursing, & Allied Health,* is an individual 65 years or older who has a functional impairment or any individual 75 years or older.

Several things should be considered when communicating with an elderly patient:

- Talk directly to the patient whenever possible (Fig. 5-3). Sometimes, a family member who accompanies the patient may have the habit of speaking for the patient when the patient is perfectly able to communicate. Sometimes, members of the patient's family may even take over the conversation when the patient is talking. An assistant should not talk to family members as though the patient were not there. The patient should remain the main focus of the conversation.
- Be sure that the patient understands all information given. Some patients may have disorders that have impaired their ability to understand and make medical decisions.
- Sometimes elderly patients develop problems with brain function. Dementias cause a patient's thinking to be confused. The patient may have trouble remembering certain things, events, and instructions given by the office staff. Written instructions may have to be given to the patient, and, in some cases, it may be necessary to communicate the instructions to a family member.
- Remember that the patient is an adult and should be treated as one.
- An elderly patient may be hard of hearing. Do not assume that a patient is hard of hearing unless you know this is so. Be careful to avoid shouting at a patient. Remember, conversations within the public areas of the clinic should be kept confidential.
- Elderly patients often suffer from visual impairment. Be certain that a patient understands written instructions that may have been given. A patient may not be able to identify locations within a health care facility and may need assistance in finding a certain location for an appointment.

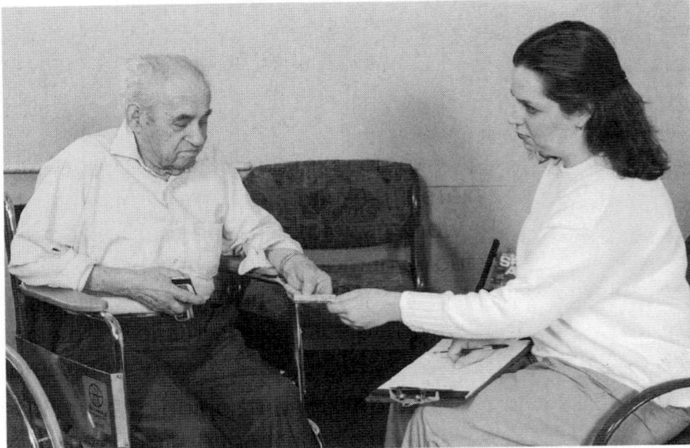

Figure 5-3 Why is it important that whenever possible, the assistant should talk directly to an elderly patient? (From Bonewit-West, K, et al. *Today's Medical Assistant.* 2nd ed. St Louis, Saunders Elsevier, 2013.)

Children

Children are frequent visitors to clinics, as patients or accompanying adults. Children may sometimes need special attention from the office staff. They may or may not be comfortable with the clinic surroundings. They may exhibit apprehension caused by previous visits; maybe they received an immunization on their last visit or experienced a painful procedure. If they are in the clinic as visitors, they may be concerned over a parent who is ill. If possible, an assistant should try to include children in conversations. Welcome them to the clinic, and leave them with a friendly impression of the office staff. If a child speaks first, continue the conversation. A pleasant conversation will assure a child that the health care staff is there to help.

Even if a child is not a patient, it is important to help them feel welcome in the medical office. Children may develop anxious feelings about medical care if the atmosphere of the office is cold and unfriendly. Every department from dermatology to cardiology should be prepared to have children present.

Occasionally, children must be left in the lobby while a parent is seeing the physician. Although it is certainly not a medical administrative assistant's job to provide daycare services, it may be necessary to supervise children and ensure their safety while a parent is receiving medical treatment. Although most offices would prefer that children are not left alone in the lobby, an assistant may have to be aware of children who have been left in the lobby while the parent is seeing the physician. Sometimes the nature of the patient's visit precludes children from being present in an examination room. Children could become apprehensive if a patient is undergoing a painful procedure or having medical care on a private part of the body.

To keep children occupied while in the clinic, activities such as storybooks, toys, videos, and coloring books can be kept in the lobby and in examination rooms. Toys should be safe for children of all ages and should be sanitized routinely by the office staff to reduce the spread of infection. If a television is present, the staff should be sure that the programming is suitable for children.

Patients With Disabilities

Patients with physical or mental disabilities may require special attention. It is important to remember to talk directly to the patient. Do not ignore the patient and talk to family members unless it is apparent that the patient is unable to communicate.

Patients who have been injured in an accident may struggle with the operation of a wheelchair and may require the assistant's aid. If appropriate, assistance should be offered to the patient (Fig. 5-4). Many patients are capable of moving around on their own, but if a patient in any situation seems to be having difficulty, an assistant may offer assistance by saying something such as "Could I offer any assistance, sir?" Then, wait for a response before proceeding. The patient may not need or desire any assistance.

CHECKPOINT

A physician who specializes in family practice often sees patients who bring their young children to the office. Explain when, how, and why the office staff might be expected to assist with children in the office.

Angry Patients

Angry patients may appear in the clinic occasionally. It is important to realize that their anger may or may not be directed toward the staff. Their anger may have been triggered earlier, and an assistant then could become the recipient of the anger. Some medical conditions, such as psychiatric disorders and illnesses or injuries involving brain function, can contribute to a patient's angry or aggressive behavior. Even healthy persons who are under a great deal of stress may become angry. Illness itself can produce a great deal of stress. Patients may be angry for a myriad of reasons, most of which an assistant may never be aware.

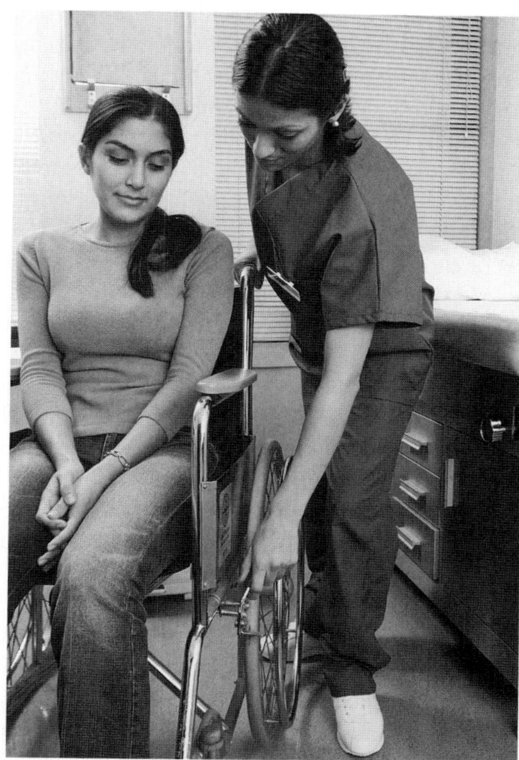

Figure 5-4 Assistance should be offered to patients who may have difficulty moving around the office. (From Young AP. *The Administrative Medical Assistant: An Applied Approach.* 7th ed. St Louis, Elsevier, 2011.)

Defusing an Angry Patient

Regardless of the reason for the patient's anger, do not avoid the anger. The anger probably will not go away by itself. Listen intently to the patient's concerns. Take notes if necessary. If the patient's concerns are not forthcoming, ask the patient what his or her concerns are. Ask the patient what he or she would like to have done about the situation. If you ask, "What can I do to help you?" people can be surprisingly reasonable and probably will not "ask for the moon." If a patient does ask for something you cannot do, he or she should be referred to your supervisor. You should offer to help the patient as much as possible without exceeding your authority in the office.

When speaking with an angry patient, remember to remain calm. Speak softly and directly to the patient. Never, ever raise your voice to a patient. Doing so would likely make the patient angrier and put the patient on the defensive. Once on the defensive, the patient probably will not listen to much more that you have to say.

When dealing with an angry patient, think of the old adage, "The customer is always right." Remember, ultimately, patients are customers. They are consumers of health care services.

It does no good to point out that a patient is wrong. The patient will remember a response, and this may make the difference in terms of how the situation is ultimately resolved. Try to resolve the situation and make sure the patient understands what can be done. Above all, be professional. Assure the patient that you will do everything that can be done to resolve the situation. Then be sure to follow through with your promise. Failing to follow through could damage patient relations with the office and may increase the chance of future litigation. Nothing should be promised that cannot be done.

When talking with an angry patient, avoid having conversations at the front desk in the presence of other patients in the office. It is a good idea to ask a patient to go into a less crowded area of the office so that you can give the patient your full attention.

Violent Patients

Depending on their skills in dealing with difficult situations, angry patients do have the potential to become violent. Although this is a rather rare occurrence in most medical offices, office staff should have plans in place and should be prepared to handle such a situation if it should arise. Some general suggestions on handling violent situations:

- Never try to handle a violent person alone.
- Remember to always remain within earshot of other staff members.

BOX 5-1

Kübler-Ross Stages of Loss

Denial
The patient cannot believe that something has happened to him or her and may feel as though "it just can't be true." The situation may seem like a bad dream.

Anger
The patient becomes very upset with the situation and may feel as though "it just isn't fair." The patient may lash out and be angry with others who are not in the same situation.

Bargaining
This stage typically has a religious connection. Faced with a situation, the patient attempts to make a deal with a higher being, saying, for example, "If I get better, I promise to ..."

Depression
In this stage, the patient may have tried many things—yelling, pleading, ignoring—and nothing is changing the situation for the better. Depression is a normal stage in the loss process. Hope for any improvement may be totally lost, and professional treatment for depression may be warranted.

Acceptance
Once the patient reaches acceptance of a situation, there is acknowledgment of the situation. The patient will likely want to say goodbye to those he or she loves and will get personal business affairs in order.

- Be careful not to back into a corner or allow the individual to position himself or herself between you and the door.
- Avoid sudden moves, as it could provoke the patient.
- Be certain to ask for help from another staff member if needed.

If an individual begins to get physical (throwing or hitting things), or if an assistant feels in danger, a call to 911 may be warranted. This, however, should be done after all else fails and should be the last resort to be used only when imminent danger is apparent.

Anxious Patients

Anxiety can manifest itself in a variety of ways. Patients may appear nervous or restless or may overreact to a situation. They may speak quickly and in a very random fashion. They may become fixated on an idea. The patient may even come right out and tell an assistant that he or she is anxious or nervous. Anxiety usually develops because of a patient's fear of the unknown.

In talking with an anxious patient, convey a calm and caring attitude. This may help to ease the patient's anxiety. If a patient is anxious about a medical condition or treatment, it is important to be careful to avoid any conversation in which you may be interpreted as giving medical advice. Listening intently and giving as much time as possible to the patient will help relieve the anxiety that a patient may be experiencing.

Depressed Patients

Depression is an illness that often is treated with medication. It is important to remember that depressed people are not weak—they are ill. Most individuals would not choose to be depressed. A depressed patient may experience a major depressive episode or may be chronically depressed over a long time. Whatever the case, the patient needs medical treatment and cannot just "snap out of it."

Depressed patients usually are not very talkative. If a patient talks of being depressed, do not dismiss the patient's complaints with a statement such as, "Oh, everything will be fine. Don't worry." If a patient makes any comments about injuring himself or herself, these comments should be taken very seriously and should be communicated directly to the physician. Because self-injury and suicide are a very real possibility with depressed patients, a medical administrative assistant must be sure to notify the medical staff of any pertinent incidents involving the patient.

Dying or Grieving Patients

Assisting patients who are dying or who are grieving the loss of a loved one presents a special challenge to everyone in the medical office. This is a very difficult time for patients and their families, and the medical office staff must be sensitive to their needs. The office staff should be prepared for a myriad of emotions from these patients and their families.

In the 1960s, Dr. Elizabeth Kübler-Ross, a physician who treated hundreds of terminally ill patients, researched the thought processes associated with the loss or grieving process and defined **five stages of loss** (Box 5-1) that often serve as the basis of caring for people suffering from terminal illness, the loss of a loved one, the loss of bodily function due to disease or injury, or even the loss of someone or something significant in their lives.

An assistant should be aware that a patient will experience the various stages of loss in a very personal way. Not all individuals experience all stages. Some may never reach acceptance; others may go back and forth between stages. Some patients spend more time in one stage than in another or may never experience one or more stages. An assistant who understands the stages of loss will be more understanding when assisting individuals who are dealing with loss.

Each person deals with loss in his or her own way. A sympathetic ear, kindness, and compassion can ease the patient's experiences in the medical office. An assistant should never avoid a patient because the assistant is uncomfortable with the situation. It is perfectly normal for the medical staff to be genuinely affected by a patient's loss, but this is also a time when patients need understanding and compassion. Strive to be kind, empathetic, and considerate of the patient's situation.

SUMMARY

A medical administrative assistant's workday consists of interactions with a wide variety of patients. Patients' beliefs are quite diverse, and an assistant must be respectful of individual differences and must take great care when communicating with patients to ensure that their needs are met. Also, patients may have special physical needs of which the assistant must be aware. Elderly patients or patients with disabilities may require additional special attention of the assistant. While in the office, patients may experience various emotions, and the assistant should strive to provide services that offer comfort to patients.

YOU ARE THE MEDICAL ADMINISTRATIVE ASSISTANT

An 18-year-old's mother is upset about her son's treatment in the medical office. Her son came in with a reaction to an antibiotic and is having difficulty breathing. The mother is upset because she knew her son was allergic to an antibiotic, but because her son is an adult, she was not asked about any allergies. The mother is talking very loudly, is becoming nearly hysterical, and is insisting on being taken back immediately to the treatment room to speak with the doctor. The treatment room is quite full of medical staff members who are working with the patient. What should you do?

Suggested Readings

A winner of the National Book Critics Circle Award for Nonfiction, *The Spirit Catches You and You Fall Down* (Noonday Press, Farrar, Straus & Giroux, 1997), by Anne Fadiman, tells the story of a Hmong child who is given the diagnosis of epilepsy and the doctors who treat her. The book includes a reader's guide that offers questions for discussion or essay topics.

The Muslim Next Door: The Qur'an, the Media and That Veil Thing by Sumbul Ali-Karamali, provides an interesting look into the life of a Muslim living in America today.

Still Alice by Lisa Genova is an engaging novel about a fictional character named Alice Howland who, at age 50, is diagnosed with early onset Alzheimer disease. The story is told from the patient's point of view. Lisa Genova has a Ph.D. in neuroscience.

REVIEW EXERCISES

Exercise 5-1 True or False

Read the following statements and determine whether the statements are true or false. Record the answer in the blank provided. T = true; F = false.

_____ 1. A patient's culture has an influence on his or her beliefs regarding health care treatment.

_____ 2. Knowledge of varying cultural beliefs can help an assistant avoid offending a patient.

_____ 3. An illness can cause a patient to be anxious.

_____ 4. The culture of the United States is easy to identify.

_____ 5. Caregivers of ill patients may act differently than usual because of stress associated with the patient's illness.

_____ 6. An assistant may have to repeat instructions for an ill patient.

_____ 7. An assistant should strive to be respectful of the patient, no matter what the circumstances.

_____ 8. Patients who are unable to speak usually communicate through an interpreter.

_____ 9. While serving an elderly patient, the assistant should be sure to phone all instructions to a son or daughter of the patient.

_____ 10. Children should not be left in a clinic's lobby, and an assistant should insist that all children accompany their parents to an examination room.

_____ 11. The best way to handle an angry patient is for the assistant to become equally angry.

_____ 12. Culture can be defined as beliefs or attitudes that are shared by a group of people and are passed from generation to generation.

_____ 13. Some cultures may object to the use of blood transfusions to treat patients.

_____ 14. Leininger's theory of culture care diversity and universality basically states that caregivers should take a patient's culture into consideration when providing health care.

_____ 15. A patient's illness can affect his or her interactions with members of the medical office staff.

_____ 16. It would be unusual for an extremely ill patient to be upset.

_____ 17. Family members are the best interpreters for patients who do not speak English.

_____ 18. An assistant should use medical terminology with all patients of the medical office.

_____ 19. It may be necessary to shout at an elderly patient who is hard of hearing.

_____ 20. Instructions for disabled patients always should be given directly to a caregiver, not to the patient.

_____ 21. A patient who has been paralyzed may experience some or all of the five stages of loss.

_____ 22. The chief focus of the caring response is the patient.

_____ 23. Failure to have an interpreter for a patient could have serious legal consequences for a health care facility.

_____ 24. The caring response means that the focus of care should be finding a cure for the patient.

Exercise 5-2 Chapter Concepts

Read the following questions or statements, and choose the answer that best completes the statement or question. Record the answer in the blank provided.

_____ 1. Which of the following is inappropriate when dealing with an angry patient?
(a) Offer to help if possible.
(b) Keep a calm voice.
(c) Ask the patient what he or she would like to have done about the situation.
(d) Record the conversation on tape.
(e) Acknowledge the patient's anger.

_____ 2. If an individual becomes violent while in the office, which of the following should **not** be done?
(a) Call the police if danger is imminent.
(b) Take the individual to a rear office, shut the door, and try to calm the individual.
(c) Ask for help from another staff member.
(d) Remain within hearing distance of other office employees.

_____ 3. Which of the following is **false** regarding anxious patients?
(a) They are dangerous.
(b) They may appear restless.
(c) They may talk fast.
(d) Anxiety may be caused by the patient's fear of the unknown.

_____ 4. Which of the following is **false** regarding depressed patients?
(a) They are ill.
(b) They usually are very talkative.
(c) An increased potential for suicide exists.
(d) Depression can be treated with medication.

_____ 5. Which of the following is **false** when patients are served in the medical office?
(a) After age 75, most elderly patients will need assistance when making health care decisions.
(b) Illness can be a stress factor for patients or caregivers.
(c) A foreign language dictionary may help an ESL patient explain a medical condition.
(d) All patients of the office should be treated with dignity and respect, no matter what their culture.

Exercise 5-3 Stages of Loss

Match each of the five stages of loss with its appropriate description. Record the answer in the blank provided.

(a) Denial
(b) Anger
(c) Bargaining
(d) Depression
(e) Acceptance

_____ 1. Patient is extremely sad about the situation and may lose hope.
_____ 2. Patient does not believe what is happening to him or her.
_____ 3. Patient is extremely upset and furious about his or her situation.
_____ 4. Patient acknowledges his or her situation.
_____ 5. Patient tries to make a deal to get out of the situation.

ACTIVITIES

ACTIVITY 5-1 PATIENT INFORMATION IN MEDISOFT

Using the following instructions, identify important patient information in Medisoft.

1. With Medisoft open, click **Lists>Patient/Guarantors and Cases.** A patient's race, ethnicity, language, or other special patient information can be included in a patient's file.
2. Using the information in the table below, open the patient's file by double-clicking the patient's name on the **Patient list** in Medisoft. Enter the information specified on the table.
3. If applicable, click the **Name, Address** tab. Select the **Race, Language or Ethnicity** information for the patients listed in the table below.
4. If applicable, click the **Other Information** tab, and in the **Flag** field, click the drop-down arrow to select the flag that corresponds with the information in the other information column in the table below.
5. As each patient's information is completed, click **Save.**

Patient Name	Name, Address tab (Race, Ethnicity, Language)	Other Information tab (Flag)
Again, Dwight	—	Medicare patient
Austin, Andrew	—	Medicare patient
Clinger, Wallace	—	Medicare patient
Doe, Jane	—	Special needs
Gooding, Charles	—	Medicare patient
Hartman, Tonya	Ethnicity–Hispanic	—
Jasper, Stephanie	—	Medicare patient
Koseman, Chadwick	Language–German	—
Sheperd, Jarem	Language–Spanish	—
Wagnew, Jeremy	Race–Pacific Islander	—
Whitmore, Ryan	—	Special needs

ACTIVITY 5-2 HEALTH CARE BELIEF SURVEY

To understand how health care beliefs can vary from patient to patient, complete the following questions regarding health care. *Do not* write your name on this assignment. Give the completed sheet to your instructor, and your instructor will tabulate the class results. Your instructor then will share the total results with the class.

1. I smoke cigarettes. Yes/No
2. I drink alcohol at least once a week. Yes/No
3. There are certain foods that I will not eat at certain times because of my religious beliefs. Yes/No
4. I use home remedies whenever possible. Yes/No
5. I would accept a blood transfusion if I needed it. Yes/No
6. I have seen a chiropractor for treatment. Yes/No
7. I have taken herbal remedies to treat a health condition. Yes/No

8. I have tried acupuncture to treat a health condition. Yes/No
9. I expect the elder of my family to make important decisions for me. Yes/No

DISCUSSION

The following topics can be used for class discussion or for individual student essay.

DISCUSSION 5-1

Have you ever been in one of the following situations?

- Seriously ill
- Caregiver of a seriously ill person
- Relative or close friend of a seriously ill person

Write a short essay or participate in a group discussion involving the following points:

- Was your life altered as a result of this experience? If so, how?
- Were the five stages of loss evident in this situation?
- Were any of the common patient beliefs identified in this chapter present in this situation?

For those who have never experienced any of these situations, listen to the discussion or read a published account of such a situation, and explain your reaction to it (verbally or in writing).

DISCUSSION 5-2

Research an issue related to health care for geriatric patients. Present a synopsis of the issue in a one- to two-page report or in a presentation to the class.

DISCUSSION 5-3

In a group, have each individual identify a health care situation in which a caring response was demonstrated by a health care professional.

Bibliography

Adams CH, Jones PD: *Interpersonal Communication Skills for Health Professionals*, , ed 2, Columbus, 2000, Glencoe McGraw-Hill.

Comak H: *New Joint Commission standard defines medical interpreters.* www.healthleadersmedia.com Accessed February 24, 2010.

O'Toole M: *Miller-Keane Encyclopedia & Dictionary of Medicine, Nursing, & Allied Health*, , ed 5, Philadelphia, 1997, WB Saunders.

Sieh A, Brentin LK: *The Nurse Communicates*, Philadelphia, 1997, WB Saunders.

U.S. Census Bureau: *Language use in the United States: 2007.* www.census.gov Accessed January 6, 2013.

Purtilo RB, Doherty R: *Ethical Dimensions in the Health Professions*, ed 5, Saint Louis, MO, 2010, Saunders Elsevier.

CHAPTER 6 Interpersonal Communications

LEARNING OUTCOMES

On successful completion of this chapter, the student will be able to

1. Describe the fundamentals of communication.
2. Identify effective and ineffective communication techniques.
3. Identify professional communication with patients and coworkers.
4. Identify professional and proper telephone communication skills.
5. Identify confidentiality issues related to patient communication.
6. Describe telephone equipment and services.
7. Apply professional written communication skills when preparing business correspondence.
8. Describe mail processing in the office.
9. Describe postal and delivery services.
10. Demonstrate use of medical practice management software to assist with patient communication.

COMMISSION ON ACCREDITATION OF ALLIED HEALTH EDUCATION PROGRAMS (CAAHEP) CORE CURRICULUM FOR MEDICAL ASSISTANTS

- Identify nonverbal communication.
- Recognize communication barriers.
- Identify techniques for overcoming communication barriers.
- Recognize the elements of oral communication using a sender-receiver process.
- Recognize elements of fundamental writing skills.
- Discuss applications of electronic technology in effective communication.
- Demonstrate telephone techniques.
- Compose professional/business letters.
- Respond to nonverbal communication.
- Describe the implications of HIPAA for the medical assistant in various medical settings.
- Explore issues of confidentiality as it applies to the medical assistant.
- Respond to issues of confidentiality.
- Apply HIPAA rules in regard to privacy/release of information.

ACCREDITING BUREAU OF HEALTH EDUCATION SCHOOLS (ABHES) COMPETENCIES FOR MEDICAL ASSISTING

Graduates

- Efficiently maintain and understand different types of medical correspondence and medical reports.
- Are attentive, listen, and learn.
- Are impartial and show empathy when dealing with patients.
- Communicate on recipient's level of comprehension.
- Serve as liaison between physician and others.
- Use proper telephone techniques.
- Use pertinent medical terminology.
- Receive, organize, prioritize, and transmit information expediently.
- Recognize and respond to verbal and nonverbal communication.
- Apply electronic technology.
- Perform basic keyboarding skills including typing medical correspondence and basic reports.
- Identify and properly use office machines, computerized systems, and medical software.
- Efficiently maintain and understand different types of medical correspondence and medical reports.
- Demonstrate professionalism by being courteous and diplomatic.
- Demonstrate professionalism by maintaining confidentiality at all times.

VOCABULARY

block style
body
closing
communication
computer file name notation
copy notation
digital sender
email
emoticon
enclosure notation

VOCABULARY—cont'd

express mail
feedback
full-block style
highly confidential information
inside address
memo
modified-block style
modified-block style with indented paragraphs
notation
Optical Character Reader (OCR)
protocol
reference initials
salutation
semiblock style
voice mail

COMMUNICATION CONCEPTS

Professional communication skills are essential for everyone in the medical office. Professional communication is courteous and respectful whether you are working as part of the administrative or clinical staff. The ability to communicate effectively with patients is vital for all medical office personnel. Communicating with patients in a professional, business-like, yet caring manner fosters trust between the medical office staff and the patient and lays the foundation for a strong, trusting, and long-lasting relationship between the patient and the practice. Even the most beautiful physical surroundings cannot make up for any staff member who lacks proper communication skills. A medical administrative assistant frequently interacts with patients, and this interaction has a great impact on the success of the practice. Whether an assistant is communicating with a patient face to face, on the telephone, or in writing, the assistant's communication must be professional and should continually reflect the image that the practice wishes to project.

Communication Basics

When applying professional communication techniques to interactions with patients, it is important to understand basic communication concepts. The *Miller-Keane Encyclopedia & Dictionary of Medicine, Nursing, & Allied Health* defines **communication** as the "sending of information from one place to another." One of the cornerstones of understanding communication is the idea that communication involves getting that information, idea, or thought from one individual to another.

Communication is an enormous topic. Entire courses and degrees are necessary to address the many nuances of this subject. This chapter addresses many of the critical components necessary in laying a foundation for effective communication within the medical office. Additional study of communication beyond this chapter would enhance your ability to communicate effectively with patients and other individuals in the medical office.

Communicating Effectively

The vast majority of people in this world can talk, but can they communicate? Are they understood?

Consider this example. If you and a friend are outside one day, and your friend remarks, "The sky is blue today," you know that your friend thinks the sky is blue and not green. But imagine if your friend says, "Look at the sky"; you may be able to guess that your friend wants you to notice that the sky is blue, but it is possible that you may be looking for something in the sky, such as an airplane or a bird, or perhaps you may notice a cloud with an interesting shape. This example illustrates how important word selection can be in the communication process.

Consider this next example. A patient enters the office and begins to speak to you in German. The patient is talking, but if you do not know German, very little communication may occur. At the very least, you will not be able to understand what the patient is saying. But if you have a very puzzled or confused look on your face and respond in English, your facial expressions and verbal response should communicate to the patient that you do not understand German.

From the examples mentioned, the basic components of the communication process are evident: a sender, a receiver, a message, and feedback. The sender and the receiver are the two parties to the proposed communication, the message is the information from the sender, and **feedback** is the information the receiver gives to the sender about the message.

Let's look at another example in a medical office setting. Suppose a patient calls the office and reports to the assistant that he or she is not "feeling well." This statement does not give the assistant a clear indication of what the problem might be. Consequently, if the assistant relayed this information to a nurse or to a physician, it would not be very helpful to either one because it is not very descriptive. If the patient reports, however, that he or she has had a sharp, stabbing-like pain in his or her lower right side for two days, this gives a much more accurate picture of the patient's condition.

Unfortunately, not every patient may describe symptoms this well, which is why medical administrative assistants benefit from cultivating good communication skills. In the previous situation, if a patient states that he or she is not "feeling well," it is the medical administrative assistant's responsibility to determine the *general* nature of the patient's problem. This is necessary to determine what type of action should be taken with the patient's call.

When communicating with a patient, it is imperative to obtain a clear picture of what the patient is trying to say. One of the most important things a medical administrative assistant can do, and one of the most essential components of effective communication, is to listen to the other person while he or she is speaking. Be attentive by giving 100% of your attention to the patient, whether the patient is in the office or on the telephone. Do not plan what you might say while the patient is speaking. Give the patient ample opportunity to say what he or she needs to say. After the patient has finished speaking, ask any questions that may be necessary to clarify the situation. Using the previous example, let's see how a medical administrative assistant might handle a patient's comment about not feeling well.

Patient: I'm not feeling well.
Assistant: What kind of symptoms are you having?
Patient: I threw up this morning.
Assistant: Is that the only symptom you've had?
Patient: I've also had a sharp pain on my lower right side.
Assistant: How long have you had the pain?
Patient: A couple of days.
Assistant: And have you had any other symptoms?
Patient: Just a slight fever.

The medical administrative assistant in this case has obtained just enough information to convey a picture of the patient's condition to the nurse or physician. It is not necessary for the assistant to get every last detail about the patient's illness from the patient. The assistant simply needs enough information to give the medical staff a clear picture of the patient's condition and to determine if the call needs immediate attention from the medical staff, if an appointment can be made, or if a message can be taken. In the preceding example, the patient might have appendicitis, which is a serious condition that must be brought to the attention of the physician immediately. If the assistant had stopped asking questions after the patient reported vomiting, the assistant would not have been given enough information to illustrate the seriousness of the situation.

When questioning a patient, an assistant must be extremely careful to identify any serious or potentially life-threatening conditions *without alarming the patient.* It is important to avoid saying anything that could be construed as attempting to diagnose the patient's problem. Patients who report serious conditions or symptoms should be referred to the physician or nurse without delay. Identifying and handling emergency calls is discussed in greater detail later in this chapter.

Previous examples clearly illustrate the importance of communication in the medical office. Because of the nature of the calls that come into the office, good communication may in some cases mean the difference between life and death to a patient.

When speaking with patients, follow these basic guidelines for effective verbal communication:

- Speak clearly. Chewing gum or eating any type of food while at the front desk is unacceptable.
- Speak loudly enough so that patients can hear but not so loud that everyone else hears.
- Pronounce words correctly.
- Speak with a caring pleasant voice. The sound of your voice conveys a message. Others can tell whether you are genuine in your responses or whether you are uninterested and uncaring. What kind of feeling does your voice convey? Is it one of caring, or is it one of indifference?
- Monitor the speed of your speech. Do not speak too fast or too slow.
- Direct your words to the individual to whom you are speaking.
- When speaking with patients, be aware that you are a representative of the practice. Patients will interpret what you say as coming directly from the physician.
- Ask enough questions to identify the needs of the patient. Do not ask so many questions that it may appear you are prying into the patient's private health matters, or it may alarm the patient.
- Be careful to protect confidentiality when speaking with a patient.
- *Never, ever* suggest to a patient what might be wrong. This is practicing medicine without a license and is punishable by law!
- Clarify the patient's needs by repeating the patient's request or statement. Clear up any misunderstandings. Say to the patient, "Let me make sure I have this right..."
- Do not interrupt. Give the patient ample opportunity to convey thoughts without interruption.
- As mentioned in Chapter 5, technical medical terms and jargon should be used only if the patient uses them in conversation, or if the patient is a health care professional.

Nonverbal Communication

Communication does not have to be a spoken or written message. Communication can occur without anyone speaking or writing anything. This type of communication is nonverbal communication and is more commonly known as body language. Nonverbal communication, or body language, is a sign or signal given by the body. These visual clues may have a greater impact on the conversation than words that are spoken.

Take a look at the interactions pictured in Figure 6-1. One of the interactions is much friendlier appearing than the other. Note how each individual in each situation is sending a strong nonverbal message with eyes, arms, and other parts of the body. An individual's appearance and body language can communicate interest or disinterest to another individual.

Individuals transmit and receive many body signals subconsciously. We may not know what gives us a certain feeling about a person, but we often get that feeling from the body signals that are being sent. A frown, slumping posture, or eyes that wander create a negative image and demonstrate disinterest toward another individual. A smile or a friendly nod creates a pleasant encounter.

Think about your own body language. What kind of nonverbal signals are you sending every day? Are they positive or negative? Cultivate positive body language habits, and you will have contributed to an inviting atmosphere for patients. Practice the following every day:

- Establish eye contact. Nothing conveys sincerity in a conversation more than a person who looks directly at someone else. Be aware that some individuals, as you learned in Chapter 5, may avoid eye contact with you because of cultural influences.

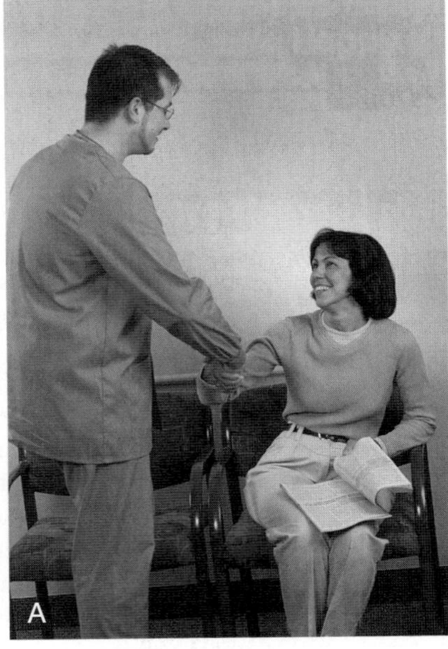

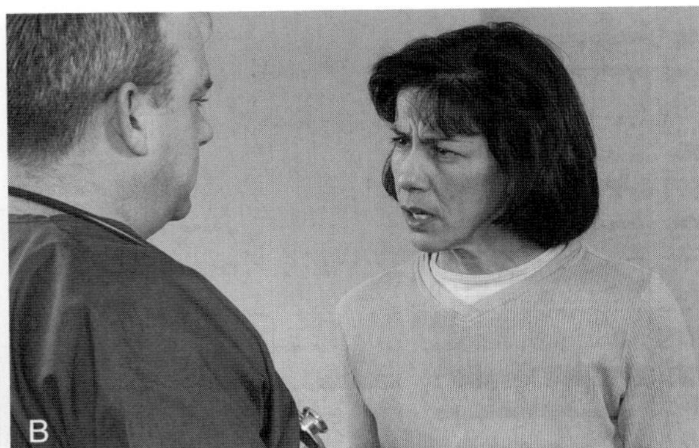

Figure 6-1 An individual's body language communicates a message. Note the different messages communicated by the patient in A versus the patient in B.

- Be conscious of your arm position. Are your arms crossed in front of your body, creating an almost protective barrier between you and another person, or are they casually at your sides or in use?
- Smile, smile, smile at all times *when appropriate.* Cheerfulness goes a long way in making the patient feel welcome in the office.
- Watch your posture. When talking with a patient, the front of your body should be directed toward the patient. Do not talk with your back to the patient.
- Watch facial expressions. Frowning sends an obvious negative message.
- Be aware of a patient's comfort zone. Leaning in too far to speak to a patient or positioning yourself closer than a few feet from a patient may invade his or her personal space and may make the patient feel uncomfortable. A distance of 18 to 24 inches is a comfortable distance when conversing with a patient.
- Be aware of the impact of personal attire and grooming. Professional appearance makes a significant impression.

HIPAA Hint

Be careful where you speak to a patient. Protected health information about a patient includes the following:

- Patient's birth date, address, telephone number, medical record number, Social Security number, and any other identifier that could specifically identify the patient
- Any information that health care providers put in the patient's medical record
- Billing information about the patient
- Patient information stored in a computer

Personality Styles

Sometimes, we can be doing everything right in communicating with others, but we may get mixed responses from various people. Have you ever noticed how people can interpret or respond to the same situation differently? These responses may be due to personality differences among individuals.

People can be introverted or extroverted. Some people love working with large groups of people, while some may be uncomfortable in a large group and may prefer working alone. Would you like working in a busy, hustle-bustle office or a quiet office? Not everyone has the same likes and dislikes, and individuals respond differently to different situations. This does not mean that one is right and one is wrong; this may just reflect personality differences. What is important is that we respect the opinions of others just as we would wish to be given the same respect in return. Think about it this way: Isn't it great that we all aren't the same, so that there are people who are well suited for different types of positions? If everyone was the same, life would get dull and boring pretty quickly.

Personality differences sometimes can lead to conflict in the office. When presented with a conflict, it is important for each individual involved to respect the rights of others. People have differing opinions or different ways of looking at things, and we need to accept those differences. Such action is a mature response to these situations and goes a long way in ensuring that the office runs smoothly.

Communication Within the Health Care Team

Every medical administrative assistant will have to work with someone during the course of employment; an assistant may work alongside someone all the time or may have only periodic interactions with coworkers. In large offices, several medical administrative assistants may be employed. These individuals need to develop a close working relationship with one another.

It is important for coworkers to treat one another with respect and courtesy. Some conflicts in the office may start because of one person's feeling of superiority or indifference to others. All members of the health care team must develop a good working relationship with one another, be tolerant of differences in others, and remember that all members of the health care team are important.

When communicating with physicians and other providers in the office, it is important for an assistant to realize that physicians and other providers (e.g., nurse practitioners, nurse midwives, physician assistants, therapists) have a tremendous responsibility in providing health care treatment, and their activities are chiefly responsible for generating the income of the practice. If an assistant can make a provider's job easier and can help office staff to be as productive as possible, everyone involved with the practice will benefit—patients included!

Communicating With Your Supervisor

The best relationships between supervisors and staff are those in which there is a healthy mutual respect. In some practices, the physician is the assistant's direct supervisor. In larger practices, an office supervisor usually is hired to oversee the business functions of the office. Regardless of who is the supervisor, it is important to remember that the supervisor is the person in charge, and the supervisor is ultimately responsible for the operation of the office.

When communicating with a supervisor, an assistant must be respectful of the supervisor's position and should strive to meet the expectations of the supervisor. It is important for you to bring to a supervisor's attention any problems or concerns that you cannot handle. Do not think that a problem will go away if it is ignored. Do not guess at what might be the solution to the problem. A supervisor and an assistant who work together will help the office run smoothly. A harmonious work environment will enhance services provided for the good of the patient and will promote a strong, successful practice. Remember the words of the Mayo Clinic founders—"The best interest of the patient is the only interest to be considered." We are all "in it" for the patient!

CHECKPOINT

A few people in the office like to gossip about other staff members. How could this affect the medical office environment?

Telephone Communication

The telephone is an indispensable piece of equipment in the office today. Most of a practice's business is conducted over the telephone. Appointments are made, patients call to inquire about health concerns, office staff members use the telephone to conduct business, and a multitude of other office activities require the use of a telephone. However, just because someone knows how to pick up the telephone and say hello, it cannot be assumed that the telephone will be used properly.

Proper Telephone Technique

The foundation of good telephone communication skills is a good telephone personality. Your choice of words, volume and tone of voice, and general expression on the telephone will have a tremendous impact on patients. A caring, pleasant-sounding, customer-friendly, service-oriented personality is essential in telephone communication in any medical office.

Many of us, at a very young age, learned to answer the telephone. What a thrill it was to hear the telephone ring and answer it! Ah, if only it were that easy! Answering the telephone in a medical office is quite different from answering a personal telephone because it carries a great deal of responsibility along with it. A patient may reveal sensitive, confidential medical information over the telephone. A patient may call the office with a potentially serious medical situation. Responsibility for answering the telephone in a medical office must be taken seriously, and as the medical administrative assistant, you will be required to continually make the right decisions when communicating on the telephone.

Many of the same rules mentioned previously for good communication apply to communicating via the telephone. When speaking on the telephone, practice the following professional telephone techniques:

- *Tone and volume of voice.* Speak in a tone that is thoughtful and caring. Speak loud enough for the patient to hear but soft enough so that others in the office will not hear. If appropriate, smile while talking on the telephone. Patients will notice the pleasantness of a smile reflected in your voice.
- *Quality of your speech.* Consider the words used in your conversation. Avoid slang, use proper grammar, and maintain professionalism while on the telephone.
- *Proper telephone posture.* You should sit upright (no slouching!), hold the handset or headset microphone one to two inches away from the mouth, and be sure to enunciate clearly (Fig. 6-2). In most medical offices, there is considerable background noise, and to be heard well, you will have to be attentive to the patient on the other end of the line and speak directly into the handset. Proper posture at the telephone will help ensure that you present your best self when you are speaking with a patient over the telephone.
- *Speed of your speech.* Be careful to speak at a rate that will be understood by the caller. Depending on your interaction with the caller, you may have to adjust your speech rate to be sure that both of you are communicating. Routine information that is repeated many times to various patients may be well understood by you, but it may be the first time the information is heard by the patient. Be sure to give information in a way that is understood by the patient.

Incoming Calls

Responsibility for managing the telephone traffic in a medical practice is an important matter. If more than one line is coming into the office, managing incoming calls can be very challenging. While an assistant is speaking on one line, one or

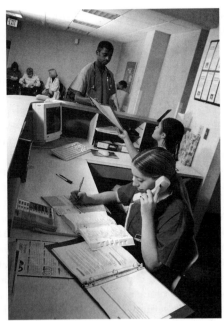

Figure 6-2 Proper posture while speaking on the telephone has a positive effect on speech. (From Young AP: *Kinn's The Administrative Medical Assistant,* ed 7, St. Louis, Saunders, 2011.)

PROCEDURE 6-1

Demonstrate Telephone Techniques

Materials Needed

- Telephone setup with two separate lines
- Pencil

1. Answer the telephone within three rings.
2. Answer the telephone using the proper greeting.
   - Welcome
   - Identification of the facility
   - Identification of the operator
   - Offer to help
3. Determine the reason for the call.*
4. Identify the caller.
5. Determine the appropriate action based on the reason for the call.
6. Confirm the call.*
7. Close the call.

Optional

8. Demonstrate holding.
9. Demonstrate transferring a call.

**Denotes a crucial step in the procedure. This step must be completed satisfactorily for the procedure to be completed satisfactorily.*

more calls may come into the office on other lines. Depending on the size of the practice, one assistant may be assigned to handle the telephone on a full-time basis. The need for telephone coverage can vary depending upon the time of day or the day of the week. Certain days of the week, particularly Monday and Friday, can have especially heavy telephone traffic. Mondays bring calls of people who were ill over the weekend, and Fridays bring calls of people who need medical care before the weekend. Because of the unpredictability of telephone traffic, any assistant or medical office employee should be ready to answer the telephone whenever needed. Procedure 6-1 details the essential components of a telephone conversation in the medical office.

In addition to learning proper telephone technique, you must be aware of some special considerations when you answer the telephone in a medical office:

- *Consider telephone location.* The office telephone should be located on the assistant's desk within an arm's reach of the office computer. Many times, you will be speaking with a patient on the telephone and will need to access information from and input information into the computer during your conversation. If the lobby is close to the front desk, you will have to be careful that patients in the lobby do not hear your voice.
- *Maintain confidentiality.* Because the office is often a busy place with patients stopping at the front desk for assistance, you will have to be sure not to divulge a caller's complete name or disclose medical information in front of another patient. All telephone conversations must be kept confidential.
- *Keep conversations brief.* Because many offices do get a tremendous volume of calls, be mindful of the time that is spent on the telephone. You must be sure to give the patient the time needed, but be sure that it is time well spent in getting information for a message or assisting the patient in another way.
- *Do not ignore a ringing telephone.* If the office is extremely busy and it is difficult to answer the telephone, some practices may be arranged in such a way as to allow other staff members in the facility to assist in answering the telephone when the telephone traffic becomes too heavy.
- *Answer incoming calls in three rings or fewer.* If the telephone cannot be answered as soon as it rings, be sure to answer within a reasonable time. If the telephone is allowed to ring four to five or even more times, many callers may begin to wonder whether the office is open, or whether the practice cares about patients who call.
- *Do not give medical advice or ask questions that may lead a patient to believe you may be diagnosing the patient's condition.* For example, if a patient calls to report severe right lower quadrant abdominal pain, *never* say, "It sounds like you have appendicitis" or "Have you ever had problems with your appendix?" Both of these statements could be interpreted as practicing medicine without a license (which is illegal) and could result in immediate dismissal from employment.
- *Do not use the telephone for personal business while on duty.* This is unprofessional behavior. Always wait for lunchtime or a break to make personal calls. With the proliferation of cell phones today, there really is not a need to tie up the office telephone line to make personal calls.

A Pleasant Telephone Greeting

If answering the telephone were as easy as it was when we were young, this chapter would have ended much earlier. However, because a practice's business is so dependent on the telephone, and because patients' lives may be at stake when the telephone is answered, it is absolutely critical that each and every call is handled with a level of professionalism that is absolutely essential in a medical office setting. It simply is not enough to say "hello" and then wait for the caller to answer. When a call is answered in a medical office, you must speak clearly and slowly. Many operators say the office greeting much too fast, and that can leave callers wondering what was really said.

Every call that comes into the office should be answered with a cheerful greeting consisting of three to four components: (1) welcome, (2) identification of facility, (3) identification of operator (assistant's name), and (4) an offer to help.

Appropriate greetings may sound like the following:

- "Good morning, Horizons Health Care; this is Annie. How may I help you?"
- "Thank you for calling Horizons Health Care; this is Mike. How may I direct your call?"
- "Good afternoon, Horizons Health Care; this is Rosa. How may I help you today?"

Welcome. The first portion of a telephone greeting is a pleasant statement, a welcome, such as "Good morning," or "Thank you for calling." These introductions are a pleasant way to start a conversation with a caller, and they help to establish a pleasant foundation for the conversation with the patient. In addition, a welcome alerts the caller that the call has been answered and helps prepare the caller to commence a conversation.

Welcomes such as "Merry Christmas" or "Happy Hanukkah" and others with obvious ties to religious holidays are not used in some office settings. The larger the organization, the more likely that greetings will be generic in nature. In a smaller office, a physician's personal preference will determine how calls may be answered. Why is such a thing even important? A simple holiday greeting could offend patients of one religion if the greeting references another religion.

Identification of the Facility or Department. After extending the welcome, the operator should identify the facility or department by name.

- "Good morning, Horizons Health Care..."
- "Good afternoon, Country Care Associates..."
- "Thank you for calling Horizons Health Care..."
- "Good afternoon, Dermatology..."
- "Thank you for calling today. This is Cardiology..."

Complete identification of the office name or department is necessary to assure the patient that the correct location has been reached. Even if the call has been received at a central switchboard and then transferred to a specific department (e.g., neurology, pediatrics), an assistant still should identify the department by name when answering, such as "Hello, Pediatrics..." or "Good Morning, Physical Therapy Services..." Identifying the facility or the department lets the caller know that the correct location has been reached.

Identification of the Operator and an Offer of Help. After identifying the facility or department, the operator states his or her name. The operator is the individual who answers the call.

In smaller facilities, very often the operator is the assistant who takes the call and performs tasks necessary to complete the handling of the call. If a patient leaves a message, schedules an appointment, or makes another request, it is likely that the assistant will directly help the patient. The assistant's name is given so the patient will be able to identify the individual who provided assistance if future questions regarding the patient's call should arise.

Larger facilities that handle a tremendous volume of calls usually have a central switchboard setup in which one or more individuals answer incoming calls. In this type of health care facility, incoming calls usually are answered with a welcome, identification of the facility, and an offer of assistance. The switchboard operator does not give his or her name because the operator does not directly deal with the call other than to transfer the call to someone who will assist the patient. A greeting such as "Good afternoon, Happy Valley Medical Clinic" or "How may I direct your call?" would be appropriate, although a facility may prefer that the operator be identified to add a personal touch to the conversation.

Telephone Protocol. Because many different types of situations can arise in the medical office, an established telephone **protocol** gives the medical administrative assistant a guide to follow when processing incoming calls. Protocol refers to instructions that should be used in response to an event. An established protocol gives an individual a guide to use when responding to a situation. Each office should establish a specific telephone protocol to be used in handling calls that come into the office. An example of a telephone protocol given in Table 6-1 provides a sample of the numerous types of calls that come into a practice and a possible response for each call. Table 6-1 is not a definitive list of calls, and before a telephone protocol is put into use in any practice, it must be reviewed and approved by the practice physician or physicians.

Reason for the Patient's Call. As mentioned previously, every call is answered with a greeting. After the greeting has been extended, the most important piece of information needed by the medical administrative assistant is the reason the caller has called the office.

In almost every other type of business, typical telephone practice is to identify the caller first. That is not the case in the medical office. Because you will be working in a medical office, the reason for the call may be a medical emergency. If a patient is calling with an emergency situation, the call must be handled quickly because seconds may make a difference. Identification of common emergency calls is addressed later in this chapter.

Caller Identification. Once the reason for the call has been identified, the assistant will ask for the caller's name. Once the reason and the caller have been identified, the assistant will be able to decide how to handle the call based on the protocol that has been established for the office.

TABLE 6-1

Sample Telephone Protocol

Type of Call	Action Taken by Medical Administrative Assistant	Call Handled by Whom
Patient requests appointment.	If not a potential emergency, schedule appointment.	Medical administrative assistant
Patient calls with a possible emergency situation.	Transfer the call immediately to the physician or nurse.	Physician or nurse
Patient requests prescription refill.	1. Take a message with medication name and patient's pharmacy name. Send message with patient's record to physician **or** 2. Patient may be instructed to call pharmacy to initiate the request for a refill.	1. Physician will call pharmacy if approved; nurse will telephone patient to inform the patient as to action taken by the physician (refilled or not refilled). 2. If patient is instructed to call the pharmacy, the patient will call the pharmacy to check on refill. If the refill is not approved by physician, the nurse or physician should notify the patient that the refill was not approved.
Patient asks to talk with physician or nurse because patient is ill or needs some medical information.	Take a message, send message with patient's record to physician or nurse. (Depending on the severity of the patient's illness, the call may need to be transferred immediately to the physician or nurse.)	Physician or nurse
Patient is returning a call to the physician or nurse.	Transfer call directly to physician or nurse as requested.	Physician or nurse
Another physician calls for the physician.	Transfer call directly to physician as requested; there is no need to ask the reason for the call.	Physician
Outside laboratory calls with test results.	Transfer call directly to individual requested by the laboratory.	Identified staff member
Patient is uncomfortable identifying the reason for calling.	Ask the patient if the call is an emergency. If not, ask the patient if you can have the nurse return a call to the patient.	Nurse
Patient calls for test results.	Take a message, send message with patient's chart to physician or nurse.	Physician or nurse
Patient calls with insurance or billing question.	After confirming the identity of the patient and whether the patient is entitled to the information, answer the patient's question. Some information may not be able to be released over the telephone and may have to be mailed directly to the patient's home.	Medical administrative assistant
Insurance company calls requesting information on a patient.	Identify requested information and name of caller. Usually, only limited information may be given over the telephone, and the caller may have to send in a written request for information that has been authorized by the patient.	Medical administrative assistant
Personal call for a member of the office staff is received.	Transfer directly to the staff member. If the call is for the physician and the physician is with a patient, notify the caller of that fact, and ask whether you should interrupt (e.g., "The doctor is with a patient right now; would you like me to interrupt?").	Identified staff member
Administration calls for a member of the office staff.	Transfer directly to the staff member. If the call is for a physician and the physician is with a patient, notify the caller of that fact, and ask whether you should interrupt (e.g., "The doctor is in with a patient right now; would you like me to interrupt?").	Identified staff member

TABLE 6-1
Sample Telephone Protocol—cont'd

Type of Call	Action Taken by Medical Administrative Assistant	Call Handled by Whom
Patient has a complaint.	Attempt to handle the situation if at all possible; otherwise, take a message or transfer the call to the appropriate individual. If necessary, notify physician of complaint.	Medical administrative assistant or identified staff member
Patient has been poisoned.	Immediately give patient telephone number of poison control center and obtain name of patient. Poison Control Centers are properly equipped to handle poisonings in a rapid manner.	Notify physician, and document call in patient's medical chart.
Pharmaceutical sales representative wants appointment to give sales talk to physician and nurse.	Make appointment under the guidelines established for the office.	Medical administrative assistant
Office supply sales representative calls.	Take message and give to staff member chiefly responsible for buying office supplies.	Identified staff member

Table 6-1 lists a sample telephone protocol that includes the various types of calls that are received in a medical office, the action an assistant should take, and who is ultimately responsible for completion of the call.

Action. After the assistant has determined why the caller is calling and who the caller is, it is time to take action. At this point, the assistant decides what needs to be done (transfer the call or assist the patient directly), and that action is then taken. Be sure to give the patient enough time to relay all concerns. Occasionally, an assistant may not be able to complete the patient's request right away, but instead may have to handle a patient's request later in the day (as in the case of release of medical records to another facility), when the business of the office has slowed down.

Call Confirmation. Once the caller has been assisted, it is important to confirm any necessary information. If an appointment is scheduled, the provider, the date, and time of the appointment should be confirmed with the caller. If a message was taken, the message written should be repeated verbatim to the caller to ensure that it accurately reflects the wishes of the caller. If appropriate, ask the caller if he or she has any questions. You should inform the caller of the action that will be taken to address this call.

Closing the Call. After action on the call has been confirmed, ask the caller if there is anything else that the caller needs. If not, you should say goodbye with an appropriate closing. Possible closings include the following:

- "Thank you for calling."
- "I'll take care of this right away."
- "Have a nice day."
- "Thank you."

Holding. Not all calls can be handled without asking a caller to hold. Of course, it would be best if no callers were ever asked to hold, but the reality is that you could be helping other patients in the office when the telephone rings. Some calls simply will not be handled without having the caller hold.

The most important thing to remember when asking a caller to hold is that the caller *must be asked* whether he or she is able to hold. As mentioned previously, some calls may be an emergency and the caller should not, of course, be placed on hold.

The appropriate way to ask a caller to hold would sound like the following:

Operator: Good morning, Horizon's Health Care. This is Amy. Are you able to hold?

At this point, the operator *must wait* for a response. Note that the caller needs to be asked if he or she is *able* to hold. If it is an emergency, this gives the caller a chance to say so. If it is not an emergency, the caller can say yes or no. The caller may say no to holding for various reasons. Maybe the caller needs only to be transferred or, possibly, the caller is calling long distance.

A caller should *never* be "told" to hold, as in "Please hold." This statement is a command and gives little opportunity for the caller to respond if he or she is not able to hold. Always give the caller a choice.

If a caller is placed on hold, a reasonable period to expect a caller to hold is no longer than one minute. One minute can seem quite long. After one minute, if the caller needs to be on hold for a little longer, the assistant should answer the line again and ask the caller whether he or she can continue to hold, or if the assistant may call the caller back. Some telephone systems even have a feature that re rings a call that has been on hold for a specific length of time. When the assistant is returning to answer a call that has been on hold, an appropriate introduction would be, "Thank you for holding. How may I help you?"

When the office is busy and incoming calls may have to hold, an assistant should wait until just after the third ring to answer the call and then should ask the caller to hold. If the assistant answers on the first ring and asks the caller to hold, that might give the impression that calls are not a big priority of the practice. By waiting just past the third ring, the caller is aware that the practice may be busy at the moment.

Two Calls at the Same Time. If a practice has a multiple telephone line system, sooner or later two lines will ring at virtually the same time. Instead of answering and holding in the order the calls are received (e.g., line one, then line two, then going back to answer line one), holding can be cut by 50% by picking up one line, asking the caller whether he or she is able to hold, and then picking up the other line and speaking with that caller directly. Either line one or line two can be picked up first. Callers will not know whether they are on line one or line two. The main objective is to minimize the number of callers who are asked to hold.

Transferring Calls. Some incoming calls will require transfer to another staff member. When transferring, the assistant should ask the caller whether he or she can hold so the call can be transferred. The assistant should let the caller know to whom he or she will be transferred. Also, when signaling the location or the person to whom you are transferring, you should announce or introduce the caller, such as "Dr. Marks, Mr. Olson is on line 1."

A proper call transfer might sound like this:

Assistant: Are you able to hold while I transfer you to Dr. Pearson's nurse, Donna?

Caller: Yes.

(Caller then is placed on hold.)

Assistant (signals nurse's station): Donna, Jane Doe is on line one.

Important things to remember when you are transferring include the following:

- Ask the caller if you may transfer the call.
- Explain to the caller what you are going to do: "Can you hold while I transfer you?"
- Announce the call: "Dr. O'Brian, Mrs. Johnson is on line one."
- When signaling the nurses' station via a speaker telephone, remember that it is possible people in the area may be able to hear. If a speaker telephone system is used, *never, ever* give sensitive information over the speaker. Something like "Mary Johnson is on line 1 for the results of her pregnancy test" is absolutely inappropriate. Obviously, this would embarrass some people, but, more important, it is a breach of confidentiality. A better way to transfer such a call is, "I have a patient on line one for the results of her lab work."

CHECKPOINT

Explain why training in proper telephone technique is important for every staff member of the medical office.

Automated Messages. In very busy offices, calls may be answered with an automated message if the telephone traffic is very heavy. Some offices prefer this to having the patient get a busy signal. Some offices may prefer to not use such a message because it may appear impersonal. Whether or not an automated system is used, it is imperative that emergency instructions be included in the message, for example, "You have reached Internal Medicine appointments. All lines are currently busy. If you are calling regarding an emergency, please hang up and call 911. Otherwise, please hold for the next available assistant."

Some automated systems can give the caller a choice to route their call to the appropriate department. For example, the following message might be used: "Press one for appointments, press two to leave a message for a health care professional."

After-Hours Calls. A practice will have patients who call when the clinic has closed. A practice must make arrangements to respond to after-hours calls. Answering services and **voice mail** systems are effective tools for handling after hours calls. The use of one of these methods is essential in helping the medical office communicate with patients regarding what they should do if they need medical attention and the office is closed.

Even though the office has voice mail or an answering service, an assistant should not rely on these alternatives to answer the telephone during business hours.

Voice Mail. A voice mail service is usually purchased along with standard telephone service. **Voice mail** plays a recorded message from the medical office staff when the telephone line is not answered after a certain number of rings. Voice mail can allow incoming messages to be recorded when the line is not answered or when a line is busy. Messages then may be played back when the assistant accesses the voice mail system. With today's technology, incoming calls are now tracked with computer programs, and these programs can store messages from patients and have the capability to recall messages almost instantly. Some offices may prefer to not allow messages to be recorded during or after hours. If a patient would call with a serious medical situation, an office may prefer to not have the patient leave a message as patients expect a return call if they are able to leave a message.

If a patient calls after hours, an outgoing message should be recorded that instructs the patient as to what should be done to get needed medical treatment until the office opens again. A message similar to the following might be used:

> *You have reached Happy Valley Medical Clinic. Our office is now closed. If you are calling about a medical emergency, please hang up and call 911. If you need immediate medical attention for a reason other than an emergency, 24-hour urgent care services are available at our facility located at 123 Main Avenue in Farmington. Our regular office hours are 9 AM to 6 PM weekdays and 9 AM to 12 PM on Saturday. Thank you for calling.*

Answering Services. An answering service is an outside company that provides individuals who answer the office telephone (at an offsite location) when the practice is closed. This alternative is used by practices that prefer to not have a machine or a recording answer the telephone. An

BOX 6-1

Potential Emergency Situations

If you receive a call regarding a patient who is experiencing any of the symptoms listed here, a medical professional should assess the situation immediately.*

- Shortness of breath
- Chest pain or pressure
- Pain in upper left arm
- Extreme dizziness or complaints of vertigo
- Loss of consciousness
- Serious injury or trauma such as broken bones or head injury
- Sudden numbness or tingling
- Blurred vision
- Slurred speech
- Severe, unrelenting headache
- Profuse, uncontrolled bleeding
- Acute abdominal pain

This list is not inclusive.

answering service answers the telephone during off hours and may give specific instructions to a patient regarding after hours care or may relay a message from a patient to an on-call provider. Answering services charge a monthly fee for services rendered.

Large group practices may prefer to provide their own staff to answer after-hours calls. Clinics, hospitals, and even insurance companies may decide to employ nursing staff who answer help lines 24 hours a day. Patients who fall ill or are injured after hours can call in and ask the nursing staff questions regarding their health situation. The staff in turn helps determine if the patient needs immediate medical treatment.

Telephone Screening. Because of the large volume of telephone traffic that most medical offices experience, screening of incoming calls is an absolute necessity in the medical office.

The screening process involves obtaining enough information about the call to handle it at the front desk or to transfer the call to the proper department. Screening actually reduces the number of calls that go back to the physician or nurse. If someone else in the office can handle a call, this makes the physician's time more productive. If at all possible, calls should be handled by the front desk.

Many patients will call a medical office and ask to speak to the physician directly. It is not often that such a call is transferred directly to the physician. Nearly all physicians prefer to have a message taken and then to have the message attached to the patient's medical record. The message and record then are forwarded to the physician. Physicians must refer to the patient's medical record so they can become familiar with the fine points of the patient's medical history and can document any call regarding medical treatment or advice given to the patient.

Identifying Emergencies Over the Telephone. Occasionally, a patient (or a relative of a patient) may telephone the clinic with a serious problem that may constitute an emergency regarding the patient's health. The person who is phoning in may or may not realize that the symptoms could pose a serious threat to the health of the patient. The medical administrative assistant must be aware of symptoms that could constitute a potentially serious health situation.

An emergency may be defined as a situation in which a patient's health might be adversely affected if immediate action is not taken. Box 6-1 outlines some critical symptoms of which an assistant should be aware. This is not an all-inclusive list but is designed to introduce you to some of the more common symptoms that may indicate an emergency situation. An assistant should review the list with the physicians in the practice to determine whether the physicians feel the list is inclusive enough for their office.

When you receive a questionable call in the clinic, you should be careful to not diagnose the patient, alarm the patient, or place the patient at undue risk. If a patient calls in with chest pain, before taking a message or making an appointment, an appropriate response by the assistant would be, "I'd like to have you speak with the nurse before I take a message" or "I'd like to have you speak with the nurse before I make an appointment."

The patient should *never* be told something like he or she might be having a heart attack. That statement may be interpreted as diagnosing the patient. The assistant also should be careful to not ask too many questions because the patient may feel that the assistant is prying, and because the number of questions asked may frighten the patient. The patient with a possible emergency also should *not* be told to go to the emergency department. Imagine what might happen if a patient gets into his or her car and drives to the emergency department. If the patient is having a heart attack, he or she could go into cardiac arrest while driving and die on the way to the hospital. Someone who is experiencing a possible heart attack or any serious medical emergency should never be behind the wheel of a car.

When the physician or nurse speaks directly to the patient and determines that the patient may be in a life-threatening situation, the physician or nurse will instruct the patient to call 911 immediately.

If you are wondering whether a situation is a potential emergency, remember this rule: *When in doubt, check it out!* Do not be afraid to check with the physician or nurse regarding any situation that you are unsure about.

Physician Out of the Office. If the physician is out of the office and is unavailable, tell the patient, "Dr. Sanchez is not in the office, but Dr. Marks is taking her calls" or "She's out of the office until (date). May I take a message or transfer you to...?" Do not mention that the physician is on vacation unless the physician approves. The physician may not want "the whole world" to know she is not at home.

Complaint Calls. No one enjoys answering complaint calls, but think of a complaint call as an opportunity to regain the patient's confidence in the office. If you should have to handle a call from a patient who is unhappy, use these suggestions for handling complaints:

MESSAGE FROM

For Dr.	Name of Caller	Rel. to pt.	Patient	Pt. Age	Pt. Temp.	Message Date	Message Time	Urgent
Lee	Susan Brimley	Mom	Elmo Brimley	14	100	8/4/xx	11:16 (AM) PM	☐ Yes ☒ No

Message: Elmo has had temp from 100–102 for 2 days – cough & thick green discharge from nose

Allergies

Respond to Phone #	Best Time To Call	Pharmacy Name/#	Patient's Chart Attached	Patient's Chart #	Initials
342-3444	any AM PM		☒ Yes ☐ No	BRIEL000	MAA

DOCTOR–STAFF RESPONSE

Doctor's/Staff Orders/Follow-up Action

Mom reports purulent nasal discharge, productive cough, ↑ temp and HA.
Instructed to make appt for today.

Call Back	Chart Mes.	Follow-up Date	Follow-up Completed–Date/Time	Response By:
☒ Yes ☐ No	☒ Yes ☐ No	8/4/xx	8/4/xx 11:45 (AM) PM	MMS

Figure 6-3 A message form (whether preprinted or electronic) may include a section for the physician or nurse to record how the call was handled. Message forms may become a permanent part of a patient's medical record. (Form courtesy of Bibbero Systems, Inc, Petaluma, California, 800-242-2376. Fax, 800-242-9330. Available at www.bibbero.com.)

- Acknowledge the patient's complaint. Even if the patient's complaint has no basis in fact, give the patient time to state his or her concerns.
- Ask the patient what you can do to help. If you can help the patient, do so. If you cannot help, find someone who can.
- Do not "pass the buck." Transferring the patient from person to person will only aggravate the patient. Help the patient if at all possible.
- Keep your cool even if the patient is angry. This can be difficult to do, but no argument with a patient was ever won.
- Do not make excuses such as "We're short-staffed today" or "The computer's down" or "We're so busy." All that these excuses convey is poor planning on the part of the practice.
- Do what you can to make sure the problem does not happen again. Take the problem and ideas for potential solutions to your supervisor if necessary.

Taking Messages. When reviewing the telephone protocol in Table 6-1, you will note that many calls require that a message be taken. When taking a message, enough information must be obtained from the caller to ensure that the call is handled properly. Remember that a message is taken to help the patient in some way, and that complete, detailed information will be needed to assist the patient as much as possible.

With today's electronic health record systems, telephone messages become part of the patient's medical record. A patient's health medical record is a legal document, and it is critical that you realize that the actual message you are writing will be a part of a patient's permanent medical record. Paper message blanks themselves can be directly adhered to the medical record. Messages are written on a full, half, or quarter sheet of paper, and the physician or nurse will document their response to the message (Fig. 6-3).

If the patient's message is recorded in an electronic health record system, these systems allow both messages to be taken and transmitted to the intended recipient electronically. No paper needs to be used at all. The same information is required for an electronic message as a written message, but instead of a slip of paper being sent to a physician, the message is created within an electronic health record system and is sent electronically to a physician via the office's computer system. Even electronic messages will become part of the patient's medical record.

When an assistant realizes that a message will have to be taken, a complete message will contain at least nine essential pieces of information necessary to process the message (Procedure 6-2):

1. and 2. *Date and time of call.* On every message, list the complete date (month, day, and year) that the call came in. AM or PM should be identified with the time. The date and time of a message are vital pieces of information should a question or problem later arise involving the patient's care.
3. *Caller's name.* The caller's complete name should be obtained.

PROCEDURE 6-2

Demonstrate Taking Telephone Messages

Materials Needed

- Telephone setup with two separate lines
- Message blanks
- Pencil

1. Determine that a message is needed for an incoming telephone call, and obtain a message blank on which to record the message.
2. Record date and time on message blank.
3. Record caller's name on message blank.
4. Record patient's name on message blank.*
5. Obtain patient's chart number. If chart number is not available, obtain patient's date of birth to help locate the chart number.
6. Record name of individual to whom the call is directed—physician or another individual.
7. Record message narrative, including action requested, on message blank.
8. Record telephone number to return call.
9. Sign the message with your name or initials.

**Denotes a crucial step in the procedure. This step must be completed satisfactorily for the procedure to be completed satisfactorily.*

4. *Patient's name.* If the patient's name is different from the caller's name, be sure to obtain the complete name of the patient. In the case of a parent who is calling on behalf of a child, the call will be returned to the parent, but the medical staff will need the child's medical record when speaking with the parent. If a caller is not the patient, the caller's relationship to the patient should always be noted.
5. *Medical record number.* If the call involves anything regarding the patient's health or medical history, the patient's medical information will be needed. The physician may have to review the patient's past medical history and/or medications and will need to make a notation in the record regarding the disposition of the call. Obtain the patient's date of birth to accurately identify his or her record. If a patient calls with a medical question and is a new patient to the practice, obtain the patient's date of birth to see whether information may have been received about the patient. It then should be noted on the message that the patient is new or does not have medical information on file with the practice.
6. *Provider name or the person who is called.* This identifies the individual to whom the call is directed, such as physician, nurse, therapist, etc.
7. *Operator (person receiving the call—assistant's name or initials).* The assistant who is taking a message must sign each message. This is done because if the medical staff has a question about the message, they may need to talk with the assistant who took the message. In most offices, the operator may be identified by his or her initials.
8. *Message narrative.* Information given to the assistant in the conversation with the patient should be listed on the message. This includes the patient's concern or reason for calling the medical office. The assistant also should include the action requested by the caller. Often, options for action are listed on the message form. A box to check in front of items such as "please return call" or "urgent" may be included on the message form. The assistant also may have to write a patient's request for action in the message narrative. An example of an action would be a request that a prescription be filled at a particular pharmacy.
9. *Telephone number.* A telephone number at which the caller can be reached should be obtained for each message. If the caller will be available only at a certain time, note the availability near the telephone number (e.g., "555-1122 after 3 PM"). Some callers may want to leave more than one number, such as a cell telephone number or a work number. Because many people have cell phones from an area of the country in which they don't live, area codes should be included with all telephone numbers to ensure that the patient will be able to be reached.

Communications Equipment

Many different kinds of telephones are readily available in the marketplace. The size of the practice will dictate just how much telephone equipment is needed. Most offices require a telephone system with speaker or intercom connections that allow calls to be transferred within the office easily.

A telephone with a minimum of two incoming and outgoing lines is necessary (Fig. 6-4) for even the smallest of practices to ensure that patients who call in are able to reach the office, and that office personnel (physicians and nurses) and communications equipment (fax machines and computers) have outside telephone access.

The telephone is not the only piece of communications equipment in the medical office. Many other devices work in conjunction with the office telephone or may operate independent of the office telephone.

Switchboard. Larger practices will likely have a switchboard system that allows calls to be answered by a central switchboard operator (Fig. 6-5). Computerized switchboard systems are now available to help track the flow of telephone traffic within the office.

Some switchboard systems allow calls to bypass the switchboard. This bypass can occur when the caller, instead of calling the main switchboard, dials an extension number directly. The call then goes directly to the intended recipient without having to be handled by the switchboard operator. Dialing an extension directly helps to reduce the number of calls handled by the switchboard. A direct dial number might be used to allow a hospital laboratory department to reach a clinic laboratory directly or vice versa. This type of call would not have to be handled by the switchboard. Using direct dial numbers greatly reduces the calls that are received at the front desk and thereby frees an assistant's time to handle other important office matters.

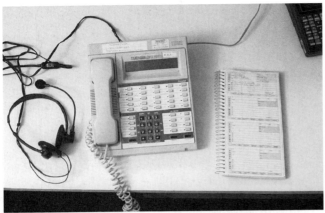

Figure 6-4 Multiline telephones are necessary for the medical office to accommodate patients calling in and staff calling out.

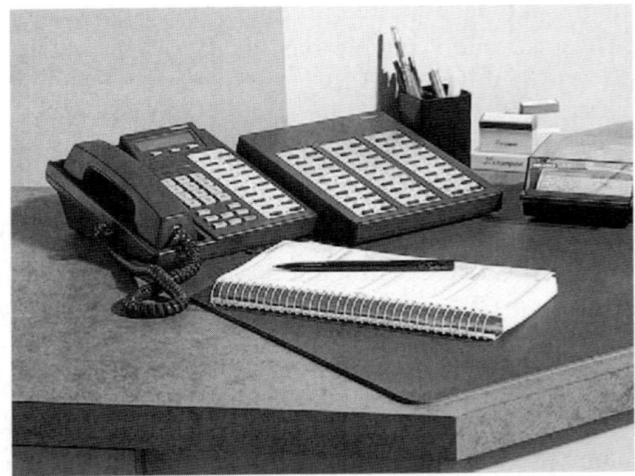

Figure 6-5 Large medical practices have a central switchboard that directs calls to the proper area in the practice. (From Young AP: *Kinn's The Administrative Medical Assistant,* ed 7, St. Louis, Saunders, 2011.)

Pager. Very often, a physician may need to be contacted when not in the clinic. A pager can be used to reach physicians in such instances.

To reach a physician using a pager, an assistant simply needs to call the pager's telephone number and leave a message. Depending on the type of pager service, the assistant may leave a verbal message or may enter a telephone number for the physician to call. An important point to remember when leaving a verbal message is to *maintain patient confidentiality.* You will not know exactly where the physician may be when the message is played, so do not leave any message that could cause embarrassment to a patient.

Cell Phone. Cell phones, too, can help the physician stay in touch with the office when the physician is away. Cell phones allow physicians to stay in immediate contact with the practice.

A major concern with cell telephone use is that calls may be intercepted or overheard by others. Obviously, for this reason, confidential information should not be discussed over a cell telephone. It is important for an office to develop a cell telephone policy that addresses how a cell telephone may be used when confidential medical information is discussed.

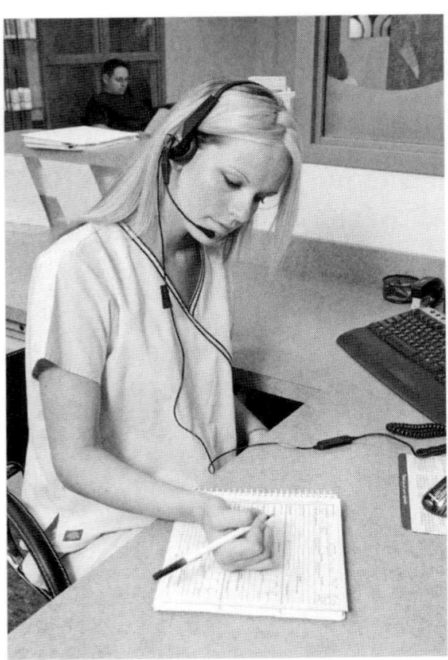

Figure 6-6 A headset allows a medical administrative assistant to write messages and operate a computer while on the telephone with a patient. (From Young AP: *Kinn's The Administrative Medical Assistant,* ed 6, St. Louis, Saunders, 2007.)

Headsets. Headsets are small devices that fit over the operator's head (Fig. 6-6) and direct sound into the operator's ears. Office headsets contain a microphone that allows the operator to carry on a complete conversation with the caller. Headsets are particularly useful because they allow operators to use their hands while on the telephone. The devices plug directly into the telephone and can allow an operator to answer the telephone with either the handset or the headset.

Using a headset is a good idea if an assistant is spending a large amount of time on the telephone. It is very difficult to balance a handset on a shoulder while trying to write a message or type information into a computer at the same time. If a headset is not used, over time, a "shoulder balancing" posture may cause an assistant to develop a neck injury as a result of repeated incorrect posture.

If a headset is used in a reception area where patients are assisted, many patients may not see that the assistant is wearing a headset and may begin to speak to the assistant while the assistant is on the telephone. When a patient approaches the desk, the assistant will have to allow the patient to see that the assistant is speaking with a patient on the telephone. Some offices even place a small sign on the receptionist's desk that lights up when the assistant is on the telephone.

Facsimile. A facsimile, or fax machine (Fig. 6-7), is a valuable piece of equipment in the medical office. Fax machines allow printed data to be transmitted almost instantly to another location anywhere in the world. A document is read electronically by one fax machine at one location and is transmitted to a fax machine at another location. Anything that is readable on a sheet of paper can be faxed; however, faxing is not the usual way to send medical information. Faxing is done only when the information must be transmitted expediently for care of the patient.

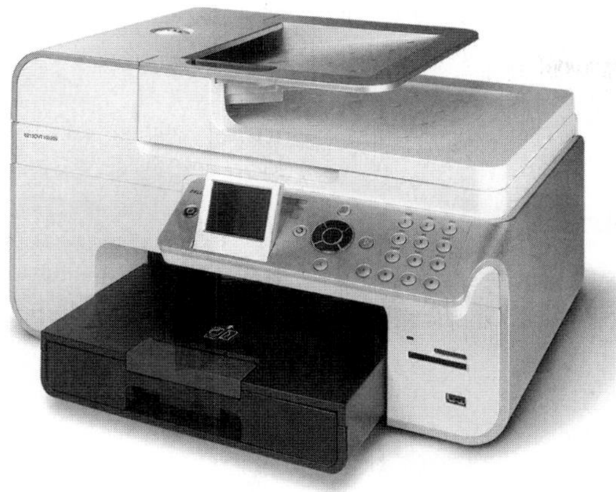

Figure 6-7 A fax machine can quickly send and receive information between health care facilities. Because of confidentiality concerns, a medical administrative assistant should use a fax machine with caution in the medical office. (From Young AP: *Kinn's The Administrative Medical Assistant.* 6th ed. St Louis, Saunders Elsevier; 2007, Fig. 9-4.)

Confidentiality concerns also exist with the use of a fax machine. A patient's medical information should not be sent via fax without the patient's expressed consent. In the case of an emergency or life-threatening situation, faxed material may be sent without the patient's knowledge if the information is needed to treat the patient; however, such a release of information occurs infrequently.

When transmitting medical information by fax, an assistant must exercise great care in entering the fax number. If one number is entered incorrectly, sensitive information may end up in the wrong hands.

New technology enables documents to be electronically sent using a device called a **digital sender**. Such equipment can scan many pages quickly and convert the pages into a pdf document. The machine then can be used to email the pdf file to any email address. Such equipment still has the same privacy concerns as a fax machine. It is critical to ensure that the information is going only where it needs to go.

HIPAA Hint

Fax machines and digital senders used for transmitting and receiving patient information must be placed in a secure area in order to safeguard this information.

Telephone Services

Several additional services may be available from local telephone companies. These services may enhance the customer service that the office staff is able to provide. The practice will have to weigh the potential benefit of the services versus their costs. The following services may be of benefit to a medical office:

- Caller ID. Caller ID features are available on many phones. Caller ID displays the number and the name of who is calling before the call is answered.
- Three-way calling. This feature allows three parties in three separate locations to speak simultaneously. This may be particularly helpful in telephone conferences among one or more physicians, a patient, and one or more family members.
- Call forwarding. Calls are forwarded from one telephone number to another. If a medical office is closed during a vacation, calls may be forwarded to another physician's office that may be taking calls for the physician.
- Conference calls. With this feature, several individuals at different locations may speak with each other simultaneously. Three or more parties at separate locations can be connected on the same call.

Communications technology is constantly changing and is growing at almost an exponential rate. Video calls over an Internet connection enable callers to see each other while talking. Texting is a common feature for cell telephone users, and this application one day may be used by medical offices to communicate with patients. At the present time, these applications are not secure; therefore, they are not used because of concerns regarding privacy. Whatever technology the future does bring, if it benefits patients, it is sure to have an impact on how business is conducted in a medical office.

Outgoing Calls

Although most of the practice's calls will be incoming calls, occasionally an assistant will have to call a patient.

Many offices have long-distance calling plans, which reduce the cost of making a long-distance call. Some practices have toll-free lines, but it may be cheaper to call long-distance and pay the per-minute charge, while reserving the toll-free line for incoming long-distance calls.

Using a Telephone Directory

Traditional printed telephone directories contain a wealth of information about telephone service, as well as information about the community. Information regarding calling features, area codes, and how to obtain services is available in most telephone directories. Community information, such as local area maps, local ZIP codes, and community services, is frequently found in many directories. An assistant should take the time to review the local telephone directory to become familiar with the type of information that is available in the directory.

Web Directories

Many online directories are readily available on the Internet. These electronic directories allow users to search for an address or telephone number for a business or a person in any state. The directories are usually available free to the user and are paid for by the advertisers who sponsor the site. An Internet search also can be used to locate contact information for other health care providers or facilities.

Developing a Personal Directory

A personal directory of frequently called numbers should be kept on hand at the front desk. It is the responsibility of the

Happy Valley Medical Group
5222 East Baseline Road
Gilbert, AZ 85234

TELEPHONE RELEASE

I hereby authorize Happy Valley Medical Group to contact me by telephone in the following manner:

Check all options that apply

Contact number (provide telephone number)	Okay to leave message with detailed information (specify names of individuals)	Leave a message with return number only	Do not leave a message
Home number			
Cell number			
Work number			
Other (specify)			
Other (specify)			

____________________ ______/______/______
Patient Name – please print month date year

____________________ ____________________
Signature of patient or authorized representative medical record number

Figure 6-8 A telephone release is absolutely necessary before you can leave messages on a patient's telephone.

front desk staff to maintain a directory of telephone numbers for physicians and other staff members, as well as for other businesses that are frequently contacted by the office. These numbers should be recorded in an easy-to-use reference, such as a computer list or a printed-paper file. The directories then should be available at the front desk and at other office telephones to allow easy accessibility for all office staff.

Frequently called numbers also can be stored in memory on many telephones. This storage can substantially reduce the amount of time it takes to dial a frequently called number. If the practice is continually calling a laboratory, such as another physician's office, a hospital, or a surgery center, storing these numbers in the telephone's memory can save a lot of time.

Leaving Messages for Patients

If a patient is not at home, the practice may prefer that the assistant leave a message for the patient. Depending on the nature of the practice and the wishes of the practice's physicians, however, a message may be left to ask a patient to return a call to the practice. Obviously, practices such as mental health clinics or other specialty treatment centers would not leave messages for patients because if the wrong person hears the message, the nature of the patient's treatment may be implied by the call.

Some offices may ask a patient to sign a telephone release (Fig. 6-8). Such a release gives a health care facility permission to leave messages with a patient's family member on an answering machine or by voice mail. Even if a telephone release has been signed by a patient, an assistant should be careful to not leave detailed embarrassing information on a message. An appropriate message to leave in such a situation would be, "This is Happy Valley Medical Clinic. Please call Taylor at 555-1234."

In the absence of a telephone release, remember not to divulge any confidential information. Even with a release, you should exercise extreme caution when leaving a message for a patient. Excessive information in a message may cause embarrassment to a patient even if a family member receives the message. There is no way of knowing who may listen to the message. Some practices prefer to never leave a message for a patient. A message as simple as "Call Amy at 555-3424 about your appointment" may seem harmless enough but actually may cause problems if the patient does not want a spouse to know about the appointment. It is best to consult with the practice's physicians to establish a policy on leaving messages.

HIPAA Hint

When leaving a telephone message with an individual, be sure to verify the individual's name, and verify that the individual has the right to the information you will leave in the message. Once the individual's identity has been verified, the individual may receive the information.

If leaving a message on an answering machine or voice mail, leave a message stating the facility from which you are calling and a telephone number for the patient to return the call. DO NOT leave lab results, medication information, or physician names in a message.

The following information is identified as highly confidential information. Never leave a message that contains **highly confidential information.**

- Mental illness or developmental disability
- HIV/AIDS treatment
- Communicable or venereal diseases
- Substance abuse
- Physical abuse
- Genetic testing

Written Communication

Not all business can be conducted over the telephone or in person, and, occasionally, an assistant will need to write a letter to a patient or a memo to office staff members. When communicating in written form, it is imperative that the assistant follow proper grammar rules. Your written word is a reflection of you and the practice.

When correspondence is written, a good set of reference materials is a must. A well-stocked office library would include medical and English dictionaries, medical word books, pharmaceutical references, and style references such as *The Gregg Reference Manual* or another office style manual. These references will be used frequently to look up spelling and appropriate usage of terms, as well as styles of written correspondence.

Many medical references are available online as well. Medical dictionaries and sites with medical information can be helpful for verifying spelling and correct usage of medical terms. Electronic medical references for computer systems also can be purchased.

Business Letters

Letters in the medical office are written on 8.5 × 11–inch office letterhead. A letterhead contains the name of the medical facility and complete mailing address, as well as the telephone number(s) of the practice, along with any logo of the practice. If the practice is small, the names of the providers may be included on letterhead. Some very large practices with many physicians may choose to print the names of the physicians in a lighter ink on the back of the stationery. Some large practices choose to not place any physician names on stationery at all because the staff may change frequently and the physician list will become outdated quickly.

All written correspondence from a medical office should be written on letterhead. This gives a professional look to the information presented within the letter. Once a letter is typewritten, it is presented to the physician for signature. A copy of every letter containing medical information written to a patient is placed in the patient's medical record, and copies of all other letters (letters pertaining to the patient's account or finances) are filed in the appropriate office file.

Components of a Letter

Many word processing packages provide templates or sample formats for easy letter and memo writing. A medical office also may choose to develop its own template to create a uniform format for all letters. Examples of letters are shown in Figures 6-9, 6-10, and 6-11, with line spacing for each type of letter noted in the left-hand margin. Even though margins may vary, letters have many of the same basic components, and these appear within a letter in the following order. See Procedure 6-3 for a summary of how to prepare a letter.

PROCEDURE 6-3

Prepare a Patient Letter

Materials Needed

- Computer with word processing software
- Printer
- Letterhead stationery
- No. 10 business envelope
- Reference materials as necessary (e.g., dictionary, grammar reference)

1. Prepare a letter to a patient using the proper components as listed below, and format as illustrated in Figures 6-9, 6-10, and 6-11.
   a. Margins
   b. Date
   c. Inside address
   d. Salutation
   e. Subject line
   f. Body
   g. Closing
   h. Notations
      i. Reference initials
      ii. Computer file name
      iii. Enclosure notation
      iv. Copy notation
2. Proofread the letter for proper grammar and punctuation.*
3. Print enough copies of the letter.
4. Address a business envelope using proper components as listed below, and format for an OCR as illustrated in Figure 6-12.
   a. Addressee
   b. Street address
   c. City ST ZIP
5. Fold and insert letter into an envelope as shown in Figure 6-13.

**Denotes a crucial step in the procedure. This step must be completed satisfactorily for the procedure to be completed satisfactorily.*

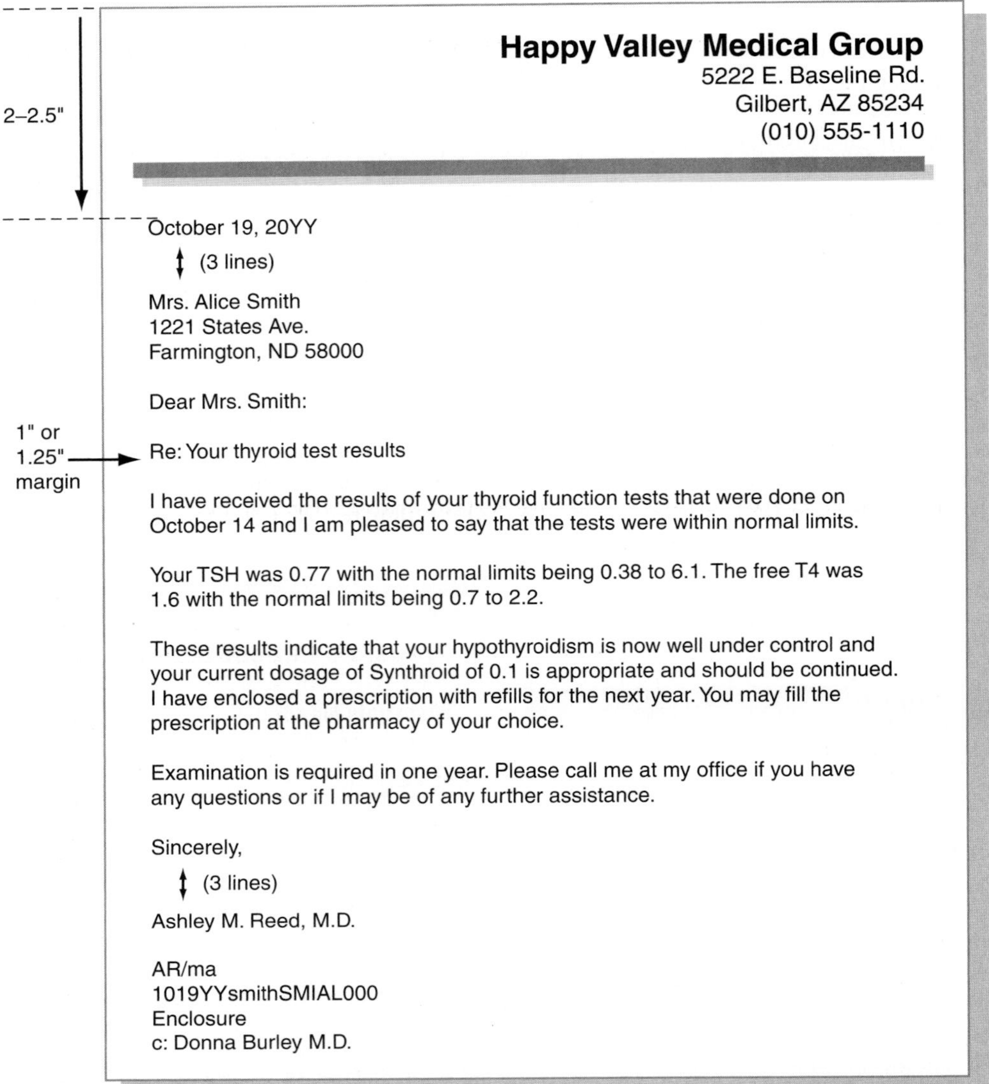

Happy Valley Medical Group
5222 E. Baseline Rd.
Gilbert, AZ 85234
(010) 555-1110

October 19, 20YY

Mrs. Alice Smith
1221 States Ave.
Farmington, ND 58000

Dear Mrs. Smith:

Re: Your thyroid test results

I have received the results of your thyroid function tests that were done on October 14 and I am pleased to say that the tests were within normal limits.

Your TSH was 0.77 with the normal limits being 0.38 to 6.1. The free T4 was 1.6 with the normal limits being 0.7 to 2.2.

These results indicate that your hypothyroidism is now well under control and your current dosage of Synthroid of 0.1 is appropriate and should be continued. I have enclosed a prescription with refills for the next year. You may fill the prescription at the pharmacy of your choice.

Examination is required in one year. Please call me at my office if you have any questions or if I may be of any further assistance.

Sincerely,

Ashley M. Reed, M.D.

AR/ma
1019YYsmithSMIAL000
Enclosure
c: Donna Burley M.D.

Figure 6-9 A block-style letter is an efficient, easy-to-use format for business letters.

Date. The date should be formatted as follows: June 15, 20xx. Some physicians may prefer to use a military date, for example, 15 June 2014. A format such as 6-15-14 is not acceptable for a business letter.

If a physician dates a letter, the date of the letter will be the date that the letter was dictated, or a date otherwise specified by the physician. If a member of the office staff is creating and preparing a letter, the date on the letter usually will be the date the letter was prepared.

The date line should start at between 2 and 2.5 inches from the top of an 8.5 × 11–inch sheet of paper. The length of the letter will determine where the date is placed. A longer letter will include the date closer to the 2-inch mark because the letter will take up more of the page. It is possible and preferable to adjust the top and side margins a bit in order to fit a letter onto one page. A one-page letter is preferable because a 2-page letter may possibly end up with the pages separated.

Inside Address. The **inside address** consists of the complete name and address of the person to whom the letter is being written. This person is known as the addressee. The correct format of the inside address is as follows:

Ms. Lydia Marten
607 Sweet Avenue
Harvester, MN 55555

In cases in which information is sent regarding a minor, the letter should be addressed to the child's parent or legal guardian.

Salutation. The **salutation** is a greeting to the addressee. An acceptable salutation for most business letters would include a title such as Mr., Mrs., or Miss, along with the patient's or the guardian's last name; this would appear as follows: Dear Ms. Marten. If the physician knows the patient well, he or she may choose to use a more personal salutation such as Dear Lydia.

Subject Line. The subject line appears below the salutation and above the body of the letter. The subject of the letter is written after the colon. In a letter to a physician regarding

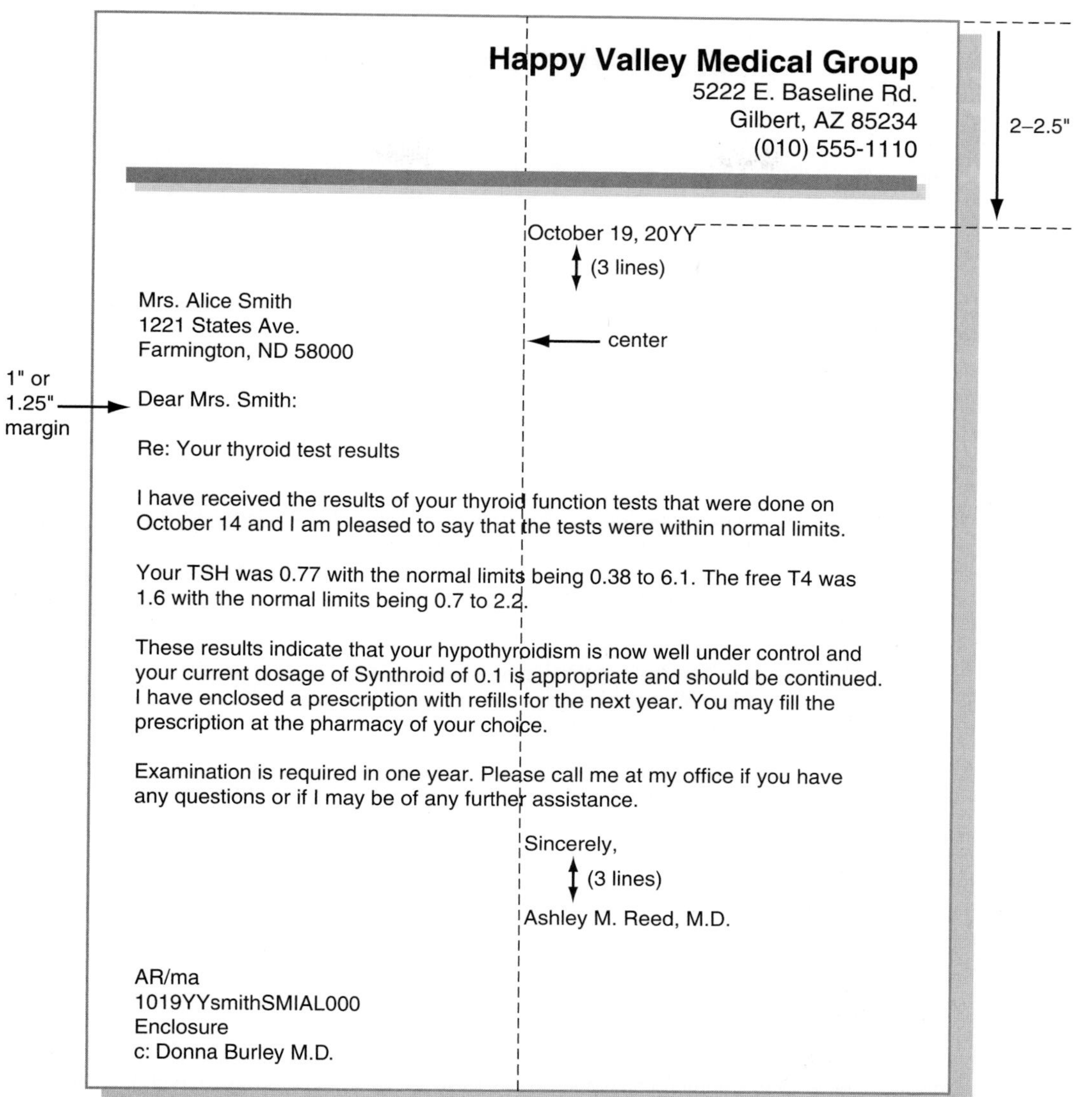

Happy Valley Medical Group
5222 E. Baseline Rd.
Gilbert, AZ 85234
(010) 555-1110

October 19, 20YY

Mrs. Alice Smith
1221 States Ave.
Farmington, ND 58000

Dear Mrs. Smith:

Re: Your thyroid test results

I have received the results of your thyroid function tests that were done on October 14 and I am pleased to say that the tests were within normal limits.

Your TSH was 0.77 with the normal limits being 0.38 to 6.1. The free T4 was 1.6 with the normal limits being 0.7 to 2.2.

These results indicate that your hypothyroidism is now well under control and your current dosage of Synthroid of 0.1 is appropriate and should be continued. I have enclosed a prescription with refills for the next year. You may fill the prescription at the pharmacy of your choice.

Examination is required in one year. Please call me at my office if you have any questions or if I may be of any further assistance.

Sincerely,

Ashley M. Reed, M.D.

AR/ma
1019YYsmithSMIAL000
Enclosure
c: Donna Burley M.D.

Figure 6-10 A modified-block style letter differs from a block style letter in that the date and the closing are indented to the center of the page.

a mutual patient, the subject line might read: Subject: Mrs. Alice Shepard. In a letter to a patient, the subject line would probably contain the main purpose of the letter (e.g., your recent thyroid test results).

The purpose of using a subject line is to enable all medical office personnel to quickly identify the chief reason for the letter. This could be a time-saving device if there are many letters within a patient's file.

Body. Information to be communicated to the patient is included in the **body** of the letter. The body often will include at least three paragraphs: an introduction, a main message, and a closing. Three paragraphs are not required; some letters are much longer, or some may consist of only one paragraph. Whatever the case, the use of smaller, shorter paragraphs makes a letter much easier to read.

If a letter is long and requires more than one page, a page notation should be used at the top of the second page to identify the addressee of the letter and other important information about the letter. This notation is absolutely necessary because a copy is made of all letters, and should the second page of the copy be separated from the first, it will be easy to identify where the second page belongs if a notation is present. A standard page notation includes the patient's name and medical record number, the page number of the letter, and the date the letter was written. The notation would look as follows:

Lydia Marten No. 12345
Page 2
June 1, 20xx

Closing. A complimentary **closing** such as Sincerely or Cordially is used to end the letter. Then the author's name is typewritten on the fourth line below the closing. This produces a blank space of three lines in which the author can sign the letter. Letters authored by physicians are signed with the use of MD and any other academic notations after the physician's name, for example, Dr. Timothy I. Marks, MD, PhD, or Dr. Kristine O'Brian, MD.

Notations. **Notations** include information written mainly for the sender of the letter. Who dictated and

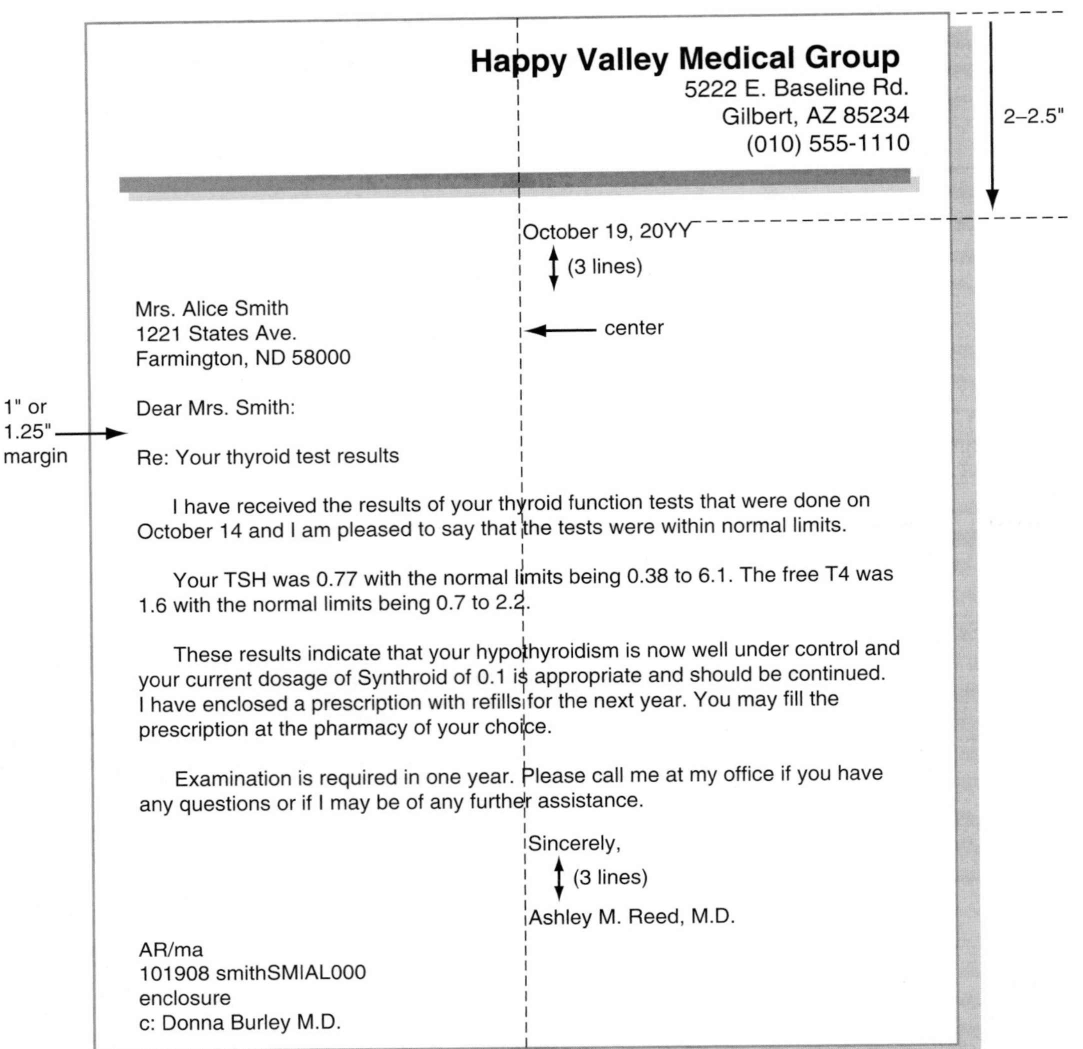
Happy Valley Medical Group
5222 E. Baseline Rd.
Gilbert, AZ 85234
(010) 555-1110

October 19, 20YY

Mrs. Alice Smith
1221 States Ave.
Farmington, ND 58000

Dear Mrs. Smith:

Re: Your thyroid test results

I have received the results of your thyroid function tests that were done on October 14 and I am pleased to say that the tests were within normal limits.

Your TSH was 0.77 with the normal limits being 0.38 to 6.1. The free T4 was 1.6 with the normal limits being 0.7 to 2.2.

These results indicate that your hypothyroidism is now well under control and your current dosage of Synthroid of 0.1 is appropriate and should be continued. I have enclosed a prescription with refills for the next year. You may fill the prescription at the pharmacy of your choice.

Examination is required in one year. Please call me at my office if you have any questions or if I may be of any further assistance.

Sincerely,

Ashley M. Reed, M.D.

AR/ma
101908 smithSMIAL000
enclosure
c: Donna Burley M.D.

Figure 6-11 A modified-block style letter with indented paragraphs is similar to the letter in Figure 6-10, with the addition of indents at the beginning of paragraphs.

transcribed the letter and who received copies of the letter and information included with the letter are examples of information included in various notations. Notations begin two lines below the author's name and appear in the following order:

- ***Reference initials***. These include the initials of the author and of the transcriptionist. The author's initials are capitalized and the transcriptionist's initials appear in lowercase letters. A slash is used to separate the initials, for example, TM/bp.
- ***Computer file name notation***. Because virtually all letters are electronically prepared with word processing software, an office can quickly store a multitude of letters in a computer system. Sometimes after a letter has been transcribed, a physician may make changes within the letter. Those changes can be made quickly if the letter has been stored. **File names** should be systematically assigned according to a uniform format and should be meaningful. For example, 091008olson28632 could be used to identify the date the letter was written and the last name and medical record number of the patient. Both the chart number and the last name would identify a specific individual to whom the letter was written. The date would be necessary to differentiate the file name from previous letters sent to the patient.
- ***Enclosure notation***. This notation identifies whether or not anything is included with the letter. This would alert a transcriptionist, an assistant, or anyone responsible for sending a letter that something should be included with the letter. If a physician has stated something in the letter such as, "I have attached a copy of your lab report" or "A prescription for Diovan is enclosed," this would indicate to the transcriptionist or the assistant that an enclosure should be noted and inserted with the letter.
- ***Copy notation***. A copy of every letter will be included in the patient's medical record. This is NOT the purpose of a copy notation. The copy notation indicates whether another individual other than the addressee is to receive

a copy of the letter. This notation is simply the letter "c" followed by a colon and the name of the party who is to receive the copy, for example, c: Donna Burley, MD. Refer to Figure 6-9 for an example of how all of the above notations are used. Historically, copy notations were identified as "cc:" which stood for carbon copy. Thankfully, the use of carbon copies is a thing of the past and the use of "cc:" has been changed to "c:".

Proper Format

A business letter can be formatted properly in various ways. Some of the more commonly used formats are the block style (see Fig. 6-9) and the modified-block style (see Figs. 6-10 and 6-11).

Most letters begin 2 inches from the top of the page. This spacing allows room for any letterhead that may be used. Occasionally, a letter may be lengthy, and you may have to alter the top and bottom margins to fit the letter on one page. Be sure to leave enough room at the top and bottom of the page to create a professional looking letter. Spacing for the various components of a letter is shown in Figures 6-9, 6-10, and 6-11.

Top and bottom margins should be set at 1 inch. Depending on the type of word processing used, default settings for side margins may range from 1 to 1.25 inches. Margins can be adjusted for both short and long letters to make the letters look more appealing on the page. You may wish to change default settings for margins to accommodate an office's letterhead.

Block Style. A **block-style** letter is probably the easiest type of business letter to produce. All letter components are flush with the left margin of the page. No indentations are used in this style, with the exception of tables or other elements that may have to be set apart in the body of the letter. An example of the block style, also known as **full-block style**, is shown in Figure 6-9.

Modified-Block Style. The modified-block style differs from the block style in that the date, complimentary closing, and author's signature begin in the center of the page. The remaining information is flush with the left margin (see Fig. 6-10). If the author prefers to indent the paragraphs in the body of the letter, this type of letter is known as a **modified-block style** with indented paragraphs or a **semiblock** style (see Fig. 6-11).

Envelopes

Standard size No. 10 business envelopes are used for business correspondence. Figure 6-12 demonstrates the proper format for addressing a business envelope. For addressing an envelope, the U.S. Postal Service has suggested these specific guidelines, which should be followed to allow envelopes to be easily read by an automated mail processing machine known as an **Optical Character Reader** (OCR). A complete list of the postal addressing standards can be found in Publication 28 by the U.S. Postal Service.

- Use all capital letters with no punctuation. Refer to Figure 6-12.
- Use black ink on white or light-colored envelopes.
- Fonts should be simple to read. Fancy fonts are difficult for machines to pick up and will cause delays in processing mail. Use at least a 10-point font.
- Left justify the address.
- Use one space between city and state and two spaces between state and ZIP.
- If using labels, be sure that labels are complete and that addresses haven't been cut off. Make sure labels are on straight.

When you are addressing a letter with an attention line, put the attention line at the top of the address, for example,

Attn Dr Maria Sanchez
Horizons Healthcare Center
123 Main Avenue
Farmington ND 58000

Release of Information
Horizons Healthcare Center
123 Main Avenue
Farmington ND 58000

- Use the free online ZIP code lookup of the U.S. Postal Service, which is located at www.usps.gov.

When the letter is placed in an envelope, the letter should be folded in thirds and inserted as indicated in Figure 6-13. This method of folding allows the letter to be removed easily when received and to be read by the recipient.

Letter Portfolio

It is a good idea to develop a portfolio of the varieties of letters written in the medical office. Simply saving copies of letters in a printed file or a computer file creates a letter portfolio. Later, when an assistant is asked to compose a letter, a portfolio provides excellent examples of letter "how-to's." A letter portfolio could contain examples for such letters as billing collection, instructions for specific procedures or tests, directions to a medical facility, or information on office procedures. When compiling a letter portfolio, an assistant must delete any patient references in the letter—name, address, chart number, and any other identifying information—that may be confidential.

> **HIPAA Hint**
>
> Health care providers must allow individuals to request an alternative means for the provider to contact the individual. An individual may request that a provider communicate through a specific telephone number or address.

Memos

Memos are internal communication pieces that are used in many offices. A memo allows information to be dispersed in an efficient format to other staff members in the office. Memos are used regularly to distribute routine information to employees regarding business procedures or occurrences. Memos may be written on blank sheets of paper or letterhead. It is inappropriate to write to a patient in a memo format. An example of a memo is shown in Figure 6-14.

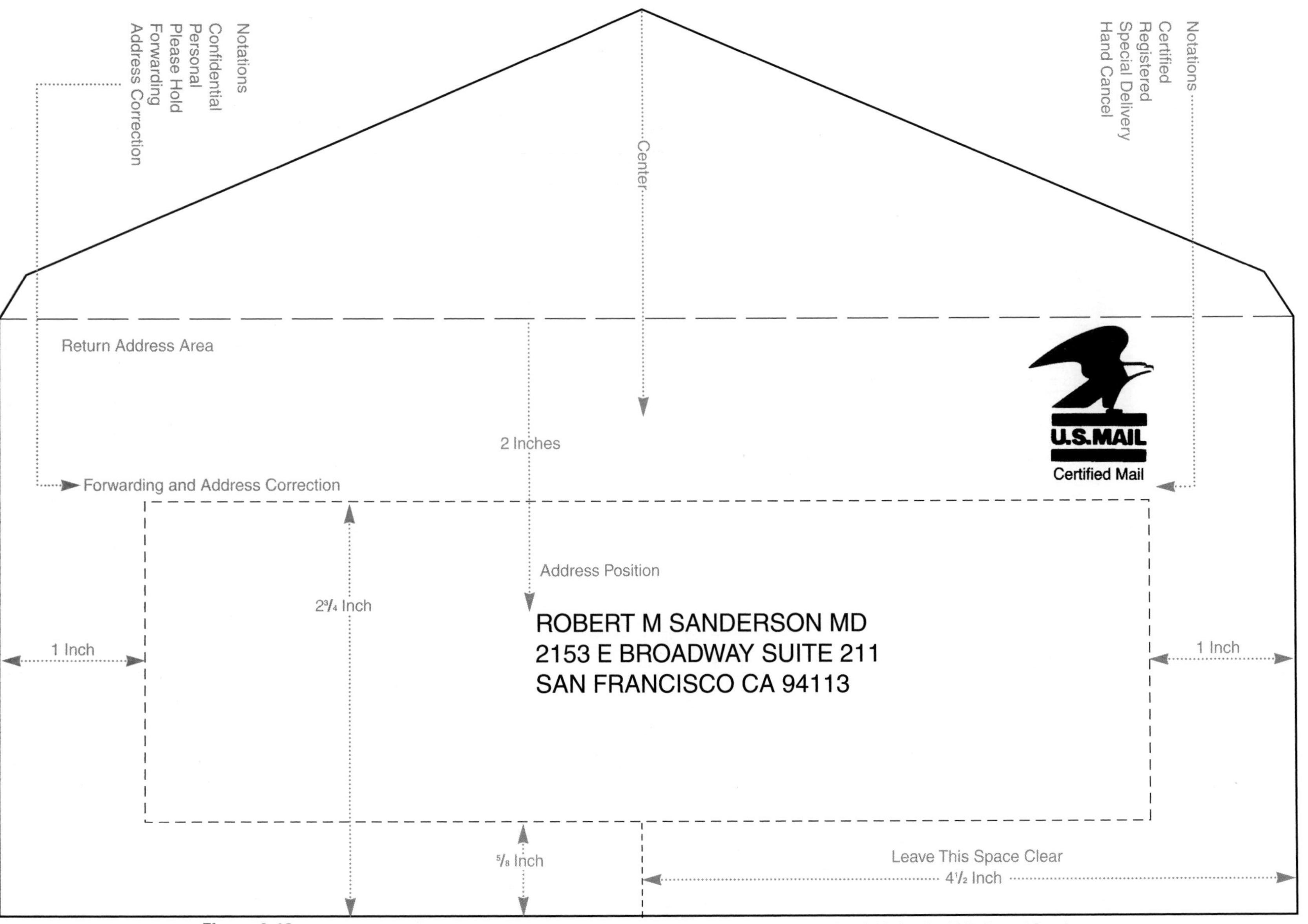

Figure 6-12 Proper format on a business envelope will ensure that a letter is processed quickly by the U.S. Postal Service.

No. 10 Envelope (9-1/2 x 4-1/8 Inches)

DO bring up the bottom third of the sheet, and crease. Fold down the upper third of the sheet so the top edge is a one-inch from the first fold, and crease. Insert the last creased edge into the envelope first.

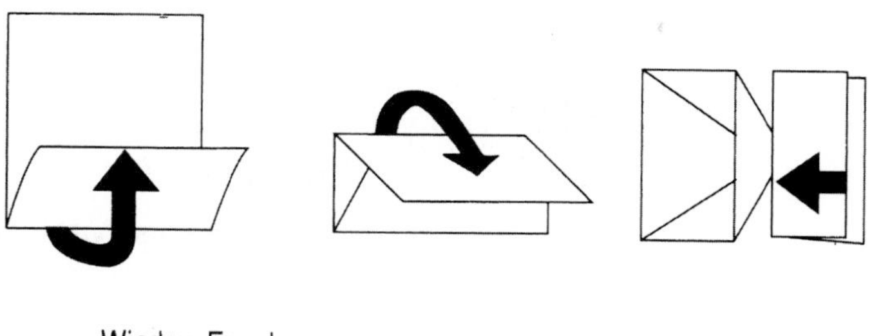

Window Envelope

DO bring up the bottom third of the sheet and fold. Fold the top of the sheet *back* to the first fold so that the inside address is on the outside, and crease. Insert the sheet so the address appears in the window.

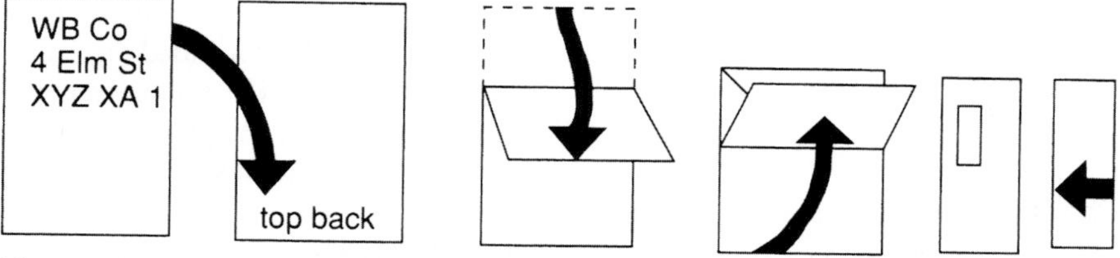

Figure 6-13 Properly folding and inserting a letter into a business envelope allows for easy reading when the letter is received. (From Diehl MO. *Medical Transcription.* 7th ed. St Louis, Saunders Elsevier, 2011.)

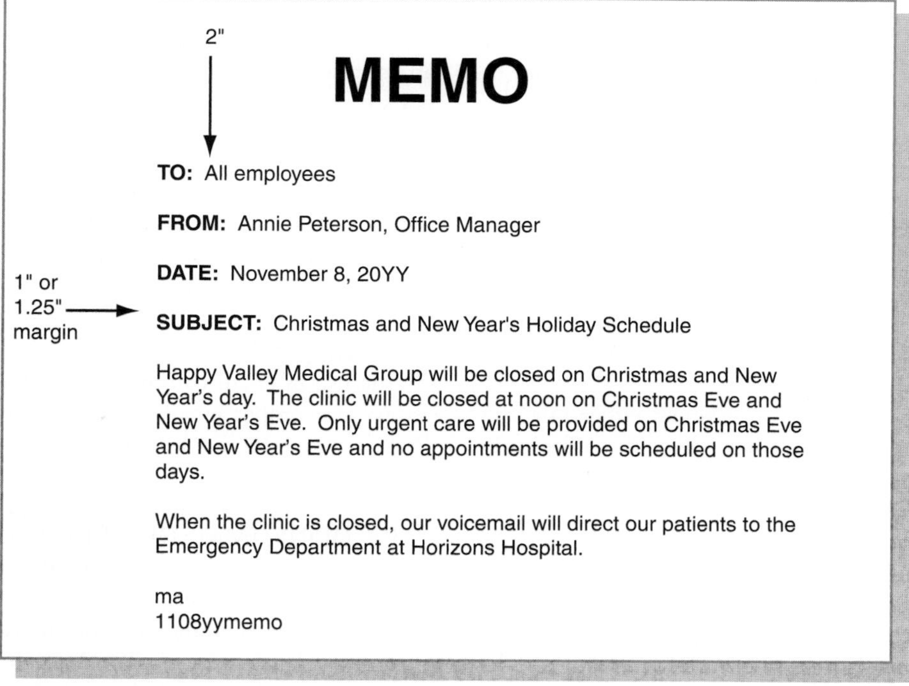

MEMO

TO: All employees

FROM: Annie Peterson, Office Manager

DATE: November 8, 20YY

SUBJECT: Christmas and New Year's Holiday Schedule

Happy Valley Medical Group will be closed on Christmas and New Year's day. The clinic will be closed at noon on Christmas Eve and New Year's Eve. Only urgent care will be provided on Christmas Eve and New Year's Eve and no appointments will be scheduled on those days.

When the clinic is closed, our voicemail will direct our patients to the Emergency Department at Horizons Hospital.

ma
1108yymemo

Figure 6-14 Following the proper format for an office memo ensures that no information will be forgotten.

PROCEDURE 6-4

Prepare an Interoffice Memo

Materials Needed

- Computer with word processing software
- Printer
- Reference materials as necessary (e.g., dictionary, grammar reference)

1. Prepare an interoffice memo using the proper components as listed below, and format as illustrated in Figure 6-14.
   a. Margins
   b. To
   c. From
   d. Date
   e. Subject
   f. Body
   g. Reference initials
   h. Computer file name
2. Proofread the memo for proper grammar and punctuation.*
3. Print enough copies of the memo for distribution.

**Denotes a crucial step in the procedure. This step must be completed satisfactorily for the procedure to be completed satisfactorily.*

Components

The heading of a memo contains four basic pieces of information. The first item is *to* whom the memo is sent, usually followed by *from* whom the memo was sent. Next, the *date* is listed, followed by the *subject* of the memo.

After the heading is completed, the body of the memo should begin on the third line below the last line of the heading. Occasionally, a signature line is added to the bottom of a memo, but it is common practice for the memo's author to initial after his or her name on the *from* line.

Reference initials belonging to the person who keyed the memo and a computer file name can be added two lines below the body of the memo.

Proper Format

Memos should begin two inches from the top of the page. If a memo is done on letterhead, sometimes the letterhead may be too large and the starting line may have to be moved a few lines down the page.

Side margins are similar to those of letters, either 1 or 1.25 inches, depending on the default settings of the office software. Margins may be adjusted to accommodate short or long memos (Procedure 6-4).

Email

An electronic mail message, or **email,** is a quick, efficient way to communicate internally in the office. Almost instantly, a printed message can be sent virtually anywhere. Email can be sent to one individual or to a group of individuals. If the medical office sends email to and receives email from patients, the message system should be checked several times daily to keep up to date with messages from patients. Email can be used to communicate information internally, just as a memo is used. Because it is so easy to use, email is sometimes overused. You should be careful not to email anything unless it is necessary. Because of the volume of email that some offices produce, it is not unusual for someone to be gone from the office for a couple of days and come back to find 50 or even 100 email messages. Reading unnecessary emails uses up valuable employee time that would be better spent assisting patients.

HIPAA Hint

Protected personal health information (PHI) can be used in a secure email system; highly confidential information cannot.

With the increased use of computers today, many patients can use email to contact a medical office. Patients may be able to contact an office with a secure email system through the office's website. Some larger health care facilities may have online forms that a patient can complete to request an appointment. Because the security of the email environment may possibly be compromised, highly confidential information cannot be included in email communication with patients. If a patient does email an office with a health-related concern, a copy of this email and the staff's response should be kept in the patient's medical record.

Email Format

Formatting an email is pretty straightforward. The message can be sent, copied, or blind copied to someone. You must be exact when typing in the address. If there is even one small error in the address, a message will not be received. If you are working in an office environment, it is better to select an address from a network address book or personal address book or reply to an email to avoid the possibility of an error in the address.

When identifying a subject for an email, be sure to be descriptive. Ever so briefly describe the purpose of the email within the subject line. If something needs immediate attention, use the term "urgent" in the subject line, or identify the email as a high-priority email.

Email Etiquette

As the use of email continues to increase, email users must always use proper email etiquette when writing messages. Proper etiquette for business use of email includes the following:

- Avoid using solid capital letters (e.g., "THIS NEEDS TO BE DONE IMMEDIATELY") or do so with extreme caution. The use of solid capital letters is equivalent to shouting at the other person.
- It has become common practice to use all lowercase letters for casual, informal email conversations. In informal messages, everything, including the beginning of sentences, may be typed in lowercase letters. This practice, however,

is not suitable for business communication in the medical office. In communicating with patients, appropriate business grammar should be used.

- Be brief, but as precise as possible. Oftentimes miscommunication may occur because each individual may react differently to the same statement. Remember, as the message is read, the sender of the statement has no opportunity to see the reaction of the receiver.
- The use of symbols to convey feeling or emotion, sometimes known as **emoticons,** may help bridge a possible communication gap. For example, a colon and right parenthesis — :) — signifies the sender's happiness during communication.
- In addition, many abbreviations are used within personal email communication. Use of such abbreviations is more casual than business-like and is best avoided in office communication.
- Above all, avoid discussing sensitive issues or serious subjects via email. The likelihood that the message will be misunderstood is great, and a more personal form of communication (in person or a telephone call) should be used to avoid misunderstanding.

CHECKPOINT

Explain the importance of deleting patient references from sample letters even though the letters remain in the office.

U.S. Postal Service Delivery Services

Most of the medical office's written correspondence is handled through the U.S. Postal Service. The more common postal delivery methods used by medical offices include city delivery and post office box delivery.

With city delivery, mail is delivered directly to the front desk or the central mailroom depending on the size of the practice. City delivery is convenient in that the postal carrier can leave the incoming mail, and outgoing mail may be picked up by the carrier to be taken to the post office. In a smaller office, mail may be exchanged with the postal carrier at the front desk or another designated location. The larger a health care facility, the more likely it is that there will be a designated mailroom within the building where outgoing mail is gathered to be sent out and incoming mail is received and distributed.

Post office box delivery service is available for a fee at most post offices. Up to five different sizes of boxes may be available from which to choose, and the size of the box determines the cost. Mail in a post office box may be retrieved at any time while the post office lobby is open.

Processing Incoming Mail

In almost all offices, mail is received every day the office is open (excluding Saturday and Sunday). As mentioned previously, it may be delivered directly to the office or picked up at a post office box. Whatever the case, once the incoming mail arrives in the office it should be handled in an expeditious manner.

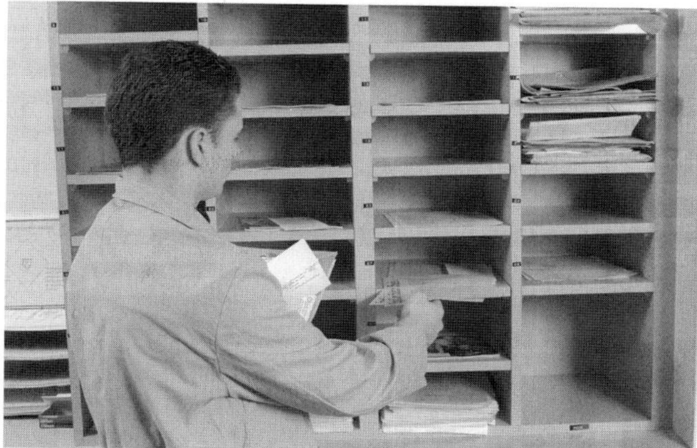

Figure 6-15 A central location for sorting mail and other office documents allows for easy distribution of all office correspondence.

Every piece of mail that comes into the office should be opened unless it is marked confidential. The exception is a confidential mailing, which should be opened only by the intended recipient.

On opening the mail, letters and other personal documents should be stamped with the date on which they were received. A machine may be used to date stamp a document or a rubber stamp may be used to easily record the date on a document. In addition to the date stamp, sometimes a physician may prefer to have the envelope stapled directly behind the letter.

After the date has been noted on the incoming mail, if the mail pertains to a patient, you should identify the patient's medical record number, and that information should be noted directly on the correspondence. The patient's medical record number can be written in black in the upper right hand corner of the document. Letters and copies of medical records from other facilities that are received will be filed eventually with the patient's medical record.

After all record numbers have been located, the correspondence is sent to the physician for review. For health care facilities that use paper medical records, the correspondence will be paper-clipped or attached in some way on the outside front of the patient's record and then sent to the physician's office. If electronic records are used, the correspondence should be sent to the physician's office as well. It is important that all received correspondence regarding patients be sent to the patient's physician for review. Frequently, physicians ask their patients to obtain another facility's records for the patient's current medical record, and a physician may be waiting for this information, which may be vital to the care of the patient.

After the mail has been dated and medical record numbers have been located, the mail is now ready for distribution inside the clinic. Because the volume of mail in most offices is considerable, it is a good idea to sort the mail into designated bins or slots for each physician or recipient (Fig. 6-15). Often, you may need to stop to assist a patient in the middle of sorting the mail. For that reason, it is a good idea to use some type of organizing receptacle for sorting the

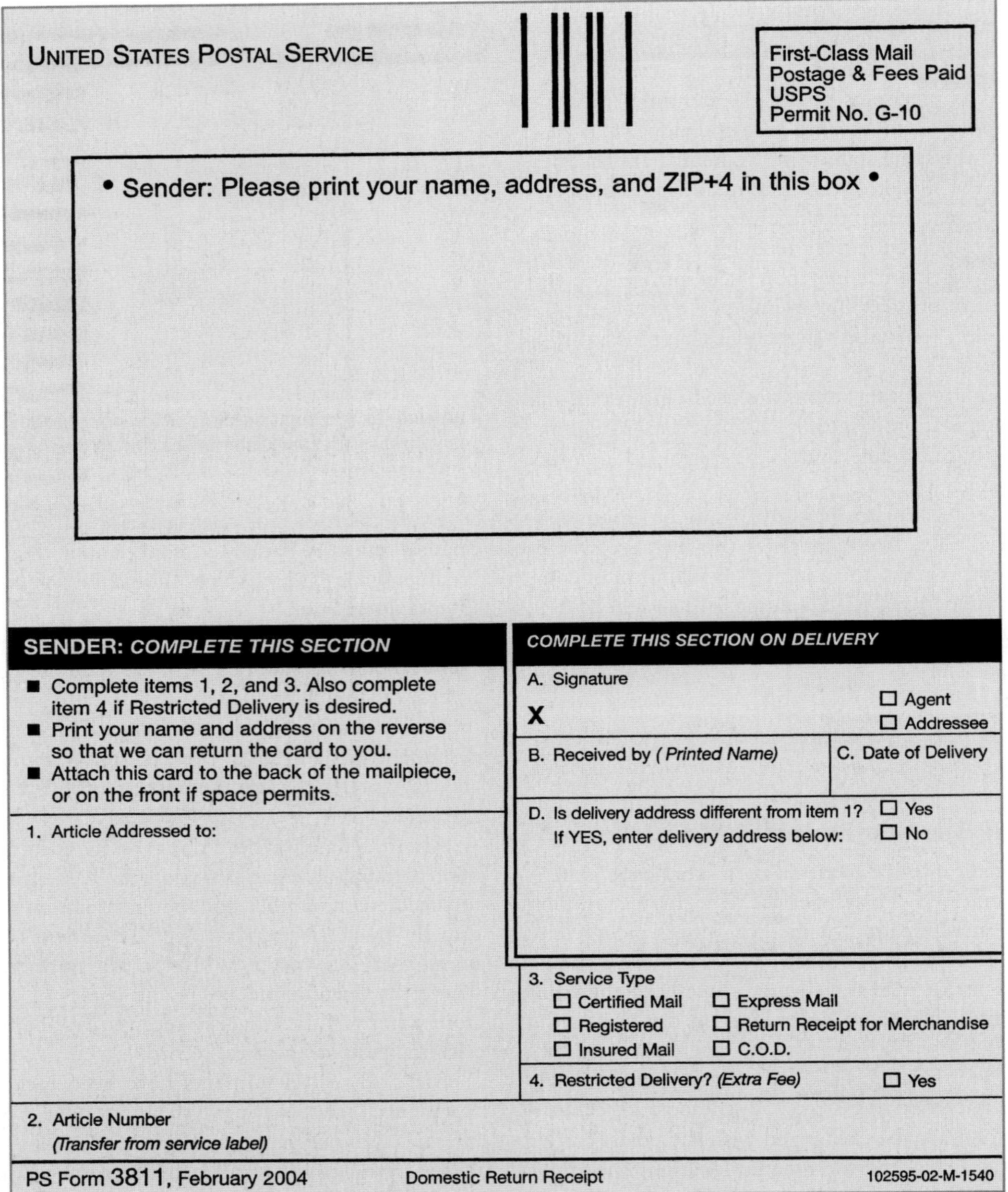

UNITED STATES POSTAL SERVICE

First-Class Mail
Postage & Fees Paid
USPS
Permit No. G-10

• Sender: Please print your name, address, and ZIP+4 in this box •

SENDER: *COMPLETE THIS SECTION*

- Complete items 1, 2, and 3. Also complete item 4 if Restricted Delivery is desired.
- Print your name and address on the reverse so that we can return the card to you.
- Attach this card to the back of the mailpiece, or on the front if space permits.

1. Article Addressed to:

COMPLETE THIS SECTION ON DELIVERY

A. Signature
X
☐ Agent
☐ Addressee

B. Received by (*Printed Name*)

C. Date of Delivery

D. Is delivery address different from item 1? ☐ Yes
If YES, enter delivery address below: ☐ No

3. Service Type
☐ Certified Mail ☐ Express Mail
☐ Registered ☐ Return Receipt for Merchandise
☐ Insured Mail ☐ C.O.D.

4. Restricted Delivery? (*Extra Fee*) ☐ Yes

2. Article Number
(*Transfer from service label*)

PS Form 3811, February 2004 Domestic Return Receipt 102595-02-M-1540

Figure 6-16 Sending a letter certified with return receipt gives the sender proof that a letter was received. (From Young AP: *Kinn's The Administrative Medical Assistant,* ed 6, St. Louis, Saunders, 2007.)

mail and not to have it strewn all over the desk. Some offices are so large that a central mailroom will sort and distribute all incoming mail to designated departments. Then assistants in each department will distribute mail to intended recipients.

Medical information about a patient received in the mail should never be filed inside the patient's chart without the physician's review of the information. If important information is filed in a patient's chart without the physician's reviewing that information, a potential legal problem could result if the received information is needed in the treatment of the patient. After reviewing the correspondence, the physician should initial and date the correspondence in a conspicuous place to indicate that the physician has reviewed the document. An assistant should check to make sure that all documents have been initialed by the physician before filing the information in the patient's record.

With an electronic records system, incoming information can be scanned into the patient's record. The scanned information can then be flagged to alert the physician to the incoming information. Once the physician has reviewed the information, the physician can electronically sign that the record has been reviewed.

Processing Outgoing Mail

Many types of services are available for sending mail. Postal rates vary considerably depending on the type of service chosen.

First Class. First class mail rates apply to almost all of the mail that is sent out by a medical office. First class mail covers letters, postcards, and the like. If mail is larger than letter size, it should be marked "First Class" to ensure proper, more expedient handling.

Express Mail. **Express Mail** is the fastest delivery service offered by the U.S. Postal Service but it is expensive. Most Express Mail packages are guaranteed delivery overnight. Usually, mail must be brought in by 5 PM to qualify for overnight Express Mail service. Delivery is made by 3 PM the next day. Express Mail may be deposited in an Express Mail delivery box, taken to a local post office, or picked up by the letter carrier. The U.S. Postal Service provides containers and mailing labels for Express Mail packages at no charge. Packages can weigh up to two pounds, and the rate stays the same no matter what the package weighs. Because of the excessive cost of Express Mail, it should be used only when a package requires expedient delivery.

Priority Mail. For documents and packages that need quick delivery, Priority Mail provides delivery service for items weighing up to 70 pounds. Copies of records may consist of many pages and can be quite heavy. Local postal offices provide Priority Mail boxes, stickers, and envelopes at no charge. Priority Mail should be well marked to ensure proper handling by the Postal Service. The U.S. Postal Service also sells boxes for mailing small packages. Boxes are sold at a flat rate and include the price of the box and postage all in one fee, regardless of what the package might weigh.

Certified with Return Receipt. Sometimes it is necessary to have proof that a letter or package has been mailed and received. In this case, the letter should be sent certified with a return receipt (Fig. 6-16). This service assigns a number to the delivery and requires that a signature be obtained at the time of delivery. This service is necessary to document important notifications to patients, such as withdrawal of medical services.

For complete information on all of the postal services that are available from the U.S. Postal Service, visit its website at www.usps.gov.

Postage Machines. Most offices today have some type of postage meter or machine (Fig. 6-17) that stamps postage directly on envelopes or on postage meter adhesive strips. These adhesive strips are affixed to larger packages that cannot fit through a machine.

Postage meters have a descending meter that tracks how much postage is left in the machine. When the postage left in the meter reaches a certain amount (sometimes less than $100), the machine automatically shuts off, and more postage must be purchased for the machine before it can be used again. Today's meters usually are connected online, and postage can be refilled online without a trip to the post office. A postage meter saves the office considerable time in that the mail may be weighed and stamped at the office and then deposited for delivery.

Presort Mail Services. For practices that process large quantities of mail to specific ZIP codes, discount rates may be available for first class delivery services if a presort mail (also known as bulk mail) service is used. Presort involves sorting the mail by ZIP code before delivering it to the post office. Offices that have a high volume of first class mail can save a few cents for each letter that is sent at the presort rate. It may not sound like much, but in the long run, the savings really do add up!

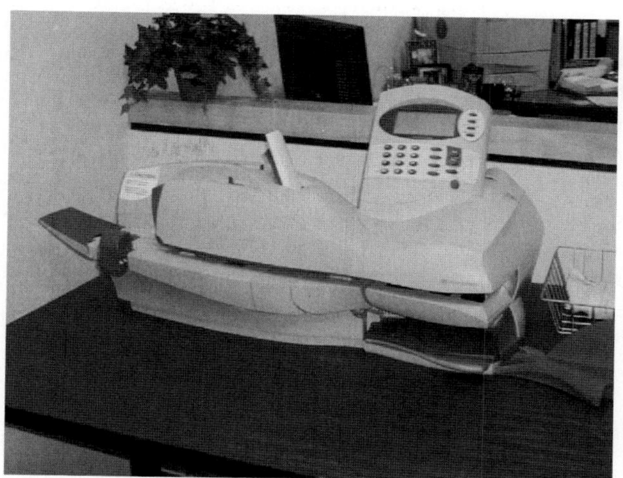

Figure 6-17 A postage machine allows postage to be affixed to letters and packages at the office. (From Young AP: *Kinn's The Administrative Medical Assistant,* ed 6, St. Louis, Saunders, 2007.)

Private Courier Services. Private courier services such as FedEx or United Parcel Service (UPS) provide alternatives to services offered by the U.S. Postal Service. Private couriers usually specialize in certain types of delivery, such as overnight delivery or package services. Different rates are available depending on what type of service is needed.

SUMMARY

As a medical administrative assistant, you will interact with patients and others every day in one way or another. It is absolutely critical that you use the proper communication skills and techniques to ensure a more effective and smooth running office.

The telephone is the central communication tool used between office staff members and patients, and professional telephone communication skills must be used by staff members to maintain the professional image of the medical office. A consistent telephone protocol will ensure that calls are handled in a professional and appropriate manner. Because the telephone is the key piece of equipment used by patients when contacting the medical office, attention must be paid to how callers are screened, asked to hold, assisted, and transferred. A variety of telephone communications equipment can be used in providing professional service to patients.

Sometimes the office needs to communicate with a patient in writing. It is normally the medical administrative assistant's responsibility to type (and sometimes compose) a letter for a patient. Proper grammar and document formatting skills must be used when business correspondence is produced. A medical office sends and receives correspondence each day that must be processed internally within the office before it is filed in a patient's chart or picked up for delivery.

Technology is also changing the way patients communicate with the office. Patients may use email to contact the office. Special care must be used when email is used to communicate with patients.

Whether conversing with a patient in person, on the telephone, or via written correspondence, an assistant must be professional at all times and should strive to meet the patient's needs whenever possible. Professional customer-oriented communication is the foundation of a long-lasting relationship between the patient and the medical office.

YOU ARE THE MEDICAL ADMINISTRATIVE ASSISTANT

Picture yourself as a medical administrative assistant in a medical practice. What would you do in the following situations?

1. A patient calls the office and complains of chest pain. The patient actually states that she thinks she is having a heart attack. How should you respond?
2. A patient calls the office and asks to speak with the physician. How should you respond?

REVIEW EXERCISES

Exercise 6-1 True or False

Read each statement and determine whether the statement is true or false. Record your answer in the blank provided. T = true; F= false.

_______ 1. An appropriate way to ask a caller to hold is to say, "Please hold."

_______ 2. A proper way to answer a call is to say, "Good morning, Skyway Medical Associates; this is Laura. How may I help you?"

_______ 3. Body language is a form of communication.

_______ 4. If the telephone traffic is very heavy, it is sufficient to answer the telephone with just "Hello."

_______ 5. Confidential information may be sent over email because it is a secure form of communication.

_______ 6. It is acceptable for an assistant to leave any message on an answering machine.

_______ 7. Announcing a transferred call means informing the recipient as to whom the call is from.

_______ 8. A medical administrative assistant may need to recognize emergency symptoms over the telephone.

_______ 9. When answering a call that is a possible emergency, an assistant should ask only those questions necessary for determining how to handle the call.

_______ 10. If a patient insists on speaking directly with the physician, you must transfer the call immediately.

_______ 11. A parent who calls to request medical information regarding his or her 25-year-old son should be given the information.

_______ 12. The office telephone should always be answered immediately after the first ring.

_______ 13. Email is synonymous with express mail.

_______ 14. A caller should never hold for longer than 20 seconds.

_______ 15. First class mail is the standard delivery service provided by the U.S. Postal Service for office letters.

_______ 16. Priority Mail service guarantees letter delivery within 24 hours.

_______ 17. A certified letter with return receipt may be used if the medical office needs a record indicating that the patient received correspondence from the office.

_______ 18. If a medical administrative assistant is responsible for entering computerized appointments for patients, a headset should be used while talking with patients over the telephone.

_______ 19. Because a medical administrative assistant is not licensed to practice medicine, an assistant who answers the telephone does not need to be able to recognize symptoms common to a medical emergency.

_______ 20. If the office is very busy, an assistant does not need to ask whether a patient can hold; the assistant can place every call directly on hold if necessary.

_______ 21. A patient can communicate a message without speaking.

_______ 22. A response to a question is known as feedback.

_______ 23. If a patient is vague about symptoms, a medical administrative assistant may need to ask the patient a few questions about his or her symptoms.

_______ 24. Personality differences can affect communication.

_______ 25. If the office is extremely busy, it is acceptable to let the telephone ring 10 times before answering.

_______ 26. If the office is extremely busy, an acceptable way to answer the telephone is to say, "Skyway Medical Associates."

_______ 27. If a caller is upset, the best thing to do is to ask him or her to call back another day when he or she is calmer.

_______ 28. A medical office needs a minimum of two telephone lines.

_______ 29. Voice mail will record a message if a telephone line is in use.

_______ 30. Screening calls is necessary to decrease the number of calls handled by the physician or other clinical staff.

Exercise 6-2 Communicating With Patients

When patients call the office, they often use laypersons' terms to describe a medical condition. Identify the appropriate medical term for each laypersons' term. Record the answer in the blank provided.

(a) Conjunctivitis
(b) Gastritis
(c) Otitis media
(d) Urinary tract infection
(e) Pharyngitis
(f) Rhinorrhea
(g) Upper respiratory infection
(h) Hematuria
(i) Sutures
(j) Laceration
(k) Epistaxis

______ 1. Stitches
______ 2. Cold
______ 3. Sore throat
______ 4. Bladder infection
______ 5. Stomachache
______ 6. Pinkeye
______ 7. Nosebleed
______ 8. Cut
______ 9. Ear infection
______ 10. Runny nose
______ 11. Blood in urine

Exercise 6-3 Telephone Screening

Identify whether or not a medical administrative assistant would be authorized or able to complete the following telephone requests. Record your answer in the blank provided. Y = yes; N = no.

______ 1. Pharmacy calls for a prescription refill for a patient.

______ 2. Patient wants to make an appointment.

______ 3. Patient has a complaint about a bill.

______ 4. Patient asks maximum dosage of ibuprofen that can be used per day.

______ 5. Patient wants to know how much the practice charges for a mammogram.

______ 6. Patient wants to know whether heat or ice should be used for an ankle sprain.

______ 7. Patient needs to cancel an appointment.

______ 8. Insurance company calls for additional information about a patient's claim.

______ 9. Patient calls asking whether two particular medications can be taken simultaneously.

______ 10. Patient calls asking for laboratory test results.

______ 11. Patient has a question about an insurance payment sent to the office.

Exercise 6-4 Chapter Concepts

Read each statement or question and choose the answer that best completes that statement or question. Record your answer in the blank provided.

______ 1. After answering a call, the first thing the assistant should do is
(a) Obtain the patient's name.
(b) Offer an appointment.
(c) Determine the reason for the call.
(d) Get the patient's chart number.
(e) Any of the above could be done first.

______ 2. A correct way to transfer a call to a physician via a speaker telephone is
(a) "Dr. Sanchez, line two."
(b) "Line two."
(c) "Kelly Garcia is on line two. She wants to know whether she should keep taking her prescription of Xanax."
(d) "Dr. Sanchez, Mrs. Garcia is on line two."
(e) None of the above

______ 3. Which of the following is not usually needed when taking a telephone message?
(a) Patient's name
(b) Patient's insurance company
(c) Reason for calling
(d) Time of message
(e) All of the above are necessary for every telephone call.

______ 4. Which of the following is inappropriate when speaking with a patient over the telephone?
(a) Speak at a moderate rate of speed.
(b) Confirm the conversation with the caller.
(c) Hold the handset one to two inches from your mouth.
(d) Use medical slang to convey your medical knowledge to the patient.
(e) Exhibit proper posture.

_____ 5. Which of the following is false regarding nonverbal communication?
(a) Nonverbal communication has little impact on communication with a patient.
(b) An assistant's posture can communicate a message.
(c) A patient's comfort zone should be respected.
(d) Lack of eye contact can communicate disinterest.

_____ 6. All of the following should be done when handling a complaint call except
(a) Offer to help the patient if at all possible.
(b) Let your supervisor know about the problem, and identify ways that the problem may be avoided in the future.
(c) Deny that a problem exists.
(d) Ask the patient what you can do, and do it if possible.

_____ 7. Which of the following may have the greatest potential for a possible breach of confidentiality?
(a) Pager
(b) Switchboard
(c) Answering service
(d) Cell telephone

_____ 8. Which of the following is inappropriate in telephone communication?
(a) Speak clearly.
(b) Maintain patient confidentiality.
(c) Confirm a call.
(d) Obtain every possible piece of information about a patient's medical condition.
(e) All of the above are appropriate when communicating over the telephone.

_____ 9. When transferring calls, the assistant should do all of the following except
(a) Explain to the patient that the call needs to be transferred.
(b) Give confidential information over a speaker telephone.
(c) Ask the patient whether he or she will hold while the call is transferred.
(d) Announce the call.

_____ 10. When handling a possible emergency call, the assistant should
(a) Tell the patient to drive to the nearest emergency department.
(b) Transfer the call only if the assistant is sure it is an emergency.
(c) Tell the patient to come to the clinic immediately.
(d) Transfer the call immediately to a doctor or nurse.
(e) Any of the above is an acceptable action when dealing with an emergency call.

Exercise 6-5 Telephone Protocol

You are working as a medical administrative assistant in a multi-physician medical office and receive the following calls. What is the best way to handle the call? Record your answer in the blank provided.

_____ 1. Mr. Stein (65 years of age) calls with indigestion and just a little shortness of breath after shoveling snow. You
(a) Transfer the call directly to Mr. Stein's physician.
(b) Take a message to give to the nurse.
(c) Tell Mr. Stein to rest and that if he doesn't feel better within 30 minutes he should call back.
(d) Give him an appointment later this afternoon.
(e) Tell Mr. Stein to hire someone to shovel his snow.

_____ 2. A physician from the hospital emergency department calls to speak with Dr. O'Brian about her patient Alice Shepard, who is currently in the emergency department. You
(a) Determine the nature of the call by asking as many questions as necessary.
(b) Never interrupt Dr. O'Brian when she is with a patient.
(c) Take a message and tell the patient the doctor will call back when she is available.
(d) Transfer the call immediately to Dr. O'Brian.

______ 3. Maggie Pinkerton reports that her daughter, Laura, has a slight fever and has been extremely tired for four days. You
   (a) Give her an appointment this afternoon.
   (b) Give her an appointment next week. She might get better before then.
   (c) Tell her to give the child two children's non-aspirin tablets and let her rest for the remainder of the day.
   (d) Tell her to call her pharmacy for advice on over-the-counter medications to give for the child's fever.

______ 4. Lisa Martin, a 20-year-old single female patient, had taken a home pregnancy test, and the result was positive. She is very upset and calls to request an appointment to see the physician about the pregnancy. She mentions that she needs to come in soon because she may wish to terminate the pregnancy. You
   (a) Tell her that no appointments are available for quite some time because you are morally opposed to abortion.
   (b) Give her the number of a local abortion clinic.
   (c) Accommodate her request for an appointment.
   (d) Tell her to come in to have another test to verify the home test.

______ 5. Nancy Martin, Lisa's mother, calls the office and asks to speak with the doctor. She is concerned that her daughter is possibly depressed. She asks if Lisa has been in the clinic lately for anything. You
   (a) Tell her Lisa called yesterday but you cannot tell her mother why Lisa called.
   (b) Tell her that information regarding a patient cannot be released without the patient's permission.
   (c) Tell her Lisa has not contacted the office for anything in the past six months.
   (d) Call Lisa and tell her that her mother called the office asking about her.

______ 6. A pharmacy calls requesting an okay for a refill of a patient's medication. You
   (a) Check the chart, and if any refills have been ordered, tell the pharmacy that another refill should be okay.
   (b) Take a message for the patient's physician.
   (c) Tell the pharmacy that all patients need to see their physician before any refills are made.
   (d) Tell the pharmacy that the patient should bring the prescription bottle into the pharmacy so it can be checked.

______ 7. Barb Baker, the practice's legal counsel, asks to speak with Dr. Marks. You
   (a) Transfer the call to Dr. Marks.
   (b) Tell Ms. Baker to telephone Dr. Marks at home this evening.
   (c) Take a message and tell Ms. Baker that Dr. Marks cannot be interrupted.
   (d) Transfer the call to the office manager.

______ 8. A patient calls to ask for results from a recent laboratory test. You
   (a) Take a message for the physician or the nurse.
   (b) Find the results and give them over the telephone to the patient.
   (c) Transfer the call to the laboratory technician.
   (d) Tell the patient that you will send the results by mail.

______ 9. Mr. O'Brian, Dr. O'Brian's husband, calls to speak with Dr. O'Brian. She is currently with a patient. You
   (a) Tell Mr. O'Brian that you must take a message.
   (b) Transfer the call directly to Dr. O'Brian.
   (c) Tell Mr. O'Brian that the doctor is currently with a patient, and ask if he would like you to interrupt.
   (d) Ask Mr. O'Brian to call back right before lunch because all patients will be gone at that time.

______ 10. Susan Walter, MD, the chief of the medical staff, calls for Dr. Sanchez. You
   (a) Transfer the call to Dr. Sanchez.
   (b) Take a message.
   (c) Ask what the call is about, and then determine whether a message should be taken.
   (d) Transfer the call to the practice manager because Dr. Sanchez is too busy.

______ 11. Eileen Smith, an obstetrics patient, calls with medical questions related to her pregnancy. You
   (a) Determine that the call is not an emergency and take a message for the physician or the nurse.
   (b) Tell her to call and ask the hospital where she plans to deliver.
   (c) Ask her whether she has consulted her prenatal guide provided by the doctor.
   (d) Check her chart to see whether you can answer her questions.

______ 12. A patient calls and is too embarrassed to say why she is calling. You
   (a) Tell her to call back when she is not so embarrassed.
   (b) Tell her that nothing will shock you.
   (c) Determine that the call is not an emergency and take a message for the physician or nurse.
   (d) Tell her to look for information on the Internet.

_____ 13. Dr. Mallard's son calls and reports that he is in trouble at school. You
(a) Take a message and tell him the doctor will call the school after school is out.
(b) Transfer the call to Dr. Mallard.
(c) Tell him to call his father.
(d) Tell him to have the teacher call back during the lunch hour.

_____ 14. A patient calls with severe vertigo. You
(a) Ask the patient whether he or she has been drinking any alcohol.
(b) Check the patient's chart to see whether he or she has had vertigo before.
(c) Transfer the call to the doctor or the nurse.
(d) Make an appointment next week for the patient.

_____ 15. An hysterical parent calls to report that her toddler has drunk half a bottle of a children's pain reliever. You
(a) Transfer the call to the pharmacy.
(b) Tell her to take the child to an emergency department.
(c) Tell her to make the child vomit the drug.
(d) Give her the number of the Poison Control Center, instruct her to call the number immediately, and obtain the patient's name before hanging up.

Exercise 6-6 Written Communication Principles

Read each statement or question, and choose the answer that best completes that statement or question. Record your answer in the blank provided.

_____ 1. The correct format for a date is
(a) Sept. 1, 2010
(b) 1 Sept 10
(c) September 1, 2010
(d) 9-10-10

_____ 2. The correct position for a date is
(a) After the salutation
(b) One inch from the top of the page
(c) Between the address and the salutation
(d) 2 to 2.5 inches from the top of the page

_____ 3. A page notation includes
(a) Date of the letter
(b) Patient's medical record number
(c) Patient's name
(d) All of the above
(e) Only b and c

_____ 4. Which of the following is true regarding business letters?
(a) The salutation in most letters would address the recipient by a first name.
(b) Shorter paragraphs make a letter easier to read.
(c) Letters regarding a minor patient should be addressed to the patient.
(d) A page notation should appear on the first page of a letter.

_____ 5. Identify the correct format for a reference notation.
(a) AB/YZ
(b) AB/yz
(c) Ab/yz
(d) AB-yz
(e) None of the above

_____ 6. Which of the following statements is false regarding notations?
(a) A computer file notation can help locate a file if a change needs to be made to a letter.
(b) A copy notation identifies individuals other than the addressee who will be sent a copy of a letter.
(c) An assistant should be alert for any enclosures that may need to be included in a letter.
(d) Notations contain important information for the addressee of a letter.

_____ 7. Which of the following is true regarding a business letter?
(a) All letters are dictated by physicians.
(b) A letter portfolio provides helpful examples of letters for the office staff.
(c) Default margins should always be 1 inch.
(d) Block-style letters are a very easy format to reproduce because everything lines up on the left margin.

_____ 8. Which of the following is false regarding addressing business envelopes?
(a) Addresses should be left justified.
(b) Any font can be used.
(c) Solid caps should be used when the address is typed.
(d) Attention lines should appear at the top of an address.

_____ 9. Which of the following is false regarding memos?
(a) Memos are communication pieces used within an office.
(b) Memos can be sent to large groups of people.
(c) Signature lines are required in a memo.
(d) Reference initials are used in memos.

_____ 10. Which of the following is false regarding email?
(a) Email can be used internally to communicate information quickly to employees.
(b) Email should be used as often as possible regardless of whether or not the information included in the email is important.
(c) Not all email may be secure.
(d) A copy of an email from a patient should be added to the patient's medical record.

Exercise 6-7 Office Emergencies

To develop a greater understanding of office emergencies and how to recognize them over the telephone, look up the following medical conditions in a medical reference and identify the symptoms commonly associated with each condition. (All of the following conditions have the potential to become critical. This list is not inclusive of all symptoms associated with the conditions or of all critical conditions that may occur with patients.)

Medical Condition	Symptoms
Myocardial infarction (heart attack)	______
Cerebrovascular accident (stroke)	______
Asthma attack	______
Appendicitis	______
Pyelonephritis	______
Migraine	______
Volvulus	______
Ileus	______
Intussusception	______
Perforated ulcer	______
Aneurysm	______
Osteomyelitis	______
Meningitis	______

ACTIVITIES

ACTIVITY 6-1 TELEPHONE MESSAGES

Perform Procedure 6-2 using the message blanks provided here. Record a telephone message for the following calls received in the office today. Some of the information required for the message will have to be obtained from the Medisoft software included with this text.

1. Open Medisoft.
2. On the main menu, click **Lists>Patients/Guarantors and Cases.** The patient list window will then open. From this window, it is possible to locate registration information for patients of Happy Valley Medical Group.
3. At the top of the Patient window, the **Patient** button should be selected and the **Field** text box should display Last Name, First Name. (If it does not, click the drop-down box to select this choice.) In the **Search for** box, begin typing the patient's name to locate the patient's registration data for the information needed below. (Because the patient list for demonstration purposes is not large, it is also possible to locate the patient's name by scrolling in the patient list window.) When the patient's name is located, double-click the patient's name, and the patient's information will appear in the **Patient/Guarantor** window. Demographic information will be listed under the **Name, Address** tab in this window.
4. After the patient's information has been located, click **Cancel** to close the patient's file. Cancel is chosen because changes have not been made to the patient's information at this time.

TELEPHONE MESSAGES: (use today's date for the date of the message)
Complete the telephone messages below using the message blanks provided with this exercise.

1. Tonya Hartman calls for results of her mammogram performed last Wednesday. She asks whether Dr. Hinckle or his nurse could call her back today after 4 PM at her home number with the results.

MESSAGE FROM								
For Dr.	Name of Caller	Rel. to pt.	Patient	Pt. Age	Pt. Temp.	Message Date / /	Message Time AM PM	Urgent ☐Yes ☐No
Message:						Allergies		
Respond to Phone #	Best Time To Call AM PM	Pharmacy Name/#	Patient's Chart Attached ☐Yes ☐No	Patient's Chart #	Initials			

(Form courtesy of Bibbero Systems, Inc, Petaluma, California, 800-242-2376. Fax, 800-242-9330. Available at www.bibbero.com.)

2. Sammy Catera has sprained her ankle and wants information on what she can do at home. She asks whether Dr. Hinckle can call her back at her home number as soon as possible.

MESSAGE FROM								
For Dr.	Name of Caller	Rel. to pt.	Patient	Pt. Age	Pt. Temp.	Message Date / /	Message Time AM PM	Urgent ☐Yes ☐No
Message:						Allergies		
Respond to Phone #	Best Time To Call AM PM	Pharmacy Name/#	Patient's Chart Attached ☐Yes ☐No	Patient's Chart #	Initials			

(Form courtesy of Bibbero Systems, Inc, Petaluma, California, 800-242-2376. Fax, 800-242-9330. Available at www.bibbero.com.)

3. Monica Peters calls to report that her son, Zach, has a fever and wants to know the correct amount of nonaspirin pain reliever to give for the fever. She asks that Dr. Mallard call her back as soon as possible at home.

MESSAGE FROM								
For Dr.	Name of Caller	Rel. to pt.	Patient	Pt. Age	Pt. Temp.	Message Date / /	Message Time AM PM	Urgent ☐Yes ☐No
Message:						Allergies		
Respond to Phone #	Best Time To Call AM PM	Pharmacy Name/#	Patient's Chart Attached ☐Yes ☐No	Patient's Chart #	Initials			

(Form courtesy of Bibbero Systems, Inc, Petaluma, California, 800-242-2376. Fax, 800-242-9330. Available at www.bibbero.com.)

4. John Bordon calls for a refill of his prescription for Flonase that he obtained from Dr. Mallard. He would like to pick up his prescription at Valley Pharmacy.

MESSAGE FROM								
For Dr.	Name of Caller	Rel. to pt.	Patient	Pt. Age	Pt. Temp.	Message Date / /	Message Time AM PM	Urgent ☐Yes ☐No
Message:						Allergies		
Respond to Phone #	Best Time To Call AM PM	Pharmacy Name/#	Patient's Chart Attached ☐Yes ☐No	Patient's Chart #	Initials			

(Form courtesy of Bibbero Systems, Inc, Petaluma, California, 800-242-2376. Fax, 800-242-9330. Available at www.bibbero.com.)

ACTIVITY 6-2 TELEPHONE TECHNIQUES

Establish a list of important telephone techniques for handling incoming calls. Call two places of business and evaluate their telephone techniques based on the list you created.

ACTIVITY 6-3 PERSONALITY STYLES

With a group of people or with a class, take a personality style inventory. Compare your answers with those of others in the group. Discuss differences in personality traits and how they could affect communication in an office environment.

ACTIVITY 6-4 EMAIL ETIQUETTE

Research email etiquette on the Internet. Locate examples of etiquette rules, emoticons, and/or slang used in email conversation.

ACTIVITY 6-5 LETTER PREPARATION

Prepare the following letter in the letter formats as given in the text: block, modified-block, and modified-block with indented paragraphs. Insert paragraphs where appropriate, and consult an office reference manual if necessary. Locate the patient information in Medisoft using the instructions given in Activity 6-1. Use Procedure 6-3 as a guide when preparing the letter. Use today's date, and type the following letter from Julia D. Mallard, MD, to Monica Peters:

> *Dear Mrs. Peters—I have received the results of your hemoglobin A1C test that was done at your recent visit, and I am pleased to inform you that the test results were within normal limits. Your test result was 6.8%. Our desired results would be a value less than 7%. Your type II diabetes seems to be well under control, and your current dosage of Glucotrol XL of 5 mg/day is appropriate and should be continued. A prescription for Glucotrol is enclosed. I recommend that you repeat this test again in 6 months. Please contact me at my office if you have any questions. Sincerely, Julia D. Mallard, MD.*

ACTIVITY 6-6 MEMO PREPARATION

Prepare the following memo for Dr. Hinckle in the memo format given in the text. Use today's date, send the memo to all employees from Wallace Hinckle, MD. The subject is employee parking. Be sure to include all of the components of a memo that are listed in the chapter. Use Procedure 6-4 as a guide when preparing the memo.

> *Next Monday, [insert date], resurfacing of our parking lot will begin. Construction will last for approximately four to five days. The construction will take place in two phases with each phase lasting one to two days. All employees are asked not to park in the lot during the construction to allow ample parking for our patients. Temporary parking during the construction is available in the church lot on Midtown Avenue.*

ACTIVITY 6-7 U.S. POSTAL SERVICE REQUIREMENTS

Identify the current U.S. Postal Service mailing requirements for

- Express Mail
- Priority Mail
- Presort Mail

ACTIVITY 6-8 TELEPHONE TECHNIQUES

Perform Procedure 6-1. Students may pair up and deliver a mock call to each other or students should prepare to receive a mock telephone call from the instructor. Review Table 6-1 to prepare to answer a call correctly.

ACTIVITY 6-9 RETURN RECEIPT FOR LETTER

Prepare a return receipt (on next page) for a certified letter that will be sent to Monica Peters. Complete the form as follows:

No. 1 Patient's information
No. 2 Article number 2364 4960 5555 0001
No. 3 Service type: certified mail

UNITED STATES POSTAL SERVICE

First-Class Mail
Postage & Fees Paid
USPS
Permit No. G-10

• Sender: Please print your name, address, and ZIP+4 in this box •

SENDER: *COMPLETE THIS SECTION*	*COMPLETE THIS SECTION ON DELIVERY*
■ Complete items 1, 2, and 3. Also complete item 4 if Restricted Delivery is desired. ■ Print your name and address on the reverse so that we can return the card to you. ■ Attach this card to the back of the mailpiece, or on the front if space permits.	A. Signature X ☐ Agent ☐ Addressee B. Received by *(Printed Name)* C. Date of Delivery
1. Article Addressed to:	D. Is delivery address different from item 1? ☐ Yes If YES, enter delivery address below: ☐ No
	3. Service Type ☐ Certified Mail ☐ Express Mail ☐ Registered ☐ Return Receipt for Merchandise ☐ Insured Mail ☐ C.O.D.
	4. Restricted Delivery? *(Extra Fee)* ☐ Yes
2. Article Number *(Transfer from service label)*	

PS Form 3811, February 2004 Domestic Return Receipt 102595-02-M-1540

(From Young AP: *Kinn's The Administrative Medical Assistant,* ed 6, St. Louis, Saunders, 2007.)

DISCUSSION

The following topics may be used for class discussion or for individual student essay.

DISCUSSION 6-1

The telephone traffic at the office has been increasing to the point that it is difficult to answer many calls within three to four rings. The office physician wants to purchase an automated system for the office that allows a computer to answer the telephone. Calls will be answered by a recorded voice that instructs the patient that his or her call will be handled by the next available assistant. How will you respond to the physician?

DISCUSSION 6-2

Refer to picture A in Figure 6-1 in the chapter. Is there anything that the assistant might correct in his interaction with the patient? Now, refer to picture B in Figure 6-1. Is there anything that the assistant might correct or change in his interaction with the patient?

Bibliography

Ballweg R, Stolberg S, Sullivan EM: *Physician Assistant: A Guide to Clinical Practice*, ed 3, Philadelphia, 2003, WB Saunders.

Diehl MO, Fordney MT: *Medical Keyboarding, Typing, and Transcribing: Techniques and Procedures*, 4 ed, Philadelphia, 1997, WB Saunders.

O'Toole M: *Miller-Keane Encyclopedia & Dictionary of Medicine, Nursing, & Allied Health*, ed 6, Philadelphia, 1997, WB Saunders.

Sabin WA: *Gregg Reference Manual*, , ed 10, New York, 2005, Glencoe McGraw-Hill.

Sieh A, Brentin LK: *The Nurse Communicates*, Philadelphia, 1997, WB Saunders.

U.S. Postal Service: *Mailing Standards of the United States Postal Service Publication 28-Postal Addressing Standards*. http://pe.usps.gov/text/pub28/welcome.htm. Accessed October 10, 2013.

University of Chicago, HIPAA Program Office: *HIPAA Best Practices Library, HIPAA Quick Reference Guide for Employees*. http://hipaa.bsd.uchicago.edu/quick_ref_guide_120806.pdf. Accessed October 10, 2013.

CHAPTER 7 Appointment Scheduling

LEARNING OUTCOMES

On successful completion of this chapter, the student will be able to

1. Explain the use of computer and manual systems for scheduling appointments.
2. Identify types of scheduling methods used in offices today.
3. Identify the common components needed for recording an appointment.
4. Explain appointment scheduling procedures.
5. Explain appropriate use of medical terminology on an appointment schedule.
6. Document no-shows and appointment cancellations.
7. Explain ancillary, referral, and surgical scheduling for patients and scheduling for pharmaceutical and other sales representatives.
8. Prepare appointment reminders.
9. Deliver verbal appointment reminders.
10. Explain proper handling of unexpected schedule interruptions.
11. Schedule appointments, and manage appointment schedules and patient information in a computerized medical practice management system.

COMMISSION ON ACCREDITATION OF ALLIED HEALTH EDUCATION PROGRAMS (CAAHEP) CORE CURRICULUM FOR MEDICAL ASSISTANTS

- Discuss pros and cons of various types of appointment management systems.
- Describe scheduling guidelines.
- Recognize office policies and protocols for handling appointments.
- Identify critical information required for scheduling patient admissions and/or procedures.
- Manage appointment schedule, using established priorities.
- Use office hardware and software to maintain office systems.
- Explore issue of confidentiality as it applies to the medical assistant.
- Respond to issues of confidentiality.
- Apply HIPAA rules in regard to privacy/release of information.

ACCREDITING BUREAU OF HEALTH EDUCATION SCHOOLS (ABHES) COMPETENCIES FOR MEDICAL ASSISTING

Graduates

- Apply electronic technology.
- Schedule and manage appointments.
- Identify and properly use office machines, computerized systems, and medical software.
- Apply computer application skills using variety of different electronic programs including both practice management software and EMR software.

VOCABULARY

ancillary appointments
chief complaint
double booking
group (block) scheduling
no-show
precertification
referral appointments
resources
triage
urgent care
walk-in

Appointment scheduling is the office activity that has, perhaps, the greatest influence on how a medical office functions. A well-managed schedule provides optimal availability of services for patients, as well as maximal utilization of facility resources such as personnel, equipment, and buildings. A well-managed schedule avoids excessive downtimes and excessive hectic times. Downtimes are times when equipment, personnel, or space is left idle or is unproductive for extended periods. Many offices prefer to use every available slot of appointment time that is available during the day. Proper scheduling of appointment times will keep everyone in the office busy at a smooth, steady pace throughout the day. A well-managed schedule reduces waiting time for patients and maximizes the number of patients the physician is able to serve each day. Most importantly, because of the reasons listed, a well-managed appointment schedule serves the best interests of the patient.

Computerized Appointment Scheduling

In most of today's medical offices, computers are used for appointment scheduling. Depending on the size of the organization, computers may be stand-alone personal computers, or they may be networked with a mainframe computer system. Even the smallest of offices will probably have a few computers that are networked.

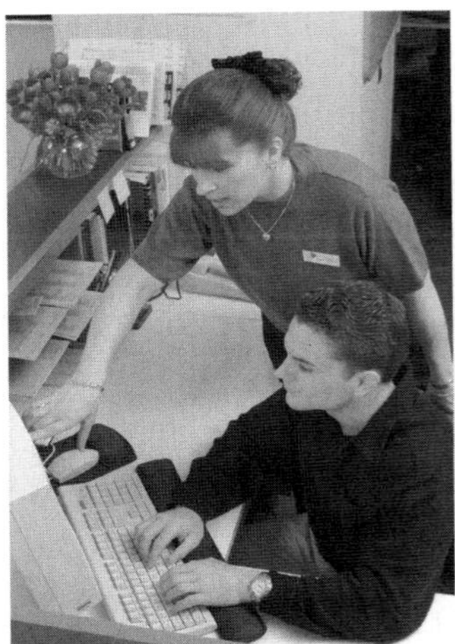

Figure 7-1 A computerized system in the medical office makes appointment scheduling efficient and easy. (From Bonewit-West K, *Today's Medical Assistant*, ed 2, St. Louis, Saunders, 2012.)

The use of a computerized appointment scheduling system has many advantages for the medical office. First and foremost is the fact that most appointment scheduling programs allow more than one user at a time to access the appointment system. This means that the office staff is able to assist more than one patient at a time, and that office productivity is increased because more than one assistant at a time can schedule or modify appointments. Even while someone is entering appointments, other staff members (e.g., physicians and nurses) can access scheduling information from the system (Fig. 7-1).

Scheduling programs prompt the user for the essential information needed to schedule an appointment. Everyone who uses the system is asked the same questions and responds to the same computer prompts. Therefore, the content of appointments entered into the computer is relatively uniform and consistent. The computer prompts for information that a user might otherwise forget to enter if using a manual or handwritten system (Fig. 7-2).

Another advantage of using a computerized system is the ability to generate updated copies of the schedule quickly (Fig. 7-3). Usually, just by entering a few simple commands, a copy of any day's schedule can be generated. Some offices even have computers at the nurses' station, in the patient care area, and within every exam room, which enables physicians or nurses to view or print, or both, the schedule on command. Some offices, through a secured computer network, even

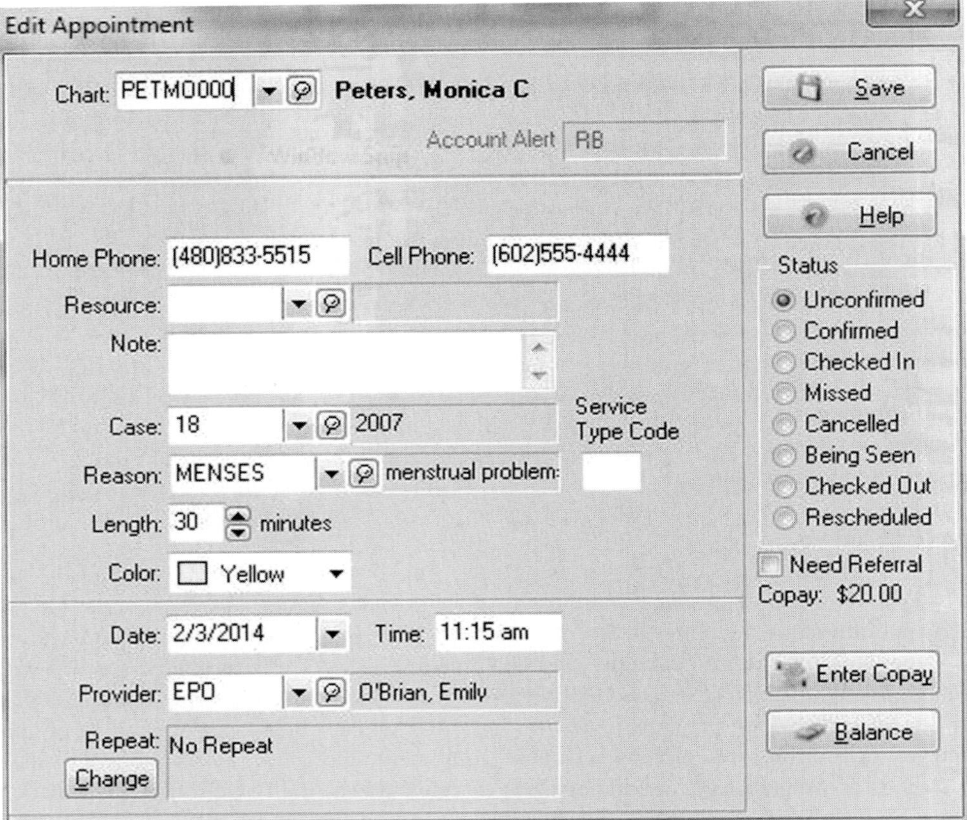

Figure 7-2 When entering an appointment in a computerized system, an assistant provides information such as patient name and the reason for the appointment; other patient information such as medical record and telephone number is automatically linked to the appointment from the computer's database. (Screenshots used by permission of MCKESSON Corporation. All rights reserved. © MCKESSON Corporation 2012.)

allow physicians to review schedules and perform other work while away from the clinic or hospital.

Another advantage of appointment scheduling is that the scheduling system interfaces with a patient database. This means that when an appointment is made, and a patient's name is entered into the schedule, other pertinent information—such as the patient's telephone number and the patient's chart number—is retrieved from the database and inserted into the schedule as well. When the schedule is printed, important information from the patient database, such as the patient's phone number, is available directly on the schedule.

Also, appointment scheduling software can provide an interface with the patient billing system. With this interface, the chance that bills may get lost or misplaced is reduced because the software is able to identify patients who have been seen for an appointment but who have not yet had charges entered for services rendered.

Happy Valley Medical Group

Lee, Robert — **Friday, October 19, 2012**

Time	Name / Chart Number	Phone / Resource	Length / Reason	Notes / Repeat Description
9:00a	Again, Dwight AGADW000	434-5777	15 COUGH	
9:15a	Brimley, Susan BRISU000	(222)342-3444	15 ALLERGY	
9:30a	Catera, Sammy CATSA000	227-7722	45 COLP	
10:15a	Jones, Suzy Q JONSU000	(480)123-4444	30 ASTHM	
10:45a				
11:00a	Doe, Jane S DOEJA000	(480)999-9999	45 LES2PLUS	
11:45a				
12:00p				
12:15p	Brimley, Elmo BRIEL000	(222)342-3444	15 EAR	
12:30p				
12:45p				
1:00p	Lunch-Lee		60	Every week on Mon, Tue, Thu and Fri
2:00p				
2:15p				
2:30p	Shepherd, Jarem SHEJA000		15 WART	
2:45p				
3:00p	Karvel, Jessica C KARJE000		45 PX4065	
3:45p				
4:00p				

Figure 7-3 An appointment schedule can be printed several times a day to keep the medical staff updated regarding changes to the schedule.

When scheduling an appointment, some programs allow the user to view several open appointment slots at one time (Fig. 7-4). The user can specify that the program should display openings for a specific provider or for a certain day. If the patient wants an appointment on a Wednesday and wants to see only Dr. Sanchez, the software will display only Wednesdays for Dr. Sanchez.

Computerized appointment scheduling enables an assistant to quickly access such information as the following:

- The time of a patient's next appointment
- All future appointments scheduled for the patient (Fig. 7-5)
- A record of a patient's previous visits to the office
- Identification of providers who have treated the patient

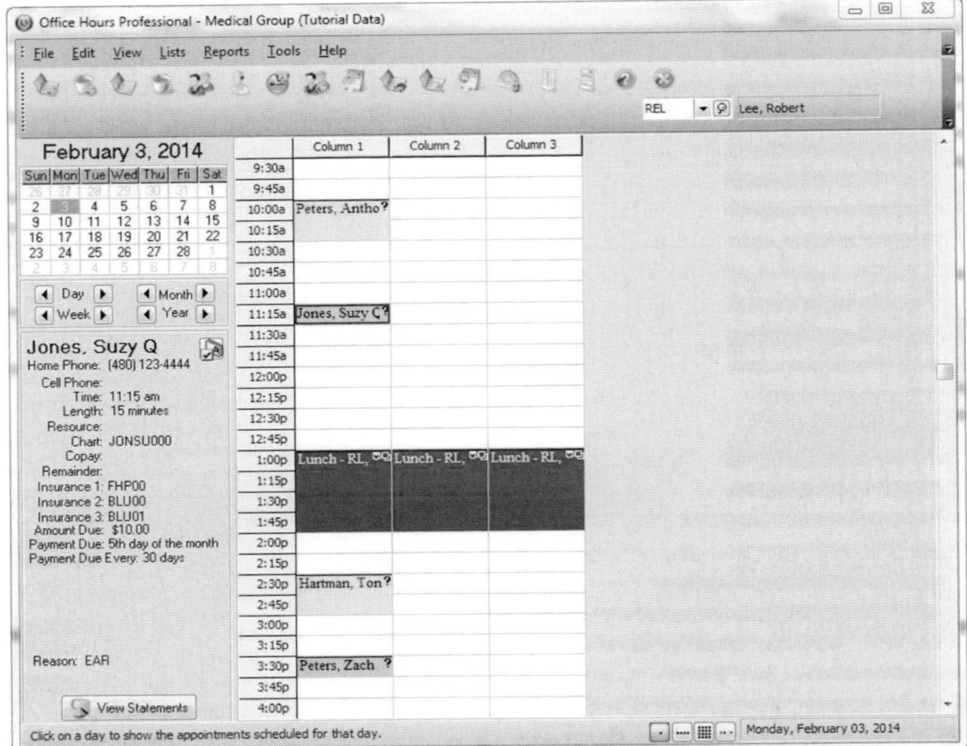

Figure 7-4 A computer scheduling program for the medical office displays appointment times that are open and scheduled for a specific day. (Screenshots used by permission of MCKESSON Corporation. All rights reserved. © MCKESSON Corporation 2012.)

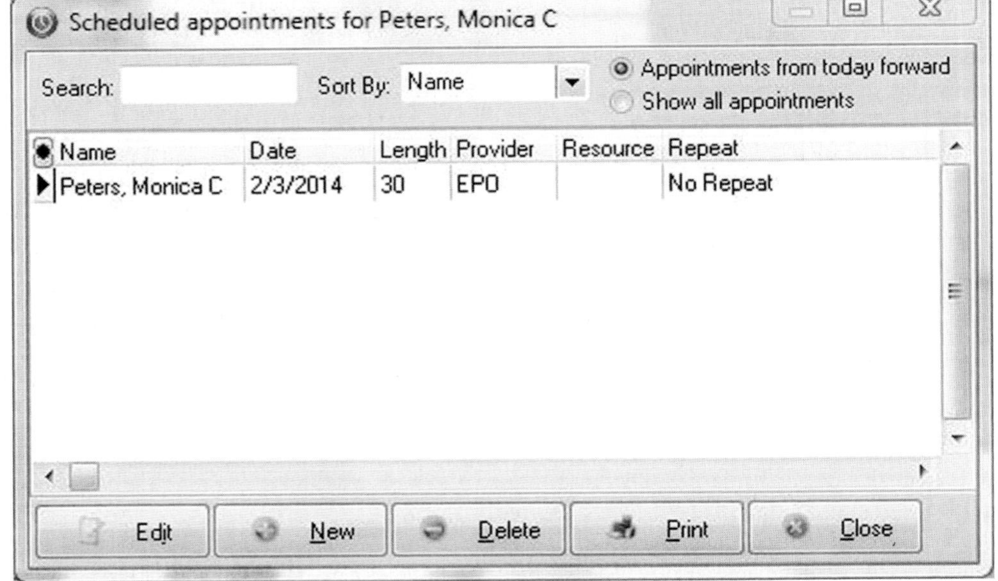

Figure 7-5 A computer printout can display all future appointments for a patient. Before the patient leaves the office, this printout can be given to a patient as a reminder of future appointments. (Screenshots used by permission of MCKESSON Corporation. All rights reserved. © MCKESSON Corporation 2012.)

Retrieving this type of information from a handwritten appointment book would be tedious and very time consuming and sometimes nearly impossible. A computerized system can have this type of information available in a matter of seconds.

Software Packages for Appointment Scheduling

Several software programs have been developed for appointment scheduling specific to the medical office. Selection and implementation of the appropriate program may be a difficult and costly process, but with the many advantages of computerized appointment scheduling, it is well worth the effort.

Implementation of appointment scheduling programs may cost several thousand dollars when the facility takes into account all the items necessary for implementation, such as

- The software itself
- Computer hardware needed to run the software
- Network cabling and other hardware necessary to connect and support the computer equipment
- Training for personnel

Although the implementation costs may seem high, computer implementation usually pays for itself by enhancing the productivity of office personnel and by providing a detailed record of the office's activities. In this day and age, a computer-based office management system that can manage appointments, patient registration information, billing, and other important activities is essential to the successful management of a busy office.

Concerns When a Computerized Appointment System Is Used

The use of a computerized system has its drawbacks. Contingency plans must be developed to handle those times when the computer system is down. Schedules should be printed often throughout the workday (every 1-2 hours if the schedule changes frequently) and distributed to physicians and nurses. Because appointment information is considered confidential, old copies of the schedule should be shredded when new copies are printed.

If a patient calls for an appointment or for information when the computer system is down, the medical office assistant should schedule an appointment manually on the computer printout. After the computer system is working again, appointment information can be entered into the system. An assistant's response should *never* be, "Our computers are down. You'll have to call back." Some patients may choose never to call back. If a patient desires an appointment for a day in the future, an assistant can offer to call the patient when the system is up and running.

Because a computer is an electronic device, an office should have a contingency plan for downtimes. Computer system failure may result from equipment or software failure or possibly a weather-related event such as a storm. Backup of computer data is vital for maintaining accurate records of office activities.

Manual System for Appointment Scheduling

Even though an overwhelming majority of medical offices use computerized appointment systems, it is important for an assistant to be familiar with how a manual system is used, just in case one is ever encountered in the workplace. In a manual system, appointments are handwritten into an appointment book (Fig. 7-6).

In looking at Figure 7-6, it is easy to spot open appointment times because they are blank. Appointments then are entered under the appropriate physician's schedule by writing in the appropriate blanks—in pencil—the patient's name, telephone number, and chart number, and the reason for the appointment. An "X" is placed in the corresponding square on the right. This allows anyone to view the weekly openings at a glance. If the patient requests an appointment at 9:30 PM sometime this week, the assistant can easily locate open slots by looking at the grid on the right.

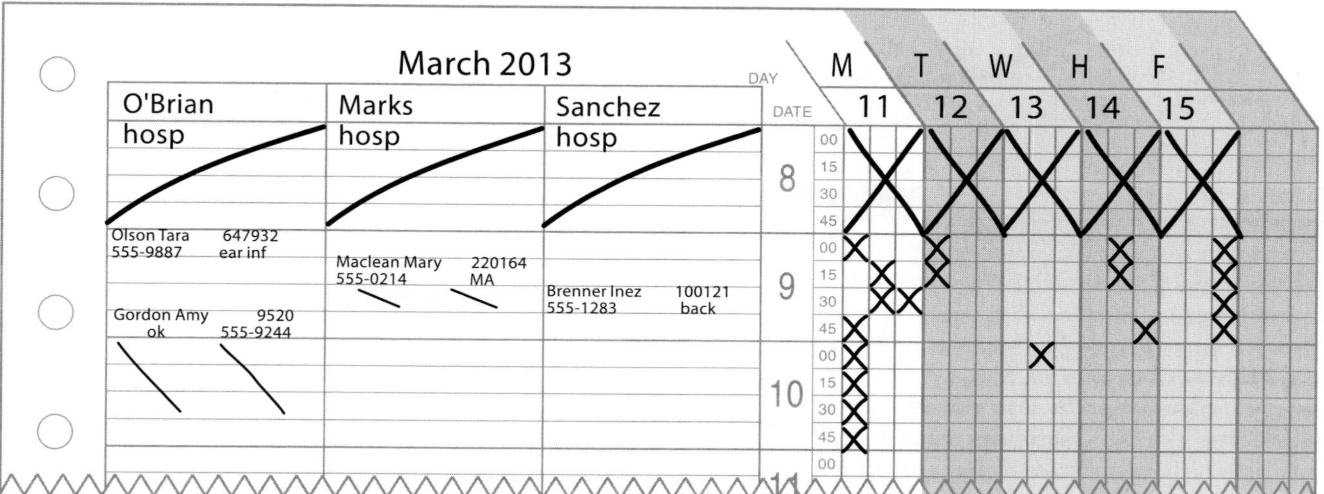

Figure 7-6 Appointment books still are used in a few medical offices. Open appointment times are indicated by the blank boxes in the grid on the right of the schedule. The lightest area of the page displays appointments available for Monday. (Form courtesy of Bibbero Systems, Inc., Petaluma, California; telephone: 800-242-2376; fax: 800-242-9330; www.bibbero.com.)

Pencils should always be used when appointments are entered in a manual system. Cancellations and rescheduled appointments are frequent occurrences in a medical office, necessitating erasures of originally scheduled appointments. Legible and accurate entries are essential so that personnel other than the assistant also may read the day's appointments. Books with entries that have been scribbled out or obliterated with correction fluid are sloppy, difficult to use, and sometimes even illegible. If ever subpoenaed, illegible records do not stand up well in court. It is a medical office assistant's obligation to keep legible and accurate appointment records.

Concerns When a Manual Scheduling System Is Used

Although appointment books are relatively inexpensive to purchase, they do have some obvious drawbacks.

First and foremost, the amount of time that a manual system takes is much more than a computerized system. It is more difficult to find open appointment times that may work with the patient's schedule. Locating information is extremely difficult because an assistant must flip through pages to look for information.

Using an appointment book means only one person at a time can schedule appointments for a specific physician. For example, you may be assisting a patient who wants to schedule an appointment with Dr. Sanchez, and another assistant may be helping another patient who also wants to schedule an appointment with Dr. Sanchez. The second patient will have to wait to schedule an appointment because the appointment book is currently in use.

In a larger practice with several providers, it is possible that more than one appointment book may be used. With several books on the desk, not only will the desk space be crowded, but an assistant may have to thumb through all the books to find an open appointment slot that meets the patient's needs. If more than one book is used, it is possible to write a patient's appointment on the wrong physician's schedule. If only one book is used for several providers, again, only one assistant can make an appointment for a patient at a given time.

A manual system for appointment scheduling can certainly get the job done, but if at all possible, a computerized system should be used to enhance productivity in the office and, ultimately, to serve patients in a more timely fashion.

CHECKPOINT

The medical office where you are employed is evaluating two pieces of appointment scheduling software for implementation in the office. Software A is cheaper but allows only one user at a time to access the appointment system. Software B is twice as expensive but allows an unlimited number of users to access the appointment system at one time. Three physicians, a nurse practitioner, three nurses, and three medical office assistants are employed at the clinic. It is your job to recommend to the providers the appropriate software package for purchase. Which software package would you recommend? Defend your answer.

Appointment Scheduling Methods

Most of today's offices have an established system for scheduling appointments. One of the first things an office staff will determine for appointment scheduling is the type of increments that will be used for office appointments. Will appointments be scheduled every 10 or 15 minutes? Or, will appointments be scheduled every half hour or every hour? The type of practice and the patients served will determine what increments are necessary. Family practice, internal medicine, pediatrics, and other providers involved in primary care usually use 10- to 15-minute intervals for appointments. Examples of appointment times necessary for specific patient complaints are shown in Table 7-1. Note that the more complicated a presenting problem is, the more time will be required for an appointment. Specialists such as neurosurgeons or psychiatrists often require lengthy examinations or interviews to assess a patient and will schedule patients for longer appointments (30- to 60-minute intervals).

Additionally, some practices request that new patients be scheduled for an additional amount of time (usually 10 to 15 minutes) because the physician will need time to get acquainted with the patient. Some practices also request that new patients report for appointments 15 minutes early to allow time for completion of a medical history questionnaire.

Double Booking (Overbooking) of Appointments

Some primary care physicians may allow the office staff to overbook their appointment schedules. This practice is known as **double booking.** Double booking involves scheduling an appointment at the same time that another appointment is scheduled. These types of appointments are usually quick, **urgent care**–type appointments that are similar to many of the 15-minute appointments shown in Table 7-1. The rationale for using double booking is that a patient's urgent care needs can be accommodated quickly. If a patient has a sore throat, he may not be able to wait a couple of days for the next available appointment. Double booking of appointments allows patients with urgent medical needs to be served sooner.

When a patient is double-booked for an appointment, the patient should be informed that the waiting time to be seen by a physician may be slightly longer than usual. *Double booking of a physician's schedule should be done only with the physician's approval.* Some physicians give blanket approval and always allow appointments to be double-booked; other physicians give their approval on a case-by-case basis.

CHECKPOINT

Which of the following appointments could be scheduled as a double-booked appointment?

(There may be more than one possible answer.)

- Wart treatment
- Headache
- Depression
- Lump
- Sinus pain
- Cough
- Ear infection
- Hearing check
- Burn

TABLE 7-1

Horizons Health Partners Appointment Scheduling Guidelines

15 Minutes	Physicals (px) (schedule by age)	30 Minutes	45 Minutes	60 Minutes
Ear pain, infection, or wash	(Pap included for female patients over 18 years)	Postoperative visit	Lesion removal (2 or more)	Initial (new) OB visit
Burn	Sports px—15 minutes	Lump	Proctosigmoidoscopy (procto)	Vasectomy
Sinus pain or infection	Younger than 18—15 minutes	Asthma	Hearing check	
URI Cough	18 to 39 years—30 minutes	Preop physical	Colposcopy	
Pharyngitis	40 to 64 years—45 minutes	Depression, any psych (use "personal")		
Wart treatment	65+ years—60 minutes	Foreign body removal		
Abdominal pain	Preop px—30 minutes	Chest pain		
Rash/urticaria		Muscle strain		
Allergies		Back pain		
Rechecks		Sprain or suspected fracture		
Recheck Pap		Menstrual problems		
Conjunctivitis		Lesion removal (1)		
Elevated temp		Ingrown toenail		
OB recheck		Headache (HA)		
UTI		Eye injury		
HTN		Laceration repair		
Diabetes				
Hemorrhoids				
Flu symptoms				

Walk-in Patients

Some providers may choose to leave occasional open spots in their schedule to accommodate acutely ill patients who walk into the clinic to be seen (hence, the name "**walk-in**"). Most practices encourage patients to make appointments, but patients occasionally may elect to drop in to the physician's office in the hope that they will be seen.

Even if the schedule is full, it is extremely important to consult the physician about any walk-in patient to find out whether the physician is able to see the patient. If the physician is unable to see the patient within a reasonable period, an appointment may have to be made for a later time. If the reason for the walk-in is a serious problem that requires immediate attention, the patient may have to be seen immediately or may have to be referred to an emergency room for treatment.

In some cases, the presenting problem is serious enough to warrant calling an ambulance to transport the patient from the clinic to the emergency department. Whatever the presenting problem, *sending a patient to an emergency department should be the decision of the physician* not of the medical office assistant. Imagine what could happen if a patient with severe indigestion is told to go to an emergency department. If the patient gets into a car, drives, and actually is experiencing a heart attack, the patient could die while driving his or her car. This, of course, would be a terrible occurrence, could additionally create potential liability on the part of the medical office, and obviously, would not serve the best interest of the patient at all.

Walk-in clinics

One of the latest trends in health care is the development of urgent care centers or walk-in clinics. These types of facilities often are open for extended hours to serve patients with health concerns that require immediate attention but that may not require the services of an emergency room. These facilities generally accept *only* walk-in patients, and patients usually are served in the order in which they arrive, with the exception of seriously ill patients who may or probably will receive top priority. Physicians should give the office front desk staff guidelines for identifying patients who need priority care. Whether or not a clinic is a walk-in facility, all assistants must be familiar with and must be able to recognize potential emergency medical situations because patients of all types will arrive at a clinic. Examples of symptoms that may indicate that a patient needs immediate medical attention are identified in Chapter 6, Box 6-1.

Group (Block) Scheduling

Sometimes, a practice will schedule several patients to come in at the same time, with the idea that these patients will be served in different areas of the clinic at that time. This practice, which is known as **group (block) scheduling,** suits some specialties very well.

For example, suppose you are working for an orthopedic practice. If four patients are scheduled at the same time, it is likely that one patient may be sent to have a radiograph taken, another may need cast removal and then a radiograph taken, one patient may see the doctor for a recheck, and the remaining patient may see the doctor for a visit that does not require a radiograph. While the third and fourth patients are waiting in examination rooms to be seen by the physician, other office personnel attend to the first and second patients. Then, when the third and fourth patients' visits are completed, the first and second patients are ready to be seen by the physician.

Series of Appointments

Sometimes a patient will need to come in for a series of appointments. A series of appointments are scheduled with the same provider, usually to address the same medical problem over and over again. This happens frequently in areas such as physical or occupational therapy, obstetrics and gynecology, or allergy and immunology. In such clinics, a patient may be seen on a regular basis for reasons such as therapy sessions, prenatal checkups, or allergy injections. It often is best to try to schedule such appointments on the same date and at the same time to reduce the possibility that the patient may miss an appointment.

CHECKPOINT

Why is it convenient for a patient to have a series of appointments established for a medical condition that needs regular attention?

Multiple Appointments

Occasionally, patients have several medical needs for which they are seeing different providers. For example, a patient who is recovering from a stroke may be seeing a neurologist, a physical therapist, an occupational therapist, and/or a speech therapist, as well as a primary care physician. It would be very inconvenient for the patient to go to the clinic several times a week or month. For the convenience of the patient, it is desirable to schedule as many appointments as possible on the same day, or to routinely schedule the patient's appointments on the same day of the week. If a patient has multiple appointments scheduled on the same day, it is important for the assistant to make sure that the patient's medical record is available for all providers who are scheduled to see the patient on that day.

Appointment Scheduling Procedures

Before appointments can be placed on the schedule, it is necessary for the assistant to identify the availability of the facility and its providers. Physicians do not work 24 hours a day and often have other work commitments, such as meetings and off-site visits to patients, such as residents of nursing homes. All of these facts must be considered when one is establishing the appointment schedule.

Establishing Appointment Parameters

When setting up the schedule, it is important for the physician to communicate his or her scheduling preferences clearly to the staff, and for the staff to understand what the physician likes and dislikes regarding the scheduling of patients.

Some providers prefer a very tight schedule to ensure that there are no downtimes during which no patient is seen. Many providers view downtime as unproductive time. Other providers may prefer to be scheduled lightly because they do not like to keep patients waiting, or they may feel pressured if several patients are waiting in the lobby at once.

Many physicians prefer variety in scheduling and restrict the scheduling of similar appointments during the day. For example, a physician may allow only two physicals to be scheduled in the morning and two in the afternoon. Physicals are routine checks of a patient's health that can be planned weeks or months in advance. This restriction in the number of physicals scheduled per day allows the practice to keep appointment slots open for acutely ill patients.

Multiphysician Practices

Scheduling gets tricky when an assistant is working in an office with several physicians. The assistant may need to remember that one physician does not see pediatric patients, but that other physicians do see pediatric patients. Some physicians prefer to be scheduled lightly, and others prefer to be scheduled heavily.

Each physician should establish his or her own guidelines for appointment scheduling; however, physicians in a larger office should try to have as much uniformity in their scheduling as possible to make scheduling of appointments easier for their staff. The office staff must remember, however, that it is necessary to respect the physicians' preferences for scheduling.

Facility Limitations

A possible complication of the scheduling process is the availability of special facilities or equipment. Perhaps the clinic has only one minor surgery room or has only one piece of equipment that is used for a special procedure. These rooms or pieces of equipment sometimes are referred to as **resources**. In such a case, room or equipment availability must be checked before the appointment is scheduled. If any room or equipment limitations are noted, office staff may choose to maintain a separate appointment schedule for the room or equipment to keep track of usage.

Setting the Schedule

The first thing an assistant must do when setting the schedule is to block off days that the facility is not open (Procedure 7-1). The facility may not be open on weekends or on certain holidays. These days must be clearly marked as closed or unavailable, so a staff member does not inadvertently schedule an appointment on a day that the clinic is closed. An assistant who is making an advance appointment may not realize that Monday, May 28, is Memorial Day that year.

Next, all vacation days and unavailable times for every physician or provider in the office must be identified. If

Dr. Mallard does not work on Tuesday afternoons, then all Tuesday afternoons on her schedule must be marked as unavailable (Fig. 7-7). If the clinic has some evening hours during the week, these slots must be made available for scheduling. And, of course, hours that the office is closed—for example, before 8:00 AM or after 6:00 PM—are marked on the schedule.

After the initial unavailable times and days have been identified and marked on the schedule, other times that the physician is unavailable then must be marked. Hospital rounds, committee meetings, personal appointments, lunch or dinner breaks, and any other commitments that prevent the physician from seeing patients should be entered on the schedule. Some physicians prefer to have all commitments during the workday entered into the schedule. That way, when the physician checks the schedule, a clear picture of commitments and appointments is presented.

PROCEDURE 7-1

Prepare an Appointment Schedule for a Medical Office

Materials Needed

- Appointment scheduling software on a computer system or
- Appointment book and pencil

1. Identify and mark off the days that the office is closed (weekends, holidays, whatever applies).
2. Identify and mark off the times of each day that the office is closed.
3. Identify and mark off the times of each day that each physician is unavailable.

Advance Booking

Most offices have the schedule established well in advance. A typical schedule shows appointments scheduled and available for at least the next 6 months. Many appointments, such as physicals, will book far in advance, some even longer than 6 months in advance. Physicians typically limit the number of such appointments per day because this type of appointment is not urgent, and physicians must leave part of their schedule available for patients with acute care needs. It is important to remember, however, that appointments made that far in advance probably will require a written reminder or a telephone reminder to the patient a short time before the appointment is scheduled. Reminders are discussed later in this chapter.

Components of an Appointment

Every appointment made in a medical facility should include five vital pieces of information:

- Patient name
- Reason for the appointment
- Telephone number at which the patient can be reached during the day
- Medical record number (if numbers are used)
- Date of birth (DOB) is required for new patients and in offices with alphabetical filing systems.

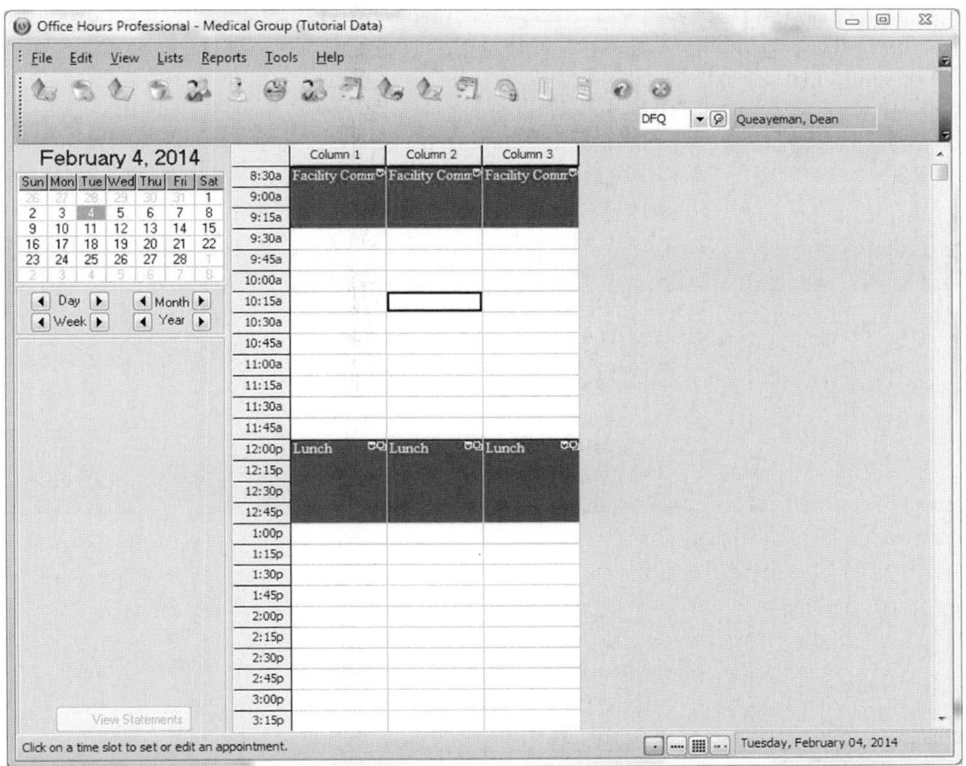

Figure 7-7 Time slots are marked off to indicate when a physician is unavailable for appointments. (Screenshots used by permission of MCKESSON Corporation. All rights reserved. © MCKESSON Corporation 2012.)

Name of Patient

The patient's name is needed, of course, to identify who is coming in to see the physician.

Reason for Appointment

The reason for the appointment, also referred to as the **chief complaint**, helps the assistant determine the amount of time needed for the appointment and allows the physician and the nursing staff to prepare for what lies ahead that day. The assistant must be very careful when listing the reason for the appointment not to diagnose the patient's condition and not to enter anything on the schedule that might be potentially damaging or embarrassing to the patient.

If a patient calls and says that he thinks he has an ear infection because he has ear pain, it is appropriate to write "ear pain" on the schedule. However, if a female patient calls and says that she has missed a period, "pregnant" should not be entered on the schedule.

When scheduling appointments a medical office assistant must constantly remember to avoid entering potentially damaging or embarrassing information (e.g., "STD," "venereal disease," "depression," "paranoid," or "nervous"). It often is best in these cases to list the reason for coming in as "personal," even if the patient states that he thinks he may have a sexually transmitted disease. It is important to remember that appointment schedules are sensitive, confidential documents because of the nature of the information contained within, and potentially embarrassing terms should not be written on the schedule.

If possible, use commonly accepted medical abbreviations when identifying the reason for the appointment. Not only will abbreviations save time and space, but they are part of a language usually known only to medical personnel, and their use will help to keep some schedule information confidential. Definitions for commonly accepted abbreviations are listed in Box 7-1. Other definitions can be found in most medical dictionaries, as well as in medical terminology books such as *Dorland's Medical Speller*. Every office should develop a list of approved abbreviations for appointment scheduling to ensure consistency of entries on the schedule.

Telephone Number

Listing the patient's daytime telephone number is useful in case the unexpected happens and the physician is unable to see that patient at the scheduled time. Situations such as a hospital emergency, a weather cancellation, or physician illness may result in the rescheduling of a large number of patients because of a physician's unavailability. The medical office assistant must try to reach the patient by telephone before the appointment time to reschedule. When telephone numbers are listed on the appointment schedule, the assistant can call patients quickly about a schedule change.

Medical Record Number

If an office uses a paper medical records system, the patient's appointment will need to include the patient's medical record number to make it easy for the office personnel to pull the medical records for the day's patients. Depending on the size of the facility, records for the day's appointments usually are pulled a day or two in advance of the patient's appointment. In multiphysician offices, the records for the day's appointments usually are grouped by physician and may be kept near the registration desk. Many assistants who are in charge of registering patients for their appointments like to then place the records for each physician in the order in which the appointments are scheduled.

Most patients will not know their medical record number, and if a manual scheduling system is used, an assistant will have to locate patients' medical record numbers by looking up each number in whatever type of manual system the office maintains. However, if a computerized system is used, medical record numbers can be automatically linked from the patient's information and included with the appointment.

Date of Birth

If a patient is new to the facility, the patient's DOB should be obtained when the appointment is booked. This will allow the

BOX 7-1

Common Abbreviations Used in Appointment Scheduling

BCP—birth control pill
BP—blood pressure
bx—biopsy
Dx—diagnosis
FB—foreign body
flex or procto—proctosigmoidoscopy
fx—fracture
HA—headache
HOH—hard of hearing
HTN—hypertension
hx—history
LLQ—left lower quadrant
LOC—loss of consciousness
LUQ—left upper quadrant
OB—obstetric
pt—patient
px—physical
RLQ—right lower quadrant
RUQ—right upper quadrant
Rx—prescription, treatment, therapy
s/p—status post
SOB—shortness of breath
Stat—immediately
Sx—symptoms
tx—treatment
URI—upper respiratory infection
UTI—urinary tract infection
x—times

medical office assistant to check the patient database to make sure a record does not already exist for the patient.

In a facility that uses alphabetical filing for medical records, knowing the patient's DOB will allow an assistant to retrieve the correct chart for the patient. It is possible for a facility to have several patients with the same name (e.g., Robert Smith). Securing the patient's DOB enables the assistant to correctly identify the patient for whom the appointment has been scheduled. A patient's address may not definitively identify a patient because an address may change—a birth date does not!

Offices that use a computerized appointment system will have the patient's telephone number medical record number, and any other necessary appointment information inserted automatically on the printout of the schedule. When computerized appointment systems are used, after the patient is identified, all necessary additional appointment information, such as medical record number, and telephone number, is automatically linked to the appointment that is made.

Once the appointment time has been secured for the patient, you should confirm the appointment by issuing a written reminder for the patient, or, in the case of an appointment made over the telephone, you should repeat all appointment information back to the caller and wait for acknowledgment of the appointment from the caller (Procedure 7-2). At that point, the appointment can be finalized and you can assist the next patient.

PROCEDURE 7-2

Schedule Appointments

Materials Needed

- List of appointments and scheduling guidelines
- Appointment scheduling software on a computer system or
- Appointment book and pencil

1. Determine the reason for the appointment.*
2. Using scheduling guidelines, determine the length of the appointment.
3. Identify the patient's name.
4. Determine the preferences for a desired appointment time.
5. Identify the date and time for the appointment, and obtain approval for the date and time from the patient (or the patient's representative).
6. Enter appointment on the schedule.
7. Confirm the appointment with the patient (or the patient's representative).*

Optional

8. If the patient is in the office, give the patient a written reminder of the appointment.

**Denotes a crucial step in the procedure. This step must be completed satisfactorily for the procedure to be completed satisfactorily.*

Prioritizing Appointments

It is often an assistant's job to decide who will get an appointment opening right away and who may need to wait to be seen. Of course, if the patient wants an appointment on the day he or she calls the office, an assistant should always try to accommodate the patient. Sometimes, however, this may not be possible.

If a limited number of openings are left for the current day, the nature and duration of the problem will likely determine whether or not a patient is scheduled for one of the remaining appointments. A patient who calls the office for treatment of warts could likely be accommodated at a later time when the schedule is not so heavily booked. If a patient calls with urinary frequency and burning, however, he or she may likely have a urinary tract infection (UTI) and cannot wait a few days to come in. A UTI left untreated could develop into a kidney infection, which can be a very serious medical condition.

In a busy primary care office, the assistant is not always able to accommodate all patients' needs for appointments. Sometimes, after a weekend or holiday, patients' needs for urgent care appointments are greater than on other days. Mondays can be particularly busy because patients may have had symptoms develop over the weekend and will call for an appointment as soon as the office opens on Monday morning. Some offices do not allow routine visits, such as physicals, to be scheduled on Mondays or on the day after a holiday, so that the office can accommodate those patients who became ill when the clinic was closed. Some offices allow acute care appointments only during evening or weekend hours.

It is important to remember that because the mission of a medical office is to serve patients, an assistant should ask a patient when he or she would like to come in for an appointment. Although the patient may not be able to get his or her first choice of appointment time, you should always try to accommodate a patient whenever possible. An assistant should not begin to suggest appointment times without considering the patient's needs.

One technique that works well is to ask the patient what day of the week he or she would prefer, and whether he or she would prefer a morning or an afternoon appointment. After listening to the patient's preference, the assistant then can let the patient know what time slots are available. With this method, the patient's needs are more likely to be met. Remember, the patient is the office's number one priority!

If a medical office assistant is unsure whether the problem needs immediate attention, the assistant should consult the physician or nurse to determine when the patient should be placed on the schedule. This decision-making process is known as **triage,** which is defined by the *Miller-Keane Encyclopedia and Dictionary of Medicine, Nursing and Allied Health* as "establishing priorities of patient care for urgent treatment while allocating scarce resources." For example, how do you decide which appointments are given to whom? If the schedule shows only five appointments left for today or for the rest of this week, you must be careful to use those appointments *only for patients with urgent medical needs.*

What if there are no appointment openings, and a patient calls with a problem that requires the attention of the physician that day? The patient should never be turned away. You should offer to take a message regarding the patient's call. The physician then may decide to overbook or, possibly, may give medical advice to the patient over the telephone.

Sometimes, a patient with a severe complaint may call to request an appointment. If the medical office assistant determines that the patient's problem is a potentially life-threatening situation, it is important for the assistant to remain calm and not alarm the patient. Instead of scheduling the appointment, an assistant should say to the patient, "Before I schedule the appointment, I'd like you to talk with the nurse." Then, the assistant can transfer the call to the nurse. The nurse will likely screen the call and, if necessary, will recommend appropriate action, possibly directing the patient to go to the nearest emergency room or instructing the patient to call an ambulance. By recognizing a potentially serious situation, the medical office assistant may help the patient avoid further harm and perhaps may even save a life.

CHECKPOINT

Why is it important for the medical office assistant to have an excellent understanding of anatomy, physiology, and disease processes in order to appropriately schedule appointments in the medical office?

No-Show Appointments

Occasionally, a patient does not arrive for a scheduled appointment. This situation is known as a **no-show.** There may be many reasons why a patient does not show up for an appointment. Whatever the reason, it is important to give the patient the benefit of the doubt and to assume that the patient inadvertently missed the appointment. A medical office assistant should never assume that the patient missed the appointment intentionally.

An assistant should give the patient sufficient time to arrive for the appointment before recording the appointment as a no-show. A simple traffic jam, a stalled vehicle, or inclement weather could delay a patient for several minutes to an hour. It is wise to wait at least 1 hour before documenting the appointment as a no-show.

Medical offices realize that from time to time patients may forget about an appointment that has been scheduled. Usually, patients are not billed for a no-show. An exception may be missed appointments at a mental health clinic, where many appointments are 1 hour in length. A missed 1-hour appointment may result in a substantial amount of unproductive time for the office. In this case, a no-show appointment may be billed to the patient. If the office has a policy of charging for missed appointments, this policy should be communicated clearly in advance to patients.

Documentation of No-shows

Once it has been determined that the patient is a no-show for an appointment, it is important that the no-show be documented in the patient's medical record. This information is documented primarily to protect the physician or provider in case of any legal action. Suppose the patient has diabetes and routinely misses appointments set up to monitor his or her disease. If the patient later develops complications and tries to place blame on the medical staff, the fact that the patient has neglected to monitor his or her disease appropriately with the physician's guidance may make the patient's claim difficult to prove in court.

When charting a no-show in the patient's record, a medical office assistant should document the no-show on the date on which the no-show occurred. If a paper record is used to document a no-show, all documentation should be written in black ink. (Documentation is discussed further in Chapter 9.) Beginning at the left-hand margin of the patient's progress notes, the current date should be entered, followed by a statement similar to "Patient failed to show for an appointment with Dr. X." The statement then should be signed at the right margin with the medical office assistant's name and job title. Any blank space between the statement and the signature should be marked out with a thin black line (Fig. 7-8). If documentation is entered into an electronic record, the date, information regarding the no-show, and the assistant's name will be entered into the patient's record.

Some medical offices may request that the assistant telephone the patient and inform him or her of the no-show appointment. As mentioned previously, the patient may have a medical condition that warrants attention and may need to reschedule the appointment. This call should be documented in the patient's medical record as well. The documentation explanation "Patient was called regarding no-show for 11-18-20xx appointment with Dr. Martin" is sufficient. A notation

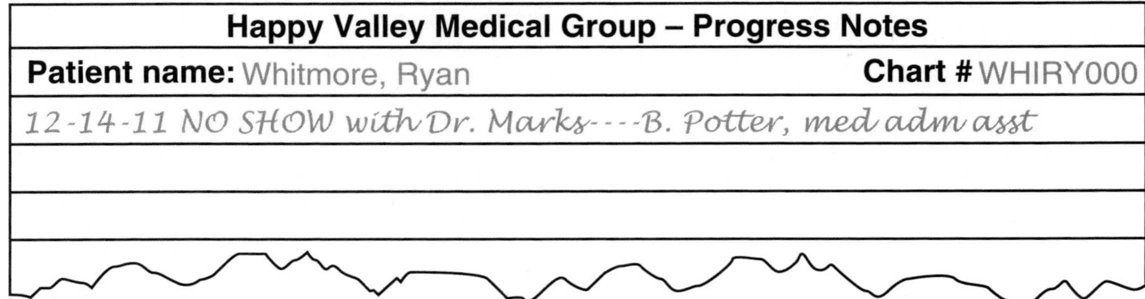
Happy Valley Medical Group – Progress Notes
Patient name: Whitmore, Ryan Chart # WHIRY000
12-14-11 NO SHOW with Dr. Marks---B. Potter, med adm asst

Figure 7-8 No-show appointments must always be documented in the patient's chart to protect the health facility from possible litigation.

also should be made as to whether or not the patient rescheduled the appointment (Procedure 7-3).

Canceled and Rescheduled Appointments

A canceled appointment occurs when a patient has made an appointment and later requests that the appointment be canceled. A canceled appointment should be removed from the schedule. If possible, an appointment cancellation should be documented in the medical record, similar to documentation for the no-show. The documentation should read something similar to "Patient canceled (date) appointment with Dr. X. Patient did not wish to reschedule" (Fig. 7-9).

A cancellation is documented for the same reason that a no-show is documented. It is important to protect the physician and the health care facility from any potential litigation whenever possible.

A rescheduled appointment occurs when a patient has made an appointment and later requests that the appointment time or, possibly, the physician be changed (Procedure 7-4). Because the patient intends to meet the physician at the rescheduled appointment, there usually is no need at that time to document the rescheduling in the patient's chart. An exception might be if the rescheduled date is far in the future.

When appointments are rescheduled, it is important for the assistant to remember to delete the first appointment from the schedule. In a busy office with a manual system, it is easy for the assistant to forget to erase the first appointment. Many computerized systems have built-in rescheduling that automatically voids the first appointment when the second is made. It is important that the schedule be accurate to reflect open time slots for other patients who may need them.

Ancillary and Referral Appointments

Sometimes, it is necessary for an assistant to schedule outside appointments for the practice's patients. **Ancillary appointments** are appointments made with departments, such as laboratory or radiography, to have special diagnostic tests performed. **Referral appointments** are appointments made with a specialist to see the patient regarding medical concerns. Insurance companies with managed care provisions usually require that referrals to a specialist must be approved

PROCEDURE 7-3

Document Appointment Changes

Materials Needed

- Patient's medical record
- Black ink pen (if paper record is used)

1. Identify appointment change (no-show, cancellation, reschedule, etc.)
2. Locate patient's medical record.*
3. In appropriate location in the patient's record, enter the date and document the appointment change.
4. Sign the record entry.*

**Denotes a crucial step in the procedure. This step must be completed satisfactorily for the procedure to be completed satisfactorily.*

PROCEDURE 7-4

Reschedule Appointments

Materials Needed

- Appointment scheduling software or
- Appointment book and pencil

1. Obtain the patient's name.*
2. Locate the original appointment.*
3. Verify the reason for the appointment. Using scheduling guidelines, determine whether the length of the appointment is correct.
4. Determine the preferences for a desired appointment time.
5. Identify the date and time for the appointment, and obtain approval for the date and time with the patient (or patient's representative).
6. Enter new appointment on the schedule.
7. Confirm the new appointment with the patient (or patient's representative).
8. Delete the original appointment.

Optional

9. Give the patient a written reminder of the new appointment.

**Denotes crucial step in the procedure. This step must be completed satisfactorily for the procedure to be completed satisfactorily.*

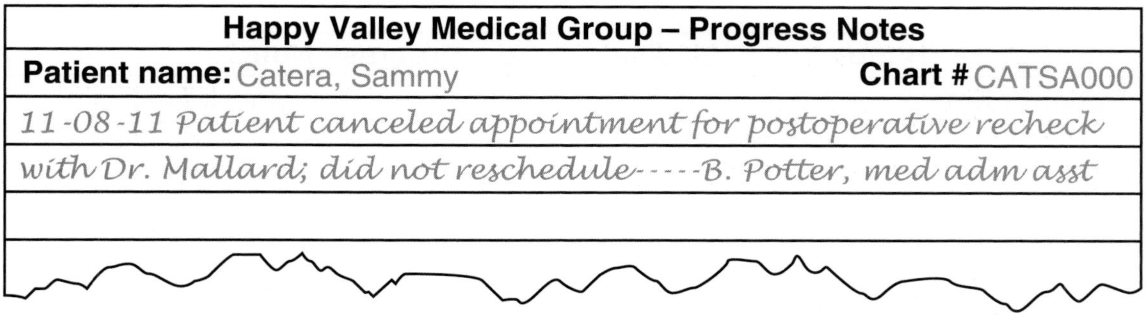

Happy Valley Medical Group – Progress Notes

Patient name: Catera, Sammy **Chart #** CATSA000

11-08-11 Patient canceled appointment for postoperative recheck
with Dr. Mallard; did not reschedule-----B. Potter, med adm asst

Figure 7-9 Cancellation of appointments by the patient should be documented in the patient's chart to protect the health facility from possible litigation.

by the patient's primary care physician before the patient can see a specialist.

When any outside appointment must be scheduled, it is important for the assistant to have all necessary information ready when calling the facility to set up the appointment. First, the medical office assistant should have already checked with the patient and obtained his or her preference for the day and time when the outside appointment could be scheduled. It is good practice also to have the patient's record on hand. When the outside appointment is scheduled, it should be recorded in the patient's record. This method of charting is similar to previous examples given in this chapter. A sample entry for these types of appointments is shown in Figure 7-10. Any instructions for the referral appointment should be obtained on behalf of the patient.

Surgical Appointments

If an assistant works for a surgeon, it will be the assistant's responsibility to schedule surgery for patients. A number of things are required for surgical appointments. First and foremost, the assistant must learn from the surgeon exactly what procedure or procedures the patient will have done. The surgeon will have established guidelines for the length of time required for each type of surgery that he or she performs. If the procedure is expected to be particularly difficult for any reason (e.g., unique circumstances of the case or age of the patient), the surgeon will inform the assistant that additional time should be scheduled for the surgical procedure.

After the procedure has been identified, the assistant must obtain the patient's current insurance information and should contact the insurance company for **precertification** or authorization for surgery. Because of the requirements of most insurance companies today, authorization must be obtained before most surgical procedures are performed, or benefits will not be paid for the procedure. (Exceptions do exist in cases of emergency treatment.) Insurance coverage must be verified and authorization obtained for the procedure, or the patient may be responsible for the entire bill. At the time of precertification, the insurance company may issue an estimate of benefits that will be paid by insurance for the surgery.

Aside from insurance company requirements, patients scheduled for surgery almost always will be required to have a preoperative physical within a week before surgery. The preoperative physical may have to be scheduled with the patient's primary care physician. This physical helps to ensure that the patient is able to undergo the surgical procedure. Of course, in emergency cases, surgery may have to be performed to save the life of the patient, regardless of whether or not a physical was done. An assistant responsible for surgical scheduling will make sure that the patient has a preoperative physical scheduled. The physician who is performing the preoperative physical conducts a physical examination of the patient and orders any necessary tests to determine whether the patient is in acceptable health to undergo a surgical procedure. After the physical has been done, copies of the results of the physical examination and tests are sent to the surgeon's office. An assistant often is responsible for making sure that the preop physical has been done, so the results may be reviewed by the surgeon prior to surgery.

At the time of initial scheduling of the patient's surgery, the patient is given a tentative date for the surgery and instructions for preoperative care. Because surgical schedules can change often, the assistant or nurse phones the patient on the day before the surgery to give the patient a time to report to the facility for surgery. Any last minute instructions are given to the patient at that time.

Pharmaceutical and Other Sales Representatives' Appointments

Many sales representatives who sell pharmaceuticals, medical supplies, and office supplies often compete for the attention of the physician.

Pharmaceutical sales representatives meet with physicians and other clinical staff members to give them information on the medications their company produces, to inform the staff about new products, and to offer free samples of many of their products. Other sales representatives may request appointments to sell medical equipment or supplies. Some offices limit the number of sales visits per representative, and some offices allow only a designated number of total appointments per week (e.g., two appointments available on Tuesday and two on Thursday). Appointments may be recorded on the patients' schedule, but it is important that they not be recorded as medical appointments; rather, they should be recorded the way meetings are recorded. Pharmaceutical representatives often are allowed, and sometimes are even encouraged, to stop in between appointments to replenish their sample stock in the office.

A medical office can receive many sales solicitations, and it is important for you to recognize sales pitches and to require

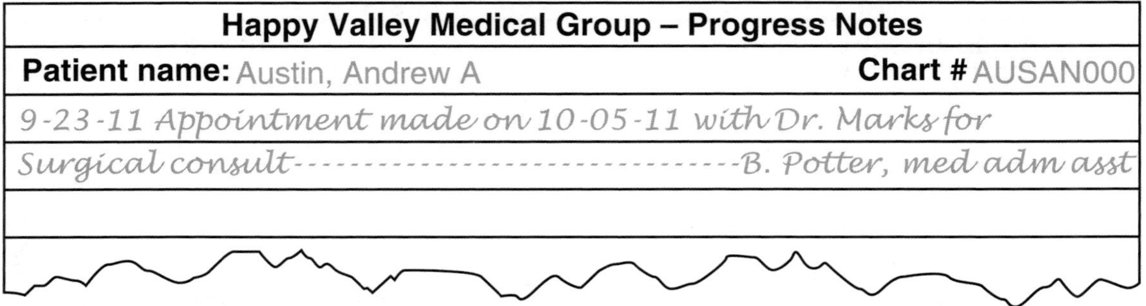
Happy Valley Medical Group – Progress Notes

Patient name: Austin, Andrew A Chart # AUSAN000

9-23-11 Appointment made on 10-05-11 with Dr. Marks for

Surgical consult------------------------------B. Potter, med adm asst

Figure 7-10 Outside appointments scheduled by the office staff should be recorded in the patient's chart.

a representative to make an appointment to see the physician and office staff. Most offices are far too busy to handle drop-in sales people. Sales representatives often bring pens, pencils, notepads, and other office supplies to the medical office staff. You should be careful to not deviate from the office policy for handling sales representatives, regardless of these "perks."

Appointment Reminders

Written Reminders

When a patient makes an appointment in person, a reminder of the appointment is given to the patient before he or she leaves the office. Electronic systems have the capability of printing appointment reminders for patients. These reminders can include only appointments with a specific department or physician or may include all appointments (not just appointments with a particular physician) that a patient has scheduled within a medical facility (Fig. 7-5).

If an office uses handwritten reminders, it is good practice to write only the patient's first name on the reminder slip. Although this slip is given directly to the patient, the medical office assistant must remember that the information contained on the slip is about a medical appointment that the patient has in the future. If the patient loses the reminder, the information on the reminder could potentially embarrass or harm the patient. A patient's name on a reminder slip for an appointment at a local mental health facility would likely identify the patient as a client of the facility, and, because of the social stigma connected with seeking some types of medical treatment, this could possibly harm the patient.

Some offices mail letters to patients 1 to 2 weeks before appointments. This is a relatively inexpensive process as letters can be automatically generated by a computer's appointment system at a preset time before each appointment. Reminders may differ in appearance from office to office, but they all contain the same basic information: (1) patient's name, (2) date, (3) time of next appointment, and (4) provider's name. Each reminder usually also contains office information, such as address and telephone number.

Telephone Reminders

Whenever the patient is present in the clinic, it is recommended that a reminder be given to the patient at that time. Many appointments, however, are scheduled over the telephone. In those cases, a telephone call should be made to remind the patient of the appointment. These telephone reminders are usually done on the day before the scheduled appointment to give the office staff enough time to reach the patient, and to give the patient notice that the appointment time is near. Telephone reminders done too far in advance might give the patient too much time to forget the appointment.

When you are working in a primary care office, a good rule to follow is to give a telephone reminder to any patient who has an appointment for 30 minutes or longer. Generally, if a primary care office is even moderately busy, a missed 15-minute appointment will not leave a huge gap in the schedule, but a missed 30- to 60-minute appointment might create a great deal of downtime. The office should establish a policy about which appointments should be preceded by telephone reminders.

The medical office assistant should use caution when leaving a telephone reminder. In no circumstance should the assistant leave the reminder with anyone but the patient, unless the patient has authorized that messages can be given to other individuals (see Fig. 6-8). When telephoning the patient, the medical office assistant should first ask for the patient by name, to verify that the message is given to the individual for whom it is intended.

A typical telephone reminder might sound like the following:

> Assistant: *Hello, may I speak with Amy, please?*
> Amy: *This is Amy.*
> Assistant: *Amy, this is Nancy calling from Happy Valley Medical Group. I am calling to remind you of your 3:00 appointment tomorrow with Dr. Martin.*
> Amy: *Oh, thank you for calling.*
> Assistant: *You're welcome. We'll see you tomorrow. Good-bye.*
> Amy: *Good-bye.*

In this conversation, you will notice that the medical administrative assistant does not identify where she is calling from until she confirms that she is talking with the patient. It is important to keep the information about the appointment confidential and to not give that information to anyone else in the household. The patient may not want information about the appointment to be shared with anyone. An exception is, of course, that parents will receive reminders for their children's appointments.

Posting the Schedule

Every day, the current day's appointment schedule is posted at or near the nurses' station for the use of the nurses and the physicians. As mentioned previously, new copies of the schedule are printed or copied throughout the day to keep the staff aware of changes in the schedule. It is extremely important to remember that the schedule should be posted out of the view of patients. The schedule should not be posted in examination rooms or in the hallway in the plain view of others.

An additional copy of the schedule sometimes is posted at the front desk where patients check in for appointments. The front desk staff may elect to do this to keep a minute-by-minute check of who has and who has not arrived for an appointment. Such a copy should be kept out of the view of patients and is used solely by the office staff. Most computer systems also can track such information.

> **HIPAA Hint**
>
> Appointment information is confidential and is protected by HIPAA, so any printed copies of appointment schedules should be disposed of properly.

Planning for the Unexpected

Even the most organized and efficiently planned schedule may be ruined when the unexpected happens. A physician may become ill and be unable to see patients. A physician could be called away to the hospital for a delivery or to see a patient for a serious problem. An emergency patient may come to the clinic. Whatever the case may be an assistant and the rest of the office staff will need to minimize the impact of the unexpected on the appointment schedule.

Patients always should be notified if the physician has been delayed. Patients currently in the office when the unexpected occurs may be given the opportunity to perhaps see another provider in the office who can accommodate them. Patients may wish to wait, or they may want to reschedule. Try to accommodate patients whenever possible. Patients usually are very empathetic in these situations. Whatever the case may be, most patients understand that emergencies do arise, and they would want the physician to be available if they were to need emergency treatment.

SUMMARY

Efficient appointment scheduling is a critical element in any medical office. A large part of the office atmosphere is determined by the office schedule. The assistant should take great care to properly schedule patients for appropriate appointment lengths and to manage no-shows, schedule changes, and unexpected occurrences. In addition, an assistant must continually try to accommodate a patient's needs when scheduling. The assistant who can successfully integrate these guidelines into everyday activities is an important asset to the medical office.

YOU ARE THE MEDICAL ADMINISTRATIVE ASSISTANT

You are working in a busy family practice office. It is midmorning, and only one appointment slot is left for an appointment today. What options might be open for accommodating patients who need to be seen today?

REVIEW EXERCISES

Exercise 7-1 True or False

Read each statement, and determine whether the answer is true or false. Record your answer in the blank provided. T = true; F = false.

____ 1. Most medical offices today use a manual system for scheduling appointments.

____ 2. A computerized system can easily identify when a patient's next appointment is scheduled.

____ 3. Offices with computerized appointment systems often are more productive than are offices with manual systems.

____ 4. If the office computers are down, the medical administrative assistant should tell callers to call back in a few hours.

____ 5. Appointment book entries in a manual system should be made in black ink to allow the schedule to photocopy well.

____ 6. Computerized systems serve patients more quickly than manual systems.

____ 7. The more complicated a patient's presenting problem is, the less time is required for the appointment.

____ 8. Primary care providers usually will require short intervals, such as 10- to 15-minute intervals, for appointments.

____ 9. A double-booked appointment is an appointment that is scheduled in two different appointment books.

____ 10. It is acceptable to leave a reminder for a patient's appointment with the patient's spouse.

____ 11. It is critical to chart a no-show for an appointment to protect the facility in case of possible litigation.

____ 12. Patients usually are billed for missed appointments.

____ 13. If a medical administrative assistant suspects that a patient is experiencing symptoms of a heart attack, the assistant should not have the patient talk to the nurse but should instruct the patient to go directly to the emergency room.

____ 14. In the absence of a medical record number, the patient's DOB should be obtained when an appointment is scheduled.

____ 15. The medical administrative assistant should always list the patient's exact words as the reason for the appointment.

____ 16. In nonemergency cases, failure to get an insurance authorization for a surgical procedure may mean that the patient may have to pay the entire bill for the procedure.

____ 17. Electronic appointment systems can print appointment reminders for patients.

____ 18. Appointment information is protected confidential information.

____ 19. A series of appointments should be scheduled on different days of the week.

____ 20. A preoperative physical is done to ensure that a patient can undergo surgery.

____ 21. Triage is done to ensure that patients with urgent care needs are given top priority.

____ 22. For a managed care plan, approval for referral to a surgical specialist probably will be required.

Exercise 7-2 Appointment Lengths

Using Table 7-1, match the appropriate length of time to schedule an appointment for patients with the following complaints. Record your answer in the blank provided. Some answers may be used more than once; some answers may not be used.

(a) 15 minutes
(b) 30 minutes
(c) 45 minutes
(d) 60 minutes

____ 1. Physical for a 62-year-old

____ 2. Abdominal pain

____ 3. Ingrown toenail

____ 4. Ear pain

____ 5. Breast lump

____ 6. Temperature of 103° F

____ 7. Plantar warts

____ 8. Physical for a 5-year-old

____ 9. Rash

____ 10. Removal of two lesions

____ 11. Sinus infection

____ 12. Cough

____ 13. Pulled muscle

____ 14. Hearing check

____ 15. Conjunctivitis

____ 16. Procto

____ 17. Urinary tract infection

____ 18. Sprained ankle

For a challenge, try the following

____ 19. A feeling of fullness in the ear

____ 20. Pain when swallowing

____ 21. Swelling of unknown cause

____ 22. Severe sunburn

____ 23. Twisted ankle

____ 24. Red, watery eyes

____ 25. Feeling of pressure between the eyes, stuffy nose

____ 26. Toe is red, is oozing pus, and is painful on touching

____ 27. FB eye

____ 28. Cold

____ 29. Px to play football

____ 30. Med recheck

____ 31. Migraine

____ 32. Wheezing

____ 33. Px before surgery

____ 34. Irregular menstrual periods

____ 35. Poison ivy

____ 36. Dysuria

Exercise 7-3 Prioritizing Appointments

In each group, choose the symptom of the patient who should receive the first available appointment on the schedule today.

____ 1. (a) Warts
(b) UTI
(c) Leg lump that has been present for 2 months

____ 2. (a) Possible fx
(b) px for 10-year-old
(c) New OB visit

____ 3. (a) Lesion removal
(b) Sports px so student can practice this evening
(c) Pain in the lower right quadrant of the abdomen

____ 4. (a) Seasonal allergies
(b) Recheck Pap
(c) Asthma flare-up

____ 5. (a) Proctosigmoidoscopy
(b) Grease burn at work today
(c) Recurrent cough

____ 6. (a) Bleeding between menstrual periods
(b) Ear wash
(c) Pink eye

____ 7. (a) Warts
(b) Cough for past 2 weeks
(c) Migraine

____ 8. (a) Lump
(b) FB—eye
(c) Painful menses

____ 9. (a) Physical for 65-year-old
(b) Procto
(c) Vasectomy

____ 10. (a) Recheck Pap
(b) Lesion removal
(c) Ingrown toenail

Exercise 7-4 Appointment Reasons

Identify whether the following items should appear on the schedule as a reason for an appointment. Y = yes; N = no.

____ 1. Abdominal discomfort

____ 2. Recheck STD

____ 3. HIV test

____ 4. Pain with coughing

____ 5. Feeling suicidal

____ 6. Venereal warts

____ 7. Light-headedness

____ 8. Recheck rash

____ 9. Paranoid

____ 10. Herpes

____ 11. Rash

____ 12. Nervous

____ 13. Lump

____ 14. Headache

____ 15. Depressed

____ 16. Genital warts

Exercise 7-5 Abbreviations for Appointment Scheduling

List the meaning of these common scheduling abbreviations.

1. fx ____________________
2. tx ____________________
3. px ____________________
4. bx ____________________
5. hx ____________________
6. HA ____________________
7. FB ____________________
8. URI ____________________
9. UTI ____________________
10. OB ____________________
11. SOB ____________________
12. HOH ____________________

ACTIVITIES

ACTIVITY 7-1 MANAGE A COMPUTERIZED APPOINTMENT SYSTEM

Using the Medisoft software provided with this text, you will establish parameters for the appointment system at Happy Valley Medical Clinic. You will be working in the month of February 2014 for the exercises in this text. (Reminder: If you experience difficulty at any time while performing these exercises, click **Help>Medisoft Help>Contents** for information on scheduling appointments.)

This exercise must be completed before any other appointment exercises are completed. All computer exercises should be completed in the order they appear in the text because much of the information included within the exercises is sequential.

To access the Medisoft appointment system, do the following:

1. Open **Medisoft>Medical Group** as instructed in previous chapters.
2. On the main menu, click **Activities>Appointment Book.** The **Office Hours Professional** window will open on today's date. You will be working in the separate part of the Medisoft software entitled **Office Hours Professional** for all appointment exercises.

To establish appointment parameters for the appointment system, do the following:

1. In the **Office Hours Professional** window, click **File>Program Options**. Make sure the **Options tab** is open. Note that the following choices will be established as a default and will be applied to the entire calendar:
   a. **Start time** and **End time**: The starting and ending times for the appointment book can be set. Set the **Start time** to 9:00 and the **End time** to 5:00.
   b. **Interval**: Appointment lengths can be set to accommodate the type of medical practice. Family practice might prefer 10-minute appointments; neurosurgery might prefer 30-minute appointments. Set the interval to 15.
   c. **Default colors**: This identifies the colors used for appointment display. Set the default colors as follows:
   - Appointment—Silver
   - Conflict—Red
   - Break—Purple

d. Remaining fields within **Options** tab should be set as illustrated below:

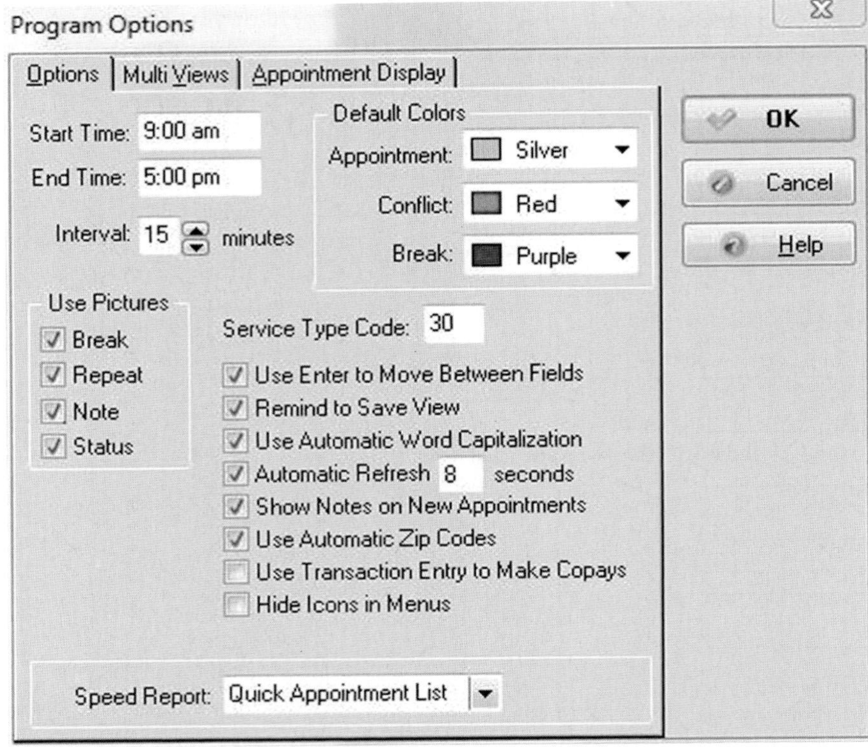

e. Leave **Multi Views** tab and **Appointment Display** tab as they are.

ACTIVITY 7-2 MANAGE A COMPUTERIZED APPOINTMENT SYSTEM—BREAK LISTS

1. To establish weekly time off for each provider, do the following:
   a. In the **Office Hours Professional** window, click **Lists>Break Lists**. You will create a new break for each different break on the list below.
   - Melvin Morris—out of office every Wednesday from 12-5
   - Emily O'Brian—out of office every Tuesday from 12-5

   b. Click **New**.
   c. Name the break **Out of Office—Wednesday Afternoon**.
   d. **Date** should be 2/1/2014.
   e. Insert beginning **time** of the break (12:00 PM). **Length** of break is 300 minutes (5 hours).
   f. Click **Change**. The repeat change window will open. Wednesday afternoon occurs once each week. Click **Weekly.** Specify **Every 1 Week(s)** in the blank provided. Wednesday should be checked. Remove the check from Monday. The **End On** box should read 2/9/2014. Click *OK* to close the repeat change window.
   g. **Some** should be selected under Providers because this break does not apply to all providers. Click **Save**.
   h. The **Provider Selection** window will appear. Click (highlight) the names of the providers for whom the break applies, in this case, Melvin Morris, DC. Click **OK**.
   i. To create time off for Emily O'Brian, repeat the steps above, substituting the information listed for her afternoon off. When you have finished entering the information, click **Close.**
2. To establish lunch breaks for the providers, do the following: Breaks for lunch are as follows:
   - Hinckle, Martinez, O'Brian —12:00 PM to 1:00 PM each day
   - Lee, Morris, Marks—1:00 PM to 2:00 PM each day (If breaks are entered for a group, lunch breaks will appear on days that Dr. Morris and Emily O'Brian have the afternoon off. Don't worry that this will happen.)

   a. In the **Office Hours Professional** window, click **Lists>Break List**.
   b. Click **New** to create a **New** break for each **different** provider.
   c. Name the break lunch—WH, JM, EO.
   d. Date should be 2/1/2014.
   e. Insert beginning time of lunch break. Length of break is 60 minutes.
   f. Click **Change**. Specify **Weekly** and **Every 1 Week(s)** in the blanks provided. Check M, T, W, T, F. The **End On** box should read 2/9/2014. Click **OK**.

3. To establish regular meetings for the physicians, do the following:
   Weekly meetings for physicians are as follows:
   - Dr. Lee has a weekly board meeting every Thursday from 8 AM to 9:30 AM. (Using the **Break List** option will override the 9:00 AM opening time.)
   - Dr. Hinckle has nursing home rounds scheduled from 3:00 PM to 5:00 PM every Tuesday.

   a. In the **Office Hours Professional** window, click **Lists>Break List**. Create a **New** break for each **different** meeting. Name the break for the meeting name and provider (e.g., Board Meeting—Lee).
   b. **Date** should be 2/1/2014.
   c. Insert beginning **time** of the meeting and specify the **length** of the meeting.
   d. Click **Change**. Specify the frequency of the meeting (normally weekly) and the day of the week for the meeting (break). The **End On** box should be 2/9/2014. Click **OK**.
   e. Schedule all meetings identified above. When you have finished entering the information, click **Close.**

(Note: Dr. Mallard will not be used for these exercises because the tutorial has repeating appointments and breaks entered on her schedule.)

ACTIVITY 7-3 MANAGE A COMPUTERIZED APPOINTMENT SYSTEM—REASON LIST

Medisoft has the capability to link a reason for an appointment with the length of time needed for the appointment. Use the table below to complete the exercise below.

To establish reasons for appointments, do the following:

1. In the **Office Hours Professional** window, click **Lists>Reason List**.
2. Click **New**. The **Appointment Reason Entry** window will open.
3. In the **Code** box, enter the appointment abbreviation from table below.
4. In the **Description** box, enter the complete description associated with the abbreviation.
5. Identify the appointment length associated with the appointment in the **Default Appointment Length** box. The **Default Appointment Color** should remain the same unless otherwise specified. Click **Save.**
6. Enter the entire list of appointment abbreviations. These abbreviations will be used in the next exercise. When done entering reasons, close the reason list.

Appointment Reason List

Code	Description	Length (minutes)	Color
ABDPAIN	Abdominal pain	15	silver
BURN	Burn tx	15	silver
EAR	Ear pain, infection or ear wash	15	silver
FLU	Flu-like sxs	15	silver
HTN	Hypertension, high blood pressure	15	silver
PNKEYE	Pink eye, conjunctivitis	15	silver
RASH	Rash, urticaria	15	silver
RECK	Recheck	15	silver
SINUS	Sinus pain or infection	15	silver
TEMP	Elevated temperature	15	silver
THROAT	Sore throat, pharyngitis	15	silver
URI	Upper respiratory infection, cough	15	silver
UTI	Urinary tract infection	15	silver
WART	Wart tx	15	silver
ASTHM	Asthma	30	yellow
BACK	Back pain	30	yellow
EYE	Eye injury	30	yellow
FB	Foreign body removal	30	yellow
FX	Suspected fracture	30	yellow
HA	Headache	30	yellow
LAC	Wound repair	30	yellow
LES	Lesion removal	30	yellow
LUMP	Lump, swelling	30	yellow
MENSES	Menstrual problems	30	yellow
MUSC	Muscle sprain/strain	30	yellow
PERS	Personal	30	yellow
POSTOP	Postoperative visit	30	yellow
TOENAIL	Ingrown toenail	30	yellow
COLP	Colposcopy	45	aqua
HEAR	Hearing check/problem	45	aqua
PROCTO	Proctosigmoidoscopy	45	aqua
NEWOB	Initial (new) OB visit	60	aqua
VAS	Vasectomy	60	aqua
PREOPPX	Preoperative physical	30	green
PX039	Physical 0-39 years	30	green
PX4064	Physical 40-64 years	45	green
PX65	Physical 65 and older	60	green
PXSPTS	Sports physical	15	green

ACTIVITY 7-4 MANAGE A COMPUTERIZED APPOINTMENT SYSTEM—ENTER APPOINTMENTS FOR EXISTING PATIENTS

Using Medisoft software, schedule the appointments in the table below by following the instructions below. (Be sure that the **Office Hours Professional** application is open [as described previously] to begin scheduling appointments.) All appointments will be scheduled for February 3 and 4, 2014.

1. In the **Office Hours Professional** window, click the drop-down arrow in the provider box on the upper right side of the Office Hours window. Click on the provider's name – Dr. Lee (for the first appointment). Once selected, the provider's name will appear in the provider box.
2. Select the appointment date by clicking arrows in the calendar displayed on the left side of the **Office Hours Professional** window. The appointment date should be highlighted. For the first appointment, select February 3, 2014.

3. Verify that the appointment time is available on the schedule. To schedule an appointment, double-click the box in column 1 next to the desired time slot. For the first appointment, select 3:30 PM. The **New Appointment Entry** window will open. Be sure to double-check the name of the provider in the lower portion of the **New Appointment Entry** window to make sure you are on the correct provider's schedule.
4. In the **New Appointment Entry** window, click the magnifying glass on the right of the **Chart** box. The **Patient Search Window** will open. Patient information can be located a number of ways: chart number, last name, social security number, etc. In the **Field** box, specify that the patient search should be **Last Name, First Name**. (Click the drop-down arrow to select this choice if necessary.) Locate the patient's information by typing the patient's last name in the **Search for** box or by using the scroll bar on the patient list. If the practice has a large number of patients, the most expedient way to locate a patient would be to input the first three to four letters of the patient's last name in the **Search for** box. (The drop-down arrow on the text box will reveal the list of patients in chart number order.)
5. Select the correct patient by double-clicking on the patient's name. The patient's name then will appear in a **New Appointment Entry** window. Press the tab key. You will note that the information for the patient now appears in the window.
6. Use the tab key to move to the **Reason** box. Select the reason from the reason list you created. For the first appointment, select **RASH.** The length of the appointment will be automatically adjusted based on the reason for the appointment. If the reason does not appear on the list, you may right click on the reason box and enter a new reason on the reason list.
7. Any additional information about the patient's appointment may be entered in the **Notes** box. Notes will print on the appointment report that will be printed later in the chapter activities.
8. Click **Save.** The patient's appointment should appear on the physician's schedule with time slots color coded for the required time for the appointment.
9. Enter all appointments from the table by following the instructions above.

Appointments to be Scheduled

Physician	Patient Name	Appointment Time	Reason/Notes
Lee	Zach Peters	2-3-14 3:30	Rash
Hinckle	Elmo Brimley	2-3-14 4:45	Rash (poison ivy?)
Lee	Tonya Hartman	2-3-14 2:30	Ingrown toenail
Hinckle	Michael Youngblood	2-3-14 2:30	Headache
Morris	Jay Brimley	2-3-14 4:00	Neck pain
Martinez	Anthony Zimmerman	2-3-14 11:00	Laryngitis
Lee	Anthony Peters	2-3-14 10:00	Finger laceration
Hinckle	John Bordon	2-3-14 2:00	Stomach upset
Martinez	Jane Doe	2-3-14 10:00	Chest congestion
Morris	Charles Gooding	2-3-14 9:00	Neck pain
O'Brian	Monica Peters	2-3-14 11:15	Menstrual problem
O'Brian	Susan Brimley	2-3-14 9:30	Sinus
Lee	Suzy Jones	2-3-14 11:15	Ear pain
Lee	Chadwick Koseman	2-3-14 4:15	Finger injury (possible fx)
Marks	Wallace Clinger	2-3-14 10:45	High blood pressure
O'Brian	Tanus Simpson	2-3-14 10:30	Pre-op px
Marks	John Doe	2-3-14 10:15	Fever
Hinckle	Lindsey Nielsen	2-4-14 9:15	Menses problem
Hinckle	Ryan Whitmore	2-4-14 10:30	Low back pain
Lee	Sammy Catera	2-4-14 3:00	Depression
Marks	John Doe	2-4-14 10:30	Recheck (feeling worse)
Martinez	Andrew Austin	2-4-14 1:00	Sinus
Marks	Dwight Again	2-4-14 9:45	Flu
Morris	Charles Gooding	2-4-14 10:15	Recheck
O'Brian	Tonya Hartman	2-4-14 9:15	Physical

ACTIVITY 7-5 MANAGE A COMPUTERIZED APPOINTMENT SYSTEM—ENTER APPOINTMENTS FOR NEW PATIENTS

Enter the following appointments for the patients who are new to Happy Valley Medical Group. Use the instructions below to enter new patient information at the time an appointment is made.

- William Frost, cell 010-555-1088, Dr. Morris, 2/3/14 10:00, back spasms
- Deanne Olson, cell 010-555-3233, Emily O'Brian, 2/4/14 10:30, ear pain

1. In the **Office Hours Professional** window, select the provider's schedule and locate the appointment day and time.
2. Open the desired time slot. In the **Chart** box, right click and select **New Patient.** Enter patient's **last name, first name**, and **cell phone number.** Click **Save.**
3. Enter the reason for the appointment. Click **Save.** The remainder of the patient's information will be entered when the patient registers for his or her appointment.

ACTIVITY 7-6 MANAGE A COMPUTERIZED APPOINTMENT SYSTEM—LOCATING APPOINTMENTS

Practice locating appointments that you have already made. Appointments can be located quickly by completing the following:

1. In **Office Hours Professional**, click **Lists>Patients/ Guarantors and Cases**.
2. Determine which patient's appointments you wish to locate and open the patient's file. In the **Name, Address** tab, click the **Appointments** button on the right. The patient's appointments will appear in a new window. If needed, click **Print**, then **Preview>print**, or **Export** to save a list of the patient's appointments. Then click **Close** to close the appointment list window, **Cancel** to close the patient information and **Close** to close the patient list.
3. Practice looking up the first five appointments from the table used in Activity 7-4. Verify that the appointments are placed on the correct date and time and are scheduled with the correct provider.

ACTIVITY 7-7 MANAGE A COMPUTERIZED APPOINTMENT SYSTEM— RESCHEDULING APPOINTMENTS

Reschedule the appointments in the table listed below.

Patient	Provider	Original Time	Rescheduled Time
Anthony Zimmerman	Martinez	2-3-14 11:00	2-3-14 2:30
Sammy Catera	Lee	2-4-14 3:00	2-4-14 9:00
Susan Brimley	O'Brian	2-3-14 9:30	2-4-14 11:00

To reschedule appointments, do the following:

1. Locate the patient's appointment on the provider's schedule. Right-click the patient's appointment and click **Cut.**
2. Locate a new time slot for the appointment. Make sure that enough time is available to reschedule the original appointment. Right-click on the new appointment slot and click **Paste.**

ACTIVITY 7-8 MANAGE A COMPUTERIZED APPOINTMENT SYSTEM— PRINTING AND SAVING APPOINTMENT SCHEDULES

To print an appointment schedule:

1. Open **Office Hours Professional**.
2. Click **Reports> Appointment List**. Select **Preview** report on screen. Click **Start.**
3. In the **Data Selection** window, enter first date to be printed (2/3/2014) and last date to be printed (2/4/2014). In the provider fields, identify the first provider (Emily O'Brian) and last provider (Wallace Hinckle) to be printed. (If no selection is made in the provider window, all providers will be printed.) Click **OK.**
4. Click the arrows on the toolbar to advance through the report. If the report is correct, click **Print Report** on the toolbar.

To save an appointment schedule file:

1. Click **Reports>Appointment List**.
2. Click **Export** the report to a file. Click **Start.** Specify which dates and providers should be saved. Name the file and save it to a location on your hard drive or on an external storage device. The file will be saved as a text file and can be electronically handed in to your instructor. (Before handing in your file, open the file to verify that the desired schedules are in the file.)

ACTIVITY 7-9 DOCUMENT APPOINTMENT INFORMATION

Using the Progress Notes sample pages located below, document the following appointment events. All entries are made today.

1. Today, Mrs. Peters calls to cancel an appointment scheduled for next Tuesday with Dr. Mallard.

Happy Valley Medical Group – Progress Notes	
Patient name:	**Chart #**

2. Yesterday, Anthony Zimmerman failed to show for the appointment that was scheduled with Dr. Lee.

Happy Valley Medical Group – Progress Notes	
Patient name:	**Chart #**

3. You have scheduled an appointment for Timothy Palmdale at Valley View Radiology Associates for an IVP next Monday at 8:00 AM.

Happy Valley Medical Group – Progress Notes	
Patient name:	**Chart #**

ACTIVITY 7-10 MEDICAL OFFICE SCENARIOS

Read each situation and role-play with a partner to show how the situation should be handled.

1. A patient's wife calls to request an appointment for her husband. They live out of town, and she would like the appointment for tomorrow because they have planned a trip to town. The patient's wife states that her husband is complaining of upper arm pain and a feeling of indigestion that is rather uncomfortable. What do you say?
2. Dr. Mallard has been called to the hospital to attend a delivery of one of her patients. She will be gone approximately 1 hour. No other providers are able to handle any of her appointments during the time she is gone. Explain the delay to her patient in the lobby, and offer alternatives to the patient.
3. A patient comes in at the wrong time for an appointment. The patient's appointment is a 15-minute appointment, but it is scheduled for tomorrow. What do you do?
4. Call your instructor or another student in the class, and practice giving a telephone reminder for an appointment scheduled with Dr. Hinckle at 9:30 AM tomorrow.

ACTIVITY 7-11 MANAGE A COMPUTERIZED APPOINTMENT SYSTEM— ELECTRONIC APPOINTMENT REMINDER

Using the skills you have acquired from the computer exercises in this chapter, print an electronic appointment reminder for Charles Gooding using **Office Hours**.

Bibliography

The Medical Management Institute: *The Medical Office Policy Handbook*, Salt Lake City, 2007, The Medical Management Institute.

University of Chicago, HIPAA Program Office. *Telephone message guidelines.* http://hipaa.bsd.uchicago.edu/Telephone_Message_Guidelines_FINAL_20081219.pdf. Accessed March 2, 2008.

CHAPTER 8 Patient Reception and Registration

LEARNING OUTCOMES

On successful completion of this chapter, the student will be able to

1. Explain the concept of exceptional patient service.
2. Describe activities associated with getting the office ready to receive patients.
3. Explain appropriate methods for welcoming a patient.
4. Explain considerations for medical office reception area.
5. Explain common medical emergencies, the use of protocol for those situations in the office, and other concerns for medical office emergencies.
6. Perform registration procedures in a computerized medical practice management system.

COMMISSION ON ACCREDITATION OF ALLIED HEALTH EDUCATION PROGRAMS (CAAHEP) CORE CURRICULUM FOR MEDICAL ASSISTANTS

- Recognize office policies and protocols for handling appointments.
- Describe various types of content maintained in a patient's medical record.
- Use office hardware and software to maintain office systems.
- Use Internet to access information related to the medical office.
- Describe the implications of HIPAA for the medical assistant in various medical settings.
- Explore issue of confidentiality as it applies to the medical assistant.
- Respond to issues of confidentiality.
- Apply HIPAA rules in regard to privacy/release of information.

ACCREDITING BUREAU OF HEALTH EDUCATION SCHOOLS (ABHES) COMPETENCIES FOR MEDICAL ASSISTING

Graduates

- Demonstrate professionalism by:
  - Exhibiting a positive attitude and sense of responsibility.
  - Maintaining confidentiality at all times.
  - Being courteous and diplomatic.
  - Conducting work within scope of education, training, and ability.
- Serve as liaison between physician and others.
- Receive, organize, prioritize, and transmit information expediently.
- Apply electronic technology.
- Apply computer application skills using variety of different electronic programs including both practice management software and EMR software.
- Prepare and maintain medical records.

VOCABULARY

code team
guarantor
Notice of Privacy Practices
referral

Aside from the telephone communication a patient has with the medical office staff, the moment at which the patient walks into the medical facility creates a lasting impression of the professionalism and competency of the staff members who work in the medical office. Providing exceptional patient service is essential to establishing a good first impression and communicates to the public the level of caring and concern to which the facility is committed. Not only are first impressions important, but patients deserve outstanding service at all times from all members of the health care team.

A good first impression and consistent quality customer service will help make patients more comfortable with and confident about the services provided in a medical office and will keep patients loyal to the medical office.

Exceptional Patient Service

The concept of exceptional patient service in health care has close ties to the concept of customer service in the business world. The business world has long known the importance of meeting the customer's needs, and the health care industry recognizes that patients expect their needs to be met as well.

The health care industry has become extremely competitive, and it is increasingly apparent to health care providers that more is required of them than providing patients with the latest and greatest health care procedures. Today's patients are true consumers of health care, and as such, they must be treated as other consumers in the marketplace are treated. Patients demand quality health care service and staff members who are genuinely concerned about their welfare; the health care industry must be concerned about retaining their customers (patients) as would members of any other industry.

Over the past 30 years, the health care industry has increased its focus on when and where services are provided. In the past, patients who needed to see a physician did so according to the physician's schedule, usually between 9 AM and 5 PM from Monday through Friday. A patient who needed immediate care at other times had to go to an emergency department. Now, many medical offices are open during the evenings and even on weekends. Also, large group clinics have extended their services to additional locations in the hope of attracting more patients. Health care services are available in shopping malls, grocery stores and other nontraditional locations. This shift in the offering of health care services has occurred in response to growing consumer demand for services outside the traditional method of delivery.

Today, the health care industry even promotes its services to patients. Patients are targeted by advertisements and public relations materials in the hope that they will be persuaded to use a particular medical facility. Rarely do these promotions focus on price; rather they focus on quality of care and the caring and concern of the staff, and they place a tremendous emphasis on serving patients' wants and needs. Promotions also might be targeted to a particular group of insurance policyholders. If patients are given exceptional service every time they enter a medical office, they will be very loyal and will not be likely to switch health care providers; thus, a strong customer base is established for the office.

What, then, is exceptional patient service? It is providing the best possible assistance to or for the patient. Patient service becomes exceptional when staff members consistently "go the extra mile," when they contribute above and beyond what is expected of them. A guiding concept in providing exceptional patient service might be to ask yourself how you would like to be treated, or how you would like your loved ones to be treated. All activities of the medical office have an impact on the patient in some way, and even those staff members who do not have direct patient contact are involved in patient service because their activities support the health care organization (Fig. 8-1).

To provide exceptional patient service, staff members must always focus on what is best for the patient. Sometimes, doing what is best for the patient is not the easiest thing to do. But we must remember that the patient is the primary reason for the work of the medical office staff and will always be the number one focus of our work.

To illustrate this point, let's look at some examples of exceptional patient service.

1. A patient stops by the desk and asks where the nearest public phone is located. Instead of answering the question by identifying the location of the public phone, a staff member can provide exceptional patient service by offering the office telephone for the patient's use.
2. An elderly patient is fumbling with her coat and is having trouble putting it on. A simple offer to help ("May I help you with your coat?") might be greatly appreciated and will be long remembered.
3. It's 4:55 PM. The phone rings. The patient who is calling states that she has just cut her finger while working in the garage. She is going to need a tetanus shot and, most likely, stitches. The clinic closes at 5:00. You check with the physician, and the physician wants the patient to come in. The physician, nurse, and assistant stay late to care for the patient.

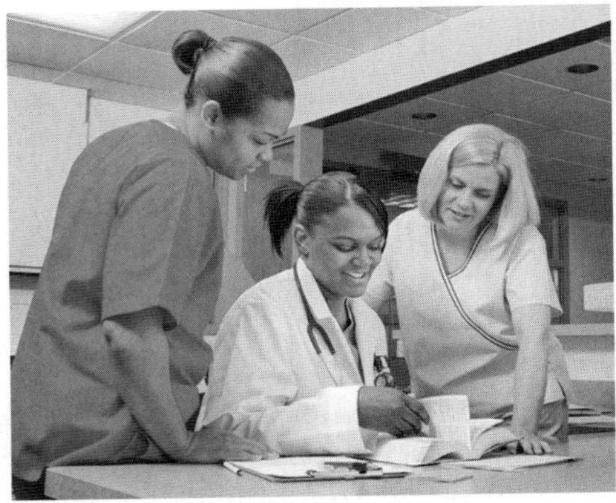

Figure 8-1 To achieve exceptional patient service, all staff members believe that the patient is always number one, and that belief is put into practice daily. (From Young AP. *Kinn's The Administrative Medical Assistant*, ed 7, St. Louis, Saunders, 2011.)

For this type of service to be effective, *all* members of the health care team, including the office staff, doctors, nurses, administrators, building services staff, and everyone in between, must be committed to always delivering exceptional patient service. This concept should serve as the foundation for all activities of the medical office. If one or more employees do not believe in and provide exceptional service, the patient will not know what to expect of the office staff because employee behavior is unpredictable.

Patient Informational Materials

Many medical offices develop informational and promotional materials for distribution to patients. Whether these materials are available online or in printed form, an office must be able to inform patients of the various services the medical facility has to offer. In addition to information about available services, these materials may provide a directory of addresses and telephone numbers and detailed maps to assist patients in locating specific areas of the facility.

Patients who are new to a facility need a resource to obtain information related to services provided by the office. Of course, such materials cannot serve as a substitute for one-on-one interaction with a staff member of the office, but they can supplement verbal information given to a patient. For example, if a patient has never been to the office before, a map can provide easy instructions for locating the office building.

Getting the Office Ready

Every day, even before the medical office is opened, certain activities must be performed to get the office ready for the day. Opening activities vary depending on the size of the office, but in most practices, several activities must be completed before the medical office is open to receive patients. Most of these activities must be done early because once the office opens, patients will need your complete attention. An office may establish an opening and/or closing checklist to help remind office staff of everything that must be done at these times. Typical opening activities include the following:

Unlock the Door

This may seem rather obvious, but more is usually involved than simply turning a key.

To begin with, the office probably will have more than one entrance. Staff members responsible for opening activities usually enter the office through a back entrance or an employee entrance—one not used by the general public. The front desk staff may be responsible for unlocking the office door when the staff is ready to receive patients for the day.

Most medical facilities are equipped with alarm systems to guard against vandalism and theft. After the door is unlocked, the alarm system will have to be deactivated. Usually, there is only a short amount of time—typically, 30 to 60 seconds—during which to turn off the alarm. Most alarm systems are deactivated by entry of a numerical code on a keypad located inside the door. These systems usually are connected to the local police department, and if the alarm system is not deactivated within the necessary length of time, the police may be summoned to the facility. If excessive false alarms are received, the medical office may have to reimburse the police department for expenses related to the false alarms.

Some offices may require that employees use a secured entrance to the medical office. Access is gained through this entrance by swiping a magnetic name badge, which will record when an employee enters and leaves an office. When such systems are used, it is unacceptable for one employee to allow another into the building without each employee swiping his or her name badge.

Obtain Charts for the Day

If the office uses paper medical records, a record must be pulled for every patient who has an appointment on that day. Usually, charts for one day will be gathered on the day before, but occasionally, an assistant may have had difficulty locating one or more of the charts. Each morning, the assistant must verify that all charts for the day's appointments have been located. Physicians and other providers dislike seeing a patient without having the patient's chart because vital information needed for the office visit may be included in the chart. Ordinarily, a medical record will be created for new patients on the day of their first appointment.

If the office uses an electronic health care record, information will always be accessible to any employee at the moment the patient arrives for his or her appointment.

Start and Check Office Equipment

A variety of equipment that is used to support office activities must be turned on early in the morning to be ready for use. Some large volume copiers require several minutes for warm-up in order to be ready for copying. Computer equipment also will have to be started to ensure that the equipment is working properly and is ready to conduct the day's work. Email and fax machines should be checked for messages that have been sent during the night.

Switch on Television or Music System

Most offices have some type of electronic media for entertainment. Television sets generally are present in the lobby, whereas music systems play throughout the facility. When a television is present in the lobby, be sure that the channel or program selected is appropriate for all visitors in the office. In every medical office, there is the possibility that children may be present, either as patients or accompanying patients. Many television programs are not suitable for children.

Television or music systems provide a pleasant distraction for patients while they are waiting for an appointment. If these systems are not turned on right away in the morning, they generally are forgotten once the hectic pace of an office begins.

Count Cash Drawer

Most offices have a cash drawer for receiving payments for services on the day they are rendered. Patients may choose to write a check or use a credit card to charge visits to the doctor. Occasionally, patients may even pay with cash. For that reason, a small amount of change is needed in the office to handle cash payments. The change fund in the cash drawer should remain at a consistent amount and will have to be counted at regular intervals to verify that the original amount of the change fund is still there.

Welcoming Patients

Once the opening activities have been completed, it is time to receive the day's patients. When a patient approaches the registration desk, an assistant should welcome the patient immediately. If the assistant is working with another patient, a simple acknowledgment, such as "I'll be right with you," conveys to the patient that you know the patient has arrived and that you will help the patient as soon as you are able. Patients should always be acknowledged on their arrival to the office to assure them that their presence has been recognized.

An assistant can greet a patient with a cheerful remark, such as "Good morning" or "Hello." Be careful to use a patient's name in the greeting. Most patients are pleased when the office staff can remember them by name, but you must be careful that others do not overhear your conversation. Even in some of the largest practices, many patients are repeat patients, and staff members are able to easily remember many patients by name.

When greeting patients, an assistant must be careful to not comment personally on the patient's medical experiences.

The following statements are examples of inappropriate and uncaring comments:

- "Oh, you're looking so much better than last week." (A medical judgment should not be made about a patient's health.)
- "It's nice to see you again." (Are we really glad the patient is in the clinic again?)
- "You don't look so good." (This is a very personal comment about the patient's appearance.)

If you are at a loss for words, it is best to simply welcome the patient with an acknowledgment such as "Hello. Let me verify your registration information for your appointment today" or "Good morning. Isn't the weather beautiful today?"

Patient Registration

The registration process involves gathering information about the patient to begin or update the patient's medical record and financial account. During registration, the assistant asks the patient a series of questions to obtain information for inclusion in the patient's medical record and to accurately bill for services rendered on that day.

The registration process is performed for all patients—existing patients (those who have been seen previously in the office) and new patients (those who have not been seen previously in the office). Registration for existing patients usually takes only a few minutes and involves updating the patient information by asking the patient to verify whether certain registration information is still correct (Procedure 8-1). Registration for patients who are new to the clinic may take several minutes because a new patient record must be created (Procedures 8-2 and 8-3).

PROCEDURE 8-1

Update Existing Patient Registration Information

Materials Needed

- Patient information
- Computer software for the medical office

1. Ask the patient for his or her full legal name, and locate the information in the patient database. Verify the patient's DOB to ensure that the correct record is updated.*
2. Verify that the following information for the patient is current:
   - Address
   - Telephone number
   - Employer
   - Insurance company name, address, policy number, and group number (copy insurance card if necessary)
   - Record any changes given by the patient.
3. Thank the patient for the information, and ask the patient to be seated in the reception area.
4. Record any changes in registration information in the patient's medical record (as applicable).

**Denotes crucial step in procedure. Student must complete this step satisfactorily to complete procedure satisfactorily.*

PROCEDURE 8-2

Obtain New Patient Registration Information

Materials Needed

- New patient registration form
- Patient medical history form
- Clipboard and pen or pencil
- Photocopier

1. Ask the patient for his or her full legal name, and check the patient database to determine whether the patient is new to the medical office.*
2. Attach a registration form and patient history form to the clipboard and give them to the patient, asking that he or she complete the forms and return them to you.
3. After the patient returns the forms, review completed forms to determine whether they are complete. Ask the patient for missing information if the forms are incomplete.
4. Ask the patient for his or her insurance card, and make a photocopy of it.
5. Thank the patient for the information, and ask the patient to be seated in the reception area.

**Denotes crucial step in procedure. Student must complete this step satisfactorily to complete procedure satisfactorily.*

PROCEDURE 8-3

Record New Patient Registration Information

Materials Needed

- Completed new patient registration form
- Medical office management computer software

Check the computer database to determine whether a record of the patient exists.*

Once the patient has been verified as a new patient to the medical office, assign a medical record number to the patient.

Enter all pertinent data for the patient into the database.

Save the new record.

**Denotes crucial step in procedure. Student must complete this step satisfactorily to complete procedure satisfactorily.*

HIPAA Hint

Remember that a patient's information that is gathered at registration (e.g., name, address, phone number, birth date, social security number) is part of Protected Health Information (PHI) and must be kept confidential.

Registration Information

During the registration process, patients are asked for demographic information, including full legal name, address, telephone number, place of employment, emergency contact information, and insurance coverage information. For established patients, this information is verified by reviewing a patient's information in a computer record or in the patient's medical record.

When patients are new to the medical office, patient registration information usually is gathered by asking the patient to complete a registration form, such as the one pictured in Figure 8-2. Information from this form then is transferred to the medical record and will be entered into the office's computer system (Fig. 8-3).

The registration process is, perhaps, one of the most critical functions performed by the medical administrative assistant. It is at this point that current information about the patient is obtained. This registration information is used to generate computerized forms for the medical record, schedule appointments for the patient, and process statements and insurance claims.

The following information is documented on the patient registration information form (see Fig. 8-2).

Patient's Personal Information

Patient information gathered during the registration process includes basic demographic data about the patient (e.g., name, address, telephone, date of birth [DOB], social security number). It is necessary to obtain the complete legal name of the patient to identify the medical record. No nicknames or abbreviations of names should be used because these can lead to confusion if at some point the patient uses a different form of his or her name. Using different forms of a name could cause another medical record to be created for a patient. If the patient lists a nickname (e.g., Timmy, Sue, Butch) or an abbreviation (e.g., Wm., Chas.), the assistant should ask the patient for a complete legal name. In many offices today, patients are asked to provide a government-issued form of identification when a new medical record is created. This helps reduce the possibility that a patient may have duplicate records. Also, if a patient is required to show identification, this reduces the possibility that a false record may be created for an illegal purpose, such as obtaining prescriptions under a false name.

Information about where the patient works (e.g., name, address, and telephone number of employer) and about the patient's occupation is obtained and may be used for various reasons. Occasionally, for such things as notification of a change in an appointment time or of results of tests, the patient may have to be contacted while at work. Also, some physicians make it a special point to know the occupation of a patient because the nature of the patient's employment may have an impact on the patient's health status.

Patient's or Responsible Party's Information

Sometimes, the patient and the person responsible for paying the medical bill are not the same person. A patient who is younger than 18 years of age, for example, usually cannot be held responsible for a bill. Instead, the bill is sent to a responsible party, or **guarantor**, usually a parent. A guarantor, the individual responsible for a patient's bill, may be the patient or someone other than the patient.

During the registration process, demographic information about the guarantor is gathered for use at a later time in the billing process. Full legal name, address, telephone number, and place of employment constitute the minimum amount of information required of a guarantor. This guarantor information *must* be gathered because, occasionally, the guarantor does not live at the same address as the patient. One example of such a situation is one in which a divorced parent pays for a child's health services but does not live with the child. Another may be a college student whose bills still are paid by a parent.

Patient's Insurance Information

Complete information regarding the patient's insurance coverage is needed at the point of registration. The name and address of the insurance company, as well as the name and address of the policyholder (the insured), policy number, group number, and relationship of the patient to the insured, are gathered to be used for an insurance claim submission after the patient's visit. If the patient's insurance is new or has changed, an assistant should copy both sides of the patient's insurance card for use by the billing department at a later time should any billing questions arise.

Patient's Referral Information

Many physicians want to know if a patient has been referred to their office. With a **referral**, a patient may be referred by another patient of the medical office or by another health care professional. Physicians often make it a point to acknowledge their appreciation of referral patients to those who have referred patients. If a patient is referred to the office by another physician, be sure that this information is given to the physician who will see the patient.

Emergency Contact

From time to time, a medical facility will need to contact a patient's family member because of an emergency involving the patient. An emergency contact is included in the patient's registration information for use should an emergency situation arise.

Sometimes more than one emergency contact is listed for a patient. The first contact would be a close family member, such as a spouse, parent, or adult child. It is preferred that a second emergency contact be named who does not live with the patient. This may seem odd at first, but imagine what would happen if the patient is in an accident along with a spouse. If the spouse is the patient's emergency contact, there would not be anyone else listed in the registration information who could be notified. An alternative contact provides another person to call should the first contact be unreachable.

In the case of an emergency involving only the patient, the patient's first contact is called first and, if there is no answer, attempts are made to reach other contacts. Emergency contact information also may be used occasionally, if necessary, for account collection.

Happy Valley Medical Group

5222 Baseline Road, Gilbert AZ 85234

REGISTRATION INFORMATION

Please print the following information. Ask the front desk to assist with any questions you may have regarding the information requested.

Patient Information

Patient Name ______________________________ Date of Birth ____/____/____ Sex M F
Last First MI month day year

Address ______________________ City ______________ State ______ ZIP ______

Telephone – Home (____)______–________ Cell (____)______–________ Work (____)______–________

Employer ______________________ position ______________________

Employer Address ______________________ City ______________ State ______ ZIP ______

Social Security number ______/______/______

Guarantor Information

Responsible Party Name ______________________________ Date of Birth ____/____/____ Sex M F
Last First MI month day year

Address ______________________ City ______________ State ______ ZIP ______

Telephone – Home (____)______–________ Cell (____)______–________ Work (____)______–________

Employer ______________________ position ______________________

Employer Address ______________________ City ______________ State ______ ZIP ______

Social Security number______/______/______

Primary Insurance Information (please present card to receptionist)

Insurance Company Name ______________________________

Policy # ______________ Group # ______________ Policyholder ______________

Address ______________________ City ______________ State ______ ZIP ______

Telephone (____)______–________other phone (____)______–________

Secondary Insurance Information (please present card to receptionist)

Insurance Company Name ______________________________

Policy # ______________ Group # ______________ Policyholder ______________

Address ______________________ City ______________ State ______ ZIP ______

Telephone (____)______–________other phone (____)______–________

Insurance Authorization & Assignment

I hereby authorize Happy Valley Medical Clinic and Medical Group Ltd. to release medical information pertaining to my medical encounters to my insurance company and to file insurance claims on my behalf. I also agree to assign any benefits payable for those claims directly to Happy Valley Medical Clinic. I understand that I am responsible for charges on my account regardless of payments made or due from my insurance company.

Patient Name (print) ______________________________ Date ______________

Signature ______________________________ Relationship (if other than patient) ______________

Figure 8-2 The patient registration information form is used to document important information that is used for registration and billing activities in the medical office.

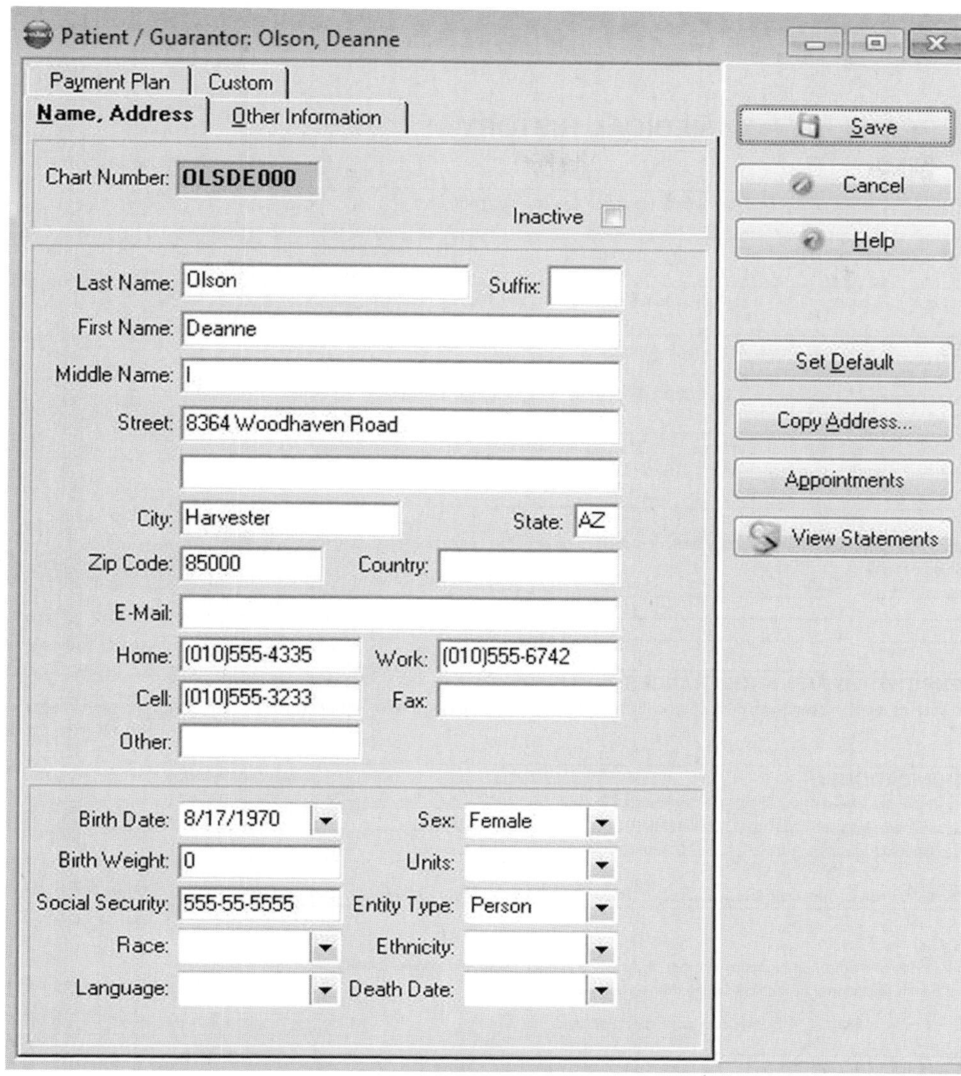

Figure 8-3 A computer database usually is used to store information for a patient's encounters with a medical office. (Screenshots used by permission of MCKESSON Corporation. All rights reserved. © MCKESSON Corporation 2012.)

Authorizations

The registration form often contains statements near the bottom of the form that authorize the practice to release information to the patient's insurance company for billing, and that authorize any payments of benefits to come directly to the practice. Also included in the authorization section may be a statement that the patient is ultimately responsible for the charges that are incurred. If the patient's signature is not obtained in the authorization section, insurance claims cannot be filed directly from the medical office, and the responsibility for filing claims will rest with the patient. Failure to have these authorizations signed means that the patient must file insurance claims, which likely will cause a delay in receipt of payment for services rendered.

Patient History Form

At the time of registration, new patients are asked to complete a medical history form (Fig. 8-4) that asks for information regarding their past illnesses, surgeries, hospitalizations, drug allergies, family medical history, and other pertinent medical information. This form becomes a part of the patient's medical record and is reviewed by the physician when the patient is examined. Because of all the information that must be obtained from new patients, new patients take more time to register and should be asked to arrive 15 minutes earlier than the scheduled appointment time to complete the registration process.

> **HIPAA Hint**
>
> A patient's medical history and any information about future treatment constitute protected health information.

Notice of Privacy Practices

When a patient is new to the office, the Health Insurance Portability and Accountability Act (HIPAA) requires that a patient be notified about how the patient's demographic information and information pertaining to his or her visit will be used. Such information is included in a document

ADULT PATIENT'S CHECK LIST FOR MEDICAL HISTORY

NAME: DATE OF BIRTH: / / DATE:

PAST SURGERIES: None ☐ – or, list here any past surgeries with approximate age at which performed.

OTHER HOSPITALIZATIONS: List reason and date(s).

ACCIDENTS: No injuries of consequence ☐ — or, list any serious type injuries, with approximate age.

PAST MEDICAL ILLNESSES: List any serious illness, with approximate age: No serious past illnesses ☐

List any major childhood diseases:

Sexually Transmitted Diseases (past or current): ☐ Gonorrhea ☐ HIV/AIDS ☐ Herpes ☐ Chlamydia ☐ Syphilis ☐ Other

Any blood transfusions: ☐ Yes ☐ No

FAMILY HISTORY: If any of the following have run in your family, check appropriate block:

Allergies ☐; Cancer ☐; Tuberculosis ☐; Diabetes ☐; Heart Disease ☐; Strokes ☐; Hypertension ☐;

Any deaths below age of 55? ☐

CURRENT MEDICATIONS:

Please list all medications you are now taking, including those you buy without a doctor's prescription (such as aspirin, cold tablets or vitamin supplements) List name, dosage and times per day.

1. ______ 4. ______ 7. ______
2. ______ 5. ______ 8. ______
3. ______ 6. ______ 9. ______

CURRENT ALLERGIES, SENSITIVITIES AND INTOLERANCES:

List anything that you are allergic to such as foods, medications, dust, chemicals, household items, pollens, bee stings, etc., and indicate how each affects you:

RECENT TRAVEL AND IMMUNIZATIONS:

Have you traveled out of the country in the last 2 years? ... ☐ No ☐ Yes, traveled in ______

Write in the dates for the shots you have had: Measles / Mumps / Rubella (MMR) ______ Polio ______

Tetanus / diphtheria (dt)______ Typhoid ______ Flu ______ Pneumococcal/Pneumonia ______

Other ______

Have you had a tuberculin (TB) skin test: ☐ No ☐ Yes Date ______ Result ? ☐ Pos. ☐ Neg. ☐ BCG ______

OTHER MEDICAL CARE:

Living Will/Durable Power of Attorney: ☐ Yes ☐ No

If you are being treated for any other illness or medical problems by another physician or mental health practitioner, please describe the problems and write the name of the physician, health practitioner or medical facility treating you.

Illness or Medical Problem	Physician or Medical Facility	City

REVIEW OF SYMPTOMS: Place a check mark in the appropriate blocks in the following list of current (within past 3 months) symptoms:

1. HEAD AND NECK

	YES	NO		YES	NO		YES	NO
Severe headaches	☐	☐	Severe hearing loss	☐	☐	Frequent colds	☐	☐
Dizzy spells	☐	☐	Ringing in ears	☐	☐	Sinus trouble or hayfever	☐	☐
Wear glasses	☐	☐	Pain in ears	☐	☐	Chronic nose obstruction	☐	☐
Failing vision	☐	☐	Discharge from ear	☐	☐	Persistent sore gums	☐	☐
Eye pain	☐	☐	Repeated nosebleeds	☐	☐	Prolonged hoarseness	☐	☐
Double vision	☐	☐	Teeth problems	☐	☐	Swelling in neck	☐	☐

2. HEART AND LUNGS

	YES	NO		YES	NO		YES	NO
Heart problems	☐	☐	Ankles swell	☐	☐	Smoking history	☐	☐
Chest pain on effort	☐	☐	Have chronic cough	☐	☐	Past ☐ Present ☐		
Skipping/irregular heart beats	☐	☐	Difficult breathing	☐	☐	Type ______ Qty ______		
Hypertension	☐	☐	Spit up blood	☐	☐	If currently smoking are you		
Cholesterol	☐	☐	Have night sweats	☐	☐	interested in quitting?	☐	☐

Continued on back page

Figure 8-4 All new patients complete a medical history form for inclusion in their medical record. (Courtesy of Bibbero Systems, Inc., Petaluma, California 94954; telephone: 800-242-2376; fax: 800-242-9330; e-mail: info@bibberosystems.com; available at www.bibberosystems.com.)

2. HEART AND LUNGS (cont.)

	YES	NO		YES	NO		YES	NO
Cholesterol	☐	☐	Have night sweats	☐	☐	Wheezing	☐	☐
Lab test date ______			Frequent chest colds	☐	☐			
Results ______			Sit up to breathe easier	☐	☐			

3. STOMACH AND INTESTINES

Chronic Abdominal Pain	☐	☐	Any chronic diarrhea	☐	☐	Sigmoidoscopy	☐	☐
Persistent nausea	☐	☐	Any black tarry stools	☐	☐	Date ______		
Heartburn	☐	☐	Any blood from rectum	☐	☐	Results ______		
Appetite loss	☐	☐	Clay colored stools	☐	☐	______		
Vomit blood	☐	☐	Habitual constipation	☐	☐			
Skin turns yellow	☐	☐	Have hemorrhoids	☐	☐			

4. URINARY TRACT / GENITAL

Frequent urination	☐	☐	Hard to start urinary flow	☐	☐	Weak stream/scanty urination	☐	☐
Any blood in urine	☐	☐	Frequent night urination	☐	☐	Pain with urination	☐	☐
Any leakage of urine	☐	☐	Passed any stones	☐	☐	Any bedwetting	☐	☐
Any retention of urine	☐	☐						

5. OB GYN (For Women Only)

Last menstrual period ______			Previous Pap smear	☐	☐	Any breast lumps	☐	☐
If currently having periods			Date of most recent Pap			Mammography	☐	☐
do you have:			______			Date ______		
Painful menstruation	☐	☐	Results ______			Results ______		
Excess menstruation	☐	☐	Current birth control	☐	☐	______		
Bleed between periods	☐	☐	Type: ______					
Any missed periods	☐	☐	Number of pregnancies ______					
Any vaginal discharge	☐	☐	Number of living children ______					

6. MUSCLES — JOINTS

Physically handicapped/limited	☐	☐	Shoulder pain	☐	☐	Red or swollen joints	☐	☐
Joint or muscle problems	☐	☐	Back pain	☐	☐	Limitation of motion	☐	☐
Varicose veins	☐	☐						

7. NEUROLOGICAL

Numbness	☐	☐	Any dizzy spells	☐	☐	Any shaking/tremors	☐	☐
Disturbance in walking	☐	☐	Any paralysis/weakness	☐	☐	Any falls	☐	☐
Trouble with balance			Any strokes	☐	☐	Speech disturbance	☐	☐
or coordination	☐	☐	Any seizures	☐	☐	Any memory loss	☐	☐

8. PSYCHOLOGICAL

Psychological/emotional /			Excessive fears	☐	☐	History of:		
stress problems	☐	☐	Nervous breakdown	☐	☐	Alcohol problems	☐	☐
Psychotherapy/counseling	☐	☐	Depression	☐	☐	Total drinks consumed		
Currently	☐	☐	Sexual problems	☐	☐	for last week ______		
In past	☐	☐	Serious marital problems	☐	☐	Drug problems	☐	☐
						Any mood changes	☐	☐

GENERAL HEALTH .... Good ☐ .... Fair ☐ .... Poor ☐

Do you eat a balanced diet: Yes ☐ No ☐ Explain ______

Do you have a lot of stress: Yes ☐ No ☐ Explain ______

Do you get regular exercise: Yes ☐ No ☐ Explain ______

Any exposure to environmental hazards such as chemicals, dust or fumes? ☐ Yes ☐ No

If yes, please explain:

IF THERE ARE ANY ADDITIONAL HEALTH FACTORS IN YOUR HISTORY
OR IF ANY OF THE ABOVE POINTS NEED CLARIFYING,
USE THIS SPACE FOR ADDITIONAL COMMENTS.

FORM # **25-8092** • 1974 BIBBERO SYSTEMS, INC. • PTETALUMA, CA. TO REORDER CALL TOLL FREE: (800) BIBBERO (800-242-2376) OR FAX (800) 242-9330 (REV 6/95)

Figure 8-4, cont'd

known as a **Notice of Privacy Practices**. This document provides the patient with details on how the patient's information may be used and disclosed to others. A patient also is informed as to what his or her rights are regarding his or her own health information and whom to contact when a complaint, request, or question is raised about this information. A patient is asked to sign a form acknowledging receipt of the Notice of Privacy Practices. Such an acknowledgment is shown in Figure 9-1.

Confidentiality When Registering Patients

When greeting patients, it is important to remember to keep your voice at a volume that cannot be heard by others who are seated in the lobby or elsewhere in the clinic. Protecting the confidentiality of the patient's visit is crucial, and you must pay special attention to protecting the confidentiality of all information given by the patient.

When registering a patient, do not repeat the reason for the patient's visit. Imagine the embarrassment if a patient were to be asked, "And you're being seen for a urinary problem today?" while others are standing behind the patient. If it is necessary for the assistant to conduct a question-and-answer interview with the patient to obtain information, this should be done in a private setting away from other patients. Some facilities have separate desks (apart from appointment check-in) that are used for registration interviews. To provide greater privacy for patients, these desks may include multiple stations with glass or solid partitions that separate the area from the lobby and the reception desk.

HIPAA Hint

Information about a patient's treatment is protected health information.

If an office is using a computerized appointment system, part of the registration process usually includes updating the status of appointments. This process involves documenting where the patient is in the appointment process. Depending on how an office wishes to use such a feature, a patient may be listed as checked in, may have missed an appointment, may be currently in with a physician, or may have already left the office. Also, the larger the facility, the more important it is to document the status of a patient's appointment because a patient may be more difficult to locate in a larger facility.

After a patient has been registered, any paperwork related to that registration should be moved to another part of the desk, so that the next patient in line does not see the previous patient's information.

HIPAA Hint

Protected health information must be protected in any form—whether in paper, electronic, or oral form.

CHECKPOINT

An assistant who is new to the office likes to help make a new patient feel more welcomed to the practice by sitting next to the patient in the lobby to answer any questions the patient may have about completing the paperwork for registration. Is this a good idea?

Reception Area

The reception area (Fig. 8-5), or lobby, of the medical office is the area in which the patients are seated as they await their appointment. You will notice that the area is not called the "waiting room." The very use of the term "waiting room" has a negative connotation and implies that patients will have to *wait* to see the doctor.

Layout and Design of the Reception Area

Much thought and consideration are necessary in planning a functional and useful layout of the reception area of a medical office. This area consists of more than chairs and a few fixtures. Let's take a look at all of the items found in a well-planned reception area.

Welcoming Atmosphere

The basic elements of the room—floor covering and wall treatments, for example—should be color coordinated and inviting. The services of an interior designer may be valuable in coordinating all the basic elements of the room. Floors usually are covered by a multicolored, industrial carpet that is easy to clean and does not show wear too quickly. Walls usually are covered with a high-quality wallpaper or paint that is scrubbable. In addition, artwork, plants, and even an aquarium might be purchased to furnish the room.

When selecting colors for the reception area, keep in mind the structural components of the room. Are there windows to let in sunlight, or is this area enclosed? Deep, dark colors may be depressing to some patients, and bright, vivid colors can be nauseating and dizzying to others. A light- to medium-toned color palette is probably the best choice for decorating this area.

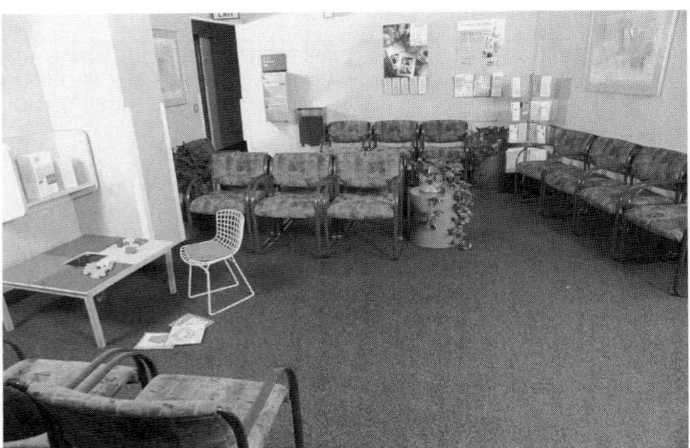

Figure 8-5 A well-planned reception area is important for the smooth, efficient handling of patients in a medical office.

Traffic Patterns

The entire reception area should be planned to allow traffic to flow easily throughout. Tight spaces and areas that handle all of the traffic that is coming and going may cause problems if many patients are in the office at the same time.

Be sure to allow adequate space in all walkways and other areas to accommodate patients who use a wheelchair. Doors must have automatic openers, and all office amenities such as restrooms and water fountains must be accessible to patients who have a disability. The Americans with Disabilities Act (ADA), a federal law, has mandated specific requirements for accessibility.

The reception desk should be located near the front entrance but separate from the main lobby (Fig. 8-6). This area must be private to ensure that patients cannot hear the activities of the office staff or the assistant's interactions with patients. When the assistant picks up the telephone at the front desk, patients who are sitting in the lobby should not hear the conversation.

Seating Arrangement

The best type of seating arrangement is a well-cushioned modular chair, as in Figure 8-5, that can be rearranged in a variety of groupings. Patients should have a comfortable place to sit before an appointment. If a television set is present in the lobby, a group of chairs should be positioned around the set and a group positioned away from the set to provide a quiet space for patients.

Chairs should be covered with commercial-grade upholstery that is easy to clean in the event that furniture becomes soiled. Sofas generally are not used in a reception area because patients may not wish to sit near other patients because of illness. In addition, sofas can be very difficult to keep clean.

Television or Music System

As was mentioned previously, most clinics provide some type of electronic entertainment for their patients. Some facilities may have both television and music.

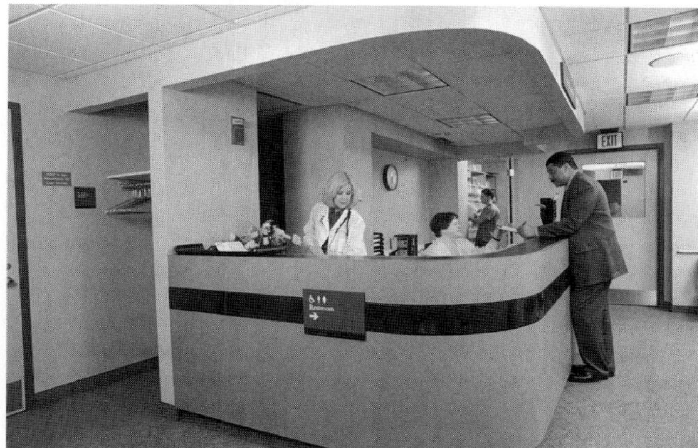

Figure 8-6 The front desk in a medical office should be positioned off to the side of the reception area to help protect the confidentiality of patient information.

The type of music often heard in a health care facility is background music (frequently known as "elevator music") played at a very low volume. This music helps to mask some of the noise of the office's everyday activities and is a nice addition to the office's atmosphere.

Television is common in many medical office reception areas. Even with background music playing, the music and the television usually do not "compete" with each other.

If a television is present in the lobby, the assistant must pay close attention at all times to what is being shown on the television. Many pediatric reception areas post signs on television sets asking patients to consider the children present, and to ask the front desk whether the channel may be changed. Many offices will not change the channel unless the programming is suitable for children. Even if you are working in a family practice or a multi specialty clinic, the chances are good that children may be present, and it is wise to monitor what is appearing on the set. Many parents find soap operas, prime time shows, and many talk shows unsuitable for children, and some programming may simply be unsuitable for a public place.

Reading Material

Nearly all physicians' offices have something available for patients to read. Magazines and medical pamphlets help patients to pass the time. Professional medical journals, meant for physicians and nursing staff, are not placed in the lobby. Similar to the television situation mentioned earlier, some clinics are very careful to supply only those magazines and pamphlets that are appropriate for all ages. Some materials, because of their content, are highly inappropriate for children.

Something for Kids

As was mentioned previously, children may be present in almost any reception area. They may be patients, or they may accompany a parent or grandparent to the clinic. Whatever the case, in every lobby, a few items should be available to keep children busy. Aquariums can help pass the time, as can children's magazines or books. Toys may be available but should not be a choking hazard. Sometimes, a small table and chairs with coloring books and crayons are available. In addition, an assistant should take special precautions to protect children who may visit the facility. Electrical outlets should be covered, and cords should be placed out of a young one's reach.

Refreshments

All offices should have a drinking fountain or water cooler available for anyone who may need a drink of water. Some offices even supply coffee for patients and others in the reception area. If coffee is provided, the coffee machine should be located in an area that is not accessible to children but must be visible to the front desk staff. Patients who may have NPO orders—nothing by mouth such as food or drink—may have to be stopped from having coffee.

Wheelchair

Every reception area should have a wheelchair located near the front door and easily accessible to the front desk staff.

Patients entering the clinic with a variety of medical concerns may need transportation in a wheelchair. Wheelchairs can and should be used for many different emergency or acute care situations. These situations are discussed later in this chapter.

Other Reception Area Fixtures

No reception area is complete without a few more items.

Wastebasket. Without a wastebasket, waste materials may be left on the furniture or the floor. Providing a wastebasket simply encourages patients to use it.

Coat rack. Without a coat rack, a coat may be left on a chair, taking up space while the patient is with the physician.

Clock. Some offices are uncomfortable with a clock in the reception area. If the practice believes in and practices exceptional patient service, however, a clock should be almost a nonissue—patients will not be in the lobby long enough to watch it!

Restroom. The restroom usually is positioned close to the front desk. When a patient asks the location of the restroom, the assistant should check the reason for the patient's appointment to determine whether a urine specimen may be necessary for the patient's visit. If a specimen is necessary, the assistant may have to direct the patient to the appropriate location in the office where a specimen can be left.

CHECKPOINT

Explain why music or television or both are important additions to a reception area.

Reception Area Maintenance

Because the reception area has such heavy use during the day, it is the responsibility of the medical administrative assistant to make sure the area stays neat and clean. The assistant will need to continually monitor the area and periodically walk through the lobby and straighten anything that is out of order.

At the End of the Day

Just as certain activities are done at the beginning of each day, there are activities that may need to be performed at the end of each day.

- Computer systems need to be locked and/or shut down at the close of business each day. Equipment may or may not be turned off or powered down as well.
- A cash drawer will need to be counted and any receipts from the day may be deposited or placed in a secure location for later pickup.
- The office alarm system may need to be set and doors locked as the last employees leave the building.

Emergency Situations

Chapter 6 discusses how to recognize some common emergency situations over the telephone, but what happens when an emergency presents itself in the medical office? No matter where the office is or what type of medical specialists (e.g., cardiologists, dermatologists, orthopedists) work in the office, this is a very real possibility. The assistant must be able to recognize and react to common medical emergencies. How you respond to such a situation may be critical to the health and welfare of a patient. To provide the patient with the best possible service, it is important for you to recognize a common emergency (Fig. 8-7) when it occurs in the reception area, or when a patient in an emergency situation walks right through the front door!

Every office should prepare adequately for emergencies by establishing protocol for handling emergencies and by offering training to all staff in the medical office on such things as cardiopulmonary resuscitation (CPR) and first aid. Before any emergency procedures are implemented, it is always necessary to obtain physician approval for any emergency procedures that will be used. It is not the assistant's responsibility to treat the patient, but the assistant should be able to recognize signs and symptoms of common emergencies and must be able to get the patient to the medical staff as quickly as possible.

What Is an Emergency?

An emergency is a situation in which a patient's health may be adversely affected if immediate action is not taken. Some emergency situations may even be life threatening. Heart attacks are obvious emergency situations. Other serious medical problems may be an emergency in that if action is not taken, the patient may be irreparably harmed. For example, a patient with a chemical splash to an eye may suffer permanent eye damage if immediate medical attention is not received.

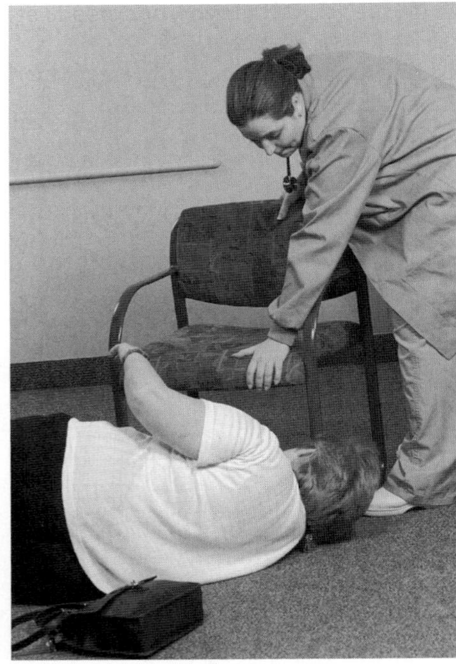

Figure 8-7 A medical administrative assistant must be able to recognize common medical emergencies and get help for the patient as quickly as possible.

Common Medical Emergencies

Following are examples of medical emergencies and common responses to these situations. Again, the emergency protocol used in a medical office *must* be reviewed and approved by the physicians of the practice before it is used.

Chest Pain

Chest pain may have various causes. Chest pain due to myocardial infarction, or heart attack, may have a predominant symptom of a painful crushing sensation or severe pressure to the chest. Pain may travel down the arms, throat, or back and may persist for several hours. The patient may appear pale, diaphoretic (sweating profusely), nauseated, and short of breath and may complain of indigestion. It is important to note, however, that not all victims of a heart attack have the same symptoms. Only some of these symptoms may be present. Heart attack pain can be experienced and described quite differently from patient to patient.

If a patient enters the clinic with complaints of any of these symptoms, the patient should be placed in a wheelchair and immediately escorted to an examination area of the office. The medical staff can be notified via intercom that a patient is on the way to an examination room. A patient with heart attack symptoms should never be seated in the lobby. In any emergency situation, a patient's name can be obtained after the patient has reached an examination room.

Seizure

Someone may experience a seizure while seated in the lobby. A grand mal seizure is evidenced by a sudden loss of consciousness and sudden involuntary movements of voluntary muscles. The patient's muscles may relax and contract in rapid succession. Some or all of the patient's body may jerk or twitch, or the patient may vomit or become incontinent.

When a seizure occurs, it is important to try to prevent further injury to the patient. Attempts should *not* be made to restrain the patient, however. If the patient is near any hard objects, such as furniture, these objects should be moved, if possible, out of the patient's way. If a hard object is struck repeatedly, the patient could awaken with multiple bruises and much discomfort over the injured region. Cushion the patient's head, if possible, with a pillow or another soft object.

Hard objects should *never* be inserted into the patient's mouth. Serious injury could occur if the object is broken by the patient's jaw and swallowed. The patient should be rolled onto one side to prevent aspiration of any vomitus that may occur. The assistant should summon the medical staff as quickly as possible and should be ready to communicate to the physician any specific signs, if known, that occurred just before and at the time of the seizure, as well as the parts of the body involved.

Most grand mal seizures are short lived, lasting only about 5 minutes. On rare occasions, a grand mal seizure may not stop, and the patient may continue to convulse. This occurrence, known as status epilepticus, is a serious, life-threatening situation.

If a patient experiences a seizure while in the clinic, a physician should always be notified as quickly as possible, even if the patient has a known history of seizures.

Respiratory Distress

Respiratory distress may be caused by a wide variety of conditions, such as a cardiac problem, a pulmonary problem, an allergic reaction, and even a panic disorder. A patient with respiratory distress exhibits dyspnea or wheezing and may even appear cyanotic.

Patients who experience respiratory distress as the result of an allergic reaction may have urticaria or edema, or both, on the face, although this is not always apparent.

Occasionally, patients with asthma may experience an episode known as status asthmaticus. This type of asthma attack is ongoing and very severe and can result in death if not treated promptly.

It is important to obtain a wheelchair for a patient with respiratory distress because loss of consciousness may occur quickly. Should the patient's symptoms accelerate, it will be much easier to transport the patient if he or she is in a wheelchair. The medical staff should be alerted, and the patient should be escorted to the examination area of the office immediately.

Diabetic Emergencies

Two types of emergencies are related to a patient's blood sugar level—hyperglycemia and hypoglycemia. In both instances, a patient does not have to be a known diabetic to experience one of these occurrences.

Hyperglycemia is a blood sugar level that is too high. Patients with hyperglycemia have a rapid pulse, warm dry skin, and decreased perspiration.

In an episode of hypoglycemia (low blood sugar), the patient may appear confused, may hallucinate, or may even go into a coma. The patient exhibits an increased pulse, a rapid heartbeat, and sweating and may appear anxious. As with many of the previous situations, you should obtain a wheelchair for any patient with a diabetic emergency and should escort the patient to the clinical area of the facility.

Both hypoglycemic and hyperglycemic patients may exhibit difficulty walking, may be irritable, and may complain of headache. The condition the patient is suffering from may not be readily apparent; thus, when a patient presents with a diabetic emergency, it is important for the assistant to not give the patient anything to eat or drink unless authorized by the physician. Even if the patient asks for a beverage, you cannot give one to the patient unless the physician approves. Supplying a beverage in this type of situation would constitute medical treatment, and the physician must decide what treatment is appropriate for the patient's condition.

Profuse, Uncontrolled Bleeding

Sometimes, when injured, a person will grab the closest thing to wrap around the wound and will head out the door to the nearest doctor's office. When the patient arrives at the clinic, his or her clothes may be soaked with blood, and the patient may need supplies to soak up additional blood.

In preparation for these emergencies, a clean supply of towels and gloves should kept at the front desk. When a bleeding patient walks through the door, the assistant can grab a towel quickly and offer it to the patient to wrap around the wound. Be careful to hand the towel to the patient and let the patient apply it to the wound. Use the towels, if at all possible, to avoid a blood spill in the reception area.

When you are dealing with a patient who is bleeding profusely, it is important to realize that the patient could go into shock as a result of loss of blood. A patient with these types of wounds should be escorted immediately to the examination area via wheelchair to avoid harm to the patient in case of collapse.

Because of the potentially hazardous nature of bodily fluids such as blood, any bloody cloths must be disposed of properly. Do not throw blood-stained cloths into the trash can in the reception area. These cloths should be disposed of properly in a designated container within the office. It is important to avoid any direct exposure to the patient's blood. If it is necessary to pick up bloody cloths that have fallen on the floor, it is absolutely essential to put on protective gloves before picking up these materials. More information on dealing with bodily fluids is included in the Standard Precautions section of Chapter 13, Business Operations of the Medical Office.

Head Injury

All head injuries should be taken seriously. Patients with a head injury may appear dazed, may vomit, may have uneven pupils, or may be unable to move an extremity.

All head injuries are potentially dangerous because there is a chance that bleeding may occur in or around the brain. Patients who report a head injury should be escorted via wheelchair to the examination area of the office immediately.

Syncope

Syncope (fainting) involves a sudden loss of consciousness. Syncope should be taken seriously because it may indicate a more serious problem occurring within the patient. If a patient faints while in the reception area of the clinic, the medical staff must be summoned immediately to assess the situation.

Psychotic Episode

An individual who experiences a psychotic episode has a sudden break with reality and is not capable of rational thought at that time. It is important to realize that this individual is irrational, and that attempts to reason with the individual will likely be futile. Psychotic individuals appear irritable and confused and may hallucinate, may have increased respirations, and may become violent. If you are confronted by a psychotic individual, it is important to be calm and to speak calmly. Be sure to consider the protection of yourself and others in the building. There is no need to be heroic to protect the physical contents of the office. Physical contents can be replaced—people cannot. If a psychotic individual makes demands for medical supplies, money, or other items in the office, comply with the individual's wishes. In such a situation, it is important to remember that a call to 911 may be warranted.

Eye Injury

Patients with eye injuries usually need the immediate attention of the medical staff. The eye may have to be washed to remove an irritant. Patients with an eye injury should be escorted to an examination room as quickly as possible and should not be seated in the lobby.

Burns

Patients who have been burned also need the immediate attention of the medical staff. Treatment may have to be instituted immediately to diminish blistering and peeling of the wound. Treatment may range from immersing the area in cool water to applying a moist or a dry dressing. No treatment should be given without the permission of the physician.

What a Medical Administrative Assistant Should Do

When dealing with an emergency situation, an assistant should always alert the medical staff (physician or nurse, or both) as soon as possible. In some cases, depending on the status of the patient, it may be necessary to assist the patient first to prevent further injury. For example, if a patient enters the office in some type of respiratory distress, the assistant may have to help the patient into a wheelchair before the patient collapses to the floor. As was mentioned in many of the previous examples, emergency situations often warrant the use of a wheelchair. In these types of situations, it is much easier and safer to transport patients in a wheelchair.

Whatever the emergency may be, it is imperative that the dignity and the privacy of the patient are protected as much as possible, and that any embarrassment to the patient is avoided.

Depending on the medical services available in the medical office, you may need to call 911 for an ambulance, or you may have to call a **code team** for an emergency situation. Code teams consist of personnel such as physicians, nurses, and anesthesia and pharmacy staff who are ready to drop everything when an emergency occurs within a health care facility to rush to the scene to administer life-saving treatment. Large facilities have preestablished code teams that can be called to respond to situations such as cardiac arrest and other life-threatening situations. Even when physicians are working everywhere within a large facility, a code team will be called to respond to an emergency situation because the team is specifically trained to respond to such events. In a smaller office, a code team may not be available, and if all physicians are out of the office, it may be necessary to call 911 for emergency help.

An assistant's main goal in assisting a patient with a medical emergency is to transfer the patient to the physician and nursing staff as quickly as possible.

After care of the emergency patient has been transferred to a member of the medical staff, you are not finished dealing with the situation. It may be necessary to locate a family member for the patient. Family members usually are contacted by the nursing staff, who may be able to give more information about the patient's condition. It may be your responsibility, however, to locate a family member by telephone and to transfer the call to the nurse. When contacting a family member for this reason, it is best to locate the individual and to choose a statement that will not alarm the family member (e.g., "This is Dr. Anderson's office calling. Could you hold for a moment to speak with the nurse?").

After an emergency situation has occurred in the lobby, patients who were present will be aware that appointment times are likely going to be delayed. Patients who arrive for appointments after the situation has cleared the lobby, however, may have to be told that there was an emergency situation, and that their appointment may be delayed. These patients should be simply told that there was an emergency, and the assistant should keep the nature of the emergency confidential.

CHECKPOINT

Explain why CPR and basic first aid training are good ideas for all medical office staff.

Other Situations

Fractures

Although most patients with fractures who present to the clinic are not medical emergencies, the medical administrative assistant should be sure to provide special attention to the patient with a fracture. If at all possible, a patient with a fracture should be placed in a treatment room immediately and should not be expected to sit in the lobby. If a patient hobbles or hops in because of a leg injury, insist that the patient sit in a wheelchair to allow easier transfer to a treatment room. Nothing would be more embarrassing to a medical office than to have a patient fall and incur further injury while hopping to a treatment room.

Acutely Ill or Uncomfortable Patients

Whether or not a situation is a true emergency, no patient in distress should be left in the reception area. Patients who are acutely ill, vomiting, or experiencing severe headache and those who are obviously uncomfortable should be transported to an examination room. Leaving the patient in the lobby conveys a feeling of uncaring and a lack of concern by members of the entire health care team. An assistant should pay attention to the overall appearance of all patients who enter the office and, if necessary, should ask whether a patient needs to lie down.

Planning for Emergencies

No one ever really expects an emergency to occur, but all medical offices must be prepared to handle emergencies when they do occur. Sometimes, the only thing the staff will be able to do is to stabilize the patient while they wait for an ambulance to arrive.

Whatever the case, it is critical for the office staff to keep calm and to carry out the practice's approved protocol for emergencies. It is important that the staff follow the established protocol exactly to avoid any possibility of litigation involving the office or the office staff.

SUMMARY

The moment a patient enters a medical office, a lasting impression of the office's commitment to patients is formed. Continually providing exceptional service conveys a high level of commitment and caring toward patients.

Not only is exceptional service important, but the office should have a pleasing and comfortable atmosphere. The medical office's reception area should be well planned and should accommodate all of the practice's patients. Great care should be paid to the design of the room as well as to amenities necessary to serve the needs of patients.

An integral part of receiving patients each day is the patient registration process. The information gathered during this process is critical to many of the other important activities of the office. When registering patients, an assistant should be aware of various symptoms that may indicate a potential emergency situation. If a patient enters the clinic with an alarming symptom, the assistant should be ready to act to prevent further injury to the patient.

Many things contribute to a patient's overall experience with a medical office, and how the patient is treated by the practice contributes a great deal to the patient's experience.

YOU ARE THE MEDICAL ADMINISTRATIVE ASSISTANT

The medical office where you work is looking to trim operating costs. One of the physicians has suggested that the front desk staff come in 15 minutes before the first appointment instead of 1 hour before the first appointment. Is this a good idea?

REVIEW EXERCISES

Exercise 8-1 True or False

Read each statement, and determine whether the statement is true or false. Record the answer in the blank provided. T = true; F = false.

______ 1. A patient's first impression of the medical office will be affected by the service given by the medical office staff.

______ 2. Because many insurance companies specify which physician a patient must use, the medical office staff need not be concerned about customer service.

______ 3. Medical offices have been responsive to patients' needs by offering extended office hours.

______ 4. Medical offices advertise their services to patients.

______ 5. An alarm system can be used to protect a medical office against vandalism and theft.

______ 6. After the office is opened for the day, the assistant will pull the records for patients who will be seen for an appointment that day.

______ 7. If an alarm system has been accidentally set off, the assistant may need to notify the police department of the false alarm.

______ 8. To make a patient feel more welcome to the office, a medical administrative assistant is encouraged to make personal comments about a patient's health.

______ 9. An assistant should greet a patient by name, if possible.

______ 10. A patient's full legal name is required during registration to prevent the creation of duplicate medical records.

______ 11. The chief reason why a patient's employer's name and telephone number are obtained is to track the patient in case a bill is unpaid.

______ 12. A guarantor is another name for an insurance company.

______ 13. Emergency information sometimes is used for account collection.

______ 14. A medical history form asks questions about the health of the patient's family members.

______ 15. If patients in the lobby can overhear the office staff discussing information about another patient's appointment, this is a breach of confidentiality.

______ 16. The physicians of the medical office must approve any emergency protocol used by the medical office staff.

______ 17. An assistant should be prepared to call 911 if necessary to provide medical care for a patient in the office.

______ 18. The negative actions of one single employee can affect the overall reputation of a medical office.

______ 19. Resources such as maps and informational items for a medical office can be made available online for quick, easy access for patients.

______ 20. Because medical offices are public places, there is no need to provide secure entrances for employees.

______ 21. Government-issued identification sometimes is required for patients to prove their identity.

______ 22. If a patient is older than 18 years of age, no guarantor information is required.

______ 23. If a patient is referred to the office by another physician, the treating physician does not need to be aware of the referral.

______ 24. Children in a reception area are a matter of concern only for assistants who work in a pediatric office.

______ 25. Some medical offices have code teams that are available to respond to medical emergencies.

Exercise 8-2 Chapter Concepts

Read each question, and choose the answer that best completes the question. Record the answer in the blank provided.

_______1. Which of the following is not done by the assistant every day in the medical office?
(a) Pull medical records for the next day's appointments.
(b) Count cash drawer.
(c) Order supplies.
(d) Check fax for overnight transmissions.

_______2. Which of the following greetings would not be acceptable when greeting a patient who has arrived in a medical office?
(a) "Good morning. Has there been any change in your address or insurance company?"
(b) "Hi, Lila. How can I help you this morning?"
(c) "Good afternoon. How may I help you today?"
(d) "Hello, Mrs. McDonald. I hope you're feeling better than yesterday."

_______3. What insurance information is not required during registration?
(a) Name of company
(b) Amount of deductible
(c) Policy number
(d) Address of company

_______4. What is false regarding authorizations on a registration form?
(a) Can authorize release of information to an insurance company
(b) If not signed, can delay receipt of payment for services
(c) If not signed, insurance claims can still be filed by medical office
(d) Can authorize payments from insurance companies to come directly to the medical office

_______5. Why are new patients asked to arrive early for appointments?
(a) The assistant must check the credit history of new patients with the local credit bureau.
(b) Extra time is needed to complete the registration and medical history forms.
(c) Extra time is needed for laboratory tests to be run.
(d) None of the above

_______6. Which of the following usually is not found in the reception area of a medical office?
(a) Professional journals for physicians
(b) Television set
(c) Magazines for a general audience
(d) Wheelchair

_______7. Which of the following is a concern when children are present in the reception area of a medical office?
(a) Location of the coffee maker
(b) Large toys that do not present a choking hazard
(c) Children's books and magazines
(d) Television playing children's videos

_______8. Which of the following should never be done for a patient who is having a seizure in the lobby?
(a) Get help from the physician immediately.
(b) Move hard objects out of the patient's way.
(c) Insert a hard object into the patient's mouth.
(d) Roll the patient to one side to prevent aspiration of vomitus.

_______9. Which of the following medical emergencies could be aided by the use of a wheelchair?
(a) Chest pain
(b) Respiratory distress
(c) Profuse, uncontrolled bleeding
(d) All would be aided by the use of a wheelchair.
(e) Only a and b would be aided by the use of a wheelchair.

_______10. Which of the following does not pertain to customer service in the medical office?
(a) Patients are health care consumers.
(b) The health care industry has been responsive to patient needs.
(c) Health care promotions usually focus on the price of services.
(d) Exceptional customer service keeps patients loyal to the office.

ACTIVITIES

ACTIVITY 8-1 ENTERING NEW PATIENT INFORMATION

Using Medisoft, practice entering the new patient registration information for William Frost and Deanne Olson, as shown in Figures 8-8 and 8-9 after this activity.

To enter registration information for a new patient, complete the following:

1. Open Medisoft. On the main menu, click **Lists>Patients/Guarantors and Cases.** The **Patient List** will open. From this window, it is possible to enter a new patient by clicking **New Patient** at the bottom of the window. (If **New Patient** is not visible, click the **Patient** radio button at the top of the **Patients/Guarantors and Cases** window.)

(When registering a new patient, it is extremely important to check the existing patient list to determine whether the patient has already been registered. Always begin a new patient registration by searching the existing patient databases. In the **Field** box, select **Search by Last Name, First Name**. In the **Search for** box, type the first three letters of the patient's last name. The patient list will display any names beginning with the letters you typed.)

2. If there is no existing patient file with the new patient's name, create a new patient record by clicking **New Patient** at the bottom of the window.
3. In the **Name, Address** tab, enter the new patient registration information from the Registration Information forms on pages 165-166. Press the tab key to move between fields. Follow the instructions below for each field in the **Name, Address** tab. If information is not available for a field, leave it blank.
   a. **Chart Number:** Leave blank. Medisoft will assign the chart number.
   b. **Last Name:** Enter patient's last name. If the patient's last name contains punctuation, omit the punctuation and omit the space where the punctuation was located.
   c. **Suffix:** If the patient has Junior or Senior or a number as part of their name, enter that information without punctuation.
   d. **First Name:** Enter the patient's complete legal name. Do not enter a nickname.
   e. **Middle Name:** Enter the patient's middle name or initial.
   f. **Street:** Two lines exist for the address. If there is only one line for a patient's address, use the first line. If there are two lines for the patient's address, the second line should be used for the street address and the first line should be used for an apartment number, building location, or name of a company.
   g. After entering the address, press **tab** and the cursor will move to the ZIP code. Once a ZIP code is entered, Medisoft will recognize the ZIP when it is entered again and will enter the City and State information automatically.
   h. **City:** Enter the patient's city.
   i. **State:** Enter the patient's state.
   j. **ZIP:** Enter the patient's ZIP if necessary.
   k. **Email:** Enter the patient's email address.
   l. **Home:** Enter the patient's home phone number.
   m. **Work:** Enter the patient's work phone number. Enter the number where the patient can be reached at work, NOT the employer's main number.
   n. **Cell:** Enter the patient's cell phone number.
   o. **Other:** Enter any other phone number.
   p. **Birth Date:** Enter the patient's birth date in the following order: MMDDYYYY.
   q. **Sex:** Identify the patient's gender.
   r. **Birth Weight:** Leave blank.
   s. **Units:** Leave blank.
   t. **Social Security Number:** Enter the patient's Social Security Number if available.
   u. **Entity Type:** If a patient record is being completed, enter **person.** If a company or business information is being completed, enter **non-person.**
   v. **Race:** Enter if known. Enter this information ONLY if provided by the patient. Do not guess as to what this information might be.
   w. **Ethnicity:** Enter if known. Enter this information ONLY if provided by the patient. Do not guess as to what this information might be.
   x. **Language:** Enter if known. Enter this information ONLY if provided by the patient. Do not guess as to what this information might be.
   y. **Death Date:** If the patient is deceased, enter the date of death.
4. In the **Other Information** tab, enter the remaining patient registration information from the Registration Information forms on pages 165-166. Insurance information will not be added until patients check in for their appointments. (Press the tab key to move between fields. If information is not available for a field, leave it blank.)
   a. **Type:** If the individual is a patient, choose **patient** from the drop-down list. If the individual is a guarantor for a patient's bill, choose **guarantor.**
   b. **Assigned Provider:** If known, identify the patient's primary care physician.
   c. **Patient ID #2:** If patient has a maiden name or previous name, enter the name in this blank.
   d. **Patient Billing Code:** Leave default as A.
   e. **Patient Indicator:** Leave blank.
   f. **Flag:** If patient is a minor, choose **minor** flag from drop-down list.
   g. **Healthcare ID:** Leave blank
   h. **Signature on File**: Leave blank at this time.
   i. **Signature date:** Leave blank at this time.
   j. **Emergency contact:** Enter information if given by patient.
   k. **Employment Information:** Enter patient's employer information if known. If there are two employer phone numbers, enter the work phone for the employer in this blank, not the patient's work phone.
5. Leave the **Payment plan** and **Custom** tabs blank.
6. When the patient's record is completed, click **Save** to save changes to the patient's record.

Happy Valley Medical Group

5222 Baseline Road, Gilbert AZ 85234

REGISTRATION INFORMATION

Please print the following information. Ask the front desk to assist with any questions you may have regarding the information requested.

Patient Information

Patient Name Frost (Last) William (First) C (MI) Date of Birth 8 / 14 / 40 (month day year) Sex [M] F

Address 1764 Vermont Avenue City Harvester State AZ ZIP 85000

Telephone – Home (010) 555 – 1234 Cell (010) 555 – 1088 Work (010) 555 – 9019

Employer retired position ______

Employer Address ______ City ______ State ______ ZIP ______

Social Security number 121 / 00 / 0012

Guarantor Information

Responsible Party Name same (Last, First, MI) Date of Birth ___/___/___ (month day year) Sex M F

Address ______ City ______ State ______ ZIP ______

Telephone – Home (___)____–______ Cell (___)____–______ Work (___)____–______

Employer ______ position ______

Employer Address ______ City ______ State ______ ZIP ______

Social Security number ____/____/____

Primary Insurance Information (please present card to receptionist)

Insurance Company Name Medicare

Policy # 121-00-0012A Group # ______ Policyholder self

Address ______ City ______ State ______ ZIP ______

Telephone (___)____–______ other phone (___)____–______

Secondary Insurance Information (please present card to receptionist)

Insurance Company Name ______

Policy # ______ Group # ______ Policyholder ______

Address ______ City ______ State ______ ZIP ______

Telephone (___)____–______ other phone (___)____–______

Insurance Authorization & Assignment

I hereby authorize Happy Valley Medical Clinic and Medical Group Ltd. to release medical information pertaining to my medical encounters to my insurance company and to file insurance claims on my behalf. I also agree to assign any benefits payable for those claims directly to Happy Valley Medical Clinic. I understand that I am responsible for charges on my account regardless of payments made or due from my insurance company.

Patient Name (print) William C. Frost Date 4-11-YY

Signature *William C. Frost* Relationship (if other than patient) ______

Figure 8-8 New patient registration form for use with Activity 8-1.

Happy Valley Medical Group

5222 Baseline Road, Gilbert AZ 85234

REGISTRATION INFORMATION

Please print the following information. Ask the front desk to assist with any questions you may have regarding the information requested.

Patient Information

Patient Name Olson (Last) Deanne (First) I (MI) Date of Birth 8 / 17 / 70 (month day year) Sex M [F]

Address 8364 Woodhaven Road City Harvester State AZ ZIP 85000

Telephone – Home (010) 555 – 4335 Cell (010) 555 – 3233 Work (010) 555 – 6742

Employer News Channel 11 position station manager

Employer Address ______ City Washington State DC ZIP ______

Social Security number 555 / 55 / 5555

Guarantor Information

Responsible Party Name same (Last First MI) Date of Birth ___/___/___ (month day year) Sex M F

Address ______ City ______ State ______ ZIP ______

Telephone – Home (___)___–___ Cell (___)___–___ Work (___)___–___

Employer ______ position ______

Employer Address ______ City ______ State ______ ZIP ______

Social Security number___/___/___

Primary Insurance Information (please present card to receptionist)

Insurance Company Name BCBS231

Policy # HK3740234 Group # ______ Policyholder self

Address 88 W Bell Road City Phoenix State AZ ZIP 85021

Telephone (800) 555 – 5555 other phone (___)___–___

Secondary Insurance Information (please present card to receptionist)

Insurance Company Name ______

Policy # ______ Group # ______ Policyholder ______

Address ______ City ______ State ______ ZIP ______

Telephone (___)___–___ other phone (___)___–___

Insurance Authorization & Assignment

I hereby authorize Happy Valley Medical Clinic and Medical Group Ltd. to release medical information pertaining to my medical encounters to my insurance company and to file insurance claims on my behalf. I also agree to assign any benefits payable for those claims directly to Happy Valley Medical Clinic. I understand that I am responsible for charges on my account regardless of payments made or due from my insurance company.

Patient Name (print) Deanne E. Olson Date 4-12-YY

Signature *Deanne E. Olson* Relationship (if other than patient) ______

Figure 8-9 New p atient registration form for use with Activity 8-1.

ACTIVITY 8-2 PATIENT CHECK-IN/ REGISTRATION

In chapter 7, appointments were made for patients. The next step in the patient process is patients arrive at the clinic and are checked in, or registered, for their appointments.

Using the information included with this exercise, check in each patient for their respective appointments, edit their registration information and enter their insurance information in Medisoft. Insurance information will be entered in a **Case.** Using the **Case** option allows you to assign specific information such as an insurance plan or treatment information to a specific appointment with a specific provider. (Cases are numbered and it is possible that the case numbers will vary from student to student.)

1. Open **Office Hours Professional.** Using the following information, locate Charles Gooding's appointment on 2/3/2014 with Dr. Morris. Go to February 3, 2014, and display Dr. Morris's schedule. Double-click Charles Gooding's appointment to open the appointment.
   Appointment Information 2/3/2014 9:00 Dr. Morris
   Registration information
   Patient Name: Charles Michael Gooding
   Address: 7612 14th Ave, Gilbert AZ 85001 Home phone: 010-555-9344 Cell Phone: 010-551-9344
   DOB: 03/27/1951 Sex: M SSN: 111-44-3223
   Provider: WH Flag: None. Employer: Bean Sprout Express Work Phone: 602-453-9988
   Case information Case Description: BLU00 020314 Guarantor: self Assigned Provider: Morris
   Insurance 1: BLU00 Policyholder: self Relationship: self Policy number: MQ6547336
2. On the right side of the **Edit Appointment** window, click the option for **Checked In.**
3. Right-click in the **Chart** box and select **Edit Patient.** Enter the information in the **Name, Address** tab and the **Other Information** tab. Each patient has signed an authorization for filing insurance claims for their visits. Select **Signature on File** for each patient and enter the **Signature date** as the date of their visit.
4. In the Chart box, **Case box** and select **New Case.** The tabs within the case window allow you to assign specific information to the patient's encounter.
   a. Under the **Personal tab**, enter the **Case Description** and **Guarantor** information. (The case description will consist of the type of insurance and date of service. Cases can be named in any way that the clinic chooses.)
   b. Under the **Account** tab, enter the assigned provider information.
   c. Under the **Policy 1** tab, enter the insurance information.
   d. Click **Save.**
5. Verify that the **Case number** appears in the **Case box** and the description is next to the case number box. Verify that you have marked "checked in" for the appointment.
6. Click **Save.** Note that a checkmark is placed next to the patient's name on the schedule.
7. As each patient enters the office, complete the remaining appointment, registration, and case information below using the previous instructions.
   a. **Appointment Information** 2/3/2014 10:00 Dr. Morris
   Registration information
   Patient Name: William C. Frost
   Address: 1764 Vermont Ave, Harvester AZ 85000 Home phone: 010-555-1234 Cell Phone: 010-555-1088
   DOB: 08/14/1940 Sex: M SSN: 121-00-0012
   Provider: MM Employer: retired Work Phone: 602-453-9988
   Case information Case Description: MED01 020314 Guarantor: self
   Assigned Provider: Morris
   Insurance 1: MED01 Policyholder: self Relationship: self Policy number: 121-00-0012A
   b. **Appointment Information** 2/3/2014 10:00 Dr. Lee
   Registration information
   Patient Name: Anthony Allen Peters
   Address: 191 Gary Way, Gilbert AZ 85234 Home phone: 480-833-5515 Cell Phone:480-882-5555
   DOB: 01/03/1977 Sex: M SSN: 221-33-2443
   Provider: JM Employer: MicroMania Inc. Work Phone: 602-746-2134
   Case information Case Description: WOR00 020314 Guarantor: self
   Assigned Provider: Lee
   Insurance 1: WOR00 020314 Policyholder: self Relationship: self Policy number: 76928
   c. **Appointment Information** 2/3/2014 10:00 Dr. Martinez
   Registration information
   Patient Name: Jane Samantha Doe
   Address: 222 East Jane St, Mesa AZ 85213 Home phone: 010-999-9999 Cell Phone: 480-888-8888
   DOB: 04/28/1962 Sex: F SSN: 123-45-6789
   Provider: WH Employer: The Computer Place Work Phone: 601-892-5120
   Case information Case Description: FHP00 020314 Guarantor: Doe, John
   Assigned Provider: Martinez
   Insurance 1: FHP00 Policyholder: Doe, John Relationship: spouse Policy number: 78-555-263
   d. **Appointment Information** 2/3/2014 10:15 Timothy Marks, PA
   Registration information
   Patient Name: John Christopher Doe
   Address: 222 East Jane St, Mesa AZ 85213 Home phone: 010-999-9999 Cell Phone: 010-999-9876
   DOB: 07/03/1972 Sex: M SSN: 123-23-2345
   Provider: RL Employer: Windham Gallery Work Phone: 602-893-4215
   Case information Case Description: FHP00 020314 Guarantor: self
   Assigned Provider: Marks
   Insurance 1: FHP00 Policyholder: self Relationship: self Policy number: 78-555-263

e. **Appointment Information** 2/3/2014 10:30 Emily O'Brian, CNP
 Registration information Patient Name: Tanus James Simpson
 Address: 3018 W 1st St, Thatcher AZ 85552 Home phone: 010-555-5555 Cell Phone:
 DOB: 04/04/1968 Sex: M SSN: 111-88-2365
 Provider: RL Employer: MicroMania Inc. Work Phone:602-746-2134
 Case information Case Description: BLU00 020314 Guarantor: self
 Assigned Provider: O'Brian
 Insurance 1: BLU00 Policyholder: self Relationship: self Policy number: GT2039453
f. **Appointment Information** 2/3/2014 10:45 Timothy Marks, PA
 Registration information Patient Name: Wallace Dale Clinger
 Address: 200 Pennsylvania Ave, Washington DC 11111 Home phone: 254-222-9111 Cell Phone: 254-234-2424
 DOB: 04/03/1965 Sex: M SSN: 123-32-4444
 Provider: RL Employer: None Work Phone:
 Case information Case Description: BLU01 020314 Guarantor: self
 Assigned Provider: Marks
 Insurance 1: BLU01 Policyholder: self Relationship: self Policy number: JUD9834
g. **Appointment Information** 2/3/2014 11:15 Dr. Lee
 Registration information Patient Name: Suzy Quinn Jones
 Address: 2273 Easy Street, Mesa AZ 85213 Home phone: 010-123-4444 Cell Phone: 010-221-4441
 DOB: 06/07/1974 Sex: F SSN: 121-22-1112
 Provider: RL Employer: News Channel 11 Work Phone:
 Case information Case Description: BLU01 020314 Guarantor: self
 Assigned Provider: Lee
 Insurance 1: BLU01 Policyholder: self Relationship: self Policy number: MLN5745
h. **Appointment Information** 2/3/2014 2:30 Dr. Martinez
 Registration information Patient Name: Anthony Thomas Zimmerman
 Address: 123 Any St, Harvester, AZ 85000 Home phone: 010-444-8855 Cell Phone: 010-444-8888
 DOB: 05/01/1963 Sex: M SSN: 993-26-2356
 Provider: RL Flag: None Employer: The Computer Place Work Phone: 601-892-5120
 Case information Case Description: AET00 020314 Guarantor: self
 Assigned Provider: Martinez
 Insurance 1: AET00 Policyholder: self Relationship: self Policy number:556-1729
i. **Appointment Information** 2/3/2014 2:30 Dr. Lee
 Registration information Patient Name: Tonya Ann Hartman
 Address: 1571 Knap Way, Portland OR 97532 Home phone: 011-847-6199 Cell Phone:
 DOB: 11/08/1972 Sex: F SSN: 333-52-3454
 Provider: MM Flag: None. Employer: US Air Force Work Phone:
 Case information Case Description: BLU00 020314 Guarantor: self
 Assigned Provider: Lee
 Insurance 1: BLU00 Policyholder: self Relationship: self Policy number: XZ6654723
j. **Appointment Information** 2/3/2014 2:30 Dr. Hinckle
 Registration information Patient Name: Michael Christian Youngblood
 Address: 73982 N 28th Ave, Phoenix AZ 85044 Home phone: 010-222-3333 Cell Phone:
 DOB: 7/5/1962 Sex: M SSN: 334-67-3847
 Provider: WH Employer: Reardons Camping Supplies Work Phone: 602-451-8686
 Case information Case Description: AET00 020314 Guarantor: self
 Assigned Provider: Hinckle
 Insurance 1: AET00 Policyholder: self Relationship: self Policy number: 572-8632
k. **Appointment Information** 2/3/2014 3:30 Dr. Lee
 Registration information Patient Name: Zach Anthony Peters
 Address: 191 Gary Way, Gilbert AZ 85297 Home phone: 010-833-5515 Cell Phone:
 DOB: 06/27/2000 Sex: M SSN: 213-12-3235
 Provider: JM Employer: Work Phone:
 Case information Case Description: BLU01 020314 Guarantor: Peters, Anthony
 Assigned Provider: Lee
 Insurance 1: BLU01 Policyholder: Peters, Anthony Relationship: child Policy number: GHP3338
l. **Appointment Information** 2/3/2014 4:00 Dr. Morris
 Registration information Patient Name: Jay Robert Brimley
 Address: 1234 W. Glendale Ave, Glendale AZ 85382 Home phone: 222-342-3444 Cell Phone:222-342-3344
 DOB: 01/23/1964 Sex: M SSN: 234-36-4433
 Provider: MM Employer: MicroMania Inc. Work Phone: 602-746-2134
 Case information Case Description: FHP00 020314 Guarantor: self
 Assigned Provider: Morris
 Insurance 1: FHP00 Policyholder: self Relationship: self Policy number: 76-562-112
m. **Appointment Information** 2/3/2014 4:15 Dr. Lee
 Registration information Patient Name: Chadwick Brian Koseman
 Address: 3278 E Joseph Way, Gilbert AZ 85297 Home phone: 010-555-6464 Cell Phone:
 DOB: 07/04/1982 Sex: M SSN: 229-83-4711
 Provider: JM Employer: Windham Gallery Work Phone: 602-893-4215

Case information Case Description: WOR00 020314 Guarantor: self
Assigned Provider: Lee
Insurance 1: WOR00 Policyholder: self Relationship: self Policy number: 77002

n. **Appointment Information** 2/3/2014 4:45 Dr. Hinckle
Registration information Patient Name: Elmo James Brimley
Address: 1234 W. Glendale Ave, Glendale AZ 85382 Home phone: 222-342-3444 Cell Phone:222-342-3344
DOB:-9/29/1997 Sex: M SSN: 888-23-3333
Provider: MM Employer: None Work Phone:
Case information Case Description: FHP00 020314 Guarantor: Brimley, Jay
Assigned Provider: Hinckle
Insurance 1: FHP00 Policyholder: Brimley, Jay Relationship: child Policy number: 76-562-112

o. **Appointment Information** 2/4/2014 9:00 Dr. Lee
Registration information Patient Name: Sammy Alexandra Catera
Address: 7214 Shape Cir, Gilbert AZ 85001 Home phone: 010-227-7722 Cell Phone:
DOB: 06/17/1964 Sex: F SSN: 934-12-0887
Provider: MM Employer: Bean Sprout Express Work Phone: 602-453-9988
Case information Case Description: BLU01 020414 Guarantor: self
Assigned Provider: Lee
Insurance 1: BLU01 Policyholder: self Relationship: self Policy number: BAR4677

p. **Appointment Information** 2/4/2014 9:15 Dr. Hinckle
Registration information Patient Name: Lindsey Jana Nielsen
Address: 341 Evergreen Terrace, Mesa AZ 85204 Home phone: 010-344-5849 Cell Phone:
DOB: 02/29/1984 Sex: F SSN: 987-65-4321
Provider: WH Employer: Army Work Phone:
Case information Case Description: CIG00 020414 Guarantor: self
Assigned Provider: Hinckle
Insurance 1: CIG00 Policyholder: self Relationship: self Policy number: 675ZXX

q. **Appointment Information** 2/4/2014 9:15 Emily O'Brian, CNP
Registration information Patient Name: Tonya Ann Hartman
Address: 1571 Knap Way, Portland OR 97532 Home phone: 011-847-6199 Cell Phone:
DOB: 11/08/1972 Sex: F SSN: 333-52-3454
Provider: MM Employer: US Air Force Work Phone:
Case information Case Description: BLU00 020414 Guarantor: self
Assigned Provider: O'Brian
Insurance 1: BLU00 Policyholder: self Relationship: self Policy number: XZ6654723

r. **Appointment Information** 2/4/2014 9:45 Timothy Marks, PA
Registration information Patient Name: Dwight Edward Again
Address: 1742 N 83rd Ave, Phoenix AZ 85021 Home phone: 010-434-5777 Cell Phone:
DOB: 03/30/1932 Sex: M SSN: 876-45-2364
Provider: RL Employer: Really Useful Trucking Work Phone: 602-457-3326
Case information Case Description: MED01 020414 Guarantor: self
Assigned Provider: Marks
Insurance 1: MED01 Policyholder: self Relationship: self Policy number: 234-23-3512X

s. **Appointment Information** 2/4/2014 10:15 Dr. Morris
Registration information Patient Name: Charles Michael Gooding
Address: 7612 14th Ave, Gilbert AZ 85001 Home phone: 010-555-9344 Cell Phone: 010-551-9344
DOB: 03/27/1951 Sex: M SSN: 111-44-3223
Provider: WH Employer: Bean Sprout Express Work Phone: 602-453-9988
Case information Case Description: BLU00 020414 Guarantor: self
Assigned Provider: Morris
Insurance 1: BLU00 Policyholder: self Relationship: self Policy number: MQ6547336

t. **Appointment Information** 2/4/2014 10:30 Dr. Hinckle
Registration information Patient Name: Ryan Michael Whitmore
Address: 2990 Power Road, Gilbert AZ 85297 Home phone: 010-444-5582 Cell Phone: 011-235-2377
DOB: 05/11/1993 Sex: M SSN: 883-34-2354
Provider: JM Employer: Reardons Camping Supplies Work Phone:
Case information Case Description: CIG00 020414 Guarantor: self
Assigned Provider: Hinckle
Insurance 1: CIG00 Policyholder: self Relationship: self Policy number: 113MPQ

u. **Appointment Information** 2/4/2014 10:30 Timothy Marks, PA
Registration information Patient Name: John Christopher Doe
Address: 222 East Jane St, Mesa AZ 85213 Home phone: 010-999-9999 Cell Phone: 010-999-9876
DOB: 07/03/1972 Sex: M SSN: 123-23-2345
Provider: RL Employer: Windham Gallery Work Phone:602-893-4215
Case information Case Description: FHP00 020414 Guarantor: self
Assigned Provider: Marks
Insurance 1: FHP00 Policyholder: self Relationship: self Policy number: 78-555-263

v. **Appointment Information** 2/4/2014 10:30 Emily O'Brian, CNP
Registration information Patient Name: Deanne I. Olson
Address: 8364 Woodhaven, Harvester AZ 85000 Home phone: 010-555-4335 Cell Phone: 010-555-3233
DOB: 08/17/1970 Sex: F SSN: 555-55-5555
Provider: EO Employer: News Channel 11 Work Phone: 0105556742
Case information Case Description: BLU00 020414 Guarantor: self
Assigned Provider: O'Brian
Insurance 1: BLU00 Policyholder: self Relationship: self Policy number: HK3740234

w. **Appointment Information** 2/4/2014 11:00 Emily O'Brian, CNP
Registration information Patient Name: Susan Marie Brimley
Address: 1234 W. Glendale Ave, Glendale AZ 85382 Home phone: 222-342-3444 Cell Phone: 222-342-3333
DOB: 05/07/1961 Sex: F SSN: 111-22-5664
Provider: MM Employer: None Work Phone: N/A
Case information Case Description: FHP00 020414 Guarantor: Brimley, Jay
Assigned Provider: O'Brian
Insurance 1: FHP00 Policyholder: Brimley, Jay Relationship: spouse Policy number: 76-562-112

x. **Appointment Information** 2/4/2014 1:00 Dr. Martinez
Registration information Patient Name: Andrew Adam Austin
Address: 199 Wallethe Way, Tempe AZ 85123 Home phone: 010-767-2222 Cell Phone:
DOB: 01/01/1950 Sex: M SSN: 999-88-7777
Provider: JM Flag: None. Employer: Really Useful Trucking Work Phone: 602-457-3326
Case information Case Description: CIG00 Guarantor: self
Assigned Provider: Martinez
Insurance 1: CIG00 Policyholder: self Relationship: self Policy number: 562HBC

ACTIVITY 8-3 COPY PATIENT REGISTRATION

One of the advantages of using software to maintain registration information is the ability to reuse this information without having to reenter the same information over and over again.

Using Medisoft, copy changes below from one record to another record:

1. On the main menu, click **Lists>Patients/Guarantors and Cases.** The Patient List will open. Make changes to the first patient's record listed below. Click **Save.**
2. Open the patient's record that needs to be changed. Click **Copy Address.** Highlight the patient's name where the correct information is stored.
3. Click **OK.** Address and telephone information will be copied to the patient's record that needs to be changed.
4. Click **Save.**

Make the changes to Jay Brimley's record first, and copy the address information over to Susan and Elmo Brimley's records as directed above.

Brimley, Jay. Change address to 3425 Sunset Lane, Glendale, AZ 85382. Telephone remains the same.

Brimley, Susan & Brimley, Elmo. Copy address from Jay Brimley's record to Susan and Elmo's records.

ACTIVITY 8-4 MISSED APPOINTMENTS

Using Medisoft, record the following missed appointments, and print a no-show report.

1. Open **Office Hours Professional.** The following patients have missed their appointments on February 3, 2014:
   a. **Appointment Information** 2/3/2014 2:00 Dr. Hinckle, John Bordon
   b. **Appointment Information** 2/3/2014 11:15 Emily O'Brian, CNP, Monica Peters.
2. Open each patient's appointment and change **Status** to **Missed.**
3. Click **Save** to save changes and close the appointment.
4. Click **Reports>No-Show Report.** Select **Export the report to a file>Start.** In the **Data Selection** window, specify the **date range 02/03/2014 to 02/04/2014.** Leave the **provider range** blank.
5. Name the file **yourlastname noshow 84** and save the report to a location you will remember. Send the report to your instructor.

ACTIVITY 8-5 PRINT PATIENT LIST

Use the following instructions to generate an alphabetic list of patients for Happy Valley Medical Clinic.

1. In Medisoft (not Office Hours Professional), click **Lists>Patients/Guarantors** and **Cases.** The **Patient List** will open. After the **Field** box, verify that the **Patient** radio button is selected. Click **Print Grid.**
2. Click **Add fields** to add the following fields: (hold CTRL key down while selecting fields) City, Sex, Signature on File, SOF date, State, Work Phone, ZIP code. Click OK.
3. Rearrange the fields by highlighting the field name and clicking the up or down arrows. Place the fields in the following order: Chart #, Name, DOB, Sex, SSN, Phone1, Work Phone, Street 1, City, State, Zip Code, Signature on File, SOF Date. If any fields are missing from the list, add them as previously instructed.
4. Delete the remaining fields from the list.
5. Click **OK.** Click **Export data to CSV file** and **Landscape** view. Click **Start.**
6. Name the file **yourlastname patient list 85** patient list and send the file to your instructor.

ACTIVITY 8-6 PREPARE AND PRINT SUPERBILLS

When a patient reports for an appointment, it is necessary to generate a superbill to record the services provided to the patient. The superbill is generated, after registration information is verified and insurance details are added to the patient's registration data.

Using **Medisoft** (not **Office Hours Professional**), print superbills by completing the following steps:

1. On the main menu, click **Reports> Superbills>Superbill (Numbered)>OK.**
2. In the **Print Report Where** window, select **Export the Report to a File/Start.**
3. Name the file **yourlastname superbills 86>Save**. Be sure to save the file to a location you will remember.
4. In the **Data Selection** window, leave **Chart Number Range** blank. Enter **Date Range** 02/03/2014 to 02/04/2014. Leave **Provider Range** blank. Leave **Beginning Superbill Number** as is. Click **OK.**
5. Open the file and verify that the information in the file is correct.
6. Send the file to your instructor.

(If a new appointment is added to the schedule after the superbills are printed, DO NOT reprint all of the superbills. If all superbills are reprinted, each superbill will have a new number assigned, and each appointment will have two superbills. This will cause problems with the tracking feature in billing. To print a superbill for an appointment that was added to the schedule, right click on the appointment in the appointment grid, and click **Print Superbill**. Only the new superbill will print.)

ACTIVITY 8-7 HEALTH CARE FACILITY INFORMATION RESEARCH

Locate on the Internet information about two to three health care facilities (local or national). What type of information is available on these Internet sites for patients?

ACTIVITY 8-8 PATIENT REGISTRATION

Using the blank registration information form, (see Fig. 8-2), perform Procedure 8-2 as identified in this chapter. You may gather information from another student in class or from another individual, as directed by your instructor.

ACTIVITY 8-9 MEDICAL OFFICE SCENARIOS

Consider the following situations. Practice giving an appro priate response to the situation given.

1. A patient enters the office in acute respiratory distress. You immediately transport the patient to an examination room. When you return to the front desk, a patient approaches the desk to inquire about what happened. How do you respond?
2. Explain to a patient the authorizations on a registration form.
3. Design a sign that might be placed near a television set to alert patients to consider young children who may be present. Be sure to communicate in a polite, considerate manner.

DISCUSSION

The following topics can be used for class discussion or for individual student essay.

DISCUSSION 8-1

A medical office has decided to streamline registration for patients and has placed a sign-up sheet at the front desk so patients can sign in as they arrive. Is this a good idea?

DISCUSSION 8-2

Discuss the importance of keeping the reception area of a medical office tidy.

DISCUSSION 8-3

The physicians of a medical office have decided that all employees should take a course in CPR. Is this a good idea?

Bibliography

Chester GA: *Modern Medical Assisting*, Philadelphia, 1998, WB Saunders.

Young AP: *Kinn's The Medical Assistant, An Applied Learning Approach*, ed 6, St. Louis, Elsevier, 2007.

Office of Civil Rights: *Summary of the HIPAA Privacy Rule, U.S. Department of Health and Human Services* May 2003, http://www.hhs.gov/ocr/privacysummary.pdf. last revised accessed 3-20-08.

O'Toole M: *Miller-Keane Encyclopedia & Dictionary of Medicine, Nursing, & Allied Health*, ed 7, Philadelphia, WB Saunders, 2005.

The Medical Management Institute: *The Medical Office Policy Handbook*, Salt Lake City, Medical Management Institute, 2007.

CHAPTER 9 Health Information Management

LEARNING OUTCOMES

On successful completion of this chapter, the student will be able to

1. Explain the role of health information management.
2. Explain confidentiality and the importance of protecting patient confidentiality.
3. Explain the role of computers in health information management.
4. Explain HIPAA.
5. Identify the components and the organization of the medical record.
6. Describe medical transcription.
7. Describe quantitative analysis.
8. Describe the necessary filing supplies and filing equipment.
9. Use methods of filing and locating medical records.
10. Demonstrate color coding of medical records.
11. Describe protection, retention, and disposal of medical records.
12. Explain procedures for releasing medical information.
13. Discuss the legal and ethical issues surrounding medical records.

COMMISSION ON ACCREDITATION OF ALLIED HEALTH EDUCATION PROGRAMS (CAAHEP) CORE CURRICULUM FOR MEDICAL ASSISTANTS

- Identify systems for organizing medical records.
- Describe various types of content maintained in a patient's medical record.
- Discuss pros and cons of various filing methods.
- Identify both equipment and supplies needed for filing medical records.
- Describe indexing rules.
- Discuss filing procedures.
- Discuss principles of using electronic medical records (EMRs).
- Identify types of records common to the health care setting.
- Organize a patient's medical record.
- File medical records.
- Use office hardware and software to maintain office systems.
- Use Internet to access information related to the medical office.
- Maintain organization by filing.
- Describe the implications of HIPAA for the medical assistant in various medical settings.
- Respond to issues of confidentiality.
- Apply HIPAA rules in regard to privacy/release of information.
- Document accurately in the patient record.

ACCREDITING BUREAU OF HEALTH EDUCATION SCHOOLS (ABHES) COMPETENCIES FOR MEDICAL ASSISTING

Graduates

- Prepare and maintain medical records.
- Demonstrate professionalism by maintaining confidentiality at all times.
- Perform basic clerical functions.
- Document accurately.
- Institute federal and state guidelines when releasing medical records or information.

VOCABULARY

accession ledger
active record
alphanumeric
assessment
breach of confidentiality
chart entries
chart notes
chief complaint
closed record
color coding
computerized patient record (CPR)
consecutive number filing
consultation
cross-referenced
diagnosis
dictation
discharge summary
electronic health record (EHR)
electronic medical record (EMR)
electronic patient record (EPR)
face sheet
health information management
history and physical (H&P)
identification sheet
impression
inactive record

VOCABULARY—cont'd

laboratory report
master patient index
medical history
medical transcription
objective
operative report
outguide
pathology report
plan
problem-oriented medical record (POMR)
progress notes
quantitative analysis
radiology report
redacted
release of information (ROI)
shingling
SOAP method
source-oriented medical record (SOMR)
subjective
summary sheet
terminal digit filing
tickler file
transposition

What is Health Information Management?

Every aspect of a patient's medical care must be documented. **Health information management** involves directing and organizing all activities related to keeping and caring for information concerning health care provided for patients. Medical administrative and health information management personnel are responsible for maintaining the medical record, preparing medical reports, releasing appropriate medical information, compiling statistics related to health care services, and coding for billing and insurance purposes.

Individuals responsible for health information management activities in the medical office ensure that patient information is documented properly, and that it is used appropriately in the business of health care. These individuals are chiefly responsible for maintaining every patient's medical record and ensuring that the record is complete and accurate.

Purposes of Record Keeping

Medical records are kept in a health care facility for a variety of reasons. One of the most important uses of a medical record is to document the care given to a patient. Without the record to chronicle the various treatments administered to a patient, health care providers would not be able to provide continuing care for the patient. The record contains documentation of a patient's health status, history, and details regarding treatments provided to the patient. It would be impossible for the physician or any other health care provider to remember everything that had been done for a patient. Even patients themselves would likely not be able to remember absolutely everything in their medical history. The medical record is an essential document that is needed by every health care provider to deliver the best possible care to a patient.

Medical records also are used for legal purposes. If a patient suffers an injury because of an accident and makes a claim against a third party, the patient would seek a medical professional's advice for treatment of that injury. The medical record would contain documentation as to the extent of the patient's injury. In this type of case, the health care provider would testify as to the patient's injuries, and the patient's medical record would be entered as evidence in court. Sometimes, a health care provider is the defendant in a malpractice suit. The medical record then provides proof of the treatments and advice the patient was given and may be used as evidence in support of or against the health care provider.

The medical record serves as documentation for insurance claims that are filed on behalf of the patient. In essence, the medical record supports what is billed to the insurance company. An insurance company may request a copy of a patient's record to determine whether charges were medically necessary or whether services provided were a covered benefit. Workers' compensation agencies require periodic reporting about a claimant's condition, and the medical record authenticates a patient's condition and treatment.

Data from medical records also may be used in a variety of ways for planning. Many of the following examples do not require identification of a patient's name, but the information contained in a patient's medical record can lead to various improvements in the provision of health care.

- The gathering of treatment data from medical records enables health care providers to offer better and more effective treatments for their patients.
- Medical information might be used for business planning when a health care facility is considering future expansion of services offered.
- Records are reviewed to ensure that treatment provided by a physician or other health care professional meets the facility's standards of quality.
- Students involved in medical education routinely review case histories to learn more about the practice of medicine.
- Medical research also requires the use of medical records to track the progress of disease or injury and patients' responses to treatment.

Types of Records

At this moment, we are at an interesting crossroads in health care record keeping. Previously, for the most part, records have been kept in paper form. With the surge of information and computer technology, we are now seeing a transition from the paper record to an electronic health record. An **electronic health record (EHR)** includes the same type of patient information as a paper record, but the information is stored digitally on a computer. The American Health Information Management Association (AHIMA) has selected EHR as the preferred identifier for this type of record. Other organizations may use the term **computerized patient record (CPR), electronic medical record (EMR),** or **electronic patient record (EPR),** but all terms refer to the same type of information.

In 2005, the Mayo Clinic made the transition from paper to electronic records. This clinic system has more than 16,000 computer terminals that make all data related to patient care—appointments, patient histories and examinations, operative reports, diagnostic studies—available to caregivers whenever needed. An electronic record enables providers and other caregivers to have immediate access to the most up-to-date patient data when providing care to patients.

When studying the information in this chapter, keep in mind that the purposes of the record keeping remain the same, whether the information is kept on paper or in a computer. Occasionally, there will be differences in how those systems function, and, where necessary, those differences will be identified.

HIPAA Hint

Protected Health Information (PHI) includes all individually identifiable health information in any format—electronic, paper, or oral. Written reports, spoken information, and pictures are examples of protected health information if they contain information that reveals the patient's identity.

Confidentiality

Many treatments in the office are of a highly personal nature, and the confidentiality of every patient's medical information is a legal requirement of all employees of the office. Patients need to be able to trust that their medical histories and treatments will be held in the deepest confidence. If that level of trust does not exist, patients may not share important information with their health care providers.

Day after day in the medical office, an assistant deals with this personal information about patients. All information encountered in the process of working in the medical office must be kept private unless the patient or someone with the proper authority has approved disclosure of the information. Everything that is seen, heard, or done in the medical office is confidential. A patient's name, diagnoses, procedures, bills, laboratory tests—essentially everything about the patient's interaction with the office—are confidential. Thus, health information includes (but may not be limited to) information that is written, is stored electronically, is spoken, or is an image (pictures such as radiology studies).

Information about a patient's medical treatment should not be released unless the release is authorized. Releasing medical information that should *not* be released is known as a **breach of confidentiality,** and anyone involved in breaching confidentiality may be subject to termination of employment, legal penalties, or both. A medical administrative assistant must do everything possible to protect all patients' medical information.

Confidentiality Agreements

Individuals who begin employment in any type of health care facility are required to sign a confidentiality agreement. No matter where employees may work within a health care facility, they may come into contact with a patient's medical information. Front desk and nursing staff are privy to a patient's diagnoses and procedures. Even building maintenance staff may be responsible for proper disposal of medical information. To emphasize the importance of confidentiality, all employees, as well as volunteers, are required to sign a confidentiality agreement. Such an agreement should include a definition of confidential information and the expectation of keeping information confidential, as well as the consequences of breaching confidentiality. Consequences often include termination of employment. A sample of a typical confidentiality agreement appears in Figure 3-2 in Chapter 3.

Confidentiality and Computerized Medical Records

A computer is present in almost every medical office. It assists the staff in a variety of office tasks, one of which is health information management. A computer system contains health information about patients, their appointments, and the diagnoses and procedures that will appear on patients' insurance claims. Medical reports and results of diagnostic studies such as laboratory tests and radiographs frequently are stored in a computer system at one location and are retrieved by a physician at another location. Computers allow easy retrieval of medical information. Portions of a medical record can be placed in a computer system, or an entire medical record can be stored in a computer system. With the increasing use of computers in health care, the latter approach is becoming commonplace in health care organizations.

Protecting the confidentiality of the health information contained in a medical record is one of the chief concerns with regard to EHRs. Computer systems must be secure and protective of the health information contained within. An organization can do several things to protect electronic health information, such as the following:

- Restrict employees' access to only those parts of a computer system necessary to do their job. Front desk staff could be limited only to the appointments and registration portion of a computer system. Laboratory results may be accessible only to physicians, nurses, and laboratory personnel.
- Require employee use of a password to access a computer system. Employees should be cautioned to never allow one employee to use another's password to access the computer system.
- Track employees' use of the computer system. A computer system can keep track of the dates and times that an employee accesses a system and can track the files that the employee has accessed. Employees should be warned that accessing a patient's information for no apparent reason can result in termination of employment. Employees are often warned that they are not allowed to access their own health record as well.
- Provide a secure environment for the computer system. Screensavers should be activated after a short period of

inactivity to keep displayed information confidential. Systems may even log the employee off after a specified period of inactivity.

As the use of computers in health care continues to grow, medical offices will have to be increasingly vigilant in ensuring the confidentiality of medical information. Electronic information is just as confidential as written information.

Health Insurance Portability and Accountability Act of 1996 (HIPAA)

The U.S. Department of Health and Human Services developed national medical record privacy standards as part of the Health Insurance Portability and Accountability Act of 1996 (HIPAA). This law became effective in April 2003 and applies to all personal health care information. These regulations (introduced in Chapter 3) include the following:

- Requirements for protecting patients' medical records
- The patient's right to know how personal health information is used
- The patient's right to obtain a copy of his or her medical record. However, there is an exception to this part of the regulation: If the patient has received psychotherapy and those notes are kept separately from the patient's other health information AND the treating provider has decided that access to psychotherapy notes should be denied, the patient does NOT have the right to obtain a copy of the psychotherapy notes.
- Restrictions on how health information can be used
- Civil and criminal penalties for violating a patient's privacy

In 2009, the Health Information Technology for Economic and Clinical Health (HITECH) Act became law. The purpose of the act was to promote the meaningful use of electronic technology for health information. Part of the HITECH Act addressed concerns about security of electronic transmission of health information. An important part of the act significantly increased monetary penalties for security violations of HIPAA.

Notice of Privacy Practices

As mentioned, each patient of a health care facility has the right to know how his or her health information will be used. Chapter 8 mentioned that a patient must be given a Notice of Privacy Practices at his or her first appointment. The Notice of Privacy Practices delineates how the patient's protected health information may be used, what the patient's rights are to his or her health information, and what responsibility the health care provider has to the patient in regard to the health information. An acknowledgment of this notice (Fig. 9-1)

Happy Valley Medical Group
5222 E. Baseline Rd.
Gilbert, AZ 85234
(010) 555-1110

NOTICE OF PRIVACY PRACTICES ACKNOWLEDGMENT

I do hereby acknowledge that I have received a copy of the Happy Valley Medical Group Notice of Privacy Practices.

I understand that I have a right to

- request restrictions on disclosure of my protected health information;
- request that communication regarding my protected health information be conducted in a specific manner;
- know what disclosures have been made of my protected health information;
- see and receive a copy of my protected health information;
- request correction of errors in my protected health information;
- make changes to this acknowledgment.

I understand that under certain circumstances Happy Valley Medical Group may be required to release a portion of my protected health information where release may be required by law.

____
Please print patient name (last, first, MI)

____________________ ____________________
DOB (MMDDYY) Medical record number

____________________ ____________________
Signature of patient or authorized representative Date

Figure 9-1 A Notice of Privacy Practices must be signed at a patient's first appointment.

must be signed and dated by the patient and retained by the health care facility.

Failure to Comply with HIPAA

HIPAA has established civil and criminal penalties for cases in which health information is not protected as required. Penalties can start at $100 per violation for general noncompliance with privacy, security, and transaction regulations. They also can become quite harsh—up to a $250,000 fine and up to 10 years' imprisonment—for obtaining or disclosure of protected health information with the intent to use the information for monetary gain.

Components of the Medical Record in a Medical Office

In a health care facility that provides any type of care for a patient, information related to the patient's condition or treatment is kept in some form of medical record. Whether in paper or electronic form, a patient's record in a medical office contains documentation related to the patient's office visits and medical tests, along with correspondence pertaining to the patient's treatment. When the components of the medical record are discussed in this chapter, keep in mind that these components can be kept in paper or electronic form. But regardless of what form the information is kept in, the content is still the same.

The medical record in the medical office contains information about a patient's office visits; medical history; immunizations; and laboratory, radiology, and other diagnostic testing, as well as any correspondence sent or received by the office. The record chronicles the history of medical treatment in the physician's office. If a patient is hospitalized, copies of hospital reports are sent from the hospital to the office for inclusion in the patient's medical record. A home health agency keeps a record of physicians' orders for patients, services, and even equipment supplied to a patient. A medical record is a record of *all* aspects of a patient's care in a health care facility.

The basic medical record, medical chart, or patient chart may contain some or all of the following: (1) summary sheet, (2) medical history, (3) progress notes, (4) medication records, (5) immunizations, (6) laboratory and pathology reports, (7) radiology reports, (8) other specialized reports or documents, (9) correspondence, and (10) hospital reports.

Summary Sheet

The summary sheet is usually the first page or the top sheet that appears in the record. It is an introductory page. The **summary sheet** (sometimes called the **identification sheet** or **face sheet**) (Fig. 9-2) contains the patient's insurance information and basic demographic data such as the patient's complete name, address, date of birth, telephone number, employer, and next of kin. The summary sheet also may contain a brief section for recording significant diagnoses, and it may contain a release-of-information statement or other necessary medical information.

Medical History

When establishing a relationship with a health care provider, every patient should be asked to complete a **medical history** (Fig. 9-3). A medical history includes questions about the patient's history of disease and injury, questions about the family medical history, and perhaps even a summary of current symptoms. If a patient cannot complete a medical history, a family member or caretaker may be asked to provide the information for the patient. If an individual other than the patient provides the medical history, that individual's name should be noted on the form. A history is normally completed at the patient's first visit, and the patient may be asked to update the information from time to time.

Progress Notes

Information regarding the patient's visits to the health care provider is listed in **progress notes** (Fig. 9-4). Every time the patient sees a physician for an appointment, the patient's condition and treatment are documented in a chart note or progress note. All activity regarding the patient—office visits, telephone calls, and documentation of outside appointments—is documented in progress notes. To identify the patient and the date of the office visit, every chart note includes some required information, such as patient name (last, first), medical record number, or date of birth.

One of the most common methods of documenting patient visits in a chart note involves use of the **SOAP method** (Fig. 9-5). This is an easy method to learn and use. Each letter stands for the type of information that is included in that section of the chart note.

S = Subjective

This portion of the chart note is the patient's account of the reason for the visit. **Subjective** information is the patient's account of his or her illness. In the subjective section, the physician identifies the patient's chief reason for the office visit. This reason is known as the **chief complaint** or the patient's primary reason for seeing the physician.

Subjective information includes such things as how the patient describes his or her illness (e.g., "I can't sleep at night"; "I feel a sharp stabbing pain in my lower back when I bend over") and includes a patient's review of body systems. In a subjective review of body systems, the physician asks whether the patient is experiencing any problems with vision, hearing, bowels, stomach, muscles, or any portion of the body that may be related to the complaint. The physician then makes a note of any comments the patient makes, such as complaints about coughing at night or about excessive urination.

Although subjective information sometimes cannot be proved by the physician, it is very important to the physician because subjective information describes the history of the patient's illness. The physician uses the subjective information supplied by the patient along with the objective information gathered during the examination to determine what is wrong with the patient. In addition to information

Happy Valley Medical Clinic
Patient Face Sheet
3/30/2008

Patient Chart #:	BRIEL000	D.O.B.:	09/29/1997	Age:	10
Patient Name:	Elmo J. Brimley	Sex:	Male		
Street 1:	3425 Sunset Lane	SSN:			
Street 2:		Mar Status:			
City:	Glendale, AZ 85382	S.O.F.:			
Phone:	(010)342-3444	Assigned Provider:	Melvin Morris		

Employer Name:	
Street1:	
City:	
Phone:	

Case Information

Case Desc:	110512	Diagnosis 1:	
Last Visit:	11/5/2012	Diagnosis 2:	
Referral:		Diagnosis 3:	
Guarantor Name:	Jay R. Brimley	Diagnosis 4:	
Street 1:	3425 Sunset Lane		
City:	Glendale, AZ 85382		
Phone:	(010)342-3444		
SSN:			

Ins Co #:	FHP00	Insured 1 Name:	Elmo J. Brimley		
Insurance 1:	FHP Health Plan	Street 1:	3425 Sunset Lane		
Street 1:	4576 E. W. Power Rd.	Street 2:			
Street 2:		Phone:	(010)342-3444		
City:	Mesa, AZ 85208	D.O.B.:	09/29/1997	Sex:	Male
Phone:		Policy Number:	76-562-112		
Ins-Start:		Group Number:			
End:					

Ins Co #:		Insured 2 Name:			
Insurance 2:		Street 1:			
Street 1:		Street 2:			
Street 2:		Phone:			
City:		D.O.B.:		Sex:	
Phone:		Policy Number:			
Ins-Start:		Group Number:			
End:					

Ins Co #:		Insured 3 Name:			
Insurance 3:		Street 1:			
Street 1:		Street 2:			
Street 2:		City:			
City:		Phone:		Sex:	
Phone:		D.O.B.:			
Ins-Start:		Policy Number:			
End:		Group Number:			

Figure 9-2 A summary sheet, face sheet, or identification sheet lists important information about the patient. Screenshots used by permission of McKesson Corporation. All Rights Reserved. © MCKESSON Corporation 2012.

Welcome to our practice. As a new patient, please fill out the information found below to the best of your ability.

Date: ______________

Patient Name ______________________ **Birthdate** __________ **Patient #** ______________

Chief Complaint: ______________________________

History of present illness:

Location: ______________ (Where is the pain/problem?)

Severity ______________ (How severe is the pain/problem on a scale of 1-5 with 5 being the most severe?)

Timing ______________ (Does the pain/problem occur at a specific time?)

Associated signs/symptoms ______________ (What other associated problems have you been having?

Quality ______________ (Example: normal versus abnormal color, activity, etc.)

Duration ______________ (How long have you had this pain/problem?, or, When did it start?)

Context ______________ (Where were you at the onset of this pain/problem?)

Modifying factors ______________ (What makes the pain/problem worse or better?, or, Have you had previous episodes?)

Past Medical History

Have you ever had the following: (Circle "no" or "yes", leave blank if uncertain)

Measles	no	yes	Anemia	no	yes	Back trouble	no	yes	Hepatitis	no	yes
Mumps	no	yes	Bladder Infections	no	yes	High Blood Pressure	no	yes	Ulcer	no	yes
Chickenpox	no	yes	Epilepsy	no	yes	Low Blood Pressure	no	yes	Kidney Disease	no	yes
Whooping Cough	no	yes	Migraine Headaches	no	yes	Hemorrhoids	no	yes	Thyroid Disease	no	yes
Scarlet Fever	no	yes	Tuberculosis	no	yes	Date of last chest x-ray ______			Bleeding Tendency	no	yes
Diphtheria	no	yes	Diabetes	no	yes	Asthma	no	yes	Any other disease	no	yes
Smallpox	no	yes	Cancer	no	yes	Hives or Eczema	no	yes	(please list):		
Pneumonia	no	yes	Polio	no	yes	AIDS or HIV+	no	yes	______		
Rheumatic Fever	no	yes	Glaucoma	no	yes	Infectious Mono	no	yes			
Heart Disease	no	yes	Hernia	no	yes	Bronchitis	no	yes	______		
Arthritis	no	yes	Blood or Plasma			Mitral Valve Prolapse	no	yes			
Venereal Disease	no	yes	Transfusions	no	yes	Stroke	no	yes	______		

Previous Hospitalizations/Surgeries/Serious Illnesses When? Hospital, City, State

____

Medications: (Include nonprescription) ______________________________

Patient social history:

Marital status	Single:____	Married: ____	Separated: ____	Divorced:____	Widowed:____
Use of alcohol:	Never:____	Rarely:____	Moderate:____	Daily:____	
Use of tobacco:	Never:____	Previously, but	quit:____	Current packs / day: ____	
Use of drugs:	Never:____	Type/Frequency:	____		
Excessive exposure at home or work to:	Fumes:____	Dust:____	Solvents:____	Air-borne Particles:____	Noise:____

Family medical history:

	Age	Diseases	If Deceased, Cause of Death
Father	____	____	____
Mother	____	____	____
Siblings	____	____	____
	____	____	____
	____	____	____
Spouse	____	____	____
Children	____	____	____
	____	____	____
	____	____	____

ITEM 29011

HEALTH HISTORY

Figure 9-3 A patient's medical history plays an important role in treating the patient. (Form courtesy of Bibbero Systems, Inc., Petaluma, California; telephone: 800-242-2376; fax: 800-242-9330; www.bibbero.com.)

Review of Systems: Please indicate any personal history below:

☐ **Constitutional Symptoms**
Good general health lately . . . . . No Yes
Recent weight change . . . . No Yes
Fever . . . . No Yes
Fatigue . . . . No Yes
Headaches . . . . No Yes

☐ **Eyes**
Eye disease or injury . . . . No Yes
Wear glasses/contact lenses . . . . No Yes
Blurred or double vision . . . . . . No Yes

☐ **Ears/Nose/Mouth/Throat**
Hearing loss or ringing . . . . No Yes
Earaches or drainage . . . . No Yes
Chronic sinus problem or rhinitis . No Yes
Nose bleeds . . . . No Yes
Mouth sores . . . . No Yes
Bleeding gums . . . . No Yes
Bad breath or bad taste . . . . No Yes
Sore throat or voice change . . . . No Yes
Swollen glands in neck . . . . No Yes

☐ **Cardiovascular**
Heart trouble . . . . No Yes
Chest pain or angina pectoris . . . No Yes
Palpitation . . . . No Yes
Shortness of breath w/walking or lying flat . . . . No Yes
Swelling of feet, ankles or hands No Yes

☐ **Respiratory**
Chronic or frequent coughs . . . . No Yes
Spitting up blood . . . . No Yes
Shortness of breath . . . . No Yes
Wheezing . . . . No Yes

☐ **Gastrointestinal**
Loss of appetite . . . . No Yes
Change in bowel movements . . . No Yes
Nausea or vomiting . . . . No Yes
Frequent diarrhea . . . . No Yes
Painful bowel movements or constipation . . . . No Yes
Rectal bleeding or blood in stool No Yes
Abdominal pain . . . . No Yes

☐ **Genitourinary**
Frequent urination . . . . No Yes
Burning or painful urination . . . No Yes
Blood in urine . . . . No Yes
Change in force of strain when urinating . . . . No Yes
Incontinence or dribbling . . . . . No Yes
Kidney stones . . . . No Yes
Sexual difficulty . . . . No Yes
Male - testicle pain . . . . No Yes
Female - pain with periods . . . . No Yes
Female - irregular periods . . . . . No Yes
Female - vaginal discharge . . . . No Yes
Female - # of pregnancies . . . . ________
Female - # of miscarriages . . . . ________
Female - date of last pap smear. ________

☐ **Musculoskeletal**
Joint pain . . . . No Yes
Joint stiffness or swelling . . . . . . No Yes
Weakness of muscles or joints . . No Yes
Muscle pain or cramps . . . . No Yes
Back pain . . . . No Yes
Cold extremities . . . . No Yes
Difficulty in walking . . . . No Yes

☐ **Integumentary (skin, breast)**
Rash or itching . . . . No Yes
Change in skin color . . . . No Yes
Change in hair or nails . . . . No Yes
Varicose veins . . . . No Yes
Breast pain . . . . No Yes
Breast lump . . . . No Yes
Breast discharge . . . . No Yes

☐ **Neurological**
Frequent or recurring headaches No Yes
Light headed or dizzy . . . . No Yes
Convulsions or seizures . . . . No Yes
Numbness or tingling sensations No Yes
Tremors . . . . No Yes
Paralysis . . . . No Yes
Head injury . . . . No Yes

☐ **Psychiatric**
Memory loss or confusion . . . . . No Yes
Nervousness . . . . No Yes
Depression . . . . No Yes
Insomnia . . . . No Yes
Suicidal Thoughts . . . . No Yes
Violent or Unusual Thoughts . . . No Yes

☐ **Endocrine**
Glandular or hormone problem . No Yes
Excessive thirst or urination . . . . No Yes
Heat or cold intolerance . . . . . . No Yes
Skin becoming drier . . . . No Yes
Change in hat or glove size . . . . No Yes

☐ **Hematologic/Lymphatic**
Slow to heal after cuts . . . . No Yes
Bleeding or bruising tendency . . No Yes
Anemia . . . . No Yes
Phlebitis . . . . No Yes
Past transfusion . . . . No Yes
Enlarged glands . . . . No Yes

☐ **Allergic/Immunologic**
History of skin reaction or other adverse reaction to:
Penicillin or other antibiotics . . No Yes
Morphine, Demerol, or other narcotics . . . . No Yes
Novocain or other anesthetics . No Yes
Aspirin or other pain remedies No Yes
Tetanus antitoxin or other serums . . . . No Yes
Iodine, Merthiolate or other antiseptic . . . . No Yes
Other drugs/medications: ____________
____
Known food allergies: ________________
____
Environmental allergies: ______________
____

To the best of my knowledge, the questions on this form have been accurately answered. I understand that providing incorrect information can be dangerous to my health. It is my responsibility to inform the doctor's office of any changes in my medical status. I also authorize the healthcare staff to perform the necessary services I may need.

________________________ ________________
Signature of Parent or Guardian Date

Doctor's Review

________________________ ________________
Signature of Doctor Date

HEALTH HISTORY

Figure 9-3, cont'd

about the patient's current illness, the subjective portion of a chart note includes information on the patient's past medical history, pertinent family medical history, social habits (e.g., drinking, smoking, use of illicit drugs), and current medications.

O = Objective

After interviewing the patient, the physician conducts a physical examination to investigate the patient's complaint. This is known as the **objective** portion of the examination.

Happy Valley Medical Group – Progress Notes

Patient Name: *Pearson, Steven* Chart number: *230184*

1-5-02 Patient calls in today regarding three-day history of 102°F temp, congestion and cough. Patient to make an appointment for sometime later today. ----- J. Mason, R.N.

Pearson, Steven #230184

Visit Date: 1-5-02

Chief complaint: Three-day history of elevated temp, congestion and cough.

S: Patient reports to the office today with a three-day history of temperature ranging from 100-102º, sinus congestion and cough. Review of systems: Patient reports the above-mentioned symptoms and mild frontal headache. Remainder of review of systems is unremarkable.

O: Patient is a well-developed, well-nourished 39-year-old male in no acute distress, appearing his stated age. Ht: 5'10", Wt: 170 lbs. HEENT: Head is normocephalic. Eyes: Pupils equal, round react to light and accommodate. Ears: TMs are clear. Nose: Nasal passages are boggy with purulent yellowish discharge. Throat is erythematous with thick PND. Chest: Clear to percussion and auscultation.

A: Sinusitis.

P: Amoxicillin 250 tid for 10 days. Patient also instructed to use an OTC decongestant as per package instructions. Return to clinic if condition does not resolve.

T.I. Marks, M.D.

Timothy I. Marks, M.D.

D: 1-5-02/TM

T: 1-6-02/mt

Figure 9-4 Office visits, telephone calls, and other interactions with a patient are documented in the progress notes section of a patient's medical record.

In this portion of a chart note, factual information about the patient is recorded. In other words, information that can be proved or demonstrated by the physician is recorded in this section.

Objective information can include some or all of the following items:

- The patient's sex
- Observations about the patient's general appearance
- Vital signs, including temperature, blood pressure, pulse rate, and respiration
- Physician's examination findings for each body area and/or organ system warranted by the patient's presenting symptoms. This objective review differs from the subjective review in that here, the physician's observations (e.g., "There is a moderate swelling over the patellar tendon"; "Chest is clear to auscultation and percussion") are noted. The statements made in the examination section can be demonstrated by actual physical evidence observed by the physician or obtained from diagnostic studies.
- Results of laboratory and radiologic tests or any other specialized testing

A = Assessment

In this part of the chart note, the physician, having considered the subjective and objective information gathered during the examination, arrives at a conclusion. This conclusion is known as the **diagnosis, assessment,** or **impression.** The history (subjective) combined with the following physical examination (objective) allows the physician to arrive at a diagnosis.

Patient name: Smith, Alice
Chart #483920
Date: 10-17-01

Chief complaint: Pain, left elbow.

S: The patient is a 28-year-old female who has a two-week history of tenderness over the lateral aspect of the left elbow. Patient is left-hand dominant. She has had lateral epicondylitis in the past, approximately five years ago. At that time she reports receiving injections for pain relief.

O: Examination of the left elbow reveals full range of motion with a mild amount of swelling, no erythema and elbow is slightly warm to the touch. She has a negative Tinel's. There is tenderness to palpation over the lateral epicondyle and mild tenderness with resisted wrist dorsiflexion.

A: Left lateral epicondylitis.

P: Patient will be sent to Physical Therapy for ultrasound with hydrocortisone treatments and should return to the clinic if pain does not resolve or worsens.

Brian H. Anderson, M.D.

D: 10-17-01/BA
T: 10-19-01/mt

Figure 9-5 SOAP notes document a patient's office visit. Each of the letters in the word *SOAP* represents the type of information included in the report.

Patient name: Olsen, Amy
Chart #: 110878
Date: 4-12-01

Patient is progressing nicely. There is still a small amount of swelling in the left knee. Patient will continue anti inflammatory medication and we will continue with physical therapy. Return in one week.

Brian H. Anderson, M.D.
D: 4-12-01/BA
T: 4-14-01/mt

Figure 9-6 A record of a patient's treatment may be documented in a chart note in the progress notes section of the medical record.

If the patient has more than one condition, each diagnosis is listed in order of significance, with the most significant diagnosis mentioned first. It is possible for only one diagnosis to appear in this section, or a patient may have several ongoing illnesses or conditions, and the diagnosis list can be quite lengthy.

P = Plan

Once the physician has determined a diagnosis, he or she recommends a treatment **plan.** This consists of instructions given to the patient regarding actions the patient should take, such as "Patient is to call the office if not feeling better in 3 days or before then if symptoms worsen" or "Apply warm moist pack to the affected area 3 times a day." Any medications prescribed for the patient are listed in this section under the name of the medication, strength, dosage, and duration of treatment. Additional tests or even hospitalization also may be part of the plan.

Sometimes, the physician may document information about the patient that does not fit into the SOAP format. In this instance, the physician dictates essential information about the visit but does not use a clearly defined format. Instead, the chart note is written in paragraph form (Fig. 9-6).

Happy Valley Medical Group – Progress Notes	
Patient Name: Stevens, Evan D.	Chart number: 689723
5-8-xx Patient's mother phones in today regarding patient's immunization status. Told	
mother that patient is up-to-date with immunizations and should return to the clinic in one	
year for additional immunizations. --J. Mason, R.N.	

Figure 9-7 A chart note (handwritten or entered electronically) is used by the medical office staff to document the details of interactions with the patient or other activities performed on behalf of the patient.

BOX 9-1

Guidelines for Handwritten Medical Record Entries

- Write legibly. No one should have to guess at what was written.
- Use black ink only. No colored markers, pens, or pencils should be used in a chart.
- Every entry in the record should be signed and dated by the individual who makes the entry. Never make, sign, or date an entry for someone else.
- Make entries promptly.
- Leave no gaps or empty lines when making an entry.
- Make any necessary corrections in an appropriate manner.
- Be objective, specific, and complete when making entries.

Entries about interactions with patients that are not office visits must be made in the record by the physician, nurse, assistant, or other medical office staff members. These entries, also known as **chart notes** or **chart entries** (Fig. 9-7), are included in the progress notes section of the medical record. Only those persons authorized to make entries can make these types of entries. Entries regarding telephone calls, outside appointments, or other information related to the patient's medical care are recorded in the chart, and these entries must be done in a certain manner as shown in Figure 9-7.

Recording Information in a Patient's Medical Record

A medical office should establish specific guidelines as to who may document in a patient's record and how that documentation should be done (Box 9-1). Entries do not always use an entire page. When entries are made in a patient's paper chart, the medical office staff should be careful to not skip lines or leave any large gaps on the progress notes page. Any extra space should be crossed out so as to not allow information to be inserted in an incorrect order.

Persons making handwritten entries in a patient's paper chart should write with black ink only. Blue ink is not an appropriate substitute. Black ink is preferred because it will appear darker than will any other color when photocopied.

PROCEDURE 9-1

Document an Event in a Patient's Chart

Materials Needed

- Patient's medical record
- Black ink pen (if entering information in a paper medical record)

1. Obtain the patient's medical record. Locate the next available place for documentation in the progress notes section.*
2. Determine the information to be written in the patient's chart. Be sure that you are authorized to enter such information.
3. Record the date and information regarding the patient.*
4. Sign the entry with your first initial, last name, and employment position in the medical office.

**Denotes crucial step in procedure. The student must complete this step satisfactorily to complete the procedure satisfactorily.*

Pencils, colored pens, markers, gel pens, and the like are inappropriate for use in a medical record. Pencil marks could be erased, ink from colored pens may not copy well, and markers may smear if a page becomes damp (see Procedure 9-1).

Each entry includes the date of the entry, a narrative about the interaction with the patient, and the signature and title of the employee who made the entry.

Medication Records

A common practice in many records is to create a medication list (Fig. 9-8) that delineates all medications taken by the patient. This includes not only prescription medications but also substances such as vitamins, over-the-counter medications, and herbal supplements. This list should be updated each time the patient sees a health care provider. It provides a valuable reference for health care personnel who are treating the patient.

Immunizations

Information regarding a patient's immunization history may be present on the medical history or may be included on a separate page or section in the record. The immunization form often includes a place for the patient's signature for consent to receive the vaccine. The form also includes information

Happy Valley Medical Group
Medication List

Patient: Peters, Anthony A
Medical Record No.: PETAN000
DOB: 1/3/1977
Date Printed: April 3, 2013

Medication Name	Strength	Instructions
Cardizem CD	180 mg	Take 3 capsules by mouth daily
Isosorbide Mononitrate	30 mg	Take 1 ½ tablets by mouth daily
Metformin HCl	500 mg	Take 2 tablets by mouth twice a day
Omeprazole	20 mg	Take one capsule by mouth daily
Rosuvastatin Calcium	20 mg	Take 1 tablet by mouth at bedtime

Figure 9-8 A medication list provides a quick summary of a patient's current medications. The list is reviewed every time the physician has an encounter with the patient.

about the manufacturer's lot number of the vaccine should there ever be a question as to what manufacturer or batch of the vaccine the patient received.

Laboratory and Pathology Reports

The laboratory section of a medical record contains the written results of a patient's laboratory tests and pathologic analyses. The pathology department is concerned with the study of disease, and the laboratory is the place in which that study takes place. A medical laboratory tests blood, urine, and other biologic specimens that are removed from the body. Urinalysis and complete blood cell count (CBC) are examples of tests typically referred to as **laboratory reports** (Fig. 9-9) or laboratory tests. **Pathology reports** (Fig. 9-10) contain descriptions of body tissue that has been sent to a medical laboratory for study. Both of these types of reports are placed in the laboratory section of a medical record.

The pathology department is also responsible for conducting autopsies and for verifying specimens that are removed from the body (e.g., the vas deferens removed during a vasectomy). Basically, anytime anything is removed from the body, a specimen usually is sent to the laboratory to be reviewed by the pathology department.

To save space in a paper chart, the office may place laboratory test results in this section of the chart through a **shingling** method. If laboratory reports measure less than a full page, shingling of the reports allows more reports to fit on one page. Shingling of reports involves placing the oldest laboratory report near the bottom of the page and laying new reports slightly above and overlapping the top of the previously placed report, with the reports thereby appearing in the chart in chronological order (Fig. 9-11). This method allows the physician to quickly flip through the reports to find the desired test results. Reports are often color coded to make them easier to locate in the laboratory section. For example, urinalysis may always be on yellow paper and hematology on pink paper. The lower portion of the report that is visible contains information about when the test was performed. Although shingling saves space, a disadvantage of using shingling is that reports must be removed for photocopying (because they are overlapping) when information is released.

With the increased use of computers in the medical office, it is now common for laboratory results to appear on an 8.5 × 11–inch sheet of paper, as shown in Figure 9-9. Those results then are filed in the patient's record in a specified order such as chronological order.

Radiology Reports

Radiology reports contain results of a patient's radiologic study. Examples of radiologic studies include x-ray, magnetic resonance imaging (MRI), computed tomography (CT) scanning, and nuclear medicine. Radiology reports (Fig. 9-12) include the name of the film or procedure that was performed, along with the findings of the radiologist, a physician trained in the use of radiology to diagnose and treat disease. Although there is no standard size for a radiology report, x-ray and other radiology reports may be done on a special radiology form, sometimes 8.5 inches wide × 5.5 inches high, or they may be done on a standard 8.5 × 11–inch sheet of paper. Radiology reports can be shingled to save space in the chart.

Other Specialized Reports and Documents

Sections may be included in a medical record for other specialized types of studies or other medical documents. A miscellaneous section may be used for medical reports that would not be filed elsewhere. In medicine, many different types of specialty reports, including electroencephalograms (EEGs), electrocardiograms (ECGs), and electromyograms (EMGs), may be used. Documents such as pediatric

Happy Valley Medical Group
5222 E. Baseline Rd.
Gilbert, AZ 85234

Patient Name: Olson, Deanne E — Date: 5-6-07
Med Record #OLSDE000 — Age: 36

HEMATOLOGY

Test	Result	Reference Range
CBC/WBC diff		
Hemoglobin	13.2	12.0-15.5
Hematocrit	37.9	34.9-44.5
Erythrocytes	4.32	3.90-5.03
MCV	87.8	81.6-98.3
RBC distrib width	11.9	11.9-15.5
Leukocytes	6.9	3.5-10.5
Neutrophils	4.54	1.7-7.0
Lymphocytes	1.56	0.9-2.9
Monocytes	0.62	0.3-0.9
Eosinophils	0.15	0.05-0.50
Basophils	0.03	0-0.1
Thrombocytes	362	150-450
MPV	7.9	7.4-10.9

Figure 9-9 Many laboratory reports today are accessible via a computer system.

College Hospital
2345 College Hospital Boulevard
Wood Creek, XX 98765

PATHOLOGY REPORT

Date: June 20, 200X — Pathology No. 430211
Patient: Elaine J. Silverman — Room No. 1308
Physician: Harold B. Cooper, MD

SPECIMEN SUBMITTED:

Tumor, right axilla.

GROSS DESCRIPTION

Specimen A consists of an oval mass of yellow fibroadipose tissue measuring 4 x 3 x 2 cm. On cut section, there are some small, soft, pliable areas of gray apparent lymph node alternating with adipose tissue. A frozen section consultation at time of surgery was delivered as NO EVIDENCE OF MALIGNANCY on frozen section, to await permanent section for final diagnosis. Majority of the specimen will be submitted for microscopic examination.

Specimen B consists of an oval mass of yellow soft tissue measuring 2.5 x 2.5 x 1.5 cm. On cut section, there is a thin rim of pink to tan-brown lymphatic tissue and the mid portion appears to be adipose tissue. A pathological consultation at time of surgery was delivered as no suspicious areas noted and to await permanent sections for final diagnosis. The entire specimen will be submitted for microscopic examination.

RTW:wfr

MICROSCOPIC DESCRIPTION

Specimen A sections show fibroadipose tissue and nine fragments of lymph nodes. The lymph nodes show areas with prominent germinal centers and moderate sinus histiocytosis. There appears to be some increased vascularity and reactive endothelial cells seen. There is no evidence of malignancy.

Specimen B sections show adipose tissue and 5 lymph node fragments. These 5 portions of lymph nodes show reactive changes including sinus histiocytosis. There is no evidence of malignancy.

DIAGNOSIS

A & B: TUMOR, RIGHT AXILLA: SHOWING 14 LYMPH NODE FRAGMENTS WITH REACTIVE CHANGES AND NO EVIDENCE OF MALIGNANCY.

Stanley T. Nason, MD

STN:wfr
D: 6-18-0X
T: 6-18-0X

Figure 9-10 Pathology reports are done on tissue removed from a patient's body. (From Diehl MO: *Medical Transcription: Techniques and Procedures,* ed 6, St. Louis, Elsevier, 2007.)

LABORATORY REPORTS

REMOVE ADHESIVE TAPE COVERING.
ADD 1ST REPORT TO BOTTOM
LINE AND SUCCESSIVE REPORTS
TO LINES ABOVE.

25-7210-3 ©1996 BIBBERO SYSTEMS, INC., PETALUMA, CA.
TO REORDER CALL 800-BIBBERO (800 242-2376) OR FAX (800) 242-9330

LABORATORY REPORTS

REMOVE ADHESIVE TAPE COVERING.
ADD 1ST REPORT TO BOTTOM
LINE AND SUCCESSIVE REPORTS
TO LINES ABOVE.

25-7210-3 ©1996 BIBBERO SYSTEMS, INC., PETALUMA, CA.
TO REORDER CALL 800-BIBBERO (800 242-2376) OR FAX (800) 242-9330

HEMATOLOGY

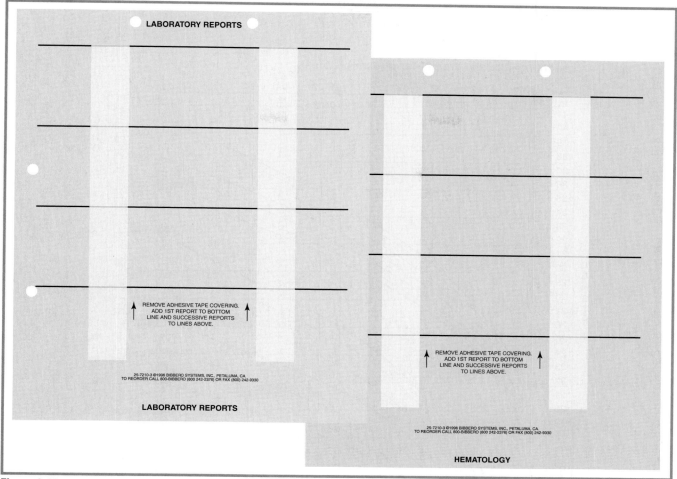

Figure 9-11 In a paper medical record, laboratory reports may be shingled to save space in a medical record. (Form courtesy of Bibbero Systems, Inc., Petaluma, California; telephone: 800-242-2376; fax: 800-242-9330; www.bibbero.com.)

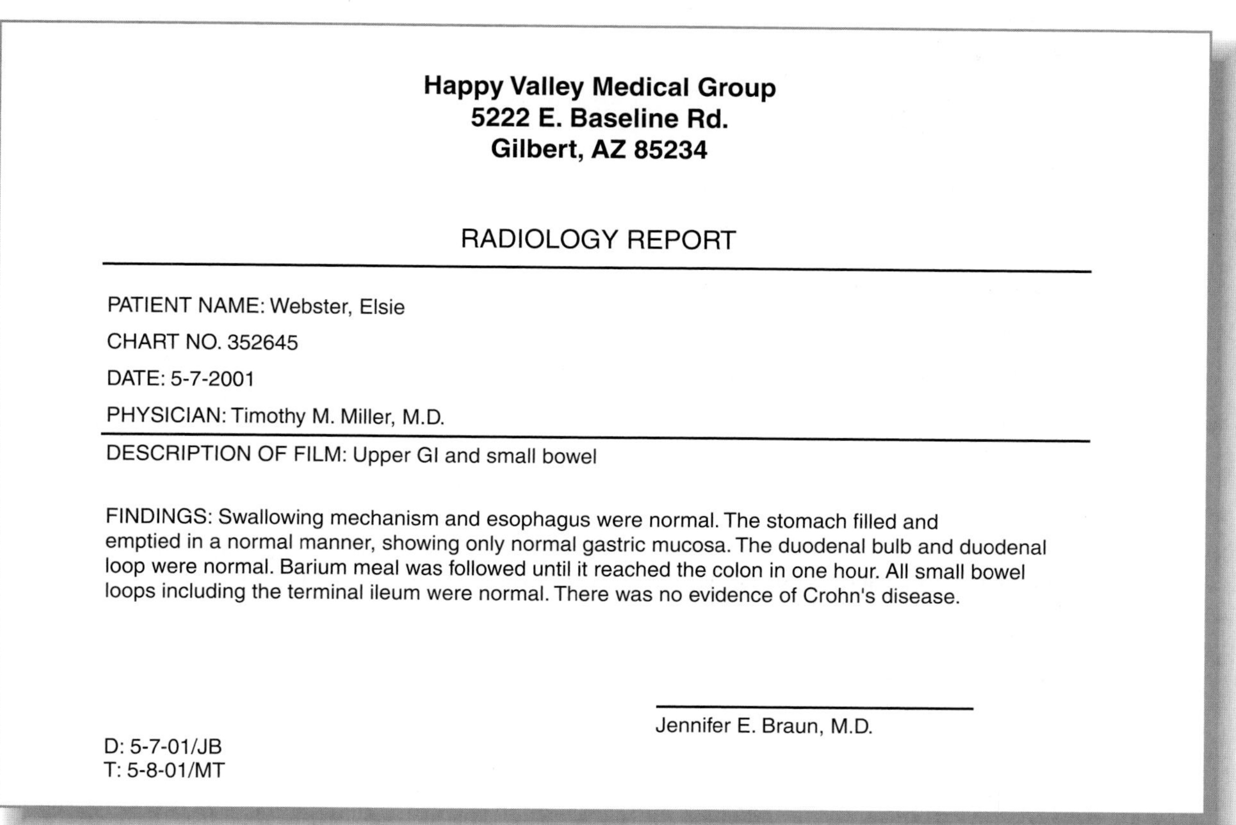

Happy Valley Medical Group
5222 E. Baseline Rd.
Gilbert, AZ 85234

RADIOLOGY REPORT

PATIENT NAME: Webster, Elsie

CHART NO. 352645

DATE: 5-7-2001

PHYSICIAN: Timothy M. Miller, M.D.

DESCRIPTION OF FILM: Upper GI and small bowel

FINDINGS: Swallowing mechanism and esophagus were normal. The stomach filled and emptied in a normal manner, showing only normal gastric mucosa. The duodenal bulb and duodenal loop were normal. Barium meal was followed until it reached the colon in one hour. All small bowel loops including the terminal ileum were normal. There was no evidence of Crohn's disease.

Jennifer E. Braun, M.D.

D: 5-7-01/JB
T: 5-8-01/MT

Figure 9-12 Radiology reports describe the radiologist's interpretation of the radiologic studies that were performed.

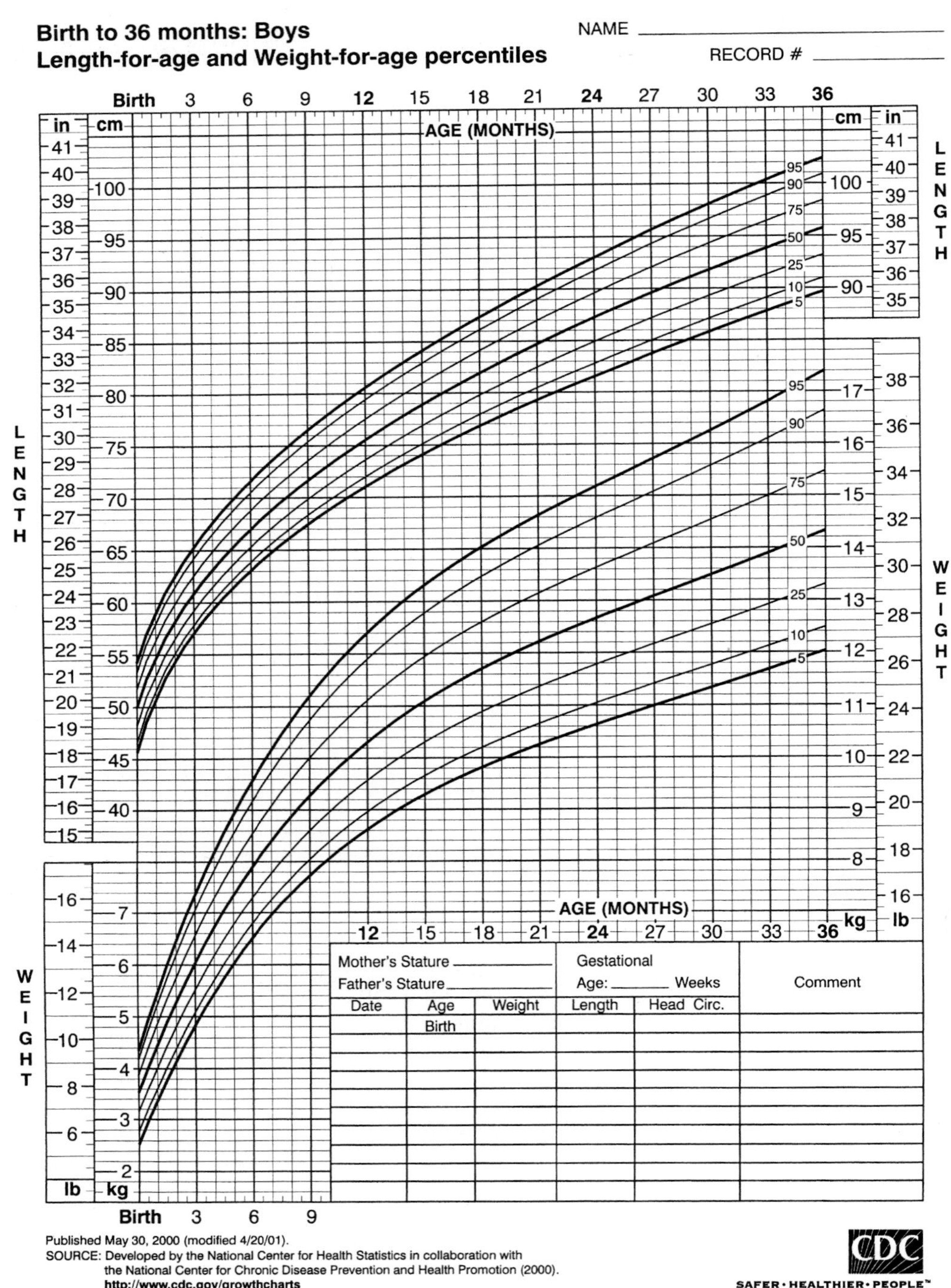

Figure 9-13 A pediatric growth chart visually presents the progression of a child's growth. (From Ballweg R, Stolberg S, Sullivan E: *Physician Assistant: A Guide to Clinical Practice*, ed 3, St. Louis, Saunders, 2003.)

growth charts (Fig. 9-13) or pregnancy flow sheets (Fig. 9-14) may be included in a patient's chart to provide a brief synopsis of certain conditions that a provider would like to follow.

Sometimes it is necessary for the physician to document patient treatment with the use of a photograph or other electronic image stored on a device such as a CD or DVD. Physicians who perform surgical procedures that involve the use of scopes (e.g., arthroscopy, laparoscopy) often archive the images of the procedure for inclusion in the patient's medical record. Photographs or videos may be taken during such a procedure or may be taken to document an injury in a case such as suspected abuse. These types of images are part of the patient's health information and require the same protection as other confidential information in the patient's record.

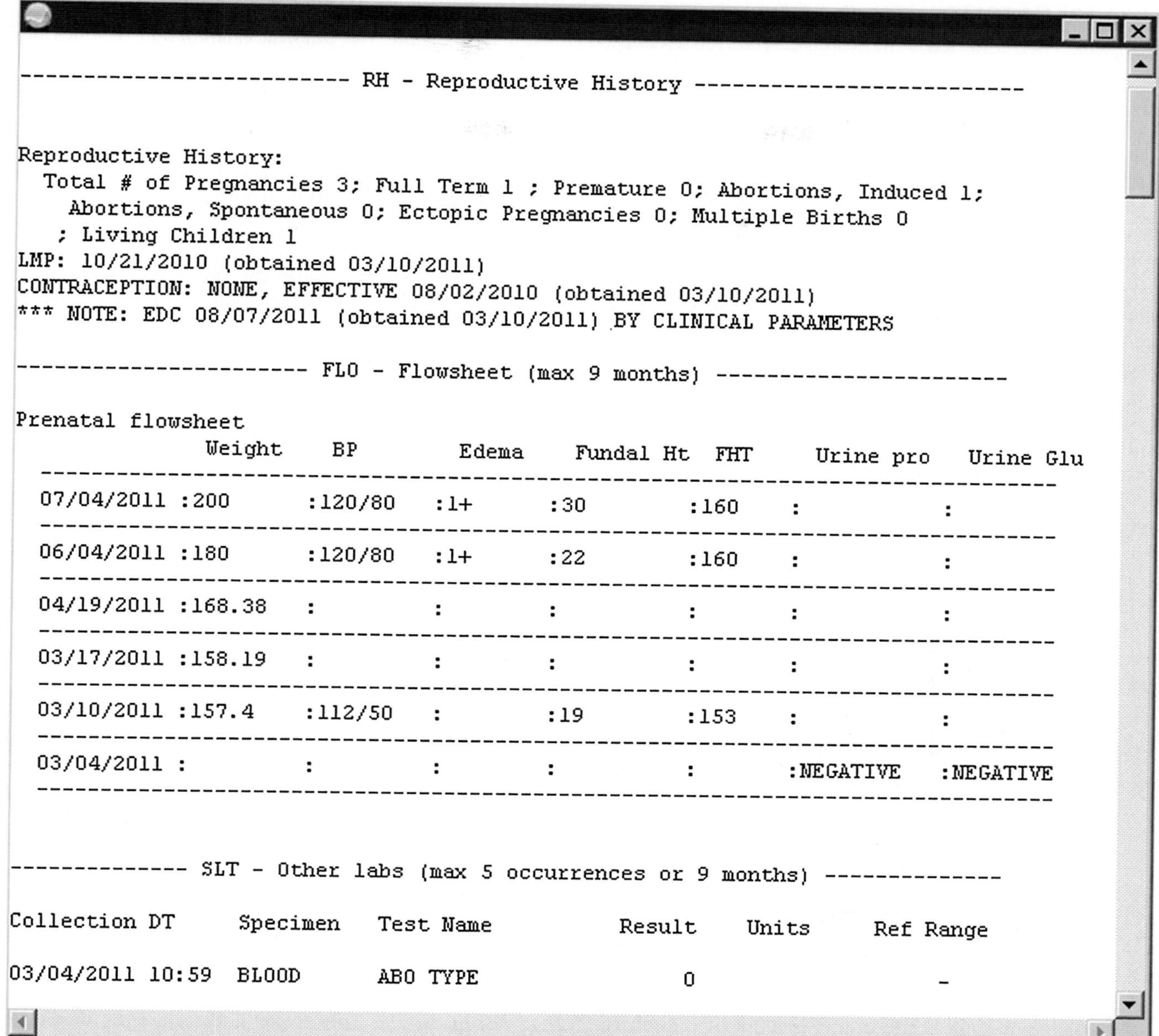

------------------------- RH - Reproductive History -------------------------

Reproductive History:
Total # of Pregnancies 3; Full Term 1 ; Premature 0; Abortions, Induced 1;
Abortions, Spontaneous 0; Ectopic Pregnancies 0; Multiple Births 0
; Living Children 1
LMP: 10/21/2010 (obtained 03/10/2011)
CONTRACEPTION: NONE, EFFECTIVE 08/02/2010 (obtained 03/10/2011)
*** NOTE: EDC 08/07/2011 (obtained 03/10/2011) BY CLINICAL PARAMETERS

---------------------- FLO - Flowsheet (max 9 months) ----------------------

Prenatal flowsheet

	Weight	BP	Edema	Fundal Ht	FHT	Urine pro	Urine Glu
07/04/2011	:200	:120/80	:1+	:30	:160	:	:
06/04/2011	:180	:120/80	:1+	:22	:160	:	:
04/19/2011	:168.38	:	:	:	:	:	:
03/17/2011	:158.19	:	:	:	:	:	:
03/10/2011	:157.4	:112/50	:	:19	:153	:	:
03/04/2011	:	:	:	:	:	:NEGATIVE	:NEGATIVE

------------- SLT - Other labs (max 5 occurrences or 9 months) -------------

Collection DT	Specimen	Test Name	Result	Units	Ref Range
03/04/2011 10:59	BLOOD	ABO TYPE	0		-

Figure 9-14 A pregnancy flow sheet details a patient's medical condition throughout her pregnancy and provides a concise picture of her history for any provider who may deliver her baby. (From U.S. Department of Health and Human Services, Indian Health Service. Resource and Patient Management System, Prenatal Care Module, Version 1.0, March 2013. http://www.ihs.gov/RPMS/PackageDocs/BJPN/bjpn010o.pdf, accessed 10/29/13)

Correspondence

The correspondence section of a medical record may contain a variety of documents. Medical records that have been received from a hospital or from other offices may be included in this section. Copies of medical record releases, consent forms, letters the patient writes to the physician, and letters the physician writes to the patient also are kept in this section. Copies of a patient's advance directives may be included here or may be kept in a specific section reserved for those directives.

Occasionally, a patient may need to be referred to a specialist for a **consultation** regarding treatment for a medical condition. For example, if a patient's physician is a family practice physician and the physician suspects that the patient has heart disease, the physician will refer the patient to a cardiologist for a consultation. After examining the patient, the cardiologist will document the findings of the examination in a consultation report. A consultation report may be filed in the correspondence section of the medical record.

Hospital Reports

When a patient is admitted to the hospital, certain reports document the treatment given while the patient is hospitalized.

History and Physical

A report known as a **history and physical (H&P)** documents the patient's condition on admission to the hospital. Because a patient's admission to the hospital is a very important event, this report must be completed for every patient within 24 hours of admission. This ensures that all information that may be necessary for treatment of the patient is available to hospital personnel. The Joint Commission, an organization responsible for accreditation of health care organizations, has established the 24-hour requirement for H&P reporting. The provider responsible for the patient's admission is responsible for completion of the H&P.

The content of an H&P (Fig. 9-15) is much like the SOAP notes described previously. An H&P contains four specific sections:

- **History.** The type of information included in this section is similar to the information included in the subjective section of a SOAP note. Depending on the severity of the patient's problem, the components of the subjective section may be brief or lengthy. Several components, including the following, make up the history:
  - ***Patient identification.*** This includes information on the patient's age, race, sex, marital status, and occupation.
  - ***Chief complaint.*** The patient's main reason for admission is included in this statement. The chief complaint could be stated something like, "Severe abdominal pain for 6 hours' duration," or "Multiple rib fracture from motor vehicle accident."
  - ***History of present illness.*** This is an account of the signs and symptoms of the patient's reason for seeing the physician. History will include information about specifics about the chief complaint, such as a description of pain or when the pain occurs, etc.
  - ***Past medical history.*** Pertinent information about the patient's previous health history is gathered as it relates to the patient's current condition.
  - ***Family history.*** If necessary to treat the patient's current condition, information is gathered from the patient regarding any family members who have a medical condition that could be related to the patient's condition.
  - ***Social history.*** Also if necessary to treat the patient's current condition, an account of the patient's personal habits, such as smoking, consumption of alcohol, or use of illegal drugs, is gathered.
  - ***Medications.*** The patient's current prescription and nonprescription medications are listed as well as vitamins and supplements taken by the patient.
  - ***Review of systems.*** The physician asks the patient questions regarding various body systems. Only those body systems related to the patient's problem are reviewed with the patient. Medicare has established documentation guidelines that describe what systems and body areas are recognized as part of the review of systems (Box 9-2).
- **Physical Examination.** Similar to the objective portion of a SOAP note, the physical examination includes the following:
  - ***General appearance.*** This section describes the patient's general appearance (e.g., "The patient is a well-developed, well-nourished female in moderate distress"). The patient's weight and height also are identified.
  - ***Vital signs.*** This includes temperature, blood pressure, pulse rate, and respirations.
    - With a hospital admission, this section is usually quite lengthy because the physician will need to document careful observation of the patient's body. The physician will document normal and abnormal findings from pertinent body areas and organ systems. Medicare has established documentation guidelines for the physical examination.
    - Results of laboratory, radiology, and any other testing are recorded under the physical examination section as well.
- **Impression.** This section identifies the physician's assessment, impression, or diagnosis of the patient's ailment. The physician considers all information gathered from the patient during the subjective portion of the visit and from the physical examination and uses that information to arrive at the patient's diagnosis.
- **Plan.** The treatment plan for the patient's condition is identified. This will include a comment about admission to the hospital, as well as information on diagnostic tests, procedures, or medications that will be ordered for the patient.

Operative Report

An **operative report** (Fig. 9-16) is a detailed account of a patient's surgical procedure. Preoperative and postoperative diagnoses are listed, and a step-by-step description of the surgical procedure itself is provided. Information is included in this report about how the patient was placed on the operating table, the type of anesthesia that was used, the type of incision that was made, and instruments and techniques that were used during the procedure, and the condition of the patient on return to the recovery room is described.

Discharge Summary

The **discharge summary** (Fig. 9-17) provides a synopsis of the patient's hospital treatment. Information is included about the patient's condition when admitted, as is information about treatments and medications administered and tests and procedures performed during hospitalization. The discharge summary also contains details about the instructions given to the patient when he or she was discharged from the hospital.

Medical Transcription

Many of the reports contained in a medical record are dictated by the physician and then are transcribed by a medical transcriptionist for inclusion in the patient's medical record. The process of **medical transcription** involves the production

Happy Valley Medical Group
5222 E. Baseline Rd.
Gilbert, AZ
(010) 555-1110

HISTORY & PHYSICAL EXAMINATION

Patient Name: Wang, Karen
Chart # 230192
Date: 6-3-02

HISTORY OF PRESENT ILLNESS: Patient is a 28-year-old Caucasian female with a history of asthma resulting in multiple hospital admissions. She had a recent upper respiratory infection that lasted approximately 10 days. She has complained of cough, chest congestion and blood-tinged sputum for the past 3 days. She was started on oral erythromycin without improvement. She presents today with increasing shortness of breath and chest discomfort. She uses only a Proventil inhaler and erythromycin at home.

PAST MEDICAL HISTORY: Noncontributory. **ALLERGIES: Aspirin**.

FAMILY HISTORY: Unremarkable.

REVIEW OF SYSTEMS: Her last normal menstrual period was approximately 1 month ago, but she denies the possibility of intrauterine pregnancy.

PHYSICAL EXAMINATION: Patient is a well-developed, well-nourished female appearing her stated age. She is in moderate distress.

VITAL SIGNS: Temp: 100.4F. She had a sinus tachycardia of 110/ BP: 110/60. Respirations: 24. HEENT: Sclerae are clear. Conjunctivae are pink and dry. Nasopharynx and TMs are clear. Oropharynx is clear. NECK: Supple without masses or lymphadenopathy. LUNGS: Coarse rales and rhonchi were heard in the right upper and left lower lobe region. There were a few scattered expiratory wheezes. HEART: Sinus tachycardia without murmur or S3. ABDOMEN: Soft with mild suprapubic tenderness without rebound, rigidity, or mass. Bowel sounds were active. EXTREMITIES: No edema; calves are benign. NEUROLOGIC: Grossly intact.

DIAGNOSTIC TESTING: Chest x-ray reveals infiltrates and atelectasis in the right upper lobe with right middle lobe and left lower lobe infiltrates.

IMPRESSION: 1. Trilobed pneumonia. 2. History of asthma with intermittent steroid use.

PLAN: Admit the patient and place her on aerosol bronchodilator, IV steroids, IV antibiotics, and oral erythromycin pending sputum gram stain C&S. Obtain arterial blood gases, WBC, and hematocrit. We will also gently hydrate her over the next 24 hours and get a follow-up chest x-ray after 24 hours.

T.I. Marks, M.D.

Timothy I. Marks, M.D.

D:6-3-02/TM
T:6-3-02/mt

Figure 9-15 An H&P documents the details of a patient's condition on admission to a hospital.

of a medical report from a physician's recording for placement in a patient's medical record. This report can be printed on paper for inclusion in a patient's record or may be stored in electronic form in an EHR and printed when necessary.

Transcribed reports are preferred over handwritten reports mainly because of concerns about legibility. Transcribed reports allow information to be easily understood by all members of the health care team, as well as by others who may review the record at other facilities. The vast majority of medical reports are transcribed, not handwritten. Dictation is also a timesaver for the physician. It takes far less time to dictate a patient's report than to write it out by hand.

Skills Needed

Individuals who do medical transcription need to be highly skilled in several areas. They must be experts in medical language and grammar who are able to decipher the physician's **dictation**, or voice recording, and to produce a readable medical report. Transcriptionists must have a high level of understanding of human anatomy, physiology, and pathophysiology to ensure that the medical reports they type are, indeed, what the physician dictated. They must possess exceptional hardware and software computer skills because virtually all transcription today is done with the use of some type of computer system. Their keyboarding skills must be

BOX 9-2

1995 Medicare Documentation Guidelines for Evaluation and Management Services

Documentation of Review of Systems (ROS) (subjective information)

Part of the patient's history includes a review of body systems (ROS) in which the provider asks the patient various questions about signs or symptoms the patient has experienced that are related to his or her chief complaint. The following systems are recognized:

Constitutional (e.g., fever, weight loss)
Eyes
Ear, nose, mouth, and throat
Cardiovascular
Respiratory
Gastrointestinal
Genitourinary
Musculoskeletal
Integumentary (skin, breasts)
Neurologic
Psychiatric
Endocrine
Hematologic/lymphatic
Allergic/immunologic

Documentation of Physical Examination

Body areas and/or organ systems are recognized in an examination.

Body Areas

Head, including face
Neck
Chest, including breasts and axillae
Abdomen
Genitalia, groin, buttocks
Back, including spine
Extremities

Organ Systems

Constitutional (e.g., vital signs, general appearance)
Eyes
Ears, nose, mouth, and throat
Cardiovascular
Respiratory
Gastrointestinal
Genitourinary
Musculoskeletal
Integumentary
Neurologic
Psychiatric
Hematologic/lymphatic/immunologic

exceptional as well; accuracy and speed are expected in the field of medical transcription.

Equipment Used

Medical transcription involves listening to the physician's dictation and creating a report (Fig. 9-18) in a computer system. Dictation involves a physician or another provider who speaks and records information about a patient's encounter. Dictation may be done through use of a tape recorder or digital system.

Digital transcription has quickly become the standard for producing medical reports. If transcription is done digitally, dictation may be done with the use of a telephone system that can hold several hundred reports from various physicians throughout the facility. The physician enters patient information by pressing buttons on the telephone, and the dictation is deposited in a digital system. The transcriptionist then accesses the reports by using a hookup with the digital system that enables the transcriptionist to listen to the dictation and type reports for a specific physician or patient.

Digital dictation equipment may be portable, similar to a handheld tape recorder. Because digital systems can electronically identify each separate piece of dictation, the use of digital systems often makes it easy to locate a specific report for transcription in a matter of seconds.

A physician may use a palm-sized tape recorder that can easily fit in a laboratory coat pocket. After seeing a patient, the physician dictates the details of the patient's visit by stating the patient's name and chart number and the contents of the medical report. Digital files then are downloaded into a computer system and then can be transcribed by a transcriptionist (Procedure 9-2).

Once the transcription is done, reports may be stored electronically for later retrieval or may be printed and inserted into a patient's paper medical record. Documents that are printed must be inserted into the patient's paper record in a specified order.

Signature

All physician dictation—whether chart notes or any report dictated by the physician—requires a space for the physician to sign the report. Dates of dictation and the initials of the person dictating, along with transcription dates and the transcriptionist's initials, are included on every report. Note the appearance of the signature and reference initials in the many reports included in this chapter.

After any dictated medical report is complete, the report is sent to the physician for authentication and signature. In an electronic record, the physician reviews the report online and then electronically signs the report with a unique password. If a paper record is used, each patient's report may be attached to the outside of his or her chart when the report is sent for signature (Fig. 9-19). This can be very useful if the physician needs the chart to verify any information included in the report.

Happy Valley Medical Group
5222 E. Baseline Rd.
Gilbert, AZ 85234
(010) 555-1110

OPERATIVE REPORT

Patient Name: Walker, Ann
Chart # 152634
Date: 9-7-02

PREOPERATIVE DIAGNOSIS: Sterile pyuria.

POSTOPERATIVE DIAGNOSIS: Normal bladder.

OPERATION PERFORMED: Cystoscopy.

PROCEDURE: The patient was taken to the urology suite and placed in the lithotomy position. The perineum was prepped with Betadine and draped in a sterile manner. Xylocaine jelly was injected into the urethra. Subsequently, the rigid cystoscope was inserted and the cystoscopy was performed. The urethra appeared normal. The bladder showed a normal trigone with normal orifices bilaterally. There was clear urine effluxing from both orifices. The mucosal pattern of the bladder was normal. No foreign bodies or stones in the bladder were seen. The bladder was drained and the cystoscope was removed.

IMPRESSION: Normal examination of the bladder.

Mary Sanchez, MD

Mary Sanchez, M.D.
D:9-8-02/MS
T:9-9-02/mt

Figure 9-16 An operative report gives a step-by-step account of a patient's surgical procedure.

PROCEDURE 9-2

Transcribe a Medical Report

Materials Needed

- Dictated medical report
- Equipment to play report (digital or tape transcriber)
- Computer with word processing software
- Printer

1. Locate the beginning of the report dictation.
2. Adjust the volume and speed of the dictation as necessary.
3. Choose the appropriate report format.
4. Type the dictated report.
5. Proofread the report and make any necessary corrections.*
6. Print the report for physician signature and insertion in the patient's medical record.

**Denotes crucial step in procedure. The student must complete this step satisfactorily to complete the procedure satisfactorily.*

Correcting Information in a Patient's Medical Record

Occasionally, a mistake may be made in the process of recording information in a patient's record. The person who makes the mistake must correct the entry. When correcting an erroneous entry in a chart, a health care professional should be careful to never obliterate the previous information. If the previous information becomes unreadable when crossed out, a court of law would not look favorably on the employee or the medical office; this action may be interpreted that someone in the office wished to hide something.

The proper way to correct an error in a paper record is to draw a single line with black ink through the incorrect information, write the correct information above it, and date and sign the entry (Fig. 9-20).

No attempt should ever be made to erase an erroneous entry or to block the error out with correction fluid. There should never be a question about what information was in the chart previously. An honest mistake most likely will be forgiven, but the courts do not look favorably upon a record if it looks as though an attempt was made to hide something.

Happy Valley Medical Group
5222 E. Baseline Rd.
Gilbert, AZ 85234
(010) 555-1110

DISCHARGE SUMMARY

Patient Name: Armstrong, Marge
Chart # 100120

ADMISSION DATE: 10-5-02

DISCHARGE DATE: 10-10-02

ADMITTING DIAGNOSIS:

1. Pneumonia.
2. Hypertension.
3. History of congestive heart failure.
4. Menopause.

HISTORY: The patient is an 80-year-old female with a complaint of chest tightness. She was seen at the emergency room at Horizons Hospital, was found to have bilateral pneumonia and hypoxemia and was admitted.

HOSPITAL COURSE: Upon admission, the patient was placed on IV antibiotics and oxgyen supplement. She improved and demonstrated gradual resolution of the hypoxemia. She was discharged in stable condition.

DISCHARGE DIAGNOSES:

1. Pneumonia.
2. Hypertension.
3. History of congestive heart failure.
4. Menopause.

PLAN: The patient was discharged in stable condition. She was placed on Ceftin 100 mg bid for 7 days. The patient is to see me for a follow-up appointment in 1 week.

Kristine G. O'Brian, M.D.

Kristine G. O'Brian, M.D.

D: 10-11-02/KO
T: 10-11-02/mt

Figure 9-17 A discharge summary reviews significant events of a patient's hospitalization.

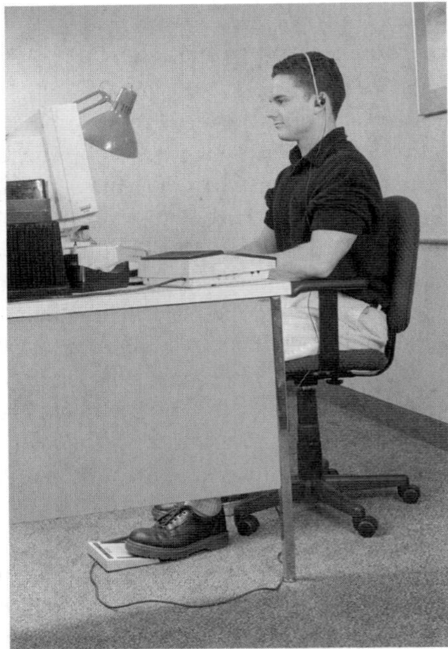

Figure 9-18 A medical transcriptionist prepares medical reports from physician dictation.

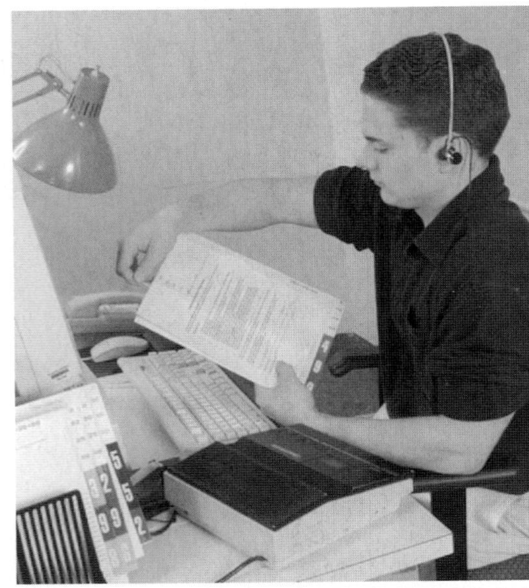

Figure 9-19 All medical reports must be reviewed and signed by the dictating physician before they can be permanently added to a patient's medical record.

Happy Valley Medical Group – Progress Notes	
Patient Name: Breckman, Jeanne N.	Chart number: 75600
10-24-xx Appointment made for consultation regarding menometrorrhagia with Dr. J. Martino	
on ~~11-1-xx~~ 11-3-xx (BF 10-24-xx) at 11:30. --B. Frost, med. admin. asst.	

Figure 9-20 When a chart entry is corrected, specific guidelines should be followed to preserve the original information that was entered in the patient's medical record.

Electronic records require specific safeguards to protect archived information. Once information has become a permanent part of the record, it will be necessary to create an entirely new entry to correct erroneous information. If an error exists in a dictated report, an addendum containing the corrected information is placed at the end of the report.

> **HIPAA Hint**
>
> A patient has the right to amend errors in his or her medical record when that information is incomplete or inaccurate.

Organizing the Medical Record

Charting Methods

Electronic and paper records in many medical offices are arranged in what is known as a **source-oriented medical record (SOMR).** In this type of arrangement, similar information is kept together or information from similar sources is grouped together. In other words, all office visits are together, all laboratory reports are together, all radiology reports are together, and so on. This method makes it easy for the physician to review a particular section of the patient's record. In a source-oriented format, each section in the record is arranged in chronological order, with the earliest document placed first on the page and the most recent placed last. Some offices may file reports in reverse chronological order with the most recent on top. Either method can be used; what is important is that everyone within an office uses the same method. This ensures that everyone who uses the record can locate the information they need.

A few practices choose to arrange the patient's chart in a **problem-oriented medical record (POMR).** This method involves grouping together all the information related to each problem. If a patient is seen for a broken leg, all information related to the leg fracture is placed in the same section. The problem-oriented format sometimes makes it difficult to compare like items in the chart, such as laboratory reports or even progress notes, because they may not be grouped together.

Chart Order

To make it easy to locate items in a paper medical record, chart dividers made of heavyweight tabbed paper should be used to section off different parts of the record. When dividers are used and the medical record is organized, all records within a medical office should be organized in the same way; that is, all dividers are placed in the same order in every record and all documents are placed in the chart in a specific order within the appropriate divider. Maintaining the same order in every record allows health care personnel to quickly locate needed patient information (Box 9-3 and Procedure 9-3).

Occasionally, depending on the setup of the health care facility, one common medical record is used for both the office and the hospital. A central health information department oversees the content of a combined record. In the case of a combined record, more than one volume may be necessary to hold all of the patient's medical information.

Documentation Guidelines

It is important that each facility establish specific policies and procedures pertaining to documentation in the medical record. Not only is this a requirement of The Joint Commission, but also it is absolutely essential to protect the patient and the facility from any possible error that could result from poor documentation.

In 1995, Medicare established documentation guidelines (Box 9-4) to ensure appropriate documentation of evaluation and management (E&M) encounters by health care providers. An E&M encounter is a visit between a patient and a health care provider (e.g., physician, therapist, nurse practitioner, physician assistant) that can occur in a variety of settings, including clinics, hospitals, nursing homes, patient homes, and so on.

In addition to the Medicare guidelines detailed in Box 9-4, there are other considerations for ensuring consistent appropriate documentation of chart entries. Note that Medicare guidelines list "The medical record should be complete and legible" as the first guideline. If entries are handwritten, the writer must use legible handwriting in the patient's record. There should *never* be a question as to the meaning of an entry.

Also, abbreviations should be used with caution in a patient's record. Each facility should develop an approved list of abbreviations, and only those abbreviations included on the list should be allowed to appear in chart documentation. The Joint Commission has developed a dangerous abbreviations list that identifies abbreviations that should not be used in handwritten chart documentation (Table 9-1). These dangerous abbreviations should never be used because they have great potential to be misunderstood, and their use could bring harm to a patient if the record is misinterpreted.

BOX 9-3

Sample Chart Order

Identification sheet (summary or face sheet)
Medication list
Medical history
Progress notes
Laboratory/pathology reports
Radiology reports
Other specialty reports
Correspondence

PROCEDURE 9-3

Organize a Patient's Medical Record

Materials Needed

- Patient's medical record
- Medical reports

1. Verify the patient's name on the reports and on the medical record.*
2. Determine where the reports should be inserted in the medical record.
3. Open fasteners that hold the chart documents together.
4. Insert the reports in the appropriate location in the patient's medical record.
5. Close the fasteners to secure chart documents.

**Denotes crucial step in procedure. The student must complete this step satisfactorily to complete the procedure satisfactorily.*

What Does Not Belong in the Record

The medical record is a compilation of data collected during the course of the patient's medical treatment. Items that contain any type of medical information about the patient should be included in the chart. Some items, however, definitely do not belong in the patient's chart.

First and foremost, no report of any kind should become a *permanent* part of the patient's medical record until the patient's physician or health care provider has reviewed the report. Even if results of a laboratory study are normal, the physician must review the report. A transcribed SOAP note or other documentation of a patient's treatment must be authenticated by the patient's physician/health care provider. If an abnormal test result were to be archived electronically or filed away without the physician's knowledge, a patient might suffer serious medical consequences. Litigation is a very real possibility if a report does not undergo physician review. Physician review is necessary whether an electronic or paper record is kept. Failure to obtain appropriate signatures demonstrates sloppy record keeping and has the potential to harm a patient.

Information regarding the patient's financial status with the health care facility does not belong in the patient's medical record. Copies of collection letters or credit arrangements, for example, or references about the patient's ability to pay should *never* be placed in the patient's chart. If a patient were to pursue litigation against the physician or the health care facility, it could be absolutely devastating to the case if the patient alleges that his or her health was compromised because certain necessary treatments were not done because of the patient's financial situation. Information regarding a patient's financial arrangements should be kept in a separate account folder in the business office of the health care facility.

Offensive, insulting, or callous comments about the patient or about another health care provider or medical office also have no place in the medical record. This would be a rarity, but if such comments appear in the record, the supervisor of

BOX 9-4

1995 Medicare Documentation Guidelines

These guidelines describe appropriate documentation for patient encounters with health care providers. These guidelines must be followed to ensure completeness of documentation for billing and other purposes.

1. The medical record should be complete and legible.
2. The documentation of each patient encounter should include the following:
   - Reason for the encounter and relevant history, physical examination findings, and prior diagnostic test results,
   - Assessment, clinical impression, or diagnosis,
   - Plan for care,
   - Date and legible identity of the observer.
3. If not documented, the rationale for ordering diagnostic and other ancillary services should be easily inferred.
4. Past and present diagnoses should be accessible to the treating and/or consulting physician.
5. Appropriate health risk factors should be identified.
6. The patient's progress, response to and changes in treatment, and revision of diagnosis should be documented.
7. The CPT and ICD-9-CM codes reported on the health insurance claim form or billing statement should be supported by the documentation in the medical record.

health information should be notified. The supervisor, in turn, will be responsible for contacting the originator of the comments to amend the offensive entry.

Records Flow

When a patient makes an appointment, a medical record number or chart number is entered into the appointment schedule. Each day, a printout of the next day's schedule is obtained, and if the office uses a paper record, the assistant uses this schedule to pull the patients' medical records for the next day.

When a patient arrives at the office for an appointment, information such as the patient's address and insurance is verified in the front of the chart as well as in any computer records. The chart and the computer records are updated if necessary. When an examination room is open, a paper record is taken along with the patient to the examination room. The nurse or clinical medical assistant then conducts a brief interview and takes vital signs such as temperature and blood pressure. The nurse or clinical medical assistant records the vital signs in the patient's record. If an electronic record is used, a computer should be available in every examination room, and a nurse or assistant will enter the patient's vital signs and history information directly into the computer at the moment the information is obtained from the patient.

After the history information is obtained, a paper record is routed to the physician; when the physician is ready to see the patient, the physician brings the chart into the examination room and begins to collect subjective and objective data from the patient. Although the patient is entitled to know the contents of his or her medical record, the record is not left in the exam room if medical personnel are not present in the room. This is to avoid alarming the patient with something in the record that may be misunderstood. Of course, if an EHR is used, the record will be accessible by means of a computer in the examination room or at the nurse's station. Medical personnel must log out of a computer when they are not in an exam room to prevent patients from accessing the records system.

At the completion of the visit, the physician may write or dictate office notes of the patient's visit, and a paper record chart is returned to the records room. After documentation is completed, all records are reviewed in a process known as quantitative analysis.

Quantitative Analysis

After a patient has seen a physician, an assistant reviews the record to ensure that all necessary components are included and completed in the record. This process, which is known as **quantitative analysis,** is described by Edna Huffman in *Health Information Management*. The main purpose of quantitative analysis is to verify that all essential pieces of the record are in place. If some portions of the record are not completed or are not included in the chart, the assistant should make sure that these items are located and completed.

A typical analysis of a record might reveal the following:

- Chart notes are not yet completed by transcription.
- A signature on a report is missing.
- A chart entry has not been dated.
- A laboratory or x-ray report is missing.

Deficient records are flagged for completion (Fig. 9-21), or the assistant may be required to locate documents needed to complete the file. Incomplete paper records should be kept in a separate holding place apart from complete records to avoid the possibility that the deficiencies are not corrected. Incomplete electronic records can be flagged as incomplete and periodic reports can be run indicating which records need completion.

It is extremely important for the medical record to be complete because:

- Delays in completing and filing reports and other information in patients' records do not serve patients well. Reliable, complete information is necessary to provide quality patient health care services.
- Accreditation standards for health care organizations require that complete and accurate records be kept on every patient.
- Records are required by many governmental agencies.
- Medical record information is necessary to obtain reimbursement from insurance companies. The record verifies the various services and level of treatment given to a patient.

TABLE 9-1

Joint Commission Dangerous Abbreviation List

Do Not Use	Potential Problem	Use Instead
u (unit)	Mistaken for 0 (zero), 4, or cc	unit
IU (International Unit)	Mistaken for IV or 10	International Unit
Q.D., QD, q.d., qd (daily); Q.O.D, QOD, q.o.d., qod (every other day)	Mistaken for each other; period after the Q mistaken for "I" and the "O" mistaken for "I"	daily every other day
Trailing zero (X.0 mg)*	Decimal point is missed	X mg
Lack of leading zero (.x mg)		0.X mg
MS	morphine sulfate or magnesium sulfate—confused for one another	morphine sulfate
MSO_4 and $MgSO_4$		magnesium sulfate

*Trailing zero may be used in laboratory reports, imaging studies reporting the size of lesions, or catheter/tube sizes. It may not be used in medication orders or other medication-related documentation. (Courtesy of © The Joint Commission, 2012. Reprinted with Permission).

Happy Valley Medical Group
Patient Record Deficiency

Provider name ____________________ Date ____________________

Patient name ____________________ Record number ______________

Please review and complete all checked items.

_____ sign report

_____ date report

_____ complete dictation ________ (date)

_____ complete diagnosis

_____ initial diagnostic study ________ (date)

_____ review flagged information

_____ other ____

____

____________________ reviewer ____________________ phone

Figure 9-21 Labels can be used to identify location and reason for deficiencies in a patient's medical record.

- The record is essential to a physician's defense. If something is not recorded or included in a record, it is assumed that it was never done. A complete and accurate record is perhaps the best defense in court should legal problems ever arise.

After all necessary information has been included in the record, a paper record may be filed with the completed records in the records room, and an electronic record will be marked as complete.

Filing Supplies

If paper records are kept, proper materials are needed to ensure that information is protected and readily accessible. Even though this next section of information may appear to pertain only to a facility that maintains paper medical records, keep in mind that all health care facilities probably will have some paper documents that must be kept. Even if a facility uses electronic records, paper records may be received from other facilities, or older archived records may have to be maintained by office staff.

Charts

A durable heavy stock folder is essential to protect the contents of the medical record. Folders may be ordered in a variety of colors, or manila folders with colored numbers along an edge of the folder may be used (Fig. 9-22). Each folder should be identified in some way with a color to expedite locating files in the medical office. Color coding and its benefits are discussed later in this chapter.

Folders must include a fastener of some type designed to hold the pages of the chart together and hold the pages to the actual chart folder. These fasteners may be located at the top of a page to allow for a flip-style chart, or fasteners may be located on the side to allow the pages to open like a book. Fasteners should be durable because pages will be added continually to the chart. It is important that fasteners be used and that papers are not just placed within a folder. If papers are not secured with some type of fastener, it is very possible that they could be lost or misplaced, thereby creating the very serious problem of an incomplete medical record.

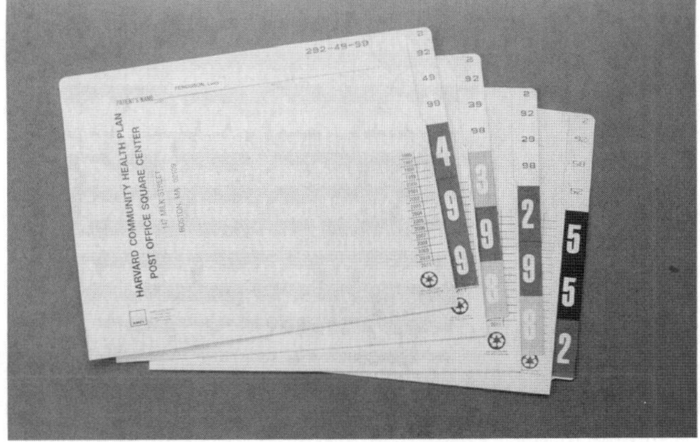

Figure 9-22 The folder for a patient's medical record may be color coded to expedite filing. The year grid on the lower right of the medical record is used to identify an active record.

Labels

Several different kinds of labels may be used on the exterior of a patient's chart (Fig. 9-23). Numerical labels that correspond to one or more of the chart numbers may be used on the side of the chart to facilitate filing. Labels that identify important information about a patient might be placed on the outside of a patient's chart. This may be done when the information may be critical to the health care provider. An example of this type of label is an allergy

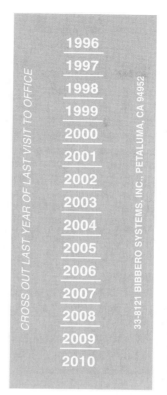

ALLERGIES:

#50320

ADVANCE DIRECTIVES

#50378

Figure 9-23 Labels may be affixed to the outside of a patient's medical record to alert the medical staff about important information. (Form courtesy of Bibbero Systems, Inc., Petaluma, California; telephone: 800-242-2376; fax: 800-242-9330; www.bibbero.com.)

label. Allergy labels may have a bright color to attract attention to the fact that the patient has an allergy to a certain type of medication.

Outguides

When a medical record is removed from the records room, an **outguide** is used to hold the place of the record. An outguide is a plastic envelope with two pockets, one of which measures about 3.5 × 5 inches and can be used to hold a note that indicates from where the chart was taken (Fig. 9-24). The larger pocket is big enough to hold reports pertaining to the patient. If reports come in regarding a patient and the chart is not in the records room, the reports are placed in the large pocket in the outguide. When the chart is returned to the records room, the reports held in the outguide can be placed into the patient's record.

Outguides are available in a variety of colors, and colors can be assigned to indicate the department or provider who has the chart. For example, if a patient had an appointment for lab work, the outguide could be green. If the patient had an appointment with cardiology, the outguide could be pink. If an employee looks for a patient's record and an outguide is in the place where the chart should be, the color of the outguide could instantly give a clue as to where the chart is. In addition, a note could be placed in the smaller pocket to indicate exactly which physician in a particular department was using the chart.

When charts are returned to filing, outguides save time because the chart's original location is marked. An assistant can easily spot the chart's location, and any newly received documents can be waiting in the outguide for inclusion in the patient's chart.

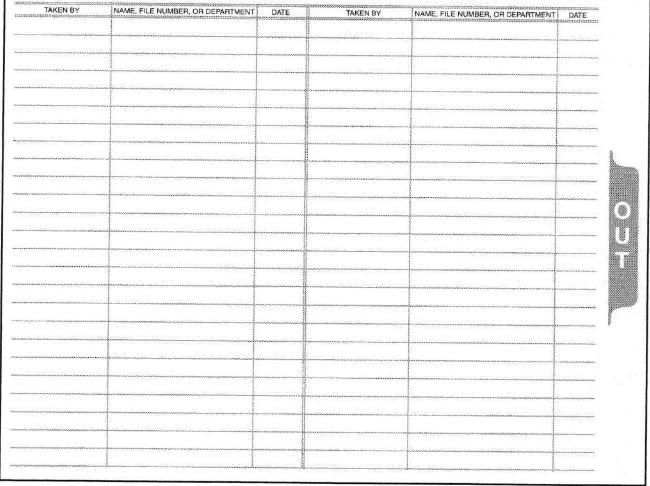

Figure 9-24 When a medical record is removed from the records room, an outguide marks a record's location. While the record is out of the records room, the outguide can be used to hold documents that need to be filed with the chart.

Filing Methods

Filing of medical records and other office documents is a very important activity in a medical facility. Filing must be kept up-to-date to allow for more expedient retrieval of

PROCEDURE 9-4

Index and File Medical Records

Materials Needed

- Medical records

1. Place the medical records in indexing order following the guidelines for the filing system adopted by the medical office.
2. Determine where the record will be filed.*
3. Verify that the filing location is correct by checking the record in front and in back of the record to be filed.
4. Complete the filing by repeating steps 2 and 3 for each record.

**Denotes crucial step in procedure. The student must complete this step satisfactorily to complete the procedure satisfactorily.*

records (Procedure 9-4). It is much easier to locate a chart or any piece of information when it is where it belongs. A wide variety of filing methods can be used in medical offices. Most health care facilities use numerical or alphabetical systems.

Numerical systems offer several advantages:

- A number provides some degree of anonymity and confidentiality for a patient. (When it pertains to records in the medical office, it may be good to be just a number!)
- The possibility of misfiling is reduced when a numerical system is used instead of an alphabetical system.
- With a numbering system, a unique number is assigned to every record. With an alphabetical system, there is a strong likelihood that there will be more than one chart with the same name. In other words, there may be more than one Mark Smith or Mark T. Smith within one records system. In the case of duplicate names, another identifier such as the patient's date of birth (DOB) will have to be used to determine the correct filing order.

Numerical Filing Systems

When a chart numbering system is begun, whether consecutive number or terminal digit, it commonly is started at a number higher than 1, such as 1000. An **accession ledger** is used to keep track of each number as it is assigned to a patient (Fig. 9-25). An accession ledger is a list of all chart numbers in numeric order and which patient is assigned to each number. In today's medical office, accession ledgers usually are accessible by means of a computerized system. The assistant merely has to type in a number, and the system will display to whom the chart is assigned.

Sometimes, numbers are automatically assigned by a computer system. No matter how the charts are filed, numbers are assigned in consecutive ascending order (1000, 1001, 1002, etc.) because this method avoids missing or skipping any available numbers. Even when numbers are assigned consecutively, the records may be filed in the records room through a different method. Two of the most commonly used numerical filing systems are consecutive number and terminal digit filing.

Consecutive Number Filing

Consecutive number filing is probably the easiest of all the filing systems. Charts are filed in the order of lowest to highest number. If chart numbers consist of a varying number of digits (e.g., 1342 and 145365), zeros can be mentally added to a number with fewer digits, if necessary, to assist with filing; thus, 1342 becomes 001342.

Use of the consecutive number filing method would place this list of chart numbers in the following order from first to last:

005365
045265
135365
145365
830308
850508

A consecutive number filing system is quite easy to learn. A drawback to this type of system, however, is that it sometimes is very easy to confuse numbers when one is looking at a large group of digits. Because of this possibility, it is common to separate longer numbers into distinct units; 850508 might be listed as 850 508 or 85 05 08.

Although everyone knows how to count, mistakes can be made in consecutive filing. A common mistake involves transposing a number. A **transposition** involves reversing the order of some of the digits. For example, 48732 becomes 47832. To avoid transposition of numbers during filing, the numbers of the records before and after the record to be filed should be checked to ensure that the record is placed in the proper sequence.

Terminal Digit Filing

The **terminal digit filing** method involves breaking a chart number into a series of groups and filing within each group. Terminal digit is the system most commonly used by hospitals today.

A chart with the number 145365 becomes 14 53 65. The assistant determines the filing order by looking at the chart number from right to left. Chart number 145365 would be indexed as follows:

primary unit—65 secondary unit—53 tertiary unit—14

The primary, or first, unit, 65, indicates that the assistant will file the chart in section 65 of the records room. Once the assistant arrives at section 65, he or she will look for the number 53 grouping within section 65. After this grouping is located, the assistant will place the chart between the numbers 13 and 15 within the grouping.

When the chart numbers previously mentioned under consecutive filing are used, the terminal digit filing method would place the numbers in the following order from first to last:

83 03 08
85 05 08
04 52 65
00 53 65
13 53 65
14 53 65

Of course, there will be many charts between those numbers, but this clearly illustrates that terminal digit filing probably would be a bit confusing for an untrained person who is trying to locate a chart. Although some extra training may be needed for new personnel, use of the terminal digit filing system usually reduces the chance of misfiling because filing personnel file the records using only two digits at a time. An added benefit of terminal digit filing is that confidentiality is enhanced; it might be very difficult for someone not familiar with this filing method to locate a patient's record.

Alphabetical Filing

Although most medical offices prefer to use some type of numerical system, some offices continue to use an alphabetical filing system. Even if a numerical system is used for filing charts, alphabetical filing may be used in other areas of the office. One example of an alphabetical system is a **master patient index.**

The master patient index is an alphabetical file of all office patients and their chart numbers. The master patient index contains the name of every patient who has ever been treated in the office. If a patient's name changes because of marriage or for another reason, the patient's previous name is **cross-referenced** to the patient's new name and vice versa (Fig. 9-26). Cross-referencing allows a patient's medical record to be easily located if a name change occurs.

Although everyone knows the letters of the alphabet and in what order the letters appear, the medical office should adopt—and strictly follow—a specific set of rules when filing alphabetically to avoid misplacing records and making them difficult to locate.

National organizations have recommended guidelines for filing alphabetically, but recommendations can differ among various organizations. The most important thing to remember about alphabetical filing is that *everyone in the office must adhere to one set of guidelines established for that office*; otherwise it might be very difficult to locate even a seemingly simple name.

In creating an easy-to-use alphabetical filing system, the following guidelines are *recommended*:

- Every name should be arranged in the following order for filing: last name, first name, middle or maiden name or initial. The last name (surname) is known as the primary unit, the first name (given name) becomes the secondary unit, and the middle name or middle initial is the tertiary unit. The names then are placed in alphabetical order. The name *Gordon Michael Smith* should be indexed as *Smith Gordon Michael.*
- An important task when registering new patients in a medical office is obtaining every patient's complete legal

Happy Valley Medical Group
Accession Ledger

Date	Chart Number	Patient Name
04-15-02	712536	Smith, Robert M.
04-15-02	712537	Smith, Tyler R.
04-15-02	712538	Jones, Kyle B.
04-16-02	712539	Carpenter, Janet T.
04-18-02	712540	Maxwell, Tana J.
04-18-02	712541	Warren, Jamie Z.

Figure 9-25 An accession ledger is a log that keeps track of chart numbers assigned and to whom and when the chart number was assigned.

Vasquez, Maria T. #621348
See Gonzales, Maria T. DOB: 10-3-77
725 West 42 Avenue
Harvester, MN 55555
010-555-9429

Figure 9-26 Cross references help track patients who have had a name change.

name. Nicknames (*Butch*) and shortened versions of a name (*Sue*) should not be used. Names such as these can lead to duplicate records in the medical office. If a patient comes in one day and gives the first name *Charles* and on a subsequent day gives the name *Chuck,* a duplicate record may be created if the patient's full legal name is not obtained. Every patient should be asked for a complete legal name.

- If a patient has a name that could be abbreviated, an abbreviation of a name should be filed as though it is spelled out (e.g., *Geo.* = *George; St. Michael* = *Saint Michael*). Here, again, the possibility exists for creation of duplicate records if a patient registers under different forms of a first name. When entering names in a computer records system, names should be entered as they are spelled out. Abbreviations of names should not be used in a computer system because a name may not be able to be located if it is abbreviated.
- In the instance of identical names, files should be arranged by patients' DOB, oldest first. Filing guidelines from some records organizations state that the address should be used to determine filing order in the case of identical names. With filing in the medical office, however, DOB should be used because a DOB never changes, but an address does.
- When initials appear as part of the patient's name, the initial should be considered a complete name (e.g., *Smith, M. Gordon* is filed before *Smith, Mark G*). The rule "nothing comes before something" applies in this case. If a patient regularly uses an initial rather than a complete name, that initial is treated as a single unit and not as an abbreviation.
- Prefixes of names should be included with the names and should be filed as one word (e.g., *Van Buren* is filed as *VanBuren; Mac Lean* is filed as *MacLean*).
- Punctuation, such as apostrophes and hyphens, should be ignored. The last name *Johnson-Smith* becomes *JohnsonSmith* for filing purposes. A computer system actually looks at a punctuation mark as a character and will try to "alphabetize" the punctuation mark.
- Professional (*Dr.*) and religious titles (*Rev., Father, Sister*) should be disregarded when filing. Patients should be listed by last name. Filing patients under the title *Sister,* for example, would be of no benefit.

Even if an office is computerized, information should be entered into the computer program in a consistent manner. A computer software program will have a specific way of recognizing all characters that are entered into the program. It is important that everyone in a computerized medical office enter every patient's information in a consistent fashion. If someone enters a punctuation mark or space in a patient's name, a computer system will identify those spaces and punctuation marks. It may be extremely difficult to search for a patient's name if it is entered correctly at a later date but had been entered incorrectly initially (see Procedure 9-4).

Alphanumeric Filing

An **alphanumeric** system combines letters and numbers to arrive at a unique identifier for each patient. The Medisoft software available with this text can be set up to use an alphanumeric system. Identifiers can be automatically assigned by a computer system, thus eliminating the possibility of duplication of numbers. Charts for the following patients would be identified as follows:

Patient Name	Chart Number
Deanne E. Olson	OLSDE000
Derek G. Olson	OLSDE001
Dewey T. Olson	OLSDE002
Delores N. Olson	OLSDE003

Charts are filed initially alphabetically and then numerically within each alphabetical section.

Color Coding

Adding color coding to a filing system is an enormous timesaver. Proper use of a color-coding system can save hours looking for paper records. **Color coding** involves assigning colors to represent letters and numbers to aid in record filing and retrieval (Fig. 9-27).

One of the main reasons for using color to identify charts is to reduce the number of misfiles that occur in the records room. An orange chart would look conspicuously out of place in the middle of hundreds of green charts. If specific colors are assigned to certain charts, it is necessary to look only for a chart assigned a particular color. Colors can be used for charts or for labels that are applied to charts.

An example of how a color-coding system could be arranged appears in Table 9-2. A color-coding system for numerical filing works well if 10 different colors are chosen. Each digit from 0 to 9 is assigned a different color. A specific digit of the medical record number (100ths or 1000ths) is used to determine the chart color. To make color coding work, specific characters are assigned to a color, and that assignment determines the color of the patient's chart.

If an office that is using a consecutive filing system were to assign the chart colors listed in Table 9-2 based on the 1000th

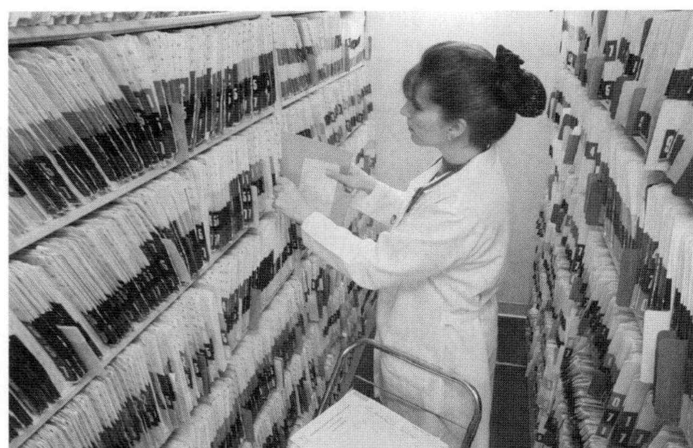

Figure 9-27 Color coding of medical records can save time when records are filed and retrieved.

place in the chart number, the charts identified here would be assigned the following colors:

Chart Number	Chart Color
194356	Tan
030383	Blue
122113	Orange
079936	Gray
173402	White

With the use of such a color scheme in a consecutive filing system, the color would change every 1000 charts. With this system, chart number 122113 could be given either an orange folder or a manila folder with an orange label applied to it.

If the office is using a terminal digit filing system, the last two numbers in the chart number would identify the section of the records room in which the chart will be located. These two numbers may be represented by colored labels that are placed on the outside edge of the medical record folder.

If the labels for each chart filed by terminal digit were chosen using the colors listed in Table 9-2, the colors of the chart labels would be listed as follows:

Chart Number	Chart Label Color
194356	red, green
030383	pink, white
122113	yellow, white
079936	white, green
173402	blue, orange

This assignment would be logical because all charts with 56 as the first unit would be filed together. Therefore, all charts in section 56 would have a red label and a green label. If a chart with a pink label and a green label were brought to that section, it would be identified as being out of place.

If color coding is adopted for alphabetical filing, an assistant may choose to assign the color by using the first two letters of the patient's last name. Using color coding with an alphabetical filing system will create a pattern in that for each successive letter of the alphabet, the folder color will change. Charts would have the colors assigned as follows:

Patient's Last Name	Chart Color
MacLean	orange, blue
Dale	white, blue
Pearson	red, tan
Rodriguez	purple, tan
Steinberg	pink, grey

Why Use Color Coding?

The use of color coding offers several advantages for the medical office. The chief advantage is that if 10 colors are used and an assistant is looking for a folder or label of a specific color, the search is reduced by approximately 90% because the nine other colors can be ignored. In other words, if an assistant is looking for a blue folder or label, he or she can ignore any color that is not blue. This can save a great deal of time when one is looking for a patient's medical record.

Another advantage is that a color-coding system can be learned easily. Let's take another look at the consecutive number filing system in which a color is assigned to the 1000th digit. The assistant will quickly learn each color and its associated number just by retrieving and filing records each day. Then, when the assistant sees chart numbers such as 131003, 841835, 471384, and 281867, the assistant will know that all of those charts are yellow because yellow represents the number 1.

The use of color coding streamlines the filing and retrieval of records and must be strictly followed for a color system to save time. Improper use of or failure to follow color-coding guidelines defeats the purpose of the system (Procedure 9-5).

TABLE 9-2

Example of a Color-Coding System

Number	Color	Letter
0	Blue	A, K, U
1	Yellow	B, L, V
2	Orange	C, M, W
3	White	D, N, X
4	Tan	E, O, Y
5	Red	F, P, Z
6	Green	G, Q
7	Purple	H, R
8	Pink	I, S
9	Gray	J, T j

PROCEDURE 9-5

Color Code Medical Records

Materials Needed

- Medical records
- Color-coding scheme
- Labels compatible with color-coding scheme

1. Obtain the color scheme for color coding medical records.
2. Affix the appropriate label to each medical record that corresponds to the filing system and associated color scheme.*
   - Alphabetical filing—use a label that corresponds to the first letter of the patient's last name.
   - Consecutive number filing—use a label that corresponds to the 1000th digit of the chart number.
   - Terminal digit filing—use labels that correspond to the two digits in the primary indexing unit.
3. Verify that the color coding is correct by placing the records for filing. Colors will appear together.

**Denotes crucial step in procedure. Student must complete this step satisfactorily to complete the procedure satisfactorily.*

CHECKPOINT

1. A medical office is using a terminal digit filing system in its records room. All chart numbers are composed of at least six digits. Charts are marked with labels that correspond to the first unit used for filing. Should the medical office use colored chart folders in addition to the colored labels, or will manila folders suffice?
2. The credit department of the medical office has asked that the assistant place a colored label on the front of a patient's chart if the patient's account has a large balance that is grossly overdue. Is this a good idea? Why?

Locating Missing Files

Although it is a rare occurrence, a paper record may be misplaced, and a missing record is a serious problem in the medical office. Careful attention should be paid to the records when filing to make sure that they are placed in the proper location. Much time can be wasted looking for a misplaced or misfiled record. When a record is missing, it is extremely important that it be found. A number of things can be done and a number of places can be checked, as shown in the following list:

- An assistant should look in the few charts preceding and after the spot in which the chart should have been filed. Occasionally, the chart may be misplaced by only a few files.
- An assistant should identify the last department or individual who used the chart. This information can be verified by checking computer records or chart requisitions. It may be necessary to double- and triple-check the physician's office, nurse's station, business office, manager's office, laboratory, and radiology areas for the file.
- If a color-coding system is in place in the records room, an assistant should scan all shelves or drawers for a color that is out of place.
- An assistant should check areas behind the shelving or drawers that hold the charts. The chart may have fallen behind or below a drawer or shelf.
- An assistant should check areas that hold inactive or closed charts.
- An assistant should check to see whether the chart has been inadvertently placed inside another chart near where it should have been filed.
- If using an alphabetical filing system, an assistant should identify another possible spelling of the patient's last name (e.g., *Larson* or *Larsen*) or should check to see if the chart may have been filed under a previous name, such as a patient's maiden name.

Every medical office should have a policy regarding removal of medical records from the office. It generally is recommended that no one—not even the physician—should ever remove a record from the office because the chance exists that it may never come back. The patient's record is invaluable for providing continued care for the patient, and it is absolutely necessary should the physician or medical office ever be involved in litigation regarding the patient.

Records Retention and Disposal

Requirements for the retention of records vary from state to state. An assistant should verify the state requirement for medical records retention. The statute of limitations for malpractice suits generally dictates the minimum amount of time that a record must be kept. Even though there may be a minimum amount of time to keep a record, keeping that record longer will benefit the patient, should the patient ever need the record.

The statute of limitations for a minor's record may not even begin until the minor is an adult. Therefore, if the statute of limitations for litigation is 2 years, a minor could have until age 20 to sue for something that occurred when the minor was 4 years old.

Records of Medicare patients must be kept for a minimum of 5 years after the patient's last treatment. Some states have enacted laws that specify the length of time a record should be kept. Some facilities have adopted policies that say that no medical records should be destroyed. Each state chapter of AHIMA should have information on requirements for retention of records within that state.

The medical office should establish a retention schedule that specifies the parameters for retaining records. Records usually are divided into three basic categories: active, inactive, and closed.

Active records are records of patients who are currently undergoing or have recently undergone treatment. **Inactive records** are records of patients who have not received treatment over a specified period of time, perhaps 6 months or 1 year. **Closed records** are records of patients who have died, who have moved from the area, or who will likely not return for treatment in the future. Closed records usually are moved to a storage location in the medical office or off the premises. Records moved to storage must be filed in a logical manner, typically using the same system as used in the office (numerical or alphabetical) and should be stored in heavy duty boxes that are clearly marked with the contents. If storage space for closed records is limited, the medical office must make arrangements for additional space or must have an alternative plan for storing the records. Electronic media, such as CD-ROM or microfilm, make possible compact storage of medical information, so that space for retaining records is not a problem.

To keep closed records up to date, names from obituaries in the local newspaper should be cross-checked on a daily, weekly, or monthly basis with the patient database in the medical office. Every name that appears in the obituaries should be checked; do not rely on memory. If a paper record exists for a deceased patient, the outer cover of the folder should be marked with the word *deceased* and the patient's date of death. A deceased record then is filed in the closed files. It should also be noted in any of the patient's information in an electronic system that the patient is deceased.

When dealing with paper records, the medical office should purge from the active files in the records room any charts that are no longer used. This should be done on a regular basis, usually yearly. To easily discern the patient's last encounter with the office, each chart folder should be marked on the outside with the last year the patient received treatment. A check mark on a grid located on the front of the chart can indicate the last year of treatment (see Fig. 9-23). The assistant then can quickly look at the cover of each chart to identify the most recent treatment of the patient. For example, if today's date is January 1, 2010, then any record without a check mark in 2009 can be assumed to be inactive.

If medical records are to be destroyed, great care must be taken to ensure that all identifiable information is destroyed completely. Records should be shredded or incinerated. Incineration services are available from outside companies. If such a service is used, a signed agreement should be obtained with the disposal company to ensure that confidential information is destroyed and is not released. However, as was mentioned previously, if at all possible, all records should be kept indefinitely.

Tickler File

Occasionally, for certain tasks, an assistant needs a reminder to do a specific activity in the office. Charts may have to be purged at a specific time, billing statements may need to be run, government reports may have to be filed, or patients may need to be reminded to set up an appointment. A **tickler file** can be used to provide these reminders for office staff.

Tickler files can be kept electronically. Computer software often includes features that allow electronic reminders to be created within the system. Calendaring features allow office activities to be scheduled far in advance. Task lists can be created to identify necessary timelines for task completion. Appointment schedules have the ability to automatically generate a reminder letter for patients at a specific time before the appointment.

Often these programs are interconnected to create one large electronic tickler file that can remind an assistant about what needs to be done daily (Procedure 9-6). The ability to have the office computer system electronically track necessary tasks and automatically perform specific activities (such as automatic letter generation) helps to ensure that nothing is forgotten.

In the absence of an electronic system, a tickler file can be easily set up in a file drawer with a separate folder for each month of the year. If a patient needs an appointment in December and it is currently only February, a reminder could be entered in October's file to call the patient to arrange an appointment. Then, at the beginning of each month, the tickler file for that month is opened and the activities completed as necessary.

PROCEDURE 9-6

Create Electronic Tickler File

Materials Needed

- Computer and scheduling software

1. Open the computer scheduling software.
2. Identify task to be scheduled.
3. Identify due date of task.
4. Identify task priority.
5. Save all changes to the task list.

File Storage and Protection

Many types of units may be purchased to hold records. Open shelving units, shelving units that have pullout drawers, and four-drawer file cabinets may be used to hold medical records. Some type of lateral shelving that allows records to be quickly inserted or retrieved works best. A four-drawer file cabinet is not recommended for charts because it is quite difficult to grasp the actual folder, and working with hundreds of charts would mean opening and closing drawers multiple times.

Whatever type of storage is used, the units should be easily accessible to all staff members. Shelves must not be too high because staff members may have trouble reaching the top shelf. The use of stepstools should be discouraged in the records room because of the hazard of falling or tripping over a stool.

In addition, files may have to be locked to protect the confidentiality of the records. Sometimes the entire records room is locked. If this is not possible, locking lateral files can be purchased. This is extremely important in highly sensitive areas such as psychiatry, but it can be done to protect records anywhere in an office.

Disaster Plan

It is the duty of the medical office to protect all records pertaining to treatment provided for patients. The office must take precautions to protect records from natural or man-made disasters. Tornado, hurricane, earthquake, and other calamities are very real possibilities in various parts of the country. Fire, flood, and theft are possibilities anywhere.

If records are placed on shelving, sufficient space must be provided between the records on the top shelf and the ceiling. Local fire departments have strict fire codes regarding the space that is required between an object such as the top of a shelf or a folder and a fire extinguishing system.

Water-based sprinkler systems generally are discouraged in a records room because water and paper do not mix. Furthermore, medical records should not be kept in the basement, although it is a common place to store records in many facilities. Even if there never is a fire, a sprinkler system can malfunction or a water main can break and destroy records in an instant. Systems that emit a gas substance to extinguish a fire are available for use in areas in which records preservation is vital. In the event of a flood, a water main break, or another catastrophic occurrence, the unintentional destruction of a record is no defense in a court of law.

Necessary steps must be taken to protect all records from damage. A record that is destroyed will provide no support for a physician involved in litigation. It is the responsibility of everyone in the office to safeguard the medical records.

Electronic records introduce a new twist to disaster planning. Electronic devices can fail or be destroyed. Backups of computer information are necessary to help protect the information should such a possibility occur.

Medical Offices with Multiple Locations

A trend in some areas of the United States today is for large health care organizations to have several branches or locations of outpatient clinics. Multiple branches or locations present a special problem in the area of medical records.

> **HIPAA Hint**
>
> A health care facility must use appropriate administrative, technical, and physical safeguards to protect PHI. Such protections include shredding documents before discarding them, preventing access to records by locking them securely, and limiting access to them by requiring a pass code.

Suppose a health care organization in a large metropolitan area has a central multispecialty clinic and five branch clinics within a 30-mile radius of one another. Patients are seen at a primary care branch clinic, and when a specialist is needed, patients are seen at the central clinic. How will medical records be coordinated? Will one record be transferred back and forth to where a patient receives medical services? This would create a comprehensive medical record for the patient but, in the case of paper records, would necessitate physically moving records from one building to another. Or, what if each clinic keeps its own record for the patient? The concern that comes with transferring records would be minimized, but it may be difficult for a comprehensive medical record to be developed for the patient.

Each health care facility faced with this decision will have to determine what works best in its organization. The advent of an electronic record would help to alleviate this dilemma. With an electronic record, a patient's medical information can be accessed from any location within the organization.

Legal and Ethical Issues

Because so many legal and ethical issues pertain to medical records, they would constitute an entire text or an entire course. Some of the more prominent issues are identified here.

Release of Information

Medical record information contains sensitive, personal details of a patient's life. It is extremely important for an assistant to remember that these details are private, and that in most cases, they should not be released to anyone without the expressed written consent of the patient. With few exceptions, it is up to patients to decide who has access to their medical information and to authorize the disclosure of medical information.

If a patient requests a copy of records to be released to a third party, such as to another medical office, hospital, or insurance company, a **release of information (ROI)** form (Fig. 9-28) is necessary. This release specifies in writing what medical information regarding the patient should be released. The release must be signed by the patient, unless the patient is a minor or is not capable of granting permission. In these cases, the patient's guardian is responsible for authorizing release of medical information. If a patient is deceased, the patient's personal representative (as appointed by the court) may request a release of medical records for the deceased.

A copy of the release should be filed in the medical record, and the fact that the release was done should be noted by the assistant in the patient's record (Fig. 9-29). The notation should be dated and signed by the individual who released the information. Patients who are seen by different providers within the same health care facility usually do not have to sign an ROI for records to be transferred within the facility. For a step-by-step guide for releasing information and for requesting information to be released from another facility, refer to Box 9-5 and Procedure 9-7.

When releasing information for a patient, an assistant should be careful to release only that information that has been requested. Occasionally, nonrequested information may be located near requested information, and the assistant should carefully review the information requested to be sure that only authorized information is released. An example of this might be if a patient requested only information about orthopedic treatment to be released and information about treatment for another illness was released.

When insurance claims are to be filed for the patient, confidential information must be sent from the office to the insurance company. This information often takes the form of procedure and diagnosis codes that identify what was done to the patient and what the patient's condition was. The patient must consent to the release of this information. A claim cannot be filed for the patient without this release. This type of release or authorization to release information can be found at the bottom of the form pictured in Figure 8-2.

Methods of Releasing Medical Information

A patient's medical information may be released in a variety of ways. If a patient requests a copy of the medical record, the assistant will either print off copies of needed reports from a patient's medical record or photocopy the paper records that are requested. After information for release is gathered, the copies are then sent to the intended recipient.

In the case of a paper medical record, the original record should never leave the health care facility from which it originated. The record is the physician's and the medical office's only protection should they ever be involved in litigation with a patient.

Currently, the use of outside services for medical records release is common. A copy service is contracted, and companies are paid by the amount of work that is done. The services actually send people directly to the medical office to copy requested records. With this type of arrangement, the original records never leave the office.

Happy Valley Medical Group
5222 E. Baseline Rd.
Gilbert, AZ 85234

REQUEST TO RELEASE MEDICAL INFORMATION

To: ______________________________
Name of facility releasing medical information

____
Address

____
City, state, ZIP

I hereby request that the following information be released from my medical record:

(Circle items requested)

complete medical record	psychiatric records (initial)
progress notes	HIV/AIDS related records (initial)
lab/x-ray studies	other ______________

Dates of Treatment ______________ to ______________
mo/day/yr mo/day/yr

The above-requested information should be sent to:

____
Name of facility to receive medical information

____
Address

____
City, state, ZIP

____
Please print patient name (last, first, MI)

____
DOB (mo/day/yr) chart number

____
Signature of patient or authorized representative

____
Date of request

1-00

Figure 9-28 A release of information form specifies what should be done with a patient's medical information.

In an EHR environment, reports or results from a patient's record can be duplicated easily by accessing the information in the computer system and simply printing the reports. The original information is still intact within the computer system, and a printout of that information then is available for release. When an EHR is used, access to reports will be restricted to personnel who are authorized to access such information.

In the case of a patient's health care emergency, critical information may be released over the telephone. The physician or nurse may ask the caller for some verification of information about the patient, such as mother's maiden name. The decision to release this information over the phone should be made by the physician or the health information supervisor.

Happy Valley Medical Group – Progress Notes	
Patient Name: St. Michael, Adam C.	Chart number: 200123
7-9-xx Request for release of medical records sent to Peaceful Valley Medical Center,	
Farmington, ND. --B. Frost, med. admin. asst.	

Figure 9-29 When a release of information has been done for a patient, the fact that the release was done should be noted in the progress notes section of the patient's chart.

BOX 9-5

Release of Medical Information

Requesting Medical Records for a Patient From Another Health Care Facility

1. Patient expresses desire to obtain records from another facility.
2. Medical administrative assistant completes ROI form and obtains patient's signature on form. If patient is a minor, a parent's or guardian's signature is obtained.
3. ROI form is photocopied, copy is placed in the patient's record, and original form is mailed. Assistant notes request for records in progress notes of patient's medical record.
4. Facility receiving the request photocopies the records that are requested and mails the records to the requesting facility.
5. Requesting facility receives the records.
6. Assistant sends the patient's chart and records received to the physician for review.
7. After the physician reviews the records, the physician initials the records and returns the chart and records to the assistant.
8. Assistant places the records in the designated section of the medical record.

Processing a Request to Send a Patient's Medical Record to Another Health Care Facility

1. Patient expresses desire for medical records to be transferred to another facility.
2. ROI form is completed and patient's signature is obtained on form. If patient is a minor, a parent's or guardian's signature is obtained.
3. Assistant photocopies records requested to be released.
4. Copy of release form is attached to the photocopied record.
5. Original of release form is placed in the correspondence section of the medical record.
6. Assistant makes a notation in the progress notes of patient's medical record that the information was released.
7. Copy of ROI and patient's medical record is sent to the other health care facility.

PROCEDURE 9-7

Process a Request to Release Medical Information

Materials Needed

- ROI form
- Black ink pen
- Patient's medical record

1. If needed, help the patient complete the release request.
2. Verify that all necessary information is included on the release.
3. Obtain the patient's medical record and confirm that the patient's name on the release is the same as the name on the medical record.*
4. Photocopy or print the requested information to be released.
5. Arrange the information in logical order.
6. Attach a copy of the ROI request on top of the release.
7. Place the original release request in the correspondence section of the patient's medical record.
8. Send the information to the medical facility identified on the release.*
9. In a chart entry, document that the release was processed.*

**Denotes crucial step in procedure. Student must complete this step satisfactorily to complete the procedure satisfactorily.*

Fax Machines

The use of a fax machine to send medical information is not recommended. A chance always exists that a fax could be sent to an incorrect telephone number. Fax machines should be used only if the record is needed quickly and there is no other way to get the information to the requesting party. Information could be mailed, if possible, or could be given directly to a patient.

Redisclosure of Medical Information

Information or records received from another health care provider may not be rereleased or redisclosed to a third party. In other words, if Happy Valley Medical receives records from Horizons Health Care, and a patient then requests ROI from Happy Valley, the assistant may send only the part of the record that originated at Happy Valley. The assistant should not photocopy the information received from Horizons Health Care. The patient must request the release of Horizons Health Care information from that facility because it has the original record.

When a Release Is Not Required

An ROI is not required from the patient if the law requires the information to be released. As was mentioned in Chapter 3, public health laws often require the reporting of certain diseases and medical occurrences, such as births, deaths, or gunshot or stab wounds. Such reporting does not require an authorization from the patient. It also is generally held that another health care provider who is treating the patient has a right to the patient's record.

If the record is being used for purposes of research or for medical education, ROI usually is not required. Records used for this type of purpose have all identifying information removed or **redacted**, and, therefore, the patient's identity is protected. Records can be used for such purposes only as long as their use is consistent with the health facility's policy on such use.

Records also may be reviewed for quality assurance purposes. A release is not required in this case. This practice allows the health facility to monitor the quality of care provided to patients in its facility.

Attorneys for a plaintiff or a defendant do not have the right to a patient's medical record without the patient's permission. Records should not be released unless the patient authorizes the release or unless a subpoena duces tecum (as mentioned in Chapter 3) is served.

An exception to this rule is that legal counsel for a medical office may review a patient's record if litigation commences regarding one of the office's patients. In this case, the record is reviewed to ascertain the office's role in the case.

In the case of a subpoena duces tecum, a medical administrative assistant or a health information employee from the medical office will likely be required to testify as to the completeness of a patient's record when it is submitted to the court. Once a record becomes involved in litigation, it is recommended that access to the record be restricted until the entire record has been copied and submitted. This action will help avoid any possible accusations of tampering with a record.

A physician may release medical information if the physician believes that the patient may harm himself or herself or another individual, or if the patient is a serious threat to society (see Box 3-3). In this case, the provider is allowed to inform the proper authorities to protect the patient or society as a whole.

Ownership

It is generally held that the medical office or physician owns the physical medical record (the paper it is printed on or the computer it is stored on), and the medical office or physician is responsible for taking care of that record. The patient owns the right to release the information contained in the record. In other words, the patient controls who gets access to the information. In lieu of the exceptions noted previously, the patient must authorize information to be released for information to go to a third party. Attorneys and private insurance companies are not entitled to a patient's medical information without the patient's consent.

Occasionally, a patient may request information from his or her record. A medical facility may want a patient to review the information in the record with a trained medical professional, but the patient is not required to. If the records are reviewed with a health care professional, the professional should remain in the room with the patient to ensure that no parts of the record are removed.

> **HIPAA Hint**
>
> A patient has a right to review and obtain a copy of his or her medical record. A reasonable fee may be charged for the copying and for any postage.

The patient also may request a copy of the record for the patient's personal use.

If the patient is to receive a copy of the record, charging the patient a nominal fee for copying is appropriate. Charging a fee is not appropriate for viewing the record. A copying charge should not be made if the patient is transferring to another facility; the copying in this case usually is done as a courtesy to the patient.

A physician, psychiatrist, or psychologist may decide that psychiatric records, because of the sensitive nature of such records, may not be released to the patient. Because of the great potential for damage to the patient if these records should accidentally become public while in the patient's hands, patients have been discouraged from obtaining copies of psychiatric records.

> **HIPAA Hint**
>
> A patient does not have the right to access the following information from his or her record: psychotherapy notes, information compiled for legal proceedings, laboratory results to which the Clinical Laboratory Improvement Act (CLIA) prohibits access, or health information from certain research laboratories.

Human Immunodeficiency Virus and Acquired Immunodeficiency Syndrome Records

Many states have enacted laws that protect the confidentiality of patients who have a diagnosis related to the human immunodeficiency virus (HIV) or the acquired immunodeficiency syndrome (AIDS). A patient who requests an HIV test may be asked to sign a consent form that stipulates to whom test results will be sent if the results are positive. Because of the social implications of HIV and AIDS, great care should be taken to protect a patient's identity when involved in HIV testing.

The AHIMA's position on handling insurance claims for patients with an HIV- or AIDS-related diagnosis is to require the patient's written consent for listing the diagnosis on the insurance claim form. Because of the sensitive nature of this type of diagnosis, it is important for patients to understand that information will be sent to an insurance company about the specific cause of their treatment.

The Future of Health Records

As identified in this chapter, we are at an interesting crossroads in managing patients' health care information. There is already an increasing presence of computer technology in every aspect of patient care. Currently, the U.S. government is providing incentive payments to Medicaid and Medicare eligible health care professionals who meet the Centers for Medicare and Medicaid Services (CMS) requirements regarding meaningful use of EHR record technology. This will provide *ever-increasing* opportunities for individuals with technical skills to excel in the medical office.

SUMMARY

Patients' medical records are the most important documents in the medical office. The ultimate purpose of maintaining medical records is to have a record that enables the physician to deliver the best possible care to each patient. Medical records are necessary for continuity of patient care and can be used to gather information for statistics related to medical treatment. They may be used in a legal case and may be reviewed to monitor quality of care and to provide documentation for billing and insurance statements. Medical records are invaluable for medical education and research. Complete, accurate records are essential for supporting all of these activities.

The medical administrative assistant may be chiefly responsible for maintaining the medical records in the office. A thorough understanding of support activities, such as transcription, filing, and quantitative analysis, is necessary to ensure a complete and accurate record. Health information management is essential for providing patients with quality health care services.

YOU ARE THE MEDICAL ADMINISTRATIVE ASSISTANT

You are the office supervisor, and the medical office in which you are working has gotten far behind in quantitative analysis of the office's medical records. How would you correct this situation?

REVIEW EXERCISES

Exercise 9-1 True or False

Read each statement, and determine whether the statement is true or false. Record the answer in the blank provided. T = true; F = false.

_______ 1. Statistics gathered from medical records can be used in planning for future health care services.

_______ 2. It is acceptable to begin to destroy all inactive and closed medical records if the records room runs out of space.

_______ 3. HIPAA is a federal law that protects the confidentiality of medical information and became effective in April 2003.

_______ 4. Anyone who can type fast can be a medical transcriptionist.

_______ 5. A consistent chart order makes it easy to locate items quickly in the patient's chart.

_______ 6. Once a patient is deceased, there is no need for the patient's medical record and it can be destroyed.

_______ 7. A surname with a prefix is indexed and filed as if it were spelled as one word.

_______ 8. White correction fluid should be used when errors in a paper medical record are corrected to ensure that the correction is done neatly.

_______ 9. All medical reports must be reviewed and initialed (or signed) by the physician before they are permanently added to a patient's record.

_______ 10. A patient's medical record may be reviewed to ensure that proper treatment was given by the patient's provider.

_______ 11. Copies of medical records are necessary for all claims filed to insurance.

_______ 12. Use of a number system for filing medical records could provide improved confidentiality over alphabetical filing.

_______ 13. An alphanumeric system is the most common filing system used in hospitals today.

_______ 14. Medical facilities must absorb the cost of photocopying records for legal cases.

_______ 15. A written consent is nice to have, but phone consent for release of information is acceptable.

_______ 16. Hyphenated names are considered as two units for filing.

_______ 17. Abbreviated names, such as *Chas.* and *Geo.*, are indexed as they are written.

_______ 18. All medical records should be saved if at all possible, but if the medical records room runs out of space, it is acceptable to begin to destroy records that have not been active for at least 4 or 5 years.

_______ 19. An insurance company may request a patient's medical record so it can determine whether the services provided to a patient were covered by insurance.

_______ 20. Medical records are reviewed to determine whether care given to patients meets the quality standards of the health care facility.

_______ 21. Federal law prohibits the unauthorized release of all patients' private medical information.

_______ 22. An employee who releases medical information that should not be released may be subject to termination of employment.

_______ 23. A problem-oriented medical record involves grouping together all like information in a chart. For example, all laboratory reports or all office visits are placed in their own individual section.

_______ 24. An outguide is used to mark the location of a record that has been removed from the records room.

_______ 25. Local obituary listings should be checked against the medical office's database to identify patients who have died.

_______ 26. A tickler file reminds an assistant of activities that must be completed at a certain time.

_______ 27. Redisclosure of medical information refers to the patient's allowing medical information to be released again without the patient's signature.

_______ 28. Public health laws may necessitate the release of certain medical information.

_______ 29. A patient's attorney has the right to view a patient's record without the patient's permission.

______ 30. A patient may not be able to obtain a personal copy of psychiatric records.

______ 31. Whenever copies of a patient's medical record are made, the patient should be billed.

______ 32. An electronic patient record contains the same type of information as a paper record.

______ 33. Digital photographs and electronic information regarding a patient's care is required to be kept confidential.

______ 34. A Notice of Privacy Practices must be signed every time the patient wants personal information released.

______ 35. If an employee is found to have violated HIPAA standards, fines and/or imprisonment is a possibility.

______ 36. A transposition involves reversing the order of a set of numbers.

______ 37. When closed medical records are moved to storage, it is recommended that the same system of filing be used that is used for the active records.

______ 38. Four-drawer file cabinets are the preferred system for filing paper medical records.

______ 39. Electronic health record, computerized patient record, electronic medical record, and electronic patient record are all synonymous.

______ 40. Digital transcription has replaced tape technology for transcription.

Exercise 9-2 Chapter Concepts

Read each statement or question, and choose the answer that best completes the statement or question. Record the answer in the blank provided.

______ 1. Health information management personnel are responsible for all of the following except
(a) Releasing medical records.
(b) Dictating medical reports.
(c) Compiling health care–related statistics.
(d) Reviewing medical records for completeness.

______ 2. A medical record can be used for all of the following except
(a) Publication in a medical journal.
(b) Planning for future health care services.
(c) Documentation in a legal case.
(d) Documentation for an insurance claim.

______ 3. All of the following are found in a medical record except
(a) Results of laboratory tests.
(b) Patient's medical history.
(c) Copy of the patient's monthly bill.
(d) A letter from the physician to the patient.

______ 4. Which of the following is not a use of the medical record?
(a) Documentation of care given to a patient
(b) Review of patient care for quality assurance standards
(c) Medical education and research
(d) All are uses of a medical record.
(e) Only a and b are uses of a medical record.

______ 5. In which of the following circumstances should medical information be released?
(a) Attorney involved in litigation regarding a patient requests the patient's medical record.
(b) An employer requests an employee's medical record.
(c) Patient's spouse requests results of a patient's laboratory testing.
(d) Patient completes release of information form requesting information to be sent to another medical facility.

______ 6. What is the purpose of quantitative analysis?
(a) To determine whether the medical record is complete
(b) To identify health care procedures that need to be improved
(c) To tally errors made by physicians and nurses when documenting patient care
(d) To penalize office staff who need to improve

______ 7. Which of the following does not belong?
(a) Diagnosis
(b) Assessment
(c) Impression
(d) Examination

______ 8. Which of the following is synonymous with face sheet?
(a) SOAP note
(b) Assessment
(c) Summary
(d) Consultation

______ 9. Color coding of medical records will
(a) Eliminate the need to perform quantitative analysis on medical records.
(b) Increase the time required to file records.
(c) Reduce the number of medical records required.
(d) Make it easier to locate records.

______ 10. The proper way to correct an entry in a medical record is to
(a) Use correction fluid to ensure that the previous information is obliterated.
(b) Draw a single line through the incorrect entry.
(c) Erase the previous entry.
(d) Have the physician initial every correction made in a chart.

______ 11. All of the following are safeguards for electronic health records except:
(a) Track electronic files that an employee has accessed.
(b) Require use of a password to access the system.
(c) Limit computer accessibility to only those areas the employee needs to do his or her job.
(d) All of the above are safeguards.
(e) Only b and c are safeguards.

______ 12. All of the following are true regarding numerical filing except:
(a) Numbers are used only once.
(b) Terminal digit filing involves breaking a chart number into different parts when determining the location for filing.
(c) There is a greater chance of misfiling with a numerical system than with an alphabetical system.
(d) A number can be more confidential than a name.

______ 13. Which of the following is false regarding disaster preparations for medical records?
(a) Water-based sprinkler systems are recommended to protect records from fire.
(b) Medical office personnel must take precautions to protect records from fire, flood, and other natural or man-made disasters.
(c) Basement storage is NOT recommended for medical records.
(d) Destroyed records spell disaster for physicians and health care facilities.

______ 14. Which of the following must be signed when a patient wants his records transferred from one health care facility to another?
(a) Notice of Privacy Practices
(b) Release of Information
(c) Confidentiality Agreement
(d) All of the above
(e) None of the above

______ 15. Which of the following can protect the confidentiality of patients' electronic health information?
(a) Allow employees to share passwords to make information more accessible.
(b) Allow all employees to access all areas of the system.
(c) Track employee use of the system.
(d) Discourage the use of screensavers and time limits if the system is inactive.

Exercise 9-3 SOAP Notes and H&P Reports

Information found in a SOAP note or H&P is listed here. Identify the part of the report in which the information would be found. Match the information with the answers listed. Record the answer in the blank provided. Each answer may be used more than once.

(a) Subjective
(b) Objective
(c) Assessment
(d) Plan

______ 1. Patient's description of present illness

______ 2. Results of a urinalysis

______ 3. Instructions on wound care

______ 4. Patient's diagnosis

______ 5. Information on prescription given to patient

______ 6. Vital signs

______ 7. Chief complaint

______ 8. Observations on patient's appearance

______ 9. Review of body systems

______ 10. Physician's observation of body systems

______ 11. Information about alcohol or drug use

______ 12. Family history

______ 13. X-ray results

______ 14. Medications the patient is currently taking

Exercise 9-4 Release of Information

Read each statement, and determine whether the medical information requested should be released. Record the answer in the blank provided.

Y= Yes, the information should be released.

N= No, the information should not be released.

______ 1. A mother is requesting the release of her minor son's medical records to an orthopedic specialist in another city.

______ 2. A 28-year-old man is requesting information about his father's medical history because a hereditary disease is suspected.

______ 3. A mother is requesting information about her 15-year-old daughter's strep test results.

______ 4. A father calls to request information about his 18-year-old son's psychiatric treatment.

______ 5. A son requests copies of his late father's medical records. He has a legal document that names him the personal representative of his father's estate.

______ 6. Wife calls to request the results of her husband's postvasectomy sperm count.

______ 7. A news reporter calls for information regarding a rumor about a patient with tuberculosis. He is calling to confirm the rumor and, if it is true, wants the patient to be identified.

Exercise 9-5 Consecutive Number Filing

Using the guidelines presented in the chapter, identify which number in each group would be first when a consecutive number filing system is used. Write the letter identifying the first number in the blank provided.

____ 1. (a) 126342
(b) 145632
(c) 126432
(d) 123642

____ 2. (a) 123642
(b) 1236
(c) 145632
(d) 142364

____ 3. (a) 81562
(b) 631795
(c) 6587
(d) 76142

____ 4. (a) 531200
(b) 62100
(c) 181200
(d) 882200

____ 5. (a) 73355
(b) 183245
(c) 93165
(d) 263054

____ 6. (a) 145177
(b) 415177
(c) 25177
(d) 235177

____ 7. (a) 432588
(b) 342588
(c) 345288
(d) 435288

____ 8. (a) 40801
(b) 10804
(c) 80201
(d) 10208

____ 9. (a) 478325
(b) 843725
(c) 523874
(d) 487235

____ 10. (a) 556565
(b) 555665
(c) 565656
(d) 555656

Exercise 9-6 Terminal Digit Filing

Using the guidelines presented in the chapter, identify which number in each group would be first when a terminal digit filing system is used. Write the letter identifying the first number in the blank provided.

____ 1. (a) 126342
(b) 145632
(c) 126432
(d) 123642

____ 2. (a) 123642
(b) 1236
(c) 145632
(d) 142364

____ 3. (a) 81562
(b) 631795
(c) 6587
(d) 76142

____ 4. (a) 531200
(b) 62100
(c) 181200
(d) 882200

____ 5. (a) 73355
(b) 183245
(c) 93165
(d) 263054

____ 6. (a) 145177
(b) 415177
(c) 25177
(d) 235177

____ 7. (a) 432588
(b) 342588
(c) 345288
(d) 435288

____ 8. (a) 40801
(b) 10804
(c) 80201
(d) 10208

____ 9. (a) 478325
(b) 843725
(c) 523874
(d) 487235

____ 10. (a) 556565
(b) 555665
(c) 565656
(d) 555656

Exercise 9-7 Alphabetical Filing

Using the alphabetic filing guidelines presented in the chapter, identify which name in each group would be first when indexed. Write the letter identifying the first name in the blank provided.

____ 1. (a) Andrew R. McKay
(b) Georgia McNeely
(c) Harvey MacKay
(d) Karen S. Martin

____ 2. (a) Maxwell Stevens
(b) Herbert Stephens
(c) Martha Stevenson
(d) Alice I. Steen

____ 3. (a) Hunter Johnson
(b) Amy Johnston
(c) Mitchell Johnson
(d) Jeanette Johnson

____ 4. (a) Louis Demarco
(b) Marco D'Leone
(c) Debra Smith-Deane
(d) Christine Dennis-DeJong

____ 5. (a) Matthew St. Andrew
(b) Olivia St. Marie
(c) Myrtle Sandborn
(d) Dora Saint James

____ 6. (a) Donald A. Meyer
(b) Donald A. Myer
(c) Donald G. Meier
(d) Donald B. Meiers

____ 7. (a) Barbara A. Nelson; DOB, 5-23-81
(b) Barbara A. Nelson; DOB, 3-4-45
(c) Barbara A. Nelson; DOB, 2-4-60
(d) Barbara A. Nelson; DOB, 10-17-92

____ 8. (a) Robert D. Smith
(b) R. David Smith
(c) Robert David Smith
(d) Robert G. Smith

____ 9. (a) Dr. Sharon T. Rose
(b) Rev. Nancy West-Richman
(c) Father Martin Turner
(d) Kelly L. St. Claire

____ 10. (a) Aaron Williams
(b) Davis Thomas
(c) Todd Weber
(d) Linda Lee

Exercise 9-8 Alphabetical Filing

Place the following names in alphabetical order in the blanks provided. Identify the primary, secondary, and tertiary units for each name.

________ Sandi J. Schmid

________ Dawn L. Johnson-Greene

________ Aubrey I. Schmit

________ Angela R. Berlin

________ Monica T. Olsen

________ Marcos L. Shmidt

________ Julie A. Johnson

________ Michelle R. Schimtke

________ James I. Bergquist

________ Gretchen K. Olson

_______ Harriet G. Schmitt

_______ Tamara A. Gregor

_______ Stanley R. Olsson

_______ Mark C. Schmidt

_______ Laura S. St. Marie

_______ Gary R. Olson

_______ Elaine D. Berg

_______ Mark T. Schmidt

_______ Steve R. Bergman

_______ Dr. Donna M. Snow

	Primary Unit	Secondary Unit	Tertiary Unit
1.	________	________	________
2.	________	________	________
3.	________	________	________
4.	________	________	________
5.	________	________	________
6.	________	________	________
7.	________	________	________
8.	________	________	________
9.	________	________	________
10.	________	________	________
11.	________	________	________
12.	________	________	________
13.	________	________	________
14.	________	________	________
15.	________	________	________
16.	________	________	________
17.	________	________	________
18.	________	________	________
19.	________	________	________
20.	________	________	________

Exercise 9-9 Components of the Medical Record

Read the description of components found in a medical record and match each description with the name of the appropriate component. Choose the answer that best completes the description. Record the answer in the blank provided.

_______ 1. Contains information about the patient's past diseases and family members' past diseases
(a) Other specialized reports
(b) Radiology reports
(c) Immunizations
(d) Medical history

_______ 2. A chronological record of a patient's visits to the physician
(a) Correspondence
(b) Summary sheet
(c) Progress notes
(d) Discharge summary

_______ 3. Contains information about patient's insurance, employer, and possibly even a release of information for insurance purposes
(a) Summary sheet
(b) Discharge summary
(c) Consultation
(d) Correspondence

______ 4. Section that contains letters written about the patient and copies of medical records from other health care facilities
(a) Consultation
(b) Correspondence
(c) Progress notes
(d) Discharge summary

______ 5. Documents the results of a study on body tissue
(a) Radiology report
(b) Pathology report
(c) Consultation
(d) Summary sheet

______ 6. When a patient is referred to a specialist, the specialist will document the encounter with the patient in a report known as a
(a) Pathology report
(b) Operative report
(c) Correspondence
(d) Consultation

______ 7. A CBC and urinalysis are known as
(a) Consultation
(b) Progress notes
(c) Laboratory reports
(d) Other specialized reports

______ 8. A report that documents a patient's condition on admission to a hospital
(a) Discharge summary
(b) History and physical
(c) Correspondence
(d) Consultation

______ 9. Report that documents a surgical procedure step by step
(a) Pathology report
(b) Consultation
(c) Operative report
(d) Progress notes

______ 10. An MRI or CT scan is an example of this type of report.
(a) Pathology report
(b) Discharge summary
(c) Other specialized report
(d) Radiology report

ACTIVITIES

ACTIVITY 9-1 ELECTRONIC TICKLER FILE (SEE PROCEDURE 9-6)

Using Medisoft, prepare an electronic tickler file.

1. Open Medisoft.
2. On the main menu, click **Activities>Launch Work Administrator.** The Assignment List will open. From this window, you will see the tasks that are currently open and each task's due date and priority level.
3. Enter a new task by clicking **New** on the bottom of the window.
4. Enter the tasks listed below. When a task is entered, click **Save** to save changes to the assignment list.

Description	Notes (white field)	Priority	Due Date
Purge inactive	Purge inactive records from medical records	1	One month from today's date
ROI	Complete release of information requests	1	3 days from today's date
Order supplies		2	Last day of this month
Telephone reminders	Call patients with appointment reminders for next week's physicals	1	Friday of this week
Statements	Run patient statements	1	3 weeks from tomorrow
Medicare	Submit Medicare claims	1	1st of next month

ACTIVITY 9-2 DATABASE MANAGEMENT

In Medisoft, identify changes to a patient's record.

Open Medisoft. Click **Lists>Patients/Guarantors and Cases.**

1. Tonya Hartman was recently married. Open Tonya Hartman's record. Change her last name to Gonzalez. Change her address and phone number to new address: 5516 Santé Fe Pkwy, Harvester, AZ 85000, and telephone: 222-555-7575. Under the **Other Information** tab, enter her maiden name in the **Patient ID #2** blank. Click **Save.**
2. Dwight Again died on February 23, 2014. Open his record and enter the **Death Date** under the **Name, Address** tab. DO NOT mark his record inactive, because inactive records cannot be billed and he has an outstanding bill from February. Click **Save.**

(Inactive records can be viewed by right-clicking on the **Patient List** window.)

ACTIVITY 9-3 CONSECUTIVE NUMBER FILING

Using the list below, place the medical records below in consecutive number order. Write a list of the medical record numbers and corresponding names in this order. (If desired, prepare a mock chart for each patient using either manila folders or 3 × 5–inch index cards and use the mock charts when completing this exercise.)

Last Name	First Name	MI	Chart Number
St. Michael	Adam	C	200123
Shepard	Alice	R	554148
Burlington	Allen	R	271911
Gordon	Amy	A	9520
Walker	Ann	F	152634
Olsen	Christian	B	401280
Olson	Christian	B	463278
Olson	Deanne	T	28632
Olsen	Derek	R	10110
Snow	Donna	M	210178
Stevens	Evan	D	689723
O'Henry	Gregory	A	320110
Brenner	Inez	N	100121
Breckman	Jeanne	N	75600
Garcia	Jose	N	120020
Wang	Karen	J	230192
French	Kirsten	M	641030
MacLean	Krista	A	348833
Stein	Margaret	I	8330
Armstrong	Marge	H	100120
Vasquez	Maria	T	621348
McLean	Mark	B	28680
McLean	Mary	K	220164
Pearsen	Michael	T	43220
Summerville	Paul	D	121087
Webster	Peggy	A	171423
Pearson	Steven	M	230184
Pearson	Susan	G	224764
Garcia	Tamara	D	364602
Olson	Tara	D	647932
O'Malley	Timothy	E	209110
MacLean	Tyler	C	649732

ACTIVITY 9-4 TERMINAL DIGIT FILING

Using the records list from Activity 9-3, place the records in terminal digit order. Write a list of the medical record numbers and corresponding names in this order.

ACTIVITY 9-5 ALPHABETICAL FILING

Using the records list from Activity 9-3, place the records in alphabetical order. Write a list of the names in this order.

ACTIVITY 9-6 CONSECUTIVE NUMBER COLOR CODING

Using the records list from Activity 9-3 and the color-coding chart in Table 9-2, color code the medical records for consecutive number filing using the thousandths place to determine the folder color and the hundredths place to determine the label color.

ACTIVITY 9-7 TERMINAL DIGIT COLOR CODING

Using the records list from Activity 9-4 and the color-coding chart in Table 9-2, color code the medical records for terminal digit filing using the primary unit to determine the color of labels used on the chart. Example: If the primary unit is 14, list the color corresponding to the number 1 first and the color corresponding to the number 4 second.

ACTIVITY 9-8 ALPHABETICAL FILING COLOR CODING

Using the records list from Activity 9-5 and the color-coding chart in Table 9-2, color code the medical records for alphabetical filing using the first two letters of the patient's last name to determine the color of labels used on the chart. Example: If the last name is Potter, list the color corresponding to the letter P first and the color corresponding to the letter O second.

ACTIVITY 9-9 CHART ENTRY

Using the progress notes page here, make a chart note entry for today regarding an appointment made for Zach Peters with Dr. Sanchez (cardiology) next Monday at 4:00 PM.

Happy Valley Medical Group – Progress Notes	
Patient name:	Chart #

ACTIVITY 9-10 MEDICAL RECORD RETENTION

Research the medical records retention laws or recommendations for your state.

ACTIVITY 9-11 CURRENT ISSUES AND TRENDS IN HEALTH INFORMATION

Research current issues and trends at AHIMA at www.ahima.org.

ACTIVITY 9-12 RELEASE OF INFORMATION

Prepare a release of information for Lindsey Nielsen, a patient of Happy Valley Medical Group. Ms. Nielson would like her complete medical record from Horizons Health Care Center, 123 Main Avenue, Farmington, ND 58000, to be sent to Happy Valley Medical. Ms. Nielsen's DOB and chart number can be located in Medisoft.

ACTIVITY 9-13 MEDICAL TRANSCRIPTION

Obtain dictated medical reports from your instructor. Listen to the reports as an example of how medical reports are dictated. Practice transcribing a complete medical report.

ACTIVITY 9-14 ELECTRONIC HEALTH RECORDS

Research the use of electronic health records at Mayo Clinic or a health care facility in your area.

ACTIVITY 9-15 ELECTRONIC HEALTH RECORDS

Research the different types of health care facilities (clinic, hospital, nursing home, home health) in your area to determine their use of electronic health records within the facilities.

ACTIVITY 9-16 MEDICAL OFFICE SCENARIOS

Consider the following situations. What is the appropriate response to the situation? Role-play your answers with another individual.

1. One of your coworkers is a personal acquaintance of a patient of the office. The patient has just undergone surgery for removal of a suspicious mass in the large intestine. Your coworker states she is hopeful that the mass was benign and then asks whether the pathology report for the patient has been received yet. What do you say?
2. A celebrity is a surprise patient in the office one day. A coworker comments about asking the celebrity for an autograph. What do you say?

ACTIVITY 9-17 NOTICE OF PRIVACY PRACTICES

Obtain a copy of a Notice of Privacy Practices and review and explain the contents of the document.

DISCUSSION

The following topics can be used for class discussion or for individual student essay.

DISCUSSION 9-1

As it pertains to this chapter, discuss why special attention should be paid to what goes into the trash can in a medical office.

DISCUSSION 9-2

Discuss the application of the AHIMA Code of Ethics (available at www.ahima.org) to the position of a medical administrative assistant.

DISCUSSION 9-3

Discuss why quantitative analysis may be one of the most important health information management activities.

Bibliography

American Health Information Management Association (AHIMA). www.ahima.org. Accessed December 10, 2007.

Burton BK: *Quick Guide to HIPAA*, St. Louis, Elsevier Science, 2004.

Clark JS: *Documentation for Acute Care. Revised*, Chicago, AHIMA, 2004.

US Department of Health and Human Services: *Health Information Privacy, HITECH Act Enforcement Interim Final Rule*. http://www.hhs.gov. Accessed February 18, 2013.

Huffman EK: *Health Information Management*, Berwyn, IL, 1994, Physician's Record.

The Joint Commission: www.jointcommission.org. Accessed February 20, 2012.

Judson K, Blesie S: *Law and Ethics for Health Occupations*, New York, Glencoe McGraw-Hill. 1994.

Lewis MA, Tamparo CD: *Medical Law, Ethics and Bioethics for Ambulatory Care*, Philadelphia, FA Davis. 1998.

Mayo Clinic: www.mayo.edu. Accessed February 24, 2012.

The Medical Management Institute: *The Medical Office Policy Handbook*, Salt Lake City, The Medical Management Institute. 2007.

Office of Civil Rights: *Summary of the HIPAA Privacy Rule, U.S. Department of Health and Human Services*. Last revised May 2003. http://www.hhs.gov/ocr/privacysummary.pdf. Accessed February 20, 2012.

CHAPTER 10 Procedure and Diagnosis Coding

LEARNING OUTCOMES

On successful completion of this chapter, the student will be able to

1. Perform fundamental concepts of procedural coding.
2. Perform fundamental concepts of diagnosis coding.
3. Identify legal and ethical concepts and issues pertaining to medical coding.
4. Identify the importance of certification in coding.

COMMISSION ON ACCREDITATION OF ALLIED HEALTH EDUCATION PROGRAMS (CAAHEP) CORE CURRICULUM FOR MEDICAL ASSISTANTS

- Use office hardware and software to maintain office systems.
- Use Internet to access information related to the medical office.
- Describe how to use the most current procedural coding system.
- Describe how to use the most current diagnostic coding classification system.
- Describe how to use the most current Healthcare Common Procedure Coding System (HCPCS).
- Perform procedural coding.
- Perform diagnostic coding.
- Respond to issues of confidentiality.

ACCREDITING BUREAU OF HEALTH EDUCATION SCHOOLS (ABHES) COMPETENCIES FOR MEDICAL ASSISTING

Graduates

- Maintain confidentiality at all times.
- Use appropriate medical terminology.
- Apply computer concepts for office procedures.
- Monitor legislation related to current health care issues and practices.
- Perform diagnostic and procedural coding.
- Update procedure and diagnosis code databases in medical practice management software.

VOCABULARY

American Academy of Processional Coders (AAPC)
Centers for Medicare and Medical Services (CMS)
Certified Coding Specialist (CCS)
Certified Coding Specialist–Physician-based (CCS-P)
Certified Professional Coder (CPC)
Certified Professional Coder–Hospital (CPC-H)
Certified Professional Coder–Payer (CPC-P)
coding
contrast medium
convention
Current Procedural Terminology (CPT)
diagnosis
encounter
first-listed diagnosis
Healthcare Common Procedure Coding System (HCPCS)
ICD-10-CM
ICD-9-CM
laterality
modifier
principal diagnosis
procedure
visit

Medical Coding

A patient's health care record documents a **procedure** that was delivered to a patient and the reason **(diagnosis)** that the procedure was performed. A patient can have more than one procedure or diagnosis in an encounter with a physician. **Coding** refers to the practice of assigning a numerical or alphanumerical code to identify a procedure (service) that has been performed and the diagnosis (condition) that has been treated. Use of standardized systems of codes in medical billing enables health care providers, insurance companies, and government agencies to "speak the same language" because each code has a specific meaning. Without a system of standardized codes, it would be difficult to establish uniformity in the description of diseases and the procedures used to treat them.

Standardized coding systems are used for a number of reasons. The use of codes means easier processing of insurance claims, which, in turn, means faster payment for the medical office. One of the chief uses of procedure and diagnosis codes is to categorize procedures and diagnoses so that statistics can be gathered. These statistics can then be used to determine whether new equipment should be purchased or new services should be made available for patients.

In a system such as Medisoft, it is possible to quickly find out how many tonsillectomies were done within a specific period of time. It is also possible to determine how many patients have had a diagnosis of myocardial infarction and even who those patients are. This enables a health care facility to, for example, send a mailing regarding new cardiac rehabilitation services to specific patients. Information from medical coding can help in planning for the health care needs of the population and can be used to further medical education and research.

In this text, emphasis is placed on outpatient coding, or coding that applies to physician professional services or services provided in a medical office setting. There is so much to know about procedure and diagnosis coding, so much so that learning to perform each type of coding well would require several courses of study. Expertise in coding can be developed only after in-depth study and actual work experience involving coding. The explanations of coding systems that follow are designed to help you become familiar with the structure and purpose of these coding systems and how they are used.

Procedure Coding—Current Procedural Terminology (CPT)

Procedures for which the physician performs and charges fees are identified by numerical codes called **Current Procedural Terminology (CPT)** codes. The CPT manual is a listing of codes assigned to medical procedures performed by physicians. The American Medical Association (AMA) publishes CPT codes annually, and an AMA editorial panel reviews proposed changes to the CPT codes when the manual is updated each year. The AMA owns the copyright for CPT codes.

CPT codes are used on a patient's insurance claim to identify procedures that the doctor performs. CPT codes are placed in box 24D on the standard insurance claim form known as the CMS-1500 (see Fig. 12-1). Complete information on this form is included in Chapter 12, Health Insurance and Health Benefits. CPT provides a structured way to categorize, track, and report medical procedures. By using CPT codes, it is possible to gather statistics on procedures performed by physicians (Fig. 10-1).

HCPCS System

CPT codes are part of a larger coding system known as the **Healthcare Common Procedure Coding System (HCPCS**, pronounced "hik-piks"). This system was established in 1978 and currently is maintained by the **Centers for Medicare and Medicaid Services (CMS)**. CMS is the agency of the federal government that is responsible for administration of Medicare, Medicaid, and the Children's Health Insurance Program.

The HCPCS system consists of the following two levels of codes:

- Level I codes are used for physician procedures and services. Level I codes are CPT codes and are copyrighted by the AMA. If a patient is treated in a medical office or in a

Happy Valley Medical Clinic
Practice Analysis

Code	Description	Amount	Units	Average	Cost	Net
11765	Wedge excision of skin of nail fold (eg,	100.00	1	100.00	0.00	100.00
36215	Lab Drawing Fee	8.00	1	8.00	3.00	5.00
43220	Esophageal Endoscopy	550.00	2	275.00	0.00	550.00
70373	X-Ray, Laryngography	45.00	1	45.00	0.00	45.00
71020	X-Ray, Chest, 2 Views	53.00	1	53.00	0.00	53.00
71030	X-Ray, Chest, Min 4 Views	65.00	1	65.00	0.00	65.00
71040	Contrast X-Ray of Bronchitis	50.00	1	50.00	0.00	50.00
72052	X-Ray, Spinal, Complete	80.00	1	80.00	0.00	80.00
73130	X-Ray, Hand, Min 3 Views	45.00	1	45.00	0.00	45.00
73562	X-Ray, Knee, Min 3 Views	45.00	1	45.00	0.00	45.00
73610	X-Ray, Ankle, Complete	55.00	1	55.00	0.00	55.00
74283	Barium Enema, Therapeutic	110.00	1	110.00	0.00	110.00
81000	Urinalysis, Routine	22.00	2	11.00	4.00	14.00
82947	Blood Sugar Lab Test	25.00	1	25.00	12.00	13.00
97010	Hot/Cold Pack Therapy	20.00	2	10.00	0.00	20.00
97128	Electro-Stimulation	15.00	1	15.00	0.00	15.00
97260	Spinal Manipulation	30.00	1	30.00	0.00	30.00
99000	Handling Fee	8.00	1	8.00	0.00	8.00
99205	Office Visit New Patient CCH	75.00	1	75.00	0.00	75.00
99211	Office Visit Est. Patient MMS	50.00	2	25.00	0.00	50.00
99213	Office Visit Est. Patient EEL	660.00	11	60.00	5.00	605.00
99214	Office Visit Est. Patient DDM	195.00	3	65.00	0.00	195.00

Figure 10-1 Medisoft can quickly generate a report identifying how many times a procedure was done within a certain time frame. (Screenshots used by permission of MCKESSON Corporation. All Rights Reserved. © MCKESSON Corporation 2012.)

TABLE 10-1
Organization of the CPT Manual

Section Name of CPT	Content of Codes
Evaluation and Management (E&M)	Physician visits, professional services
Anesthesia	Anesthetic administration
Surgery	Surgical procedures in all body systems
Radiology	X-ray, nuclear medicine, magnetic resonance imaging, computed tomography scans
Pathology and Laboratory	Laboratory and pathology services
Medicine	Various procedures and services not listed elsewhere

hospital, the physician's professional services (e.g., office or hospital visits) are billed with a CPT code.

- Level II codes are used for nonphysician services and supplies (e.g., medications and medical equipment) and procedures not included in Level I.

Format of the CPT Manual

The CPT manual is divided into six basic sections of numerical codes, identified and arranged in the order listed in Table 10-1. The manual is arranged in numerical order with the exception of the Evaluation and Management (E&M) codes, which appears first in the manual.

At the beginning of each section, guidelines alert the user to special considerations regarding selection of a code in that section. Special instructions sometimes are included at the beginning of subsections of codes within each section. For example, at the beginning of the surgery section, guidelines give instructions on various items such as the definition of a surgical package and modifiers that can be used to report the performance of more than one procedure. The musculoskeletal subsection within the surgery section also contains guidelines that apply specifically to that subsection.

In addition to the six sections of CPT codes, the manual contains an index and several appendices. When the CPT manual is used, the index is always used first. The index introduction gives instructions for locating procedures within the index. In the index, procedures are listed by:

- Condition (e.g., hematoma, cyst)
- Anatomic site (e.g., carpal bone, hip)
- Name of procedure (e.g., arthroscopy, cast)
- Synonym, eponym, or abbreviation (e.g., Burhenne procedure, Swenson procedure, WBC)

This arrangement often makes it possible to arrive at the same procedure code by using different entries within the index. For example, the procedure code for a *tonsillectomy* could be located under *tonsils, excision; tonsillectomy;* or *excision, tonsils.* However, depending on which entry you use, the number of codes listed can vary (Fig. 10-2). As you become familiar with the manual, it is a good idea to investigate other entries in the index to ensure that you arrive at the correct code.

Basics of Procedure Coding (CPT–HCPCS Level II)

When selecting CPT codes, it is very important to have a thorough understanding of the procedure that has been done. Often in the listing of codes, slight variations are listed for the procedures. Let's take the tonsillectomy example again. In CPT 2013, it matters if the tonsils were removed, or if the tonsils and adenoids were removed. If adenoids are included in a tonsillectomy code, it must be documented in the patient's record that the patient's adenoids were removed. Also, the patient's age is taken into account when this type of procedure is coded. In order to correctly code this surgical procedure, complete details of the procedure will be included in the patient's operative report, and the patient's age will be verified in the patient's medical record.

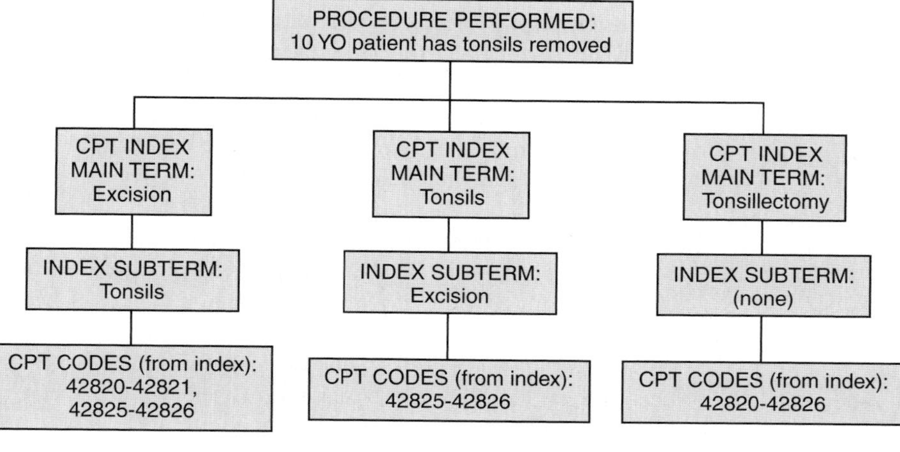

Figure 10-2 It is possible to locate a procedure in the CPT manual by looking up different main terms.

When coding procedures, information for procedures may be documented in SOAP (subjective, objective, assessment, and plan) notes, H&P (history and physical) reports, lab studies, and radiology reports, to name a few. It is imperative to code directly from the report in the patient's health record. Each report will need to be read in its entirety before coding any procedure. Only those procedures that are documented in a report can be coded. Even though a physician may indicate that a procedure was "routine," special circumstances or even additional procedures may be documented in a patient's report, and it will be up to the coder to verify any of those possible instances.

If a coder is unfamiliar with the procedure, information regarding the specifics of the procedure can be obtained from sources such as the Coders' Desk Reference. This reference provides detailed descriptions of CPT codes, and these descriptions can be compared with information contained in the patient's record. Using the previous tonsillectomy example, the Coder's Desk Reference will give a complete description of what is included in each possible tonsillectomy code. If, after reading the descriptions, a coder has difficulty choosing between codes, it is possible that a coding supervisor, another experienced coworker, the physician or even other reliable Internet resources may be able to provide information or descriptions of a procedure that will assist a coder in selecting the correct code.

When coding, procedure codes should never be chosen directly from the index. Always verify codes by reading the description of the code listed in one of the sections of the manual. Each procedure code description is almost always more detailed within that section than in the index. What may look like a good code in the index may not fit once the entire description is reviewed. It is important to read the code description carefully to ensure that the correct CPT code is selected. Procedure 10-1 illustrates the basic steps to be followed in selecting a procedure code.

PROCEDURE 10-1

Assign Procedure Codes for a Patient's Encounter

Materials Needed

- Medical records
- CPT-4 manual, current year's edition

1. From the patient's record, identify all procedures performed during a patient's encounter.
2. Locate the main term of each procedure in the index by identifying the condition, anatomic site procedure, or service provided.
3. Look in the main term for any additional modifiers. Identify all codes that may fit the procedure.
4. Locate each of the codes from number 3 in the appropriate section of the CPT manual.
5. Read the description for each code and choose the code(s) that best fits the procedure(s).*

**Denotes a crucial step in the procedure. The student must complete this step satisfactorily in order to complete the procedure satisfactorily.*

Sections of the CPT Manual

Evaluation and Management (E&M)—99201-99499

The E&M section contains codes related to procedures/services that a health care provider delivers to patients in various health care locations. These include a medical office, a hospital, a nursing home, and an emergency room, to name a few. In addition, this section includes special services that a provider may deliver in those settings, such as critical care services, telephone calls, or preventative medicine services. This section largely comprises codes that indicate that the patient is receiving the provider's expert opinion during his or her encounter with the provider.

When one is coding in this section of the CPT, many factors will need to be determined: *who was treated, what type of service was done,* and/or *where was the treatment administered.*

Who Was Treated. The status of the patient will have to be determined for many of the procedures listed in the E&M section. Status refers to whether the patient is a new or established patient. According to the E&M guidelines in CPT 2013, a new patient is described as a patient "who has not received any professional services from the physician or another physician of the same specialty who belongs to the same group practice, within the past 3 years," and "an established patient is one who has received professional services from the physician or another physician of the same specialty who belongs to the same group practice, within the past 3 years."

Status also refers to whether the patient was treated as an outpatient or an inpatient. Often this is closely associated with the place of treatment, and the place will determine whether the patient is treated as an outpatient or an inpatient.

What Type of Service Was Done. Determination of the level of service for many of the E&M services involves identifying three key components: history, examination, and medical decision-making. Each of these components is documented in a patient's encounter with a health care provider, and that documentation is analyzed to determine what level of service has been provided to the patient. Each of the key components, as well as additional components that can affect the level of service, is completely described in the E&M guidelines within CPT. The patient's record will identify what type of service was rendered. For example, did the physician provide a consultation, critical care services, prolonged care, intensive care unit care, counseling, or preventative services to the patient? The type of service provided will affect the code selection.

The guidelines in the E&M section define each type of service. For example, the guidelines before each subsection define when nursing home codes can be used, what preventative care is, and what behavioral care is.

Where the Treatment Was Administered. Another extremely important factor to note when coding an E&M service is where the service took place. A physician or other health care provider can see a patient in a variety of health care settings:

- *Medical office*—This includes many different types of offices: solo practice, urgent care center, multi-specialty group practice, etc. A clinic is a medical office.

- *Hospital*—A hospital often is associated with treating patients as inpatients, but services also can be provided in observation units within hospitals or in an emergency department.
- *Nursing home*—A nursing home is a facility that provides 24-hour-a-day skilled nursing care to residents (patients).
- *Rest home*—A rest home differs from a nursing home in that 24-hour-a-day skilled nursing care is not available in a rest home. A rest home is a facility where people pay rent for room and board. Rest homes typically have tenants who are elderly or are recovering from illness or injury or cannot live independently. Care provided in an assisted living facility often is coded as service provided in a rest home. Basic support services such as medication assistance may be available in some rest homes.
- *Patient's home*—Yes, doctors do make house calls. Services can be provided to patients within their own homes.

Anesthesia Coding—00100–01999

Many procedures done in the practice of medicine require the use of anesthesia. Anesthesia can be provided by an anesthesiologist, a nurse anesthetist, or the physician who is performing the procedure. Selection of the correct anesthesia code is based on the body location where the procedure was performed. Additionally, the method of the procedure may affect selection of the appropriate code, that is, whether the procedure was done with an incision or with a scope. For example, a hysterectomy will be coded differently depending on whether the uterus was removed through an abdominal incision or vaginally.

The important thing to remember when coding anesthesia is that the coder is coding for anesthesia services and not surgical services. When coding for anesthesia services, the CPT code will begin with a 0.

Surgery Coding—10021–69990

As mentioned earlier, the surgery section is the largest section of CPT. This section is further divided into subsections by clinical specialty. Within each specialty, additional subdivisions known as categories and subcategories often are based on the part of the body that is being treated.

The surgery guidelines provide the definition of a surgical package. Services such as local anesthesia, one related E&M visit before surgery, and typical postoperative care are included in a surgical code, hence a surgical package.

Surgical coding requires an in-depth understanding of the procedures themselves and the different ways in which they can be done. Several subsections and categories have specific instructions related to the codes contained within those sections. Some of the most common surgery coding situations are listed below.

Lesion Removal. Probably one of the most important things to know when coding a lesion removal is the pathology of the lesion that was removed. Was the lesion benign or malignant? It is also important to know how the lesion was removed. Was it excised, shaved, pared, or removed by destruction? Also, the lesion and the margin removed are measured in centimeters before the excision is performed. This measurement will be needed in order to select the correct CPT code.

Some lesion removal codes can include several lesions within one code. Other codes may require a separate code for each individual lesion. With some codes, it is necessary to know the pathology of the lesion before the removal can be coded. There are some codes in which the pathology is known because the lesion type is known, such as a corn or callus.

Wound Repair. This category of codes refers to the repair of wounds of the integumentary system. If a patient sustains a laceration, depending on the wound's severity, the repair may be included in this group of codes. Complete descriptions of types of wounds are included in the category guidelines. Wound repair is divided into three categories—simple, intermediate, and complex—with a complete description of each included in the guidelines preceding the wound repair codes. Probably one of the most often overlooked rules for coding wound repair is that the lengths of wounds within the same code group (e.g., wounds to the arm and the scalp) and with the same type of repair (e.g., simple) are added together.

Fracture Care. Guidelines at the beginning of the musculoskeletal subsection define important terms in the treatment of fractures: open and closed treatment and percutaneous skeletal fixation. Fracture care cannot be coded unless it is known what type of treatment was provided for the fracture. The type of treatment is not necessarily related to the type of fracture. For example, it is possible that a patient could sustain a closed fracture, yet open repair is required for that fracture.

Also, it is important to note that the guidelines state that application and removal of the first cast or traction device are included with the fracture treatment. If a patient should have a cast removed and another applied, the second cast would not be included in the original surgical package and the patient could be charged for the second cast application.

Cardiology. Cardiology coding is perhaps one of the most challenging areas of coding. Special instructions are given regarding pacemakers, bypass grafts, and aneurysm repairs, to name a few. For instance, to code bypasses, it must be known where the grafts for the bypass came from and how many bypasses were done. In addition, several procedures in this specialty require the use of additional codes from the radiology or medicine section of CPT.

Maternity Care and Delivery. This subsection includes codes for antepartum care, delivery, and postpartum care. Also included are codes that combine all three services. The use of a delivery code requires that the coder know how the patient delivered (vaginal or cesarean) and whether any complications occurred that required additional procedures.

Radiology Coding—70010–79999

The radiology section includes codes for x-ray, ultrasound, computed tomography (CT) scanning, magnetic resonance imaging (MRI), mammography, and radiation therapy. Vascular procedures that involve inserting a catheter into specific

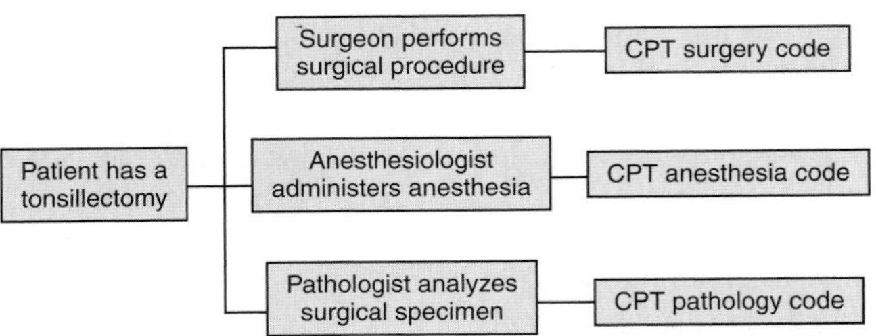

Figure 10-3 Diagram of coding for a patient's surgical procedure.

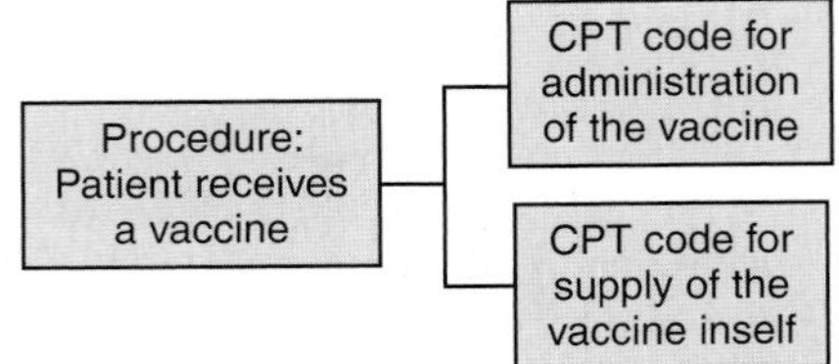

Figure 10-4 Diagram of coding for vaccine administration.

arteries, transcatheter procedures, and radiologic guidance for other procedures also are included within this section. The radiation oncology subsection includes codes on treatment planning, delivery, and management. Nuclear medicine includes studies that require administration of a radioactive substance that is traced in a patient. When coding in this section of CPT, be aware that radiologic procedures may require the use of a **contrast medium** (various substances that can be traced in a radiologic study) or a radioactive drug.

Pathology and Laboratory Coding—80048–89356

Laboratory procedures involve the testing of various substances in the body, such as blood, urine, feces, and other body substances. A series of tests included in this section are known as organ- or disease-oriented panels. These panels consist of a number of individual tests that usually are ordered together to test for a disorder or to assess overall health. For a panel to be coded, all tests within the panel must be done.

A frequently used portion of the pathology and laboratory section is the surgical pathology subsection. These codes are used to report the study of tissues that have been removed from the body during procedures that resulted in removal of part of the body. As was mentioned previously, lesion removal cannot be coded until the pathology of the lesion is known. With lesion removal, a patient may be charged for both the lesion removal and the pathology test performed on the lesion. If a patient had a surgical procedure requiring anesthesia, the patient would be charged for the anesthesia services, the surgical procedure itself and surgical pathology as well (Fig. 10-3).

Medicine Coding—90281–99602

The Medicine section contains a huge variety of codes. Vaccines and their administration are located in this section. When a vaccine is given, two codes are often necessary to code the service. Vaccine codes are used for the actual substances that are injected, and administration codes are assigned for administration of the substance (Fig. 10-4). The need for two codes to describe this one procedure can be likened to getting a car repaired. Let's say, for example, that a car needs new brakes. An auto repair shop will bill the owner for both the parts and labor for the repair. In the vaccine scenario, the parts component is the medication and the labor component is the administration of the vaccine.

Psychiatry subsection includes codes for outpatient and inpatient psychotherapy. Ophthalmology services range from examination for a specific eye problem to complete evaluation of the eyes. The medicine section also includes several different cardiology exams, such as electrocardiograms (ECGs), cardiac catheterizations, and echocardiography. Most subsections in the medicine section contain specific instructions related to that particular subsection, and, just like guidelines that are elsewhere in CPT, it is critical to be familiar with the content of the guidelines that pertain to the codes that are being selected.

CPT Appendices

Several appendices in the back of the CPT manual provide valuable information for the selection of CPT codes. It is important to be aware of the content of these appendices. This will help save time when coding and will improve the accuracy of code selection. Depending on the area of a coder's responsibility, one or more of the appendices may be frequently consulted when coding.

Appendix A–Modifiers. From time to time, procedures are performed under special circumstances. Perhaps a procedure was more complicated than usual, or maybe less was done in a surgical procedure. If special circumstances surround the patient's procedure, a **modifier** should be used with the CPT code to indicate the special circumstances. A modifier is used to communicate something different about the procedure or service that was provided. Modifiers are used with a CPT code and are included in box 24D on the CMS-1500 (see Fig. 12-1). Modifiers that are frequently used in each section are included in the section guidelines, and a complete listing of modifiers and their descriptions is located at the end of the manual in Appendix A. A quick list of modifiers is usually listed directly inside the front cover of the CPT manual.

Symbols

A series of symbols is used throughout the manual to alert the user to special considerations about certain codes. These symbols are used to identify codes that have changed since the previous edition, new codes, and codes that must be used with other codes. Meanings of symbols are found in the CPT introduction.

Special Considerations

When coding is performed for insurance claims, it is important that the current version of the CPT manual always be used. Each year, several codes change or are added or deleted. Codes are used from January 1 to December 31 of each year. If an out-of-date code is listed on an insurance claim, this will cause the insurance company to deny the claim and will lead to unnecessary delay in payment for health care services rendered.

CHECKPOINT

The office manager decides to not purchase a new edition of the CPT because there were not a lot of changes from the previous year. What impact, if any, would the office manager's decision have?

Procedure Coding—HCPCS Level II—National Codes

The second level of the HCPCS contains codes that are assigned for many different medical items and services billed by physician and nonphysician providers. HCPCS Level II codes are found in a different manual than CPT. Because HCPCS Level II codes are owned by the federal government, there may be different publishers of these manuals.

HCPCS Level II codes are used to bill for such items as:

- Medical supplies (e.g., dressings and bandages, walkers, crutches, pacemakers)
- Ambulance services
- Medications
- Medical equipment (e.g., wheelchairs)
- Vision and hearing supplies and services
- Nutrition counseling

Coding for HCPCS Level II supplies and services is done in much the same way as coding for Level I. The supply or service is located in the index and then is verified in the main section of the manual. Level II codes are easily distinguished from CPT codes in that Level II codes are alphanumerical—consisting of one letter followed by four numbers.

Medicare often requires use of HCPCS Level II codes instead of CPT codes. A listing of HCPCS II is available free online by searching for HCPCS II at www.cms.hhs.gov, or it may be purchased in one of many published manuals. If a manual is purchased, complete instructions will be available regarding specific symbols and other features that are used within that particular manual.

Modifiers

Just like CPT, HCPCS Level II uses modifiers to describe special circumstances that apply to a code assignment. Some Level II modifiers may be used in conjunction with HCPCS II or CPT codes to describe a specific part of the body (Box 10-1). Some insurance companies require that modifiers should be used to more specifically identify where on the patient's body procedures have been performed.

Table of Drugs

Occasionally, a patient will receive medications during an encounter with a health care provider. These medications may be administered in many different ways. The administration of injections can be coded with a CPT code from the Medicine section or HCPCS Level II code, but a HCPCS Level II code usually is used to identify the supply of the medication that was injected. So, when a patient receives an injection, two codes will be used to identify the procedure (similar to the previous vaccine example): an administration code and a supply code.

BOX 10-1

HCPCS Level II Modifiers for Description of Body Location

E1	Upper left, eyelid
E2	Lower left, eyelid
E3	Upper right, eyelid
E4	Lower right, eyelid
F1	Left hand, second digit
F2	Left hand, third digit
F3	Left hand, fourth digit
F4	Left hand, fifth digit
F5	Right hand, thumb
F6	Right hand, second digit
F7	Right hand, third digit
F8	Right hand, fourth digit
F9	Right hand, fifth digit
FA	Left hand, thumb
LC	Left circumflex coronary artery
LD	Left anterior descending coronary artery
LT	Left side (used to identify procedures performed on the left side of the body)
RC	Right coronary artery
RT	Right side (used to identify procedures performed on the right side of the body)
T1	Left foot, second digit
T2	Left foot, third digit
T3	Left foot, fourth digit
T4	Left foot, fifth digit
T5	Right foot, great toe
T6	Right foot, second digit
T7	Right foot, third digit
T8	Right foot, fourth digit
T9	Right foot, fifth digit
TA	Left foot, great toe

The Table of Drugs and Chemicals includes medications that may be given to patients. The table may include different entries depending on how the medication was administered to the patient or what strength of medication was used. The table includes an index, and it may be necessary to know the generic name of the drug because many entries within the table are listed by generic name. As with other sections of HCPCS II and CPT, you never should code directly from the index; instead, you will need to verify your selection in the numeric listing of codes.

Diagnosis Coding—*International Classification of Diseases*

Diagnosis coding in the medical office is done with a system of numerical codes called the *International Classification of Diseases* (ICD).

This diagnosis system is currently scheduled for a major update on October 1, 2014. Until that date, the *International Classification of Diseases, 9th Revision, Clinical Modification* (**ICD-9-CM** or **I-9**) will be used. After that date, the *International Classification of Diseases, 10th revision, Clinical Modification* (**ICD-10-CM** or **I-10**) will be required to be used.

The *International Classification of Diseases* coding system was developed and is maintained by the World Health Organization. The National Center for Healthcare Statistics, part of the U.S. Centers for Disease Control and Prevention, is responsible for the Clinical Modification (CM) of the ICD-9 system.

Diagnosis Coding—International Classification of Diseases, 9th Revision *(I-9)*

The I-9 system consists of numeric or alphanumeric codes that can consist of three, four, or five digits (numbers or a letter and numbers) depending on the nature of the code. The code length will be determined when the code is verified in the numeric listing of the I-9 manual. A coder must use all the digits specified for each code. Failure to use all required digits will mean a code is incorrect and will cause a claim to be rejected and any payments to be delayed. Diagnosis codes are listed in box 21 on the CMS-1500 (see Fig. 12-1).

Format of the ICD-9-CM Manual

The ICD-9-CM consists of the following three parts:

- Volume 1, Tabular List of Diseases—Numerical list of codes and their complete descriptions
- Volume 2, Index of Diseases—Alphabetical list of main terms and subterms used to locate diagnosis codes in the tabular list
- Volume 3, Index and Tabular List of Procedures—Alphabetical index of inpatient procedures and a numerical list of those procedures

When working in a medical office setting, Volumes 1 and 2 of the ICD-9-CM are used for coding the patient's diagnosis. Volume 3 is used for coding inpatient hospital procedures (services) provided by a facility. You will recall that a physician's professional services are coded with a CPT code. In the case of treatment provided for an inpatient, a CPT procedure code will be used to identify the procedure or service provided by the physician, an ICD procedure code (Volume 3) will be used to identify the facility services provided for that procedure or service, and an ICD diagnosis code (Volume 1) will identify the patient's diagnosis to be billed along with the CPT procedure code and the ICD procedure code.

Conventions Used in ICD-9-CM

Conventions are used throughout the ICD-9-CM manuals to point out special conditions related to codes. The ICD-9-CM codes are not copyrighted by any organization, so there are many different publishers of ICD-9-CM manuals. Depending on the publisher of an ICD-9-CM manual used in the medical office, conventions used in ICD-9-CM may appear differently. The purpose of the conventions, however, is the same in all of the manuals—to alert the coder to any special notations or conditions associated with selecting a particular code. A convention may be a symbol, such as a set of parentheses, or it may be an abbreviation, such as *NOS*.

A synopsis of some common conventions is shown in Figure 10-5. Each ICD-9-CM manual provides detailed instructions (usually at the beginning of the manual) to acquaint the user with specific conventions used in the particular code book. Instructions are almost always available in every coding manual, and anyone who performs coding should become completely familiar with the conventions and instructions for the manual that is being used.

Updates for ICD-9-CM

The ICD-9-CM is updated annually on October 1. Changes are available in the *Federal Register, Coding Clinic,* and *American Health Information Management Association Journal.* It is important to use an updated version of the ICD manual when coding, to ensure proper processing of claims. It is important to use the correct codes for the year in which the patient

ICD-9-CM Symbols and conventions with examples

NEC Not elsewhere classifiable. This category should be used only if the coder lacks the information to code to a more specific category.

Radiculitis (pressure) (vertebrogenic)
729.2
cervical NEC 723.4

NOS Not otherwise specified. The diagnosis cannot be found in another place.

723.4 Brachia neuritis or radiculitis NOS
Cervical radiculitis
Radicular syndrome of upper limbs

( ) Parentheses are used to include adjectives that may or may not be present in the diagnosis statement

Sprain, strain (joint) (ligament) (muscle)
(tendon) 848.9
abdominal wall (muscle) 848.8
Achilles tendon 845.09
acromioclavicular 840.0
ankle 845.00
and foot 845.00

[ ] Brackets are used to identify synonyms, substitute terms, or add information that clarifies the diagnosis statement.

524.60 Temporomandibular joint disorders, unspecified
Temporomandibular joint-pain-dysfunction
syndrome [TMJ]

Figure 10-5 These symbols and conventions alert an assistant to special conditions regarding a diagnosis code. They are the same for ICD-9-CM and ICD-10-CM.

encounter occurred. Failure to use codes for the correct year could result in rejection of an insurance claim, extra work for the office staff, and a delay in payment for services rendered.

Outpatient Guidelines

As was mentioned previously, emphasis in this text will be placed on coding that would be done in a medical office setting. Section IV of ICD-9-CM guidelines, Diagnostic Coding and Reporting Guidelines for Outpatient Services, provides the foundation for diagnosis coding instructions within this chapter. If a coder is working in an inpatient setting, different guidelines will apply to the coding of diagnoses for patients. If a question arises regarding how a specific diagnosis code is used, a coder should also consult the chapter specific guidelines for guidance on the proper use of a code.

Important highlights of the outpatient guidelines are described in the following subsections. Be sure to read the guidelines in the ICD-9-CM manual in their entirety.

Encounter/Visit. The terms **encounter** and **visit** can be used interchangeably. Both terms are used to refer to a meeting or contact with a health care provider, whether a physician or other nonphysician provider.

Selection of First-Listed Condition. The term **principal diagnosis** is not used in the outpatient setting. The term **first-listed diagnosis** is used instead. This term refers to the chief reason for the patient's encounter with the physician. If the patient has more than one diagnosis, additional codes for coexisting conditions can be listed after the first-listed diagnosis.

Symptoms and Signs and Uncertain Diagnoses. According to the *Miller-Keane Encyclopedia of Medicine, Nursing and Allied Health,* a sign is "any objective evidence of disease or dysfunction," and a symptom is "any indication of disease perceived by the patient." Sometimes a patient's diagnosis may not be known at the time of an encounter, and a symptom or sign can be listed as a diagnosis if the diagnosis is not confirmed (uncertain). For instance, if the patient comes in with a bad cough, lab tests could be done for pertussis (whooping cough). The diagnosis may be cough at the first visit, and if the lab test comes back positive, the diagnosis would be pertussis for a second visit. When coding in an outpatient setting, it is only possible to code what the provider knows at the time, and with the example above, whooping cough is not known at the first visit. Although it was suspected, it cannot be coded in an outpatient setting. A suspected condition, however, *can* be coded in an inpatient setting.

It is acceptable to code signs or symptoms for a patient's diagnosis if a more definitive diagnosis has not been established. However, if a diagnosis has been established, signs or symptoms that are common to that diagnosis are not coded. For example, if a patient's diagnosis is gastroenteritis, it is not necessary to code abdominal pain, as abdominal pain is a symptom associated with gastroenteritis.

Basics of Diagnosis Coding (ICD-9)

In the medical office setting, CPT assigns a numerical code to procedures, HCPCS II assigns an alphanumerical code to other procedures and services, and ICD-9-CM assigns a numerical code to a diagnosis. In coding for a patient encounter, Procedure 10-2 outlines the basic steps involved in selecting the correct diagnosis code. Review and apply the important points to remember in Box 10-2, and remember to apply the coding guidelines for outpatient coding when you are determining the correct diagnosis code.

Volume 2—The Index

Just like CPT, the ICD-9 manual has an index. As was mentioned previously, the index is Volume 2 of the manual, and this is always used first. The index should always be used to begin to locate a diagnosis code. Once a code is located in the index, the code is verified in the tabular (Volume 1) section of the manual. Coding directly from the index (without verifying the code in the tabular listing) can lead to coding errors.

Diagnosis codes are listed in the index under main terms, which can be an eponym (e.g., Alzheimer), a disease process (e.g., infection), a symptom or sign (e.g., fever), a condition (e.g., menopause), or an adjective (e.g., thrombotic). Anatomic sites usually are *not* main terms in ICD.

Once the main term is located in the index, any descriptive subterms should be located beneath the main term (Fig. 10-6). Such subterms can help narrow down the selection for the correct diagnosis code.

Table of Drugs and Chemicals

The Alphabetical Index to Poisoning and External Causes of Adverse Effects of Drugs and Other Chemical Substances, is also known as the Table of Drugs and Chemicals. This table

PROCEDURE 10-2

Assign Diagnosis Codes for a Patient's Encounter

Materials Needed

- Medical records
- ICD-9-CM or ICD-10 manual, current year's edition

1. Identify all diagnoses treated during a patient's encounter.
2. Determine the primary reason for the patient's office visit.
3. Locate the main term of the diagnosis in the index (Volume II).
4. Locate any modifiers beneath the main term.
5. Identify the numerical code referenced in Volume II.
6. Locate the code from Volume II in the tabular (numerical) listing (Volume I) in the manual.
7. Read the description of the code. Determine whether the code fits the diagnosis given for the patient.*
8. Code any additional diagnoses listed in the patient's encounter by repeating steps 3 through 7.

**Denotes a crucial step in the procedure. The student must complete this step satisfactorily in order to complete the procedure satisfactorily.*

BOX 10-2

Important Points to Remember When Performing Diagnosis Coding

1. Always use both the index and the tabular. Never code directly from the index.
2. If possible, locate each term in the diagnosis in the index. This will ensure more accurate code selection. For example, if the patient's diagnosis is chronic suppurative otitis media, you could find the diagnosis under the main term *otitis* and then locate *media,* then *chronic,* then *suppurative* within the index.
3. As was mentioned earlier, signs and symptoms can be coded if the patient has an ill-defined condition, and the physician cannot arrive at a diagnosis. However, if a diagnosis is established, signs and symptoms that are a regular part of the diagnosis are not coded. For example, if the patient's diagnosis is myocardial infarction, chest pain should not be coded because chest pain is an associated symptom of a heart attack.
4. If a patient has symptoms that are not normally associated with a condition, those symptoms can be coded. For example, if the patient's diagnosis is ankle sprain and the patient has a cough that is treated, the cough also should be coded because this is not normally associated with an ankle sprain.
5. Sometimes it is necessary to use more than one code to accurately describe a diagnosis. For example, a urinary tract infection should be coded along with the organism that caused the infection, if that organism is known.
6. Sometimes two diagnoses can be coded with only one code. For example, attention deficit disorder with hyperactivity can be coded with one code.

Be as specific as possible when coding. Code all adjectives or descriptors of a diagnosis that are listed in a patient's record.

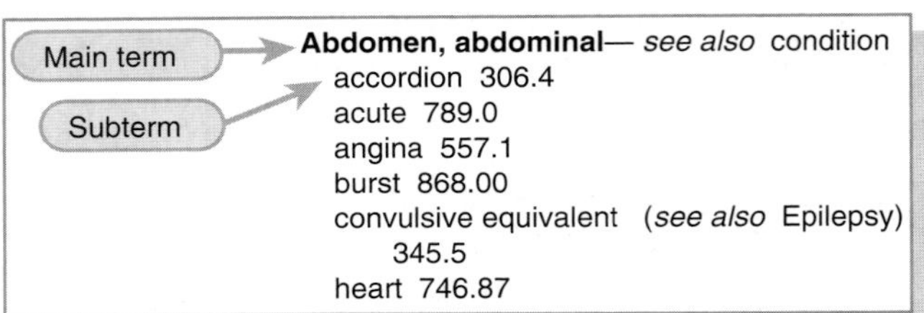

Figure 10-6 Main terms appear in bold type. Subterms are indented beneath the main term. (Modified from Buck CJ. *2013 ICD-9-CM for Hospitals, Volumes 1, 2 & 3, Professional Edition.* St. Louis: Saunders; 2013.)

provides information on codes for injury due to a drug or other potentially hazardous substances such as lighter fluid, gasoline, window cleaner, or even water. If a patient ingests such a substance or experiences an adverse event caused by exposure to that substance, a poisoning code and an E code (explained later in this chapter) can be found in the table to describe the event. Remember, the table is an index, and a coder should never code directly from an index. Always verify the code selection in the tabular portion of the manual.

Volume 1—Tabular Listing

The Tabular listing of ICD-9 (Volume 1) contains the numerical listing of all diagnosis codes. The volume contains 17 chapters and is largely organized by body systems. A listing of the chapters is located in Figure 10-7. When coding, it is important to always first consult the alphabetic index (Volume 2) and then locate the code(s) within the tabular list (Volume 1). Coding only from the tabular or the index can lead to costly mistakes in coding.

Late Effects

A late effect is something that happens to a patient after the acute phase of disease or injury has passed. Late effects can happen relatively quickly after the acute phase or may not appear until years later. There is no set time for a late effect to occur. What happens as the result of a late effect is known as a residual. An example of a late effect and residual is when a patient sustains a leg fracture and a few years later develops arthritis at the old fracture site; the residual is arthritis, and it is the late effect of the fracture. The residual code would be listed first and the late effect code would be listed second.

V Codes

Sometimes a patient may have an encounter with a physician without having any physical complaints. This type of service may be coded with a V code, which is included in the ICD-9-CM chapter titled "Classification of Factors Influencing Health Status and Contact with Health Service." V codes are located within the main index and are listed under main terms that describe the reason for the encounter (Box 10-3). The V code tabular section of the manual contains the descriptions of V codes. V codes can be used to identify encounters such as physical examinations, screenings for disease, immunizations, and follow-up or aftercare for specific injuries or diseases and many other health conditions. For example, a patient may see a physician for a routine physical examination. In this case, the code would be V70.0.

E Codes

This chapter, titled "Supplementary Classification of External Causes of Injury and Poisoning," is used to identify circumstances surrounding an injury event. Not all facilities collect E codes; in fact, many outpatient settings do not. E codes are used primarily by inpatient facilities. However, it is important to know how to use these codes should they be required by an institution in which you work.

ICD-9-CM Chapter	Chapter Contents	Code Range
1	Infectious And Parasitic Diseases	001-139
2	Neoplasms	140-239
3	Endocrine, Nutritional And Metabolic Diseases, And Immunity Disorders	240-279
4	Diseases Of The Blood And Blood-Forming Organs	280-289
5	Mental Disorders	290-319
6	Diseases Of The Nervous System And Sense Organs	320-389
7	Diseases Of The Circulatory System	390-459
8	Diseases Of The Respiratory System	460-519
9	Diseases Of The Digestive System	520-579
10	Diseases Of The Genitourinary System	580-629
11	Complications Of Pregnancy, Childbirth, And The Puerperium	630-679
12	Diseases Of The Skin And Subcutaneous Tissue	680-709
13	Diseases Of The Musculoskeletal System And Connective Tissue	710-739
14	Congenital Anomalies	740-759
15	Certain Conditions Originating In The Perinatal Period	760-779
16	Symptoms, Signs, And Ill-Defined Conditions	780-799
17	Injury And Poisoning	800-999
18	Supplementary Classification of Factors Influencing Health Status And Contact With Health Services	V01-V91
19	External Causes Of Morbidity	E000-E999

Figure 10-7 ICD-9-CM Table of Contents. (Centers for Disease Control & Prevention. ftp://ftp.cdc.gov/pub/Health_Statistics/NCHS/Publications/ICD9-CM/2011/Prefac12.rtf. Accessed October 15, 2013.)

BOX 10-3

Common Main Terms for V Codes

Absence
Contact with
Contraceptive, contraception
Examination
Exposure to
History, family
History, personal
Immunization
Screening
Status (post)
Vaccination

E codes are used to described the what, where, and how of an injury. For example, if a patient fractures a leg while falling down the stairs in his home, this case could be coded with three ICD-9-CM codes: one code for the leg fracture and two E codes—one for the fall down the stairs and another for an injury in the home.

Collection of E codes helps to provide data for injury-related research and can be used on outpatient or inpatient claims. E codes, though, are meant only to provide additional information and can never be used as the first-listed or principal diagnosis for a patient.

Volume 3—Procedures

As was mentioned previously, Volume 3 contains the index and the tabular list for procedures. This is used to code a facility's portion of a procedure or service that has been provided. It cannot be used in place of CPT because CPT codes are used to identify a physician's professional service that has been provided.

Diagnosis Coding—International Classification of Diseases, 10th Revision, Clinical Modification (ICD-10-CM)

Beginning October 1, 2014, diagnosis codes in the ICD-10-CM must be used to code diagnoses. The ICD-10 is derived from the official version of the *International Classification of Diseases*, developed by the World Health Organization. The National Center for Health Statistics is responsible for the maintenance of the U.S. Version of ICD-10 codes known as the ICD-10-CM or I-10.

A major difference between I-9 and I-10 is that there is no procedure coding system in ICD-10. Because I-10 does not include procedure codes for facility billing, the CMS is responsible for developing the procedure coding system, which is known as ICD-10-PCS (procedure coding system).

Format of the ICD-10-CM Manual

The ICD-10-CM consists of the following two parts:

- Volume 1, Tabular List of Diseases (in numerical order)
- Volume 2, Index of Diseases (in alphabetical order)

Just like ICD-9, Volumes 1 and 2 of the ICD-10-CM (Fig. 10-8) are used for coding a patient's diagnosis for encounters in health care facilities such as medical offices, nursing homes, hospitals, etc.

Coding with I-10 is not difficult. If a coder has previous experience with I-9, the ideas behind diagnosis coding are pretty much the same—it is important to consult both the index and the tabular list when coding and to code a diagnosis to the greatest level of specificity, which means it is important to code all of the components of a patient's diagnosis.

The structure of I-10 includes categories, subcategories, and codes. They are defined as follows:

Category—A category consists of three characters. A character can be a number or a letter.

Subcategory—A subcategory can be either four or five characters. Each sublevel after a category is a subcategory.

Code—A code can be three to seven characters. A code is the final level of coding.

A difference between the I-9 and I-10 systems is that a placeholder character is used in the I-10 system. The placeholder character is an "x" and does exactly that—it marks a place where another character is not required, but a subsequent character is. For example, the code for other specified disorders of the left ear is H93.8x2.

Conventions Used in ICD-10

Conventions are used throughout the ICD-10 manuals as well to point out special conditions related to codes. The purpose of the conventions is the same also—to alert the coder to any special notations or conditions associated with selecting a particular code. Many of the conventions are the same for I-10 as they are for I-9.

ICD-10-CM Chapter	Chapter Contents	Code Range
1	Certain infectious and parasitic diseases	A00-B99
2	Neoplasms	C00-D49
3	Diseases of the blood and blood-forming organs and certain disorders involving the immune mechanism	D50-D89
4	Endocrine, nutritional, and metabolic diseases	E00-E89
5	Mental, Behavioral, and Neurodevelopmental disorders	F01-F99
6	Diseases of the nervous system	G00-G99
7	Diseases of the eye and adnexa	H00-H59
8	Diseases of the ear and mastoid process	H60-H95
9	Diseases of the circulatory system	I00-I99
10	Diseases of the respiratory system	J00-J99
11	Diseases of the digestive system	K00-K95
12	Diseases of the skin and subcutaneous tissue	L00-L99
13	Diseases of the musculoskeletal system and connective tissue	M00-M99
14	Diseases of the genitourinary system	N00-N99
15	Pregnancy, childbirth, and the puerperium	O00-O9A
16	Certain conditions originating in the perinatal period	P00-P96
17	Congenital malformations, deformations, and chromosomal abnormalities	Q00-Q99
18	Symptoms, signs, and abnormal clinical and laboratory findings, not elsewhere classified	R00-R99
19	Injury, poisoning, and certain other consequences of external causes	S00-T88
20	External causes of morbidity	V00-Y99
21	Factors influencing health status and contact with health services	Z00-Z99

Figure 10-8 ICD-10-CM Table of Contents. (Centers for Disease Control & Prevention. www.cdc.gov/nchs/icd/icd10cm.htm. Accessed October 15, 2013.)

Many of the common conventions are described in Figure 10-5. There are several conventions that are the same between I-9 and I-10. Each ICD-10 manual provides detailed instructions (usually at the beginning of the manual) for all conventions used in that manual.

Outpatient Guidelines

Section IV of the guidelines is still the location for definitive instructions for proper coding of the diagnoses in an outpatient setting.

Important new highlights of the I-10 outpatient guidelines are described below. When coding in I-10, be sure to read the new guidelines in their entirety. The I-9 guidelines pertaining to selection of the first-listed condition, signs and symptoms, uncertain diagnoses are essentially unchanged in I-10.

Level of Detail in Coding

ICD-10-CM codes can be anywhere from three to seven characters long. A code must contain the complete number of characters required for that code to be a valid code. For example, if seven characters are required, seven characters must be used.

Laterality

The I-10 system is quite a bit more specific, in that a location, such as right or left side, can be identified with a unique diagnosis code. This is known as **laterality**. Some codes have a right, left, or bilateral distinction. If a location is not specified in the patient's medical record, a code for an unspecified side should be used.

Basics of Diagnosis Coding with ICD-10-CM

Coding with I-10 is very much the same as coding with I-9. When coding a patient's diagnosis, the main term of the diagnosis is first located in the alphabetic index and any modifiers (adjectives) pertaining to the diagnosis are accounted for in the index as well. Then the code obtained from the index is verified in the tabular. The index and tabular must be used; otherwise, coding errors are likely to happen if this is not done.

Volume 1—Tabular Listing

The Tabular listing of ICD-10 (Volume 2) contains the numerical listing of all diagnosis codes. The volume contains 21 chapters and is largely organized by body systems. A listing of the chapters is located in Figure 10-8. When coding, it is important to first consult the alphabetic index (Volume 2) and then locate the code(s) within the tabular. Coding directly from the tabular list can lead to mistakes in coding.

V, W, X, and Y Codes—Chapter 20 of I-10 Tabular

This chapter, titled "External Causes of Morbidity" is used to identify circumstances surrounding an injury event. The codes from this chapter are secondary diagnosis codes; they cannot be used as a first-listed diagnosis. These codes can be used when coding in any health care facility.

If a patient has sustained an injury, it is acceptable to assign multiple external cause codes in order to fully describe the injury.

Z Codes—Chapter 21 of I-10 Tabular

Sometimes a patient may have an encounter with a physician without having any physical complaints. This type of service may be coded with a Z code, which is included in the ICD-10-CM chapter titled "Factors Influencing Health Status and Contact with Health Services." The main terms for Z codes are located in the main alphabetic index (Volume 2).

Codes from the Z section of the manual are used to describe circumstances other than illness or injury. Z codes are used to identify encounters such as physical examinations, screenings for disease, immunizations, and follow-up or aftercare for specific injuries or diseases and many other health conditions. For example, a patient may see a physician for a routine physical examination. In this case, the code would be Z00.00.

Z codes can be used for coding in any type of health care facility. Most Z codes can either be used as a first-listed diagnosis or as a secondary diagnosis.

Legal and Ethical Issues in Coding

Ethics

When performing both procedure and diagnosis coding, it is important never to "overcode" or code something that did not occur. Knowingly and willingly performing such an act constitutes fraud and results in severe legal penalties. Third-party payers routinely audit medical records to validate codes. Documentation from a patient's medical record must be able to support all codes used in billing for any patient encounter.

Ethical issues can frequently arise in relation to medical billing practices. What is important to remember is that the only services that can be billed are those that are documented in the patient's record and that documentation must fully support the procedure and diagnosis code selection for the patient's visit.

The **American Academy of Professional Coders (AAPC),** the largest certifying organization in the United States, has established a Code of Ethics for medical coders (Fig. 10-9). Members of the American Academy of Professional Coders (AAPC) are expected to follow this code, and members are encouraged to report members who violate this code.

Accurate, complete, and thorough coding is a vital component to the overall financial health of an organization. Errors in coding can mean lost revenue because charges are missed or incorrect. Errors in coding can also be costly because hefty fines may be assessed for coding errors.

Compliance

The term *compliance* is used often in medical offices today. Briefly, compliance involves making sure that federal, state, and local requirements pertaining to health insurance or

AAPC Code of Ethics

Commitment to ethical professional conduct is expected of every AAPC member. The specification of a Code of Ethics enables AAPC to clarify to current and future members, and to those served by members, the nature of the ethical responsibilities held in common by its members. This document establishes principles that define the ethical behavior of AAPC members. All AAPC members are required to adhere to the Code of Ethics and the Code of Ethics will serve as the basis for processing ethical complaints initiated against AAPC members.

AAPC members shall:

- Maintain and enhance the dignity, status, integrity, competence, and standards of our profession.
- Respect the privacy of others and honor confidentiality
- Strive to achieve the highest quality, effectiveness, and dignity in both the process and products of professional work.
- Advance the profession through continued professional development and education by acquiring and maintaining professional competence.
- Know and respect existing federal, state and local laws, regulations, certifications, and licensing requirements applicable to professional work.
- Use only legal and ethical principles that reflect the profession's core values and report activity that is perceived to violate this Code of Ethics to the AAPC Ethics Committee.
- Accurately represent the credential(s) earned and the status of AAPC membership.
- Avoid actions and circumstances that may appear to compromise good business judgment or create a conflict between personal and professional interests.

Adherence to these standards assures public confidence in the integrity and service of medical coding, auditing, compliance and practice management professionals who are AAPC members.

Failure to adhere to these standards, as determined by AAPC's Ethics Committee, may result in the loss of credentials and membership with AAPC.

Figure 10-9 American Academy of Professional Coders (AAPC) Code of Medical Ethics. (American Academy of Professional Coders. http://www.aapc.com/aboutus/code-of-ethics.aspx accessed October 24, 2013.

benefits programs (such as Medicare or Medicaid) are being followed. Compliance programs ensure that this happens. As was mentioned in Box 9-4, Medicare has specific documentation guidelines that were established in 1995, and those guidelines are still in use today. Not only is documentation critical in providing quality patient care, but documentation is necessary to determine whether a procedure is medically necessary. Complete documentation of a patient's history, examination, and diagnosis will prove the medical necessity of a procedure.

When codes are submitted, the coder is ensuring that the code that was billed represents what actually happened. The circumstances of the procedure must be detailed enough to support the code choice that was made. If not, consequences can be serious. Large fines and even incarceration may apply to individuals who knowingly and willingly submit claims for payment that cannot be documented.

The Coding Profession

Help is always available for anyone responsible for coding in the medical office. Many products are published that provide detailed examples, illustrations, and explanations of codes. As was mentioned previously, there is much to know about coding. An educational program of which coding is a key component may provide several courses for procedure and diagnosis coding and insurance claims processing.

Examinations are available for individuals who wish to become certified coders. Some coding certifications require completion of specific training or work experience before a person is allowed to take a certification examination. Attainment of a coding certification demonstrates proficiency in coding and may be required by some employers who hire coders.

Currently, many different types of coding certifications are available. Two national organizations are primarily involved with the certification of coders: the AAPC and the American Health Information Management Association (AHIMA).

The AAPC awards many coding-related certifications: the **Certified Professional Coder (CDC),** the **Certified Professional Coder–Hospital (CPC-H)** the **Certified**

Professional Coder–Payer (CPC-P), and many specialty credentials. The AHIMA awards the Certified Coding Specialist (CCS) and the Certified Coding Specialist–Physician-Based (CCS-P). Certifications of both organizations are recognized by most employers who seek coding personnel.

SUMMARY

Medical coding uses widely recognized systems of codes to categorize procedures that are provided for patients and their associated diagnoses. Coding is an integral part of the billing process. Accurate and complete coding is a vital component to the overall financial health of any health care organization.

YOU ARE THE MEDICAL ADMINISTRATIVE ASSISTANT

Picture yourself as a medical administrative assistant in a medical practice. What would you do in the following situations?

1. Another medical administrative assistant has coded an encounter incorrectly. The final cost appears to be the same, but you know that the form reflects the incorrect diagnosis coding. Why is it important to correct this mistake?
2. Your office has a particular patient who comes in every 3 months. The patient routinely has several examinations or procedures. You notice that for every visit only one of these procedures is recorded. As a member of the AAPC what are you expected to do?

REVIEW EXERCISES

Exercise 10-1 True or False

Read each statement, and determine whether the statement is true or false. Record the answer in the blank provided. T = true; F = false.

____1. A patient may be charged for only one procedure per office visit.

____2. The CPT coding system assigns a numerical code to every procedure performed in the medical office.

____3. A patient's medical record serves as documentation of procedures charged to the patient.

____4. Coding is used for insurance billings in hospitals and in physicians' offices.

____5. If a patient sees a family practice physician at Happy Valley Medical Group and he saw another family practice physician at the same group practice last year, according to CPT, the patient would be a new patient.

____6. It is appropriate to code directly from the Table of Drugs in HCPCS II.

____7. Documentation in a patient's record is needed to prove the medical necessity of a billed procedure.

____8. To make coding faster, it is acceptable to code directly from an index.

____9. ICD-10 goes in to effect on October 1, 2014. After that time it will be acceptable to use ICD-9 or ICD-10.

Exercise 10-2 Chapter Concepts

Read the statement or question, and determine the answer that best fits. Record the answer in the blank provided.

______ 1. "ICD" as in ICD-9-CM stands for
(a) Information on Clinical Disorders
(b) International Classification of Disease
(c) Internal Coding of Diagnosis
(d) International Coding of Disorders

______ 2. The volume of the ICD-9-CM manual that is listed in numerical order is
(a) Volume I
(b) Volume II
(c) Volume III
(d) Volume IV

______ 3. ICD-10 codes that are used for coding routine physical examinations:
(a) V codes
(b) E codes
(c) Y codes
(d) Z codes

______ 4. ICD convention that also means "or":
(a) excludes
(b) see
(c) and
(d) NOS

______ 5. Something that happens to a patient after the acute phase of the disease or injury has passed:
(a) symptom
(b) late effect
(c) modifier
(d) guideline

______ 6. ICD-10 placeholder character:
(a) #
(b) X
(c) ^
(d) None of the above

______ 7. CPT stands for
(a) Correct Procedure Terminology
(b) Current Practice Terminology
(c) Correct Procedure Transactions
(d) Current Procedural Terminology

Exercise 10-3 Procedure Coding Concepts

Using the correct edition of the CPT manual, identify the section of the CPT manual in which the following codes are located. Record the answer in the blank provided.

(a) Anesthesia
(b) Surgery
(c) Radiology
(d) Pathology and Laboratory
(e) Medicine
(f) Evaluation and Management

______ 1. 80050

______ 2. 29819

______ 3. 99301

______ 4. 93000

_______ 5. 71020

_______ 6. 01382

_______ 7. 99213

_______ 8. 73721

_______ 9. 80100

_______ 10. 90636

Read the statements below, and determine whether each statement is true or false regarding CPT. Record the answer in the blank provided.

_____11. In coding wound repair, the lengths of two or more lacerations from the same area and of the same repair may be added together.

_____12. A panel is a series of blood tests that are commonly ordered together.

_____13. To code a lesion removal, it is not necessary to know the pathology of the lesion that has been removed.

_____14. The three key components in determining the level of E&M service are history, examination, and medical decision making.

_____15. It is possible to locate procedures in the CPT index under more than one main term.

_____16. The HCPCS system consists of four levels of codes.

_____17. The entire HCPCS system is copyrighted by the AMA.

_____18. Fracture care includes application and removal of the first cast.

_____19. A rest home is the same as a nursing home.

_____20. Local anesthesia is included in the surgical package.

_____21. A patient who has not been to a medical facility in 7 years may be charged for a new patient visit.

Exercise 10-4 Procedure Coding

Identify the correct CPT code for the following professional services, using the steps given in Procedure 10-1. Underline the main term found in the index and record the answer in the blank provided.

22. Emergency department visit, detailed history and physical examination, medical decision making moderate complexity.

 ____

23. Tubal ligation_______________
24. Removal of 10 skin tags_______________
25. Chest x-ray, complete, four views_______________
26. I&D foot bursa_______________
27. Excision of thyroid gland due to a malignant lesion_______________
28. Repair of a strangulated umbilical hernia; patient is 3 years old_______________
29. Office visit, established patient, comprehensive history and physical examination_______________
30. Total bilirubin_______________
31. Obstetric panel_______________
32. Prothrombin time_______________
33. Simple excision of nasal polyp_______________
34. Routine obstetric care with antepartum and postpartum care with a vaginal delivery_______________
35. Repair of three superficial lacerations (wounds) of the cheek—1 cm, 2 cm, 3 cm_______________
36. Uncomplicated treatment of three rib fractures_______________

Exercise 10-5 HCPCS II Coding Concepts

Read the statements below, and determine whether each statement is true or false regarding HCPCS II. Record the answer in the blank provided.

____1. Some HCPCS II modifiers can be used with CPT codes.

____2. An HCPCS II code from the Table of Drugs is used to identify the administration of a substance.

____3. HCPCS II codes are used to bill for supplies and nonphysician services.

____4. HCPCS II codes consist of five numbers.

Exercise 10-6 HCPCS II Coding

Using a current edition of the HCPCS II manual, locate the procedure code for the following supplies/services, following the steps given in Procedure 10-1. Underline the main term found in the index, and record the correct answers in the blanks provided.

5. Portable whirlpool______________

6. Pair of metal forearm crutches with tips and handgrips______________

7. Raised toilet seat______________

8. Aminophylline 250 mg injection (supply only) ______________

9. Ativan 2 mg injection (supply only) ______________

10. Flexible nonadjustable cervical foam collar ______________

11. Standard reusable bed pan______________

12. Nebulizer with compressor______________

13. Heavy duty wheelchair with fixed full-length arms, elevating leg rests______________

14. TENS unit, four leads______________

15. Adjustable height folding walker______________

Exercise 10-7 I-9 Diagnosis Coding Concepts

Read the statements below, and determine whether each statement is true or false regarding ICD-9-CM. Record the answer in the blank provided.

____ 1. Volumes 1 and 2 are used to code diagnoses in an outpatient setting.

____ 2. A diagnosis code should support the procedure code that was selected.

____ 3. Conventions are used to identify special instructions or conditions.

____ 4. *Encounter* and *visit* are synonymous.

____ 5. A sign can be observed by a physician.

____ 6. E codes are used for every patient treated for an injury in an outpatient setting.

____ 7. There is no set time limit for a late effect to appear.

____ 8. The Table of Drugs and Chemicals is used to identify the codes associated with poison from an ingested substance.

____ 9. If five digits are listed for a diagnosis code, you may omit the last two digits to make coding easier.

____ 10. The correct code for an infant born with a goiter is 240.9.

____ 11. The correct code for pneumonia is 486.

____ 12. The correct code for congestive pneumonia is 486.

Exercise 10-8 I-10 Diagnosis Coding Concepts

Read the statements below, and determine whether each statement is true or false regarding ICD-9-CM. Record the answer in the blank provided.

_____1. Volume 2 is the volume that is in numerical order.

_____2. It is possible for a three-character code to be a valid code.

_____3. All ICD-10 conventions are new.

_____4. ICD-10 is copyrighted by the AMA.

_____5. Laterality refers to coding a diagnosis to the highest level of specificity.

_____6. An ICD-10 code can be anywhere from 3 to 7 characters in length.

_____7. Overcoding means assigning a code for which there is no documentation in the patient's record.

Exercise 10-10 I-9 and I-10 Diagnosis Coding

Using the most current editions of the ICD-9-CM and ICD-10-CM manuals, locate the diagnosis codes for the following diagnoses using the steps given in Procedure 10-2. Underline the main term found in the index, and record the correct answers in the blanks provided.

	I-9 code	I-10 code
1. Menometrorrhagia	________	________
2. Pharyngitis	________	________
3. Upper respiratory infection	________	________
4. Closed fracture of three ribs	________	________
5. Dupuytren's contracture	________	________
6. Carpal tunnel syndrome	________	________
7. Psoriasis	________	________
8. Physical examination for participation in sports competition	________	________
9. Localized atopic eczema	________	________
10. Varicose veins	________	________
11. Loose body in right knee	________	________
12. Benign hypertension	________	________
13. Partially torn medial meniscus	________	________
14. Morton's neuroma	________	________
15. Chronic cholecystitis with cholelithiasis	________	________
16. Allergic rhinitis	________	________
17. Chest pain	________	________
18. Fatigue	________	________

ACTIVITIES

ACTIVITY 10-1 ENTER DIAGNOSIS CODES IN MEDISOFT

Using the diagnosis codes in table below, update the diagnosis code list in Medisoft. Enter all of the diagnosis codes given. (Once I-9 codes are obsolete, there is no need to enter those codes.)

1. Open Medisoft and click **Lists>Diagnosis Codes.** Verify that the code to be added is not on the list. In the **Field** box, select **Code 1.** In the **Search for** box, begin typing the diagnosis code to search for the code on the list. (If the code is on the list, it can be edited to update the description and amount if necessary.)
2. Click **New.** In the **Code 1** field, enter the diagnosis code exactly as it appears on the list.
3. In the **Description** field, enter the complete description for the code.
4. Leave **Code 2** and **3** blank. (Codes 2 and 3 will automatically be filled in when the code is saved.)
5. Click **Save.** (If a mistake is made while entering a code number and the mistake is saved, the code will need to be deleted. Code 1 cannot be changed once it is saved.)

I-9 code	I-9 description
V70.0	Routine general medical examination at a health care facility
V72.84	Preoperative examination, unspecified
052.9	Varicella without mention of complication
311	Depressive disorder, not elsewhere classified
346.90	Migraine, unspecified
382.9	Unspecified otitis media
401.9	Unspecified essential hypertension
464.00	Acute laryngitis without mention of obstruction
473.9	Unspecified sinusitis (chronic)
487.1	Influenza with other respiratory manifestations
490	Bronchitis, not specified as acute or chronic
626.2	Menorrhagia
703.0	Ingrowing nail
708.9	Urticaria, unspecified
723.1	Cervicalgia
724.2	Low back pain
780.60	Fever, unspecified
816.00	Closed fracture of phalanx, hand
883.0	Open wound of finger(s), without mention of complication

I-10 code	I-10 description
B01.9	Varicella without complication
F32.9	Major depressive disorder, single episode, unspecified
G43.909	Migraine, unspecified, not intractable without status migrainosus
H66.90	Otitis media, unspecified, unspecified ear
I10	Essential (primary) hypertension
J04.0	Acute laryngitis
J10.1	Influenza due to other identified influenza virus with other respiratory manifestations
J32.9	Chronic sinusitis, unspecified
J40	Bronchitis not specified as acute or chronic
L50.9	Urticaria, unspecified
L60.0	Ingrowing nail
M54.2	Cervicalgia
M54.5	Low back pain
N92.0	Excessive and frequent menstruation with regular cycle
R50.9	Fever, unspecified
S61.209A	Unspecified open wound of unspecified finger without damage to nail, initial encounter
S62.609A	Fracture of unspecified phalanx of unspecified finger, initial encounter for closed fx
Z00.00	Encounter for general adult medical examination without abnormal findings
Z01.818	Encounter for other preprocedural examination

ACTIVITY 10-2 ENTER PROCEDURE CODES IN MEDISOFT

Using the procedure codes in table below, update the procedure code list in Medisoft.

1. Open Medisoft and click **Lists>Procedure/Payment/ Adjustment Codes.** Verify that the code to be added is not on the list. In the **Field** box, select **Code 1.** In the **Search for** box, begin typing the procedure code to search for the code on the list. (If the code is on the list, it can be edited to update the description and amount if necessary.)
2. Click **New.** In the **General** tab in the **Code 1** field, enter the procedure code exactly as it appears on the list.
3. In the **Description** field, enter the complete description as listed for the code.
4. In the **Code type** field, **procedure charge** should be selected.
5. In the **Amounts** tab, enter the amount for the procedure in field **A.**
6. Click **Save.** (If a mistake is made while entering a code number and the mistake is saved, the code will need to be deleted. Code 1 cannot be changed once it is saved.)

CPT code	CPT description	Amount
A4550	Surgical tray	$15
12001	Simple wound rep, 2.5 cm	$143
26720	Closed tx phal shaft fx	$178
71020	Chest x-ray, 2 views, frontal & lateral	$53
98940	Chiro tx spinal 1-2 regions	$35
99070	Misc supplies	$12
99212	Office visit, est pt, level II	$40
99213	Office visit, est pt, level III	$60
99396	Well exam 40-64 yr	$130

Bibliography

American Academy of Professional Coders: www.aapc.com. Accessed November 27, 2012.

American Health Information Management Association: www.ahima.org. Accessed November 27, 2012.

American Medical Association: *Current Procedural Terminology*, Chicago, American Medical Association, 2012.

Buck CJ: *Step-By-Step Medical Coding*, St Louis, Elsevier, 2013.

Centers for Medicaid and Medicare Services: www.cms.hhs.gov. Accessed November 23, 2012.

World Health Organization: *International Classification of Diseases Information Sheet*. www.who.int Accessed November 19, 2012.

CHAPTER 11 Medical Billing

LEARNING OUTCOMES

On successful completion of this chapter, the student will be able to

1. Explain the steps of the billing process.
2. Explain the basic components of the billing process.
3. Explain features of a medical office computerized accounting system.
4. Identify appropriate procedures for granting credit.
5. Explain appropriate procedures for pursuing collection of accounts.
6. Describe cycle billing and accounts receivable aging.
7. Identify legal and ethical concepts and issues pertaining to billing and collection practices.

COMMISSION ON ACCREDITATION OF ALLIED HEALTH EDUCATION PROGRAMS (CAAHEP) CORE CURRICULUM FOR MEDICAL ASSISTANTS

- Use Internet to access information related to the medical office
- Perform accounts receivable procedures including
  - Post entries on a daysheet
  - Perform billing procedures
  - Perform collection procedures
- Explain both billing and payment options
- Identify procedure for preparing patient accounts
- Discuss procedures for collecting outstanding accounts
- Describe the impact of both the Fair Debt Collection Act and the Federal Truth in Lending Act of 1968 as they apply to collections
- Discuss types of adjustments that may be made to a patient's account
- Use computerized office billing systems
- Describe the implications of HIPAA for the medical assistant in various medical settings
- Respond to issues of confidentiality

ACCREDITING BUREAU OF HEALTH EDUCATION SCHOOLS (ABHES) COMPETENCIES FOR MEDICAL ASSISTING

Graduates

- Demonstrate professionalism by maintaining confidentiality at all times
- Perform billing and collection procedures
- Apply electronic technology
- Apply computer concepts for office procedures
- Comply with federal, state, and local health laws and regulations

VOCABULARY

aging
arrival
assignment of benefits
charge slip
copayment
cycle billing
diagnosis
dun
dunning messages
encounter form
Equal Credit Opportunity Act (ECOA)
Fair Debt Collection Practices Act
fee schedule
fee slip
fee splitting
fraud
service record
superbill
unbundling
upcoding

Compassion, precision, and meticulousness are expected from the medical staff when a patient receives medical care; these same qualities are expected of the entire office staff in everything they do. Great care must be taken as well when charges and payments are processed in the medical office. Patients' accounts must be kept up-to-date at all times, and charges, payments, and other adjustments made to those accounts must be accurate.

Many components make up the billing process, and an assistant must stay current on the constant changes that affect medical billing. An assistant who is thoroughly trained in billing processes is a tremendous asset to a medical office.

The Billing Process

When someone hears the term *billing process*, all that may come to mind is a slip of paper on which charges are written. The billing process is far more than a slip of paper, however. The billing process actually begins at registration and ends after every charge has been paid and includes many steps in between. Depending on the size of the practice, a medical administrative assistant may be responsible for the entire billing process or may perform only specific parts, with other parts being performed by coworkers in different departments. Even if an assistant is not responsible for the entire process, a basic understanding of the entire process will enable an assistant to help patients who have questions about their medical bills.

One of the most critical parts of the billing process takes place before the physician ever sees a patient. This critical part is the point at which a patient enters the medical office and arrives for an appointment. At this point, vital information, such as the patient's address, telephone number, and insurance company information, is gathered from the patient. Recording this information correctly is absolutely essential for billing the patient and filing insurance claims. Also, if a question should ever arise regarding the patient's bill, this information will be needed to reach the patient or the person responsible for the bill.

Registration

On entering a medical office, a patient stops at the front desk to check in or register for an appointment. This time is often referred to as an **arrival.** If a patient is new to the office, registration is the time at which the following information is obtained from the patient:

- Patient's complete name and current address
- Patient's date of birth
- Patient's home phone number
- Patient's employer's name, address, and telephone number
- Guarantor information—complete name, address, and telephone number of party responsible for payment of account
- Insurance company name and address and policy number

This information may be obtained through a verbal interview with the patient at the registration desk or by asking the patient to complete a registration form (see Fig. 8-2) that contains the information needed for the registration process. The office may even elect to mail a registration form to a new patient to allow the patient to complete the form and return the form by mail ahead of time.

If a patient is an established (returning) patient to the practice, vital billing information, such as name, address, telephone number, and insurance company information, is verified at the time of registration to be sure the office has correct information for billing.

Why is registration such an important part of the billing process? The information collected at this point is the information that will be used to generate the patient's bill and monthly statement and any related insurance claims. Even one error at this point could mean that a statement does not reach the patient, or that an insurance claim is filed incorrectly. Such billing delays can be frustrating to the patient and the physician, can create extra work for the office staff, and can cause delays in receipt of payment for services rendered by physicians in the medical office.

When the patient registers, an assistant may be required to collect a **copayment** (partial payment for services that day) before the patient sees the physician. A copayment is a fee that an insurance company requires that a patient pay for each encounter with a physician.

HIPAA Hint

Registration information, including a patient's name, address, phone number, date of birth, and medical record number, is protected health information.

Superbill

After the registration information has been obtained or verified, an assistant prepares a **superbill** (Fig. 11-1) to be included with the patient's chart during the office visit. A superbill is the document from which the patient's bill is generated. It contains the patient's diagnosis and a listing of the charges that are incurred during an office visit. Some facilities use different names for a superbill, such as **encounter form, charge slip, fee slip,** and **service record**. All of these terms denote an invoice for services rendered.

Superbills may be produced in either of three ways: they may be preprinted by a professional printing company, they may be printed via computer when the patient registers, or they may be electronic.

Preprinted superbills may be prepared with copies in duplicate, triplicate, or more. If necessary, a copy of the superbill can serve as a control copy. A control copy is kept to make sure that all bills are processed. When the physician's copy is sent to billing, it is matched with the control copy. Control copies that are not matched after a specified period of time will be researched to determine what happened to the original superbill and to discern whether charges should be billed to the patient.

On rare occasions, a patient's superbill may be inadvertently misplaced or left between the pages of a patient's chart. If the charges for a patient are significantly delayed, a physician may choose not to bill that patient. For example, a superbill that has not been processed within 3 months after the visit may be considered too old, and the physician may not wish to bill the patient. Taking action in this situation is more or less a double-edged sword: if the physician bills the patient late or does not bill the patient at all, the physician's billing practices appear careless, and if the patient is concerned about the carelessness of the practice's billing processes, this may draw attention to the physician's practice in general. A patient, therefore, might infer that the physician operates a careless practice.

Computer-generated (printed) superbills are created after the patient's registration has been verified and the assistant is ready to prepare the patient's medical record for the visit. This type of superbill may be customized to the physician's practice. A computer can track the most common reasons for an office visit and can track the illnesses and conditions that the physician treats most often. This information will be

1024

Happy Valley Medical Group
5222 E. Baseline Rd.
Gilbert, AZ 85234
(010) 555-1110

Date: 3/30/2013

BRIEL000 Brimley, Elmo 11/5/2013 8:00:00 AM

EXAM		FEE
New Patient		
Problem Focused	99201	
Expanded Problem, Focused	99202	
Detailed	99203	
Comprehensive	99204	
Comprehensive/High Complex	99204	
Initial Visit/Procedure	99025	
Well Exam Infant (up to 12 mos.)	99318	
Well Exam1–4 yrs.	99382	
Well Exam 5–11 yrs.	99383	
Well Exam 12–17 yrs.	99384	
Well Exam 18–39 yrs.	99385	
Well Exam 40–64 yrs.	99386	
Established Patient		
Minimum	99211	
Problem Focused	99212	
Expanded Problem Focused	99213	
Detailed	99214	
Comprehensive/High Complex	99215	
Well Exam Infant (up to 12 mos.)	99391	
Well Exam1–4 yrs.	99392	
Well Exam 5–11 yrs.	99393	
Well Exam 12–17 yrs.	99394	
Well Exam 18–39 yrs.	99395	
Well Exam 40–64 yrs.	99396	
Obstetrics		
Total OB Care	59400	
Obstetrical Visit	99212	
Injections		
Administration Sub. / IM	90782	
Drug		
Dosage		
Allergy	95155	
Cocci Skin Test	86490	
DPT	90701	
Haemophilus	90737	
Influenza	90724	
MMR	90707	
OPV	90712	
Pneumovax	90732	
TB Skin Test	86585	
TD	90718	
Unlisted Immun	90749	

PROCEDURES		FEE
Anoscopy	46600	
Arthrocentesis/Aspiration/Injection		
Small Joint	*20600	
Interm Joint	*20605	
Major Joint	*20610	
Audiometry	92552	
Cast Application		
Location Long Short		
Catherization	*53670	
Circumcision	54150	
Colposcopy	*57452	
Colposcopy w/ Biopsy	*57454	
Cryosurgery Premalignant Lesion		
Location(s):		
Cryosurgery Warts		
Location(s):		
Curettement Lesion w/Biopsy	CTF	
Curettement Lesion w/o Biopsy		
Single	*11050	
2–4	*11051	
>4	*11052	
Diaphram Fitting	*57170	
Ear Irrigation	69210	
ECG	93000	
Endometrial Biopsy	*58100	
Exc. Lesion w/ Biopsy	CTF	
w/o Biopsy		
Location Size		
Exc. Skin Tags (1 – 15)	*11200	
Each Additional 10	*11201	
Fracture Treatment		
Loc		
w/Reduc w/o Reduc		
Fracture Treatment F/U	99024	
I & D Abscess Single/Simple	*10060	
Multiple or Comp	*10061	
I & D Pilonidal Cyst Simple	*10080	
Pilonidal Cyst Complex	10081	
IV Therapy – To One Hour	90780	
Each Additional Hour	*90781	
Laceration Repair		
Location Size Sim/Comp		
Laryngoscopy	31505	
Oximetry	94760	
Punch Biopsy	CTF	
Rhythm Strip	93040	
Treadmill	93015	
Trigger Point or Tendon Sheath Inj.	*20550	
Tympanometry	92567	

LABORATORY		FEE
Aerobic Culture	87070	
Amylase	82150	
B12	82607	
CBC & Diff	85025	
CHEM 20	80019	
Chlamydia Screen	86317	
Cholesterol	82465	
Digoxin	80162	
Electrolytes	80005	
Ferritin	82728	
Folate	82746	
GC Screen	87070	
Glucose	82947	
Glucose 1 HR	82950	
Glycosylated HGB (A1C)	83036	
HCT	85014	
HDL	83718	
Hep BSAG	86278	
Hepatitis Profile	80059	
HGB & HCT	85014	
HIV	86311	
Iron & TIBC 83540	83550	
Kidney Profile	80007	
Lead	83655	
Liver Profile	82977	
Mono Test	86308	
Pap Smear	88155	
Pregnancy Test	84703	
Prenatal Profile	80055	
Pro Time	85610	
PSA	84153	
RPR	86592	
Sed. Rate	85651	
Stool Culture	87045	
Stool O & P	87177	
Strep Screen	86403	
Theophylline	80198	
Thyroid Profile	80091	
TSH	84443	
Urinalysis	81000	
Urine Culture	87088	
Drawing Fee	36415	
Specimen Collection	99000	

Diagnosis / ICD – 9		Total Estimated Charges:
I acknowledge receipt of medical services and authorize the release of any medical information necessary to process this claim for healthcare payment only. I ☐ do ☐ do not authorize payment to the provider Patient Signature	Tax ID Number:	Payment Amount:

Figure 11-1 Superbills may be automatically generated by billing software such as Medisoft. (Form used by permission of MCKESSON Corporation. All Rights Reserved. © MCKESSON Corporation 2012.)

printed on a computerized superbill. In an office in which physicians practice many different specialties, a computer could, essentially, customize a superbill for every physician in the practice. Including each physician's most-often-used information on a customized superbill can save a significant amount of time when a physician identifies procedures to be billed because the physician's most frequently used procedures and diagnoses are readily available on the superbill. A computer-generated superbill could be used along with a paper medical record or could be used with an electronic medical record.

A superbill can also be entirely electronic with the patient's billing information being entered directly into a computer system. This type of superbill is part of a paperless billing process. With the computerization of most medical offices, some kind of computerization of superbills is destined to be the norm.

Computerized systems can provide excellent audit control for superbills. The computer can assign a control number to an office visit or superbill, and a report can be generated detailing the superbills that have not had charges entered into the system.

CHECKPOINT

A patient calls the office to report that she has not yet received a bill for services performed a month ago. What do you do?

A superbill, no matter what form, is divided into three parts: patient information, a list of procedures, and a list of diagnoses.

Patient Information

Depending on the needs of the practice, this section can vary greatly. Complete patient information (name, address, date of birth, and insurance information) may be included on the superbill. This information may be written or printed on the form, or a computerized label may be generated that can be stuck on the form.

Some superbills are very streamlined and may include only the bare essentials needed to produce a bill for the patient. Limited information necessary to identify the patient may be all that is included on the superbill. The rest of the data needed for billing can be retrieved at a later time after entry into a computer billing system.

Procedures

A service provided for a patient in the course of medical treatment is known as a **procedure.** Many types of procedures, such as office visits, surgical procedures, laboratory and x-ray tests, and immunizations, can be performed. A patient may undergo more than one procedure during a single visit to the physician. If a patient has a procedure performed that is not on the superbill, the procedure may be handwritten or entered on the superbill and can be verified with the content of the patient's medical record.

Diagnoses

The cause of the patient's visit to the office is listed as the **diagnosis.** The diagnosis, which reflects the physician's determination of the patient's illness, provides the reason for the office visit. A patient may have more than one reason for seeing a physician; therefore, there may be more than one diagnosis for a visit. The diagnosis may be an illness, an injury, or a routine health treatment such as a physical examination or other checkup. All diagnoses pertinent to the visit should be listed on the superbill, with diagnoses numbered by importance. The chief reason for the patient's visit is listed as the first diagnosis, and any other diagnoses are listed subsequently as the second, third, or fourth diagnosis.

HIPAA Hint

If an assistant should encounter billing information of a family member, coworker, or friend, the assistant should report the encounter to his or her immediate supervisor, who will decide whether the task should be assigned to someone else.

Billing Office Processes

After the patient's encounter with the physician is over and the physician has recorded the procedures performed and the diagnosis on the superbill, the superbill is then routed to the billing office. In some situations, the physician may send the patient with the superbill to the front office. This may be bad practice because patients may forget to return the superbill to the front desk. In most instances, superbills are handled by the office staff and the patient rarely sees the superbill.

Sometimes, the physician may place the superbill in a paper chart so that the bill can be removed when the charts are reviewed for quantitative analysis in the records room. This practice also has drawbacks because bills may become lost inside a patient's chart.

Perhaps the best practice for returning superbills to the front office for billing is to keep superbills in a specific location in the room in which the physician does paperwork. Such a location may be a shelf- or wall-mounted file or a manila folder. At the end of the day, the superbills should be collected and given to the assistant for billing.

If electronic superbilling is done, the physician enters the information into a computerized billing record. No matter how the superbills are completed, they are returned to an assistant for coding. An assistant will double check the procedures and diagnoses with the information in the patient's medical record. Then after all procedures and diagnoses are coded, an assistant enters charges onto the patient's account.

Computerized Billing Systems

Once the coding of a patient's encounter is completed, the encounter then is ready to be billed (Procedure 11-1). After the charges are entered into the patient's account, the patient's insurance claim is completed, and the claim is sent to the insurance company. In some offices, claims for certain types of insurance may be done in a large batch at a certain time of the month. The insurance claim process is detailed in Chapter 12. A summary of the billing process as the superbill travels through the medical office is illustrated in Figure 11-2.

Almost all medical offices today use some type of computerized billing system (Fig. 11-3). Computerized systems are an absolutely necessity as they provide the following functions:

- A database that contains CPT codes and their associated costs can be maintained. When a code is entered, the current price of the procedure automatically appears on the patient's bill. This database is essentially the fee schedule.
- A database that contains ICD-9 or ICD-10 codes can be maintained for identifying a patient's diagnosis on an insurance claim.

PROCEDURE 11-1

Enter Patients' Charges Into a Billing System

Materials Needed

- Computer billing system

1. Gather the superbills to be recorded.
2. Assign the correct procedure code for each encounter.*
3. Assign the correct diagnosis code for each encounter.*
4. Record the encounters in the billing system. Enter the correct information in each billing category.*

**Denotes a crucial step in the procedure. The student must complete this step satisfactorily to complete the procedure satisfactorily.*

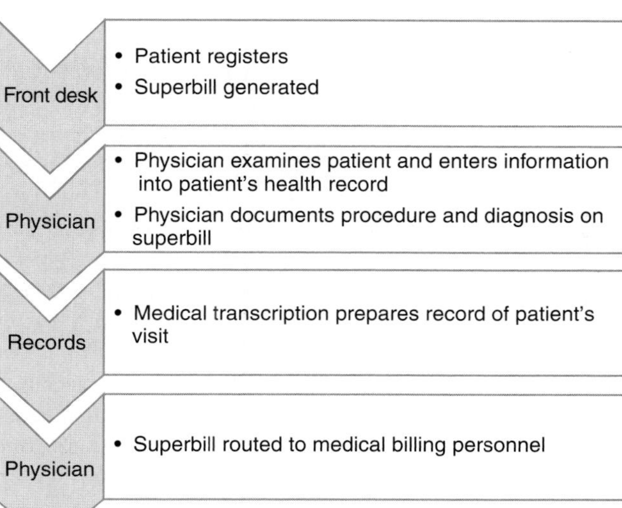

Figure 11-2 Several steps are included in the billing process.

- Statistics needed for planning can be gathered. With a computerized billing system it is possible to identify the procedures that are done most often and the diagnoses that are treated most often. This information can help the office management plan equipment purchases and can help management decide how financial resources will be allocated. Departments that produce more or generate the most income will likely receive greater financial investments.
- A patient's billing information, such as name, address, and insurance company, can be obtained from the program's database for easy billing.
- A patient's information can be accessed or updated from any computer location in the medical office if the office's computer system is networked.
- Appointments that have not been billed can be tracked to eliminate the possibility of forgotten charges.
- Past due accounts that may need attention for collection can be easily identified.
- Reports for obtaining a clear picture of the business end of the practice can be run.
- Insurance claim information can be easily obtained and claims generated. Claims may even be filed electronically from the computer system.

HIPAA Hint

A patient's billing information is protected health information (PHI).

Credit

Usually, after a patient sees a physician in the medical office, he or she will receive a bill for services at a later date. This patient has received credit.

Credit can be as simple as incurring a charge and paying for it at another time. Many patients seen in most medical offices receive credit because they are not required to pay for office charges immediately after an office visit.

The federal **Equal Credit Opportunity Act (ECOA)** of 1975 requires that consumers are treated equally and fairly when applying for credit. The law stipulates that an individual cannot be denied credit on the basis of race, color, religion, national origin, sex, marital status, or age (as long as the individual has the capacity to enter into a contract). An individual cannot be denied credit if he or she receives income from public assistance. The amount of a person's income, however, can be used to determine whether he or she will receive credit. Credit must be given equally to persons who apply for credit. For example, a business could not deny credit to single women who make less than $25,000 per year but give credit to men who make the same amount. Such action would be discrimination.

When one is considering a patient for credit, the patient's income, expenses, debt, and credit history can be reviewed to determine whether the patient is credit worthy. Not everyone who asks for credit receives credit. Credit can be refused only

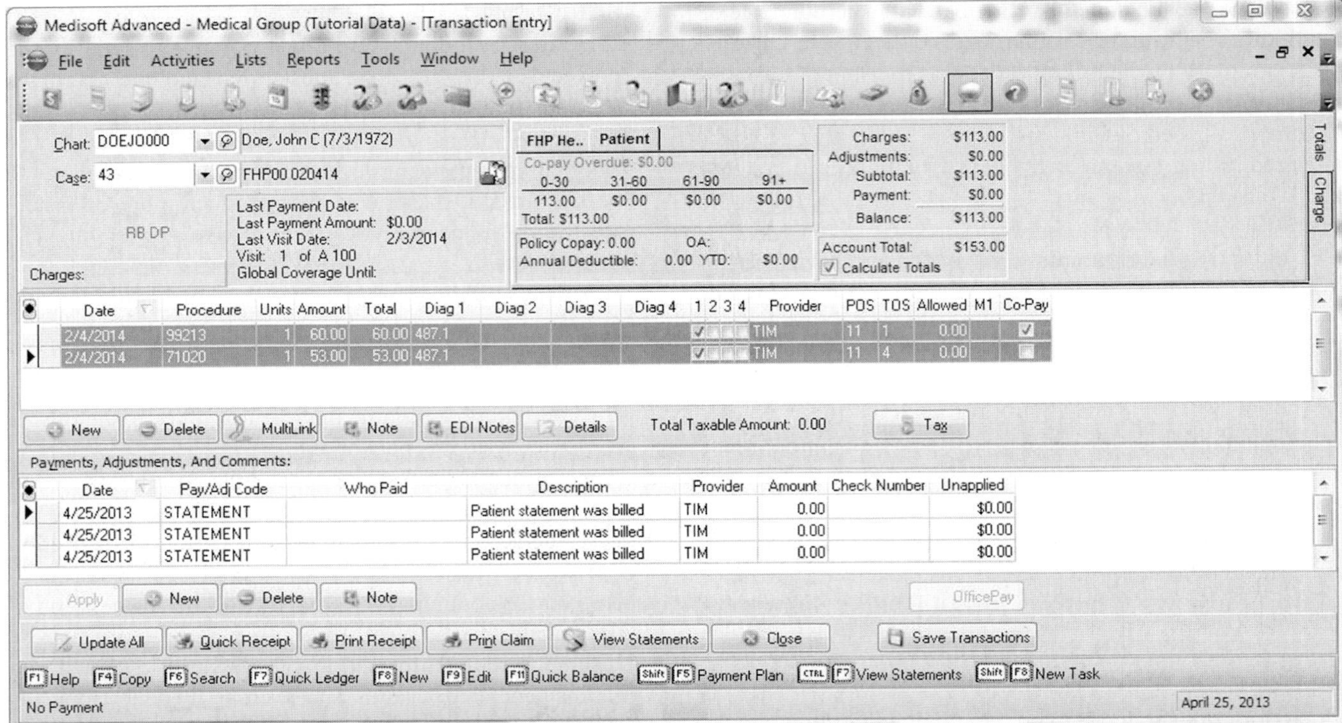

Figure 11-3 Billing software gathers an assortment of information related to the billing process. (Screenshots used by permission of MCKESSON Corporation. All Rights Reserved. © MCKESSON Corporation 2012.)

because of inability to pay. Remember to adhere to the following guidelines when determining a patient's request for credit:

- A patient's sex, race, color, national origin, or religion cannot be asked.
- A patent's marital status can be asked only if a spouse's income would be used to obtain credit. If asking about marital status, a creditor may ask whether the patient is married, single, or separated. Creditors are not allowed to ask whether a patient is divorced or widowed.
- You cannot ask for information about a patient's spouse unless the spouse will use the account, or the patient needs to rely on the spouse's income.
- You cannot refuse to consider income because of its source (e.g., public assistance, pension funds, child support).

Statements of Account

Each month, a statement of each account is generated. A statement contains a summary of charges and payments for family members on an account. Statements are printed and sent to the account's guarantor (Fig. 11-4). The guarantor is the individual who is responsible for payment of the account. A guarantor could be the patient, a parent, a spouse, or another individual (Procedure 11-2).

Statements usually are sent to guarantors monthly; the size of the practice determines when statements are generated. Small practices may elect to mail out all statements at the end of the month. For large practices that send out hundreds or even thousands of statements each month, it may be impossible to send out statements for all patients at once. A **cycle billing** process may be used to even out the medical office staff's workload. Cycle billing involves billing patients at intervals throughout the month. The practice's accounts are divided into equal groups, and each group is assigned a specific time of the month during which statements are done and sent. Statements can be sent via the U.S. Postal System or may be sent electronically, but regardless of how they are sent, it still takes considerable time to send statements.

With cycle billing, the patient's last name or account number can be used to determine the day of the month that the statement is to be billed. As an example, if a patient's name and the information in Table 11-1 are used to determine the billing date, Harriet Anderson's bill would be sent out on the 1st of every month, and Allen Williams' bill would be sent out

PROCEDURE 11-2

Produce Monthly Statements for Patient Accounts

Materials Needed

- Patient account information (computer billing information or ledger cards)

1. Establish the statement due.
2. Determine which accounts should have a statement generated. If a cycle billing system is used, only certain statements may need to be generated.
3. Post any outstanding charges to patient accounts.
4. Post any outstanding payments to patient accounts.
5. Print the statements.*

**Denotes a crucial step in the procedure. The student must complete this step satisfactorily in order to complete the procedure satisfactorily.*

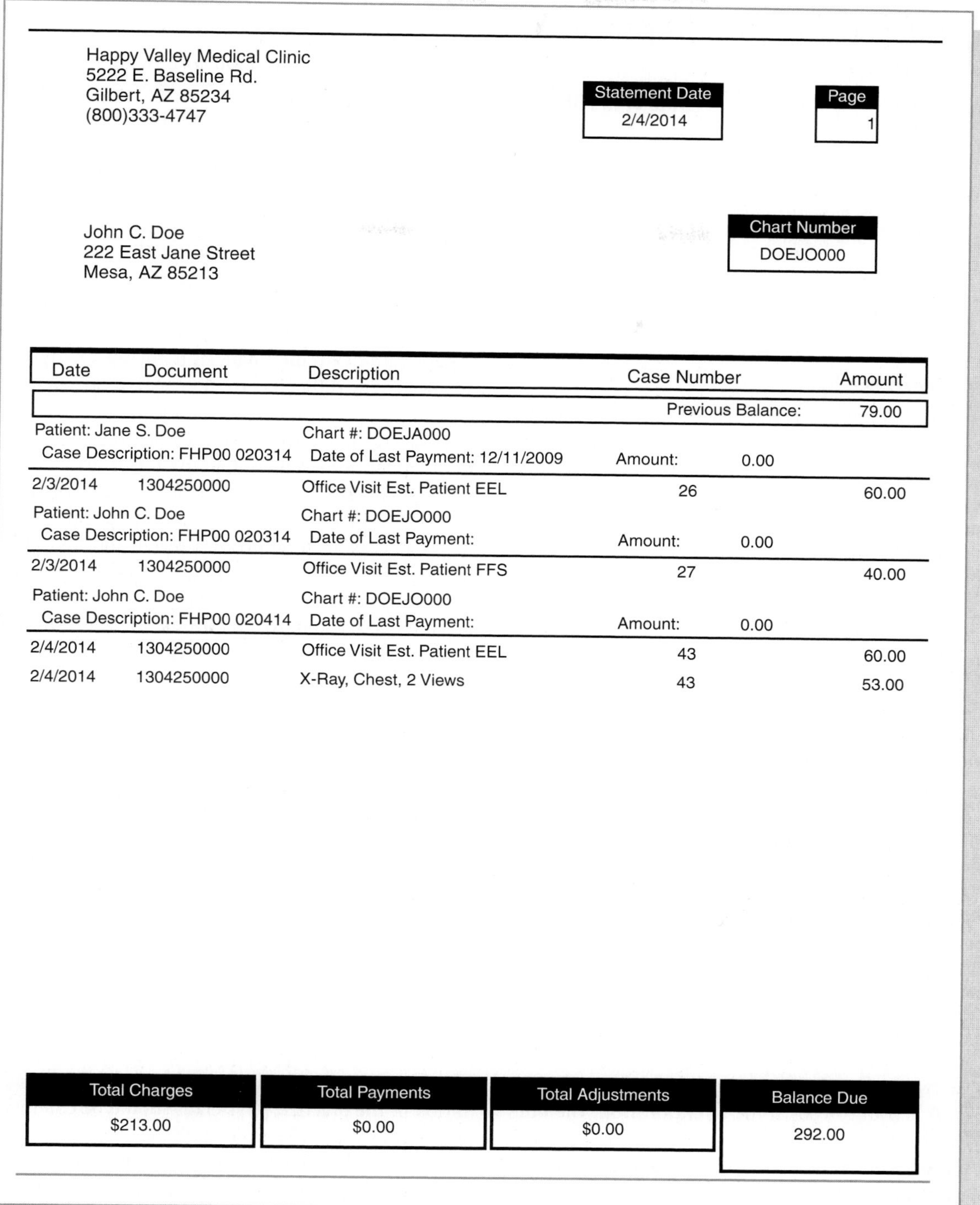

Happy Valley Medical Clinic
5222 E. Baseline Rd.
Gilbert, AZ 85234
(800)333-4747

Statement Date	Page
2/4/2014	1

John C. Doe
222 East Jane Street
Mesa, AZ 85213

Chart Number
DOEJO000

Date	Document	Description	Case Number	Amount
			Previous Balance:	79.00
Patient: Jane S. Doe		Chart #: DOEJA000		
Case Description: FHP00 020314		Date of Last Payment: 12/11/2009	Amount: 0.00	
2/3/2014	1304250000	Office Visit Est. Patient EEL	26	60.00
Patient: John C. Doe		Chart #: DOEJO000		
Case Description: FHP00 020314		Date of Last Payment:	Amount: 0.00	
2/3/2014	1304250000	Office Visit Est. Patient FFS	27	40.00
Patient: John C. Doe		Chart #: DOEJO000		
Case Description: FHP00 020414		Date of Last Payment:	Amount: 0.00	
2/4/2014	1304250000	Office Visit Est. Patient EEL	43	60.00
2/4/2014	1304250000	X-Ray, Chest, 2 Views	43	53.00

Total Charges	Total Payments	Total Adjustments	Balance Due
$213.00	$0.00	$0.00	292.00

Figure 11-4 Patient statements usually are generated monthly and are sent to the accounts' identified guarantors. (Form used by permission of MCKESSON Corporation. All Rights Reserved. © MCKESSON Corporation 2012.)

on the 25th of every month. The payment due date for each statement will depend on the time of the month the statement was sent. Use of cycle billing in a medical office enables the staff to carry on normal activities of the office and to process statements and payments as a part of everyday activity.

Imagine that a practice has 1000 active accounts. If all accounts were billed on the last day of the month, an assistant would have to send out statements in a sudden flurry of activity at the end of the month. Then, if all payments were due by the 20th of the month, the days surrounding the 20th would be spent trying to get volumes of payments recorded in the patients' accounts.

Cycle billing spreads the work out over the course of the month. With this type of billing system, statements are constantly going out and payments are constantly coming in. Cycle billing also provides a steady flow of cash coming into the office.

TABLE 11-1

Cycle Billing Schedule

Patient's Last Name	Date of Month
A–C	1st
D–G	5th
H–K	9th
L–N	13th
O–R	17th
S–U	21st
V–Z	25th

Aging Accounts

An assistant must monitor account balances each month to determine whether an account has become seriously overdue. Accounts receivable **aging** categorizes the outstanding charges on a patient's bill and identifies how long the charge has been on the patient's account. Account balances are kept on 30-day intervals (e.g., fewer than 30 days or current, 31 to 60 days, 61 to 90 days, and more than 90 days). Accounts with the same balance can have very different collection concerns based on an aging summary. Tracking aging balances demonstrates how old account charges are and enables an assistant to quickly see which balances may need attention for collection.

To understand the importance of reviewing accounts receivable aging, let's take a look at the following two accounts:

Patient's Name	Susan Pearson	Matthew Stein
Account balance	$1000	$1000
Current balance (<30 days old)	$500	$0
Balance 31–60 days old	$300	$100
Balance 61–90 days old	$100	$50
Balance >90 days old	$100	$850

Although the two account balances are the same, it is obvious that Mr. Stein's account needs some attention from the billing office. The distributions of the patients' balances are quite different. Aging accounts help an assistant identify accounts that may need some collection attention.

Collection

Occasionally, in the course of business in the medical office, some patients do not pay their account. Most medical offices do pursue some type of collection action, but the degree to which a physician or a practice pursues collection may vary widely.

An account may not be paid for numerous reasons. A patient may have moved and may not have received a bill. The patient may be unhappy with medical care received. The patient may have a change in income. The charges may be incorrect. The patient may be ill and unable to keep up with paying bills. There are likely even more reasons that an account might be unpaid.

Most physicians are used to providing some services for which they know they will never be reimbursed. Physicians provide some services on a charitable basis, but that does not mean that a physician will write off every account if the patient does not pay. Depending on the physician, overdue accounts may be targeted for collection.

Before pursuing any type of collection action on a patient's account, an assistant must consult the patient's physician to determine whether collection action is appropriate. The physician may not want to initiate any type of collection action if a patient is suffering from a serious medical condition, is experiencing extreme financial hardship, or is going through an otherwise difficult situation. Many physicians feel that pursuing collection action when a patient is in such a situation would make them appear uncaring. If a patient is currently undergoing chemotherapy for cancer, the physician is not likely to want the business office to call the patient about an overdue bill. Likewise, if a patient has other serious problems, such as an ill child or a recent job loss, the physician most likely will not want to pursue collection. In addition to consulting a patient's physician, the assistant should check a patient's account to determine whether any outstanding insurance claims or payments exist before initiating collection on the patient's account.

Collection Guidelines

Physicians in a practice should establish collection guidelines for an assistant to follow. Physicians may decide that accounts more than 60 days past due should be brought to their attention, or they may decide that only those accounts that have not had a payment for 3 months or longer should be brought to their attention. It is highly recommended that physicians provide guidance to the office staff regarding their philosophy pertaining to collection of overdue accounts. Physicians in a practice should clearly communicate their personal philosophy of account collection and the collection activities of which they approve. This ensures that the activities of the office staff are in line with the physician's business philosophies. Because the degree to which collection is pursued may affect the reputation of the practice, physicians should be chiefly responsible for establishing collection guidelines.

When collecting a patient's account, an assistant should remember that word will "get around" as to the physician's bill collecting practices. It is probably best for the reputation of the medical practice to use methods that are polite and respectful, not aggressive. Today, patients may be unable to pay because of illness, but tomorrow, they may be able to pay and will remember the empathy shown by the practice regarding the patient's medical charges. Aggressive collection practices could have a serious, detrimental effect on the image of the practice.

Fair Debt Collection Practices Act

The **Fair Debt Collection Practices Act** protects debtors against third-party debt collectors who use unfair practices when collecting a debt. This applies to outside agencies that a medical office may hire to collect its bad debts. This federal law specifies the following:

- If calling someone other than the debtor, a collector must identify themselves and state that they are searching for location information for the debtor.
- Collectors cannot use threats of violence or harm to the debtor, their reputation or personal property.
- Collectors cannot use offensive language.
- Collectors cannot misrepresent themselves.
- When a third party (e.g., a guarantor's relative or employer) is used to locate a debtor, the third party can be contacted only once.
- A debt collector cannot inform the third party that the individual is a debtor.
- A debt collector must use convenient hours—8 AM to 9 PM—to contact the debtor.
- A debt collector cannot contact the debtor at church or at special events.
- A debt collector cannot contact the debtor if the debtor states that he or she has an attorney (unless the attorney fails to respond).
- A debt collector cannot continue to contact a debtor if the debtor states in writing that he or she refuses to pay the debt, or if the debtor says not to contact him or her again.
- A debt collector cannot threaten patients with action that the collector does not intend to take. For instance, a collector cannot say, "We will turn your account over to a collection agency if you don't pay the balance in one month," and then not do so.
- A debt collector cannot harass any person by continually calling on the phone.
- A collector cannot communicate via postcard.

Even though this federal law applies to third-party collectors, most states have debt collection statutes, and state statutes often extend fair debt collection practices to all debt collectors, as well as to third-party collectors. In this instance, a medical office, as well as the third-party collectors, would have to abide by state law. It is very important for any person who conducts collection activity to follow these requirements. Failure to follow the law could cause a debtor to sue a debt collector for violating the applicable federal or state law.

In addition, some states have laws that specifically address medical debt. These laws provide more consumer protection regarding the collection of medical debt. This protection can save a consumer from losing his or her home to pay medical debt by limiting amounts that can be charged for interest.

Collection Methods

Initial Collection Methods

When collecting an overdue account, an assistant should remember to approach a guarantor sincerely and respectfully.

When an account is past due, the first collection action that probably will be used is a gentle reminder that is printed on, stamped on, or enclosed with the patient's statement. A comment such as "Your account is past due" or "Your payment is overdue" is indeed a collection action and serves as a reminder that the business office has noticed that payment has not arrived. These types of messages are known as **dunning messages**. A dunning message is any type of message that makes a request for payment on an account. If a physician decides not to pursue collection on a patient's account, the account should be marked "DO NOT DUN." **Dun** refers to repetitive action to collect.

TABLE 11-2

Examples of Dunning Messages

Age of Account Balance	Statement Message
Current	Thank you for your continued patronage.
31–60 days	Please pay your account promptly.
61–90 days	Your account is past due.
91–120 days	Finance charges are assessed on balances over 90 days.
Over 120 days	Please contact our credit office (555-1234) to arrange a payment schedule.

Many computer systems can be set up to include dunning messages automatically on statements that are overdue. Messages can differ depending on the age of an account balance (Table 11-2). If a physician has decided not to collect on a patient's account, an assistant should be very careful to make sure that the patient's statement does not include a dunning message. Even if previous arrangements have been made with the billing department, a patient could become very upset if a message is included. The excuse that "the computer automatically puts it on" is inappropriate and is simply not acceptable. Although statements may be computer generated, an assistant is still responsible for making sure they are handled correctly.

Telephone Collection

Another action that can be used to collect on an account is to try to contact the guarantor by phone. Because a patient and a guarantor are not always the same person, an assistant should always ask to speak to the individual identified as the guarantor. An assistant must speak to the guarantor and to no one else about an overdue bill.

When collecting over the telephone, an assistant should remember a few basic principles, some of which have foundation in the law:

- Be respectful.
- Do not threaten action that you do not intend to take.
- Call at a reasonable hour, that is, between 8 AM and 9 PM. Calling outside a reasonable time could constitute harassment.
- Ask the patient to establish a payment schedule; get an agreement on a monthly payment.

Collection Letters

A collection letter (Fig. 11-5) is a formal notice sent to a patient that an account is overdue. Before a collection letter

Happy Valley Medical Group
5222 E. Baseline Rd.,
Gilbert, AZ 85234
(010) 555-1110

December 21, 200x

Mr. Jonathan Martin
1642 West 53rd Avenue
Harvester, MN 55555

Dear Mr. Martin:

I am writing today regarding the status of your account. Your account balance is currently $2,565.32, all of which is over 90 days past due. We have not received a payment on your account within the past 60 days.

Please contact our office immediately to work out a payment plan for your account.

Sincerely,

Taylor Hudson
Office Manager

TH/ma
enclosure

Figure 11-5 A collection letter is sent to a guarantor to collect on an account when other informal methods have not produced a response.

is sent, dunning messages should be used on a patient's statement, and an attempt should be made to contact the patient by telephone. The content of collection letters should be in keeping with legal and appropriate debt collection practices, as mentioned previously. An assistant may want to keep a file of sample letters approved by the physician.

In-Person Collection

If a physician approves, an assistant may speak to a patient during a visit to the medical office. This type of collection practice can be difficult and uncomfortable for both the patient and the assistant and should be done only if privacy can be maintained during the conversation. It is up to the physician to decide what type of collection practices will be used in the office. Collection can be as simple as the assistant's asking a patient whether a payment could be made on the account.

Locating a Missing Guarantor

Occasionally, statements may be returned labeled *addressee unknown,* or a guarantor's phone may no longer be in service. If one of these situations occurs, it may still be possible to locate a guarantor.

In the search for a missing guarantor, helpful information may be found in the medical record of any of the patients listed on the guarantor's account. If a patient completes a registration form such as the one pictured in Figure 8-2, information regarding the patient's nearest relative and employer may be given. Remember, you cannot reveal that the guarantor is a debtor, and you can use the third party only once regarding this information; however, you could identify that you are trying to locate the individual and ask whether the third party has a new address or telephone number for the guarantor. Also, do not forget to consult a local telephone book or directory service or to conduct an Internet-based people search. The guarantor may have a new listing in your local area.

Private Agency Collection and Small Claims Court

On occasion, a physician may wish to use outside means to collect a debt. A patient's account may be sent to an outside collection agency that specializes in debt collection.

A drawback to using an outside agency for collection on a patient's account is that the agency may use means to collect the account of which the physician does not approve and of which the physician may not even be aware. If an outside agency is used, the medical office staff should be sure to communicate the importance of following the office's philosophy regarding collection. Outside collection agencies are often costly, keeping a hefty percentage (sometimes 50%) of the total amount that is collected.

Small claims court collection is also an option for an office that may wish to pursue collection on an account. For a small fee, a claim can be filed with the court. There are limits on what can be collected in small claims court, and the use of this type of collection may not be suitable for a physician.

Billing Topics

What Does the Doctor Charge?

Occasionally, patients may inquire about the physician's fee for services. A common occurrence in the medical office is for patients to ask such questions as, "How much does it cost for a strep test?" or "How much is a physical?" Patients sometimes do not realize that they cannot come into the office and order whatever they want. Some procedures may be different for some patients. An assistant might reply, "We are unable to perform only a strep test without the doctor's approval. You would need to see the doctor for an office visit, and she would need to determine whether a strep test is necessary. If a strep test is ordered, there would be a charge for an office visit and for the test. Our office visits typically range from $X to $Y, and a strep test is $Z. If the doctor sees the need for any additional tests, those would be charged separately." In the case of a physical, a patient may be told, "Charges for a physical vary based on the patient's age and any tests that may need to be done along with the physical."

When giving an estimate of physician charges, do not give an absolute amount but instead give a range of possible charges because each patient is unique and will have different needs for medical care. For example, a patient with a chronic medical condition such as diabetes may require additional time for an office visit and may need additional laboratory tests. A great deal of what is required during a patient's encounter with the physician depends on the patient's condition and medical history.

When talking to a patient about charges for medical care, be sure to clearly state that the charges given are merely an estimate. Depending on the patient's condition, a physician may decide to order additional tests or may spend extended time with the patient. Many variables exist within every patient visit.

When a patient inquires about the physician's charges, an assistant should encourage the patient to notify the physician and/or office manager of any concerns the patient may have regarding charges for medical services. If a patient has financial hardship, a physician may have sample medications for the patient in lieu of a costlier prescription. The office staff may have information regarding charitable programs for patients with high medical costs. Sometimes physicians discount a patient's bill or they may even elect to not charge for some items that the patient receives. If the patient has anxiety about the physician's charges, most offices are very willing to work with patients and to make arrangements for extended payment.

Assignment of Benefits

Patients covered by insurance usually are encouraged to have their insurance claim payments sent directly to the physician's office. Such an arrangement is called **assignment of benefits**. The assignment of benefits authorization is located at the bottom of the patient registration form (see Fig. 8-2) or may be a separate form that the patient signs. Provision for assignment of benefits also may be included on the superbill, as in Figure 11-1. Use of a superbill for authorization would require the patient to sign every superbill, rather than authorizing it just once as in Figure 8-2. A signature on such an authorization allows insurance payments to be sent directly to the medical office.

Most medical offices prefer that patients assign their health benefits directly to the office because the practice then will receive any insurance benefits directly from the insurance company. The practice thus receives payment for at least a portion of its services. Patients who do not assign benefits to the clinic instead receive the insurance payments themselves. With this alternative, the practice may have to wait to receive payment from the patient. The medical office even runs the risk that the patient may keep the payment and use the money for something else.

Fees for Medical Care

How does a dollar amount actually get on the patient's bill? Amounts for medical procedures are determined long before the patient enters the clinic. Each medical practice establishes what is called a **fee schedule**. This schedule is a listing of every procedure done by the practice's physicians and a dollar amount to be charged for each procedure. Similar to any other business, medical offices must set prices for all of its services. If an office uses a medical practice management software such as Medisoft, the fee schedule is basically the procedure or transaction code list. The fee schedule should be reviewed at least annually to determine whether any changes in fees are warranted.

Charges for medical procedures vary throughout the country. Outside factors such as the local economy, cost of living, and competition all have an impact on what the physician charges for a medical procedure. Other items that affect the cost of medical services include such variables as the length of time the physician spends with the patient and the complexity of the patient's condition. A patient seen for congestive heart failure requires an extensive history and examination and more complex decision making on the physician's part than does an otherwise healthy patient seen for an ear infection. The patient with heart failure most likely would incur a higher office charge because of the nature of his or her condition.

Sometimes insurance programs, such as government benefit programs (e.g., Medicare, Medicaid), have established maximum amounts that may be charged. If a medical office wishes to serve patients who receive these government benefits, the office may be limited in the amount that may be charged for a procedure.

Legal and Ethical Issues in Medical Billing

Medical Debt

Medical debt is a significant problem. The Centers for Disease Control and Prevention released information from the National Health Interview Survey titled "Financial Burden of Medical Care: Early Release of Estimates From the National Health Interview Survey, January-June 2011" that identified that during that time "one in three Americans lived in a family that was experiencing the financial burden of medical care." Medical debt is not a rarity; it is perhaps all too common.

Many Americans are now using credit cards, taking out mortgages, and even selling their homes to meet their medical expenses. Even if a person has insurance, huge amounts of medical debt can be incurred while he or she is trying to survive a catastrophic illness. Large insurance deductibles and 20% coinsurance on thousands of dollars in medical fees can deplete patients' finances and put people in danger of losing their homes unless they turn to credit cards or other sources to pay off their debt.

Unfortunately, many people in debt stop getting the care they need because they do not want to incur any more expense. Some elderly or disabled individuals on very fixed incomes may have to choose between buying groceries and meeting their health care needs.

In addition, to make matters worse, a credit card company can choose to change interest rates for cardholders at any time with very little notice. Moreover, if payment is late on a credit card, hefty late fees can be added to the balance.

This is an issue that has no easy solution. It is important to have compassion and empathy for patients who are struggling with medical debt. Not only are they suffering from the financial burden of medical costs, but they likely are also suffering from significant illness. Excessive medical debt represents a significant threat to the well-being of patients.

It is important that medical office staff be educated as to options that may be available for patients to handle their medical debt. Some offices may even employ special credit counselors to work with such patients. Sometimes many options are available to help patients manage the debt. Charitable sources may be able to ease a patient's medical debt. Help may be available from pharmaceutical companies. Sometimes patients may not be aware that they may qualify for Medicaid or Medicare. In addition, some health care organizations will write off a portion of a patient's medical debt if the patient requests help in negotiating their fees.

Unfortunately, bankruptcy is sometimes the only option for individuals to get out of health care–related debt. Statistics from several studies show that many individuals who are going through bankruptcy have significant medical debt that contributed to their bankruptcy.

Confidentiality

All medical billing information—whether it is a patient's superbill, monthly statement, or insurance claim—is as confidential as information in a patient's medical record. A patient's bill contains information pertaining to when a patient saw a physician and what was done at the visit. A patient's superbill contains diagnosis and procedure codes related to an office visit and to the physician who provided treatment. A patient's insurance claim also contains procedure and diagnosis information.

Information from a patient's account should never be given to anyone without the patient's written permission. An insurance company that calls the office must have the patient's authorization to release information from the patient's medical record that relates to specific charges. This release of information for billing purposes is normally obtained when a patient registers.

Billing Fraud

Fraudulent billing practices can cost consumers, insurance companies, and government agencies substantial amounts of money. **Fraud** in billing refers to knowingly and willfully billing for something that did not occur. Fraudulent billing practices are punishable by law. Medical billing fraud can be committed by a patient, a provider, or both parties.

Patient fraud can be committed by using someone else's insurance information (see the section on Identity Theft), obtaining government assistance under a false identity, or receiving and reselling medical items received under a government program.

Provider fraud can be committed by billing for services not rendered, **upcoding** a patient's charges (charging a higher code than documented), **unbundling** charges (charging individually for items that should be billed together as a package), providing treatment that is not medically necessary, billing for procedures that were not done, or using another provider's billing number for submission of insurance claims.

Provider/patient fraud occurs when kickbacks are exchanged for undergoing medical treatment or for providing insurance information for billing. There are actually individuals who try to obtain insurance numbers to submit fraudulent bills. Also, individuals may willfully sell their insurance numbers to allow them to be used to fraudulently bill an insurance company.

Personal injury mills where unscrupulous providers order unnecessary tests and treatments is another example of fraud. In a personal injury mill, doctors submit claims to insurance companies for services that are not necessary or not done and patients willingly participate in these fraudulent activities.

Fraud is theft and has severe legal consequences. When billing a patient for services rendered, a medical administrative assistant should be careful and thorough in the preparation and completion of all patient charges, making sure that documentation supports all items on the patient's bill and the insurance claim.

Identity Theft

Just how can identity theft affect a medical office? Imagine a person (we will call him Andrew) who sees a physician, is admitted to the hospital, and undergoes surgery, all the while pretending to be someone he is not. Andrew registered as John and is using John's medical insurance and even his records.

Identity theft in a medical setting involves an imposter's receiving medical services and having the services charged to another person or to his or her insurance company. The insurance company pays benefits, and the medical office bills the real patient for the remainder (in the above case, John would get the bill!). This kind of scenario has far-reaching implications:

- John's medical record was changed without John even being treated.
- John is financially responsible until proved otherwise.
- Andrew runs the risk of receiving a medical treatment that could endanger his life. What if Andrew was allergic to a drug? Because John's record was used, drug allergy information may be incorrect.

That is just one scenario. There are also instances in which people work together in identity theft. For example, let's say Mary needs medical care but does not have insurance. If Laurie has insurance, she may give her information to Mary and allow her to use her insurance card.

These are just a few of the deceptive practices that medical offices must watch for. It is possible to put simple safeguards in place. Simply asking a patient for government-issued picture identification would stop many of these instances from occurring.

Fee Splitting

Fee splitting refers to the practice of paying a physician for referral of a patient to another physician or company. The Current Opinions of the Judicial Council of the American Medical Association (AMA) states that it is unethical for a physician to receive anything of value (e.g., money, gifts) in exchange for referring a patient to another provider. In addition, a patient should not be referred to a pharmacy or other health care–related business that a physician has ownership in, without the knowledge that the physician has an interest in that business.

Charges for Minors

If a patient is a minor, the bill should always be addressed to an adult who is responsible for payment; the bill should not and cannot be addressed to the minor. Generally, a minor who is not emancipated cannot be held responsible for charges incurred. It often is very difficult, if not impossible, to hold a minor responsible for a bill.

In the case of divorce, a bill for services provided to a minor should be sent to the parent designated by the court to pay for medical expenses. In the absence of any court arrangements, the assistant should work with the minor's parents to establish a suitable billing arrangement of which both parents are aware. If there is no designation, a bill for services provided to a minor usually is sent to the parent who presents the child for treatment.

Once a minor reaches the age of 18, the minor may be billed directly for medical treatment. Due to the confidentiality of medical billing information, many health facilities now create a new account for all individuals once they turn 18.

CHECKPOINT

A minor calls the office and wishes to see a physician for information on birth control. The minor does not want her parents to know about the visit. Based on what you learned in Chapter 3 and in this chapter, what might your answer be?

Estate Claims

When a patient dies, it is important to determine whether any medical charges pertaining to the patient are owed to the office. To keep up with local deaths, an assistant should review the obituaries in local area newspapers on a daily basis. Sometimes, a physician may notify an assistant of a patient's death; sometimes, a death certificate may arrive at the office for completion by the physician.

On hearing of a patient's death, an assistant should be mindful of the need for the patient's family to grieve but also should remember that the law often dictates how and when outstanding bills of the deceased are paid. Legal notices, such as the one shown in Figure 11-6, are printed in the newspaper in the county in which the decedent's will is probated. There

IN THE DISTRICT COURT OF WALKER COUNTY
STATE OF NORTH DAKOTA

In the Matter of the Estate of
Louis F. Knox, Deceased

NOTICE TO CREDITORS

NOTICE IS HEREBY GIVEN that the undersigned has been appointed personal representative of the above estate. All persons having claims against the said deceased are requested to present their claims within three months after the date of the first publication of this notice or said claims will be forever barred. Claims must either be presented to Paula Knox, personal representative of the estate, at 2468 Meadowview Road, Farmington, ND 58000, or filed with the Court.

Dated this 3rd day of September, 2013.

Paula A. Knox
Personal Representative
2468 Meadowview Road
Farmington, ND 58000

Lisa M. Howard
Attorney at Law
P O Box 952B
Farmington, ND 58000
Attorney for Personal Representative
First publication on the 3rd day of September, 2013.
(September 3, 10, 17, 2013)

Figure 11-6 Published legal notices inform creditors when claims for payment must be filed.

may be a time limit in which any debtors of the decedent must file claims for payment against the estate. Any claim against the estate usually is sent to the personal representative of the decedent's estate and is essentially a notice to the estate that the decedent owed money.

In the example shown in Figure 11-6, the state of North Dakota allows 3 months during which claims must be filed, or they will not be allowed. Laws regarding collecting from an estate vary from state to state, and it is important for an assistant to be aware of local time limitations.

When should a bill be sent after a death? A reasonable time should elapse between a patient's death and the sending of a statement to the personal representative of the patient's estate. It would be uncaring to have a bill for medical care (especially if a patient died while under a physician's care) arrive within the first few weeks of a patient's death. If possible, an assistant should wait to send a bill until after this period has passed.

A bill should be sent, however. Failing to send a bill after a patient's death may cause family members to question the motives of the physician. They may infer that the physician feels responsible in some way for the patient's death. Therefore, a deceased patient's statements should be sent for payment, but an assistant should avoid sending a statement within the initial period after the death.

Missed Appointments—To Bill or Not to Bill

What happens if a patient misses an appointment with a physician? Should the patient be charged for the appointment?

In most practices, physicians choose not to charge a patient for missing an appointment. Physicians realize that from time to time, a patient may forget about an appointment. In a busy medical office, where a physician sees a few patients within the span of an hour, an occasional patient who forgets an appointment probably will not be noticed in the schedule.

In some practices, however, in which a physician sees only a few patients during the day (such as psychiatry, in which each patient usually is scheduled for an hour appointment), a physician may wish to charge the patient for the missed visit.

The AMA's Council on Ethical and Judicial Affairs specifies that a patient can be charged for a missed appointment if the patient has been told in advance that there will be a charge for missed appointments. Providers who charge for missed appointments should make their policy clearly known to patients and may even wish to have patients sign a notice that they are aware that a charge will be made if an appointment is missed.

A medical office should be sure to make clear to patients its policy on charging for missed appointments. Notices can be placed in monthly statements, patients may be asked to sign a notification of such a policy, and/or a prominent notice may be posted within the physician's office.

Medical Records

If a patient with a past due account requests that his or her medical records be sent to another physician, can the physician refuse to send the patient's record until the account is paid? The physician cannot refuse, according to the AMA's Council on Ethical and Judicial Affairs. The council states that it is unethical to withhold the release of a patient's medical record because a patient has an outstanding bill. Therefore, regardless of the patient's account balance, a patient's request for release of medical records should be accommodated. Withholding records could jeopardize a patient's health and could even possibly put a physician at risk for legal action.

SUMMARY

Many different activities are included in the billing process. Vital information regarding payment of a patient's charges is gathered at the point of registration. After registration, the superbill is generated and is used to document a patient's diagnosis and treatment for billing and insurance purposes. From the superbill, a patient's account is updated and insurance claims are generated. An assistant may be responsible for a portion of the billing process or may be responsible for the entire billing process in the medical office. Each month, statements are generated for each account. If an account becomes past due, it may be the assistant's responsibility to begin to collect on the account. Procedures used in the collection process should be approved by the physicians in the office and must stay within legal guidelines.

A medical administrative assistant should have a clear understanding of all of the activities involved in billing for medical services. A complete understanding of these components will enable an assistant to serve the patient in the best way possible.

YOU ARE THE MEDICAL ADMINISTRATIVE ASSISTANT

A guarantor calls you and begins to ask questions regarding the monthly statement from the medical office in which you work. There is a charge of $100 for an office visit and a related laboratory test for the guarantor's spouse. The guarantor begins to ask questions, wanting to know what kind of test was done and what the diagnosis was for the visit. How do you respond?

REVIEW EXERCISES

Exercise 11-1 True or False

Read each statement, and determine whether the statement is true or false. Record the answer in the blank provided. T = true; F = false.

_____ 1. A patient's registration information is verified at each office visit to ensure that the correct information is available for billing and insurance purposes.

_____ 2. Registration forms should not be mailed to new patients ahead of time.

_____ 3. Registration mistakes can be costly.

_____ 4. Control copies are used for superbills to ensure that all bills are accounted for.

_____ 5. Computer-generated superbills can be specialized for each physician.

_____ 6. When a patient inquires about the cost of a physician's services, the patient should be given an exact quote.

_____ 7. Delayed billing practices reflect poorly on a medical office as a whole.

_____ 8. If a medical administrative assistant is not responsible for generating patients' bills, it is not necessary for the assistant to know the components of the billing process.

_____ 9. A patient may be charged for only one procedure per office visit.

_____ 10. If a computer system is used for billing in the medical office, all information for the patient should be listed on the superbill.

_____ 11. An assistant should discourage any discussion of fees for medical services.

_____ 12. In the case of a child with divorced parents, the bill should always be sent to the patient's father.

_____ 13. If a patient has been notified in advance of charges for missed appointments, it is ethical to bill a patient for a missed appointment.

_____ 14. Most physicians will charge patients for a missed appointment.

_____ 15. It is generally preferred that patients assign their insurance benefits to a medical office.

_____ 16. If a patient does not assign insurance benefits to a medical office, payment to the office may be delayed.

_____ 17. A medical office establishes a fee for each service when the service is performed.

_____ 18. Some insurance programs have maximum amounts that are allowed to be charged for medical services.

_____ 19. Charges for medical services are the same across the country.

_____ 20. The larger the practice, the more likely it is that cycle billing should be used when patients are billed.

_____ 21. A patient's physician should always be consulted before collection activity is begun on the patient's account.

_____ 22. Physicians should establish collection guidelines for the medical office.

_____ 23. Collection procedures used by an assistant will affect an office's reputation.

_____ 24. A superbill contains a summary of charges and payments on a patient's account.

_____ 25. Cycle billing means that a patient's statement is sent out every other month.

_____ 26. Once a patient reaches 18 years of age, he or she is usually his or her own guarantor.

Exercise 11-2 Chapter Concepts

Read the statement or question, and determine the answer that best fits. Record the answer in the blank provided.

_____ 1. Which of the following is not necessary registration information when a patient visits a medical office for an appointment?
(a) Guarantor for the patient's account
(b) Patient's date of birth
(c) Patient's previous address
(d) Patient's employer
(e) Patient's insurance information

_____ 2. Which of the following is true about the billing process?
(a) After completion, superbills should be placed in the patient's chart and the chart returned to the records room.
(b) Patients should be asked to return their superbills to the front desk.
(c) The nurse is responsible for recording a patient's procedure and diagnosis on the superbill.
(d) Superbills should be collected at a specific location and returned to the front office at the end of each day.

_____ 3. Which of the following is true about billing for a missed appointment?
(a) Patients should always be charged for missed appointments.
(b) The AMA has notified physicians that it is illegal to charge for missed appointments.
(c) A medical office should establish a policy for charges for missed appointments.
(d) A physician who has only a few patients scheduled every day probably will not notice a missed appointment in the schedule.

_____ 4. To obtain credit, a patient's marital status may be asked if
(a) The patient is younger than 25 years.
(b) The income of the patient's spouse will be used to obtain credit.
(c) The patient is female.
(d) The patient is covered by Medicare.

_____ 5. A patient can be refused credit if
(a) Part of the patient's income comes from public assistance.
(b) The patient is younger than 21 years.
(c) The patient is not a natural born citizen of the United States.
(d) The patient is unable to pay because of insufficient income.

_____ 6. The first method used to attempt to collect a debt might be
(a) Calling the guarantor at work.
(b) Writing a letter to the guarantor.
(c) Adding a dunning message to the guarantor's statement.
(d) Asking the patient in person for a payment.

Exercise 11-3 Collection Practices

Read the following statements, and determine whether the statement is good or bad practice in collecting a debt. Record your answers in the blanks provided. A = good practice; B = bad practice.

_____ 1. Consult with a physician regarding a patient's account status.

_____ 2. Contact a debtor at a public event.

_____ 3. Threaten a debtor.

_____ 4. Be polite.

_____ 5. Speak harshly.

_____ 6. Use foul language.

_____ 7. Call the debtor repeatedly in the middle of the night until a payment is received.

_____ 8. Call the debtor a "deadbeat."

_____ 9. Speak only to the guarantor about the debt.

_____ 10. Send the guarantor a letter explaining what charges are owed.

_____ 11. Talk about the debt to whoever answers the guarantor's phone.

_____ 12. If all else fails, turn the account over to a collection agency.

_____ 13. Ask the patient to commit to a monthly payment.

_____ 14. Refuse to release a patient's medical records until the patient's account is paid in full.

_____ 15. Call a guarantor's employer when the guarantor is not allowed to receive calls at work.

ACTIVITIES

ACTIVITY 11-1 VERIFY PROGRAM OPTIONS FOR BILLING

1. On the Medisoft main menu, click **File>Program Options>Data Entry.**
2. Verify that the Program Options for billing are set as follows. Select or deselect all data entry options similar to the screen pictured below. Click **Save** to close program options. Click **OK** if HIPAA log off message appears.

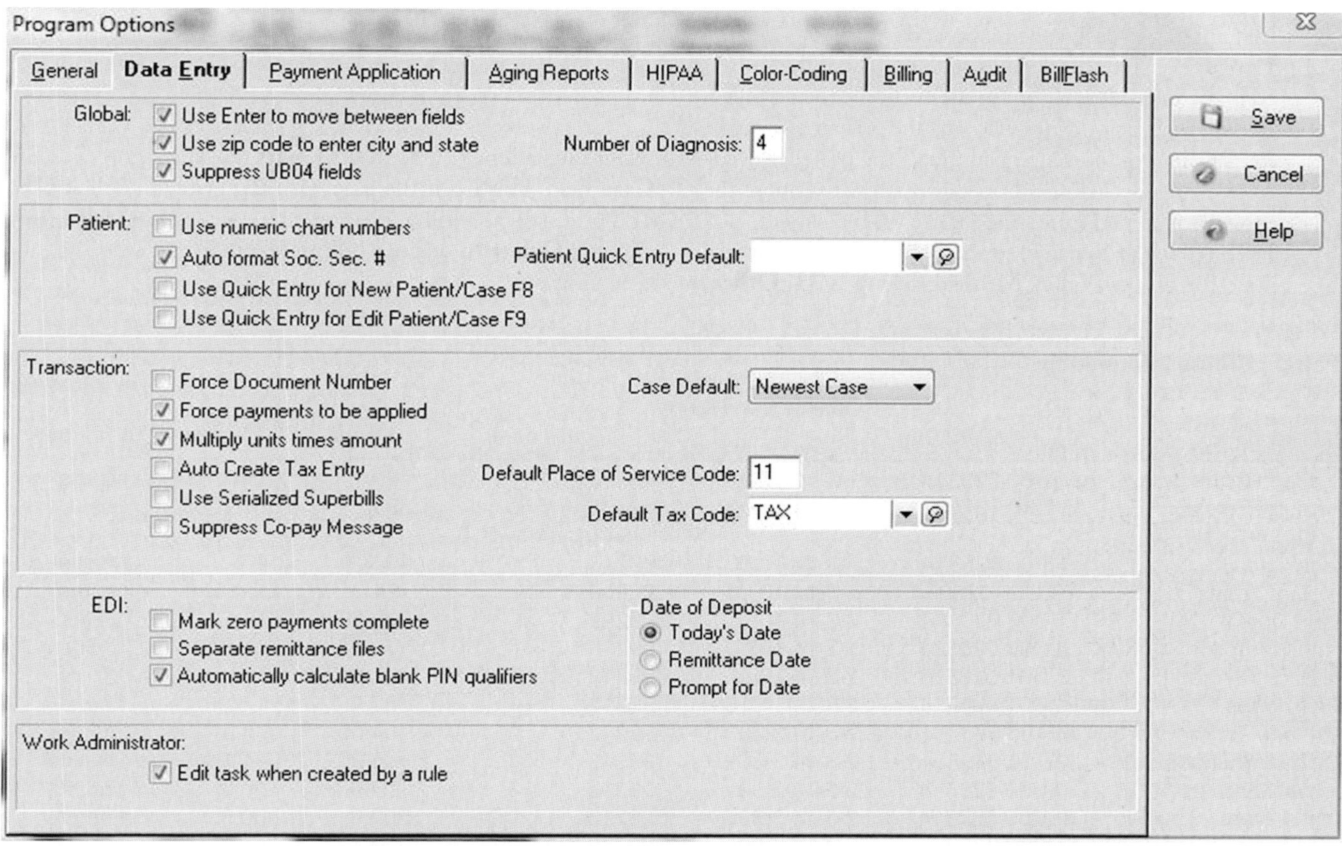

ACTIVITY 11-2 ENTERING CHARGES IN MEDISOFT

Enter billing information for patients seen on February 3 and February 4, 2014. Billing information is included in the following table. (If you experience difficulties at any time while performing this exercise, click **Help>Medisoft Help>Contents** for information on **Entering Charges**.)

1. On the Medisoft main menu, click **Activities>Enter Transactions.** The **Transaction Entry** window will open.
2. Enter billing information as follows. Billing information is contained in the table on page 256. (To move from field to field within the transaction entry window, simply press the **Enter** or **Tab** key or click on the desired field in the billing window.)
   a. **Chart**—Click the drop-down arrow on the chart field. Double-click the name of the patient to be billed.
   b. **Case**—Click the drop-down arrow on the case field. Double-click the name of the case that was assigned for the appointment to be billed.
   c. **Date**—Enter the date or click the drop-down arrow, and click the date of the patient's encounter.
   d. **Procedure**—Type the procedure code in the box or click the drop-down arrow to select the procedure code for the patient's encounter. If a new code needs to be added to the procedure code list, it can be added by right-clicking on the **Procedure** box.
   e. **Units**— This field indicates the number of times the procedure was performed. Usually this field has a value of 1. Leave the units as is unless instructed otherwise.
   f. **Amount**— This field is automatically filled in when the procedure code is selected. A price is set for almost all procedure codes.

g. **Diagnosis 1, 2, 3, 4**—Type the diagnosis code in the first box or click the drop-down arrow to select the diagnosis code for the patient's encounter. Use the type of diagnosis code that is currently required for processing claims: either an I-9 or I-10 code. DO NOT use both codes. If a new diagnosis code needs to be added to the diagnosis code list, it can be added by right-clicking on the **Diag 1** box.
h. **1, 2, 3, 4**—If more than one diagnosis is listed for an encounter, place a checkmark under each diagnosis() that applies to each specific procedure code.
i. **Provider**—Medisoft defaults to the provider that is listed in the case information for the encounter being billed. Be sure that the provider who saw the patient gets credit for the charges for that encounter. If the provider needs to be changed, click the drop-down arrow to choose the provider who performed the service for the patient.
j. **POS (Place of Service)**—The default place of service code for Happy Valley Medical Group is **11, Office.** (If a service is provided in another location, the correct code may be entered in the **POS** field.) Leave the remaining fields as is.
k. If more than one procedure was performed, click **New** near the bottom of the **Charges** portion of the window. DO NOT click the **New** button in the **Payments** area.
l. If the charges are complete, click **Save Transactions**.
m. To begin to enter billing information for another patient, click the drop-down arrow on the **Chart** field to select a new patient.
n. When all bills have been entered, click **Close** at the bottom of the window.

If a mistake is made after a transaction has been saved, select the patient's name in the **Chart** box and right-click the **Case** field. Highlight the case with the error, and click **OK**. The original case will appear, and charges can be deleted by clicking **Delete** to delete a billing line item.

Patient Billing Information

Patient Name	Case description	Date of Service (Date of Appt)	Procedure code	I-9 code	I-10 code	Provider
Charles Gooding	BLU00 020314	2-3-14 9:00	98940	723.1	M54.2	Morris
Anthony Peters	WOR00 020314	2-3-14 10:00	12001, A4550 surgical tray $15	883.0	S61.209A	Lee
Jane Doe	FHP00 020314	2-3-14 10:00	99213	490	J40	Martinez
William Frost	MED01 020314	2-3-14 10:00	98940	724.2	M54.5	Morris
John Doe	FHP00 020314	2-3-14 10:15	99212	780.60	R50.9	Marks
Tanus Simpson	BLU00 020314	2-3-14 10:30	99213	V72.84	Z01.818	O'Brian
Wallace Clinger	BLU01 020314	2-3-14 10:45	99213	401.9	I10	Marks
Suzy Jones	BLU01 020314	2-3-14 11:15	99212	382.9	H66.90	Lee
Anthony Zimmerman	AET00 020314	2-3-14 2:30	99212	464.00	J04.0	Martinez
Michael Youngblood	AET00 020314	2-3-14 2:30	99213	346.90	G43.909	Hinckle
Tonya Gonzalez	BLU00 020314	2-3-14 2:30	99212	703.0	L60.0	Lee
Zach Peters	BLU00 020314	2-3-14 3:30	99212	708.9	L50.9	Lee
Jay Brimley	FHP00 020314	2-3-14 4:00	98940	723.1	M54.2	Morris
Chadwick Koseman	WOR00 020314	2-3-14 4:15	26720, 99070 misc. supplies (finger splint) $12	816.00	S62.609A	Lee
Elmo Brimley	FHP00 020314	2-3-14 4:45	99212	052.9	B01.9	Hinckle
Sammy Catera	BLU01 020414	2-4-14 9:00	99213	311	F32.9	Lee
Lindsey Nielsen	CIG00 020414	2-4-14 9:15	99212	626.2	N92.0	Hinckle
Tonya Gonzalez	BLU00 020414	2-4-14 9:15	99396	V70.0	Z00.00	O'Brian
Dwight Again	MED01 020414	2-4-14 9:45	99213, 71020	487.1	J10.1	Marks
Charles Gooding	BLU00 020414	2-4-14 10:15	99212	723.1	M54.2	Morris
Deanne Olson	BLU00 020414	2-4-14 10:30	99212	382.9	H66.90	O'Brian
John Doe	FHP00 020414	2-4-14 10:30	99213, 71020	487.1	J10.1	Marks
Ryan Whitmore	CIG00 020414	2-4-14 10:30	99213	724.2	M54.5	Hinckle
Susan Brimley	FHP00 020414	2-4-14 11:00	99212	473.9	J32.9	O'Brian
Andrew Austin	CIG00 020414	2-4-14 1:00	99212	473.9	J32.9	Martinez

ACTIVITY 11-3 PATIENT STATEMENTS—COMPUTERIZED

To print statements of patients' accounts, do the following:

1. On the Medisoft main menu, click **Reports>Patient Statements.** Click **Patient Statement** (30, 60, 90). Click **OK**.
2. Specify **Export the report to a file** and click **Start.**
3. Name the file **yourlastname statements,** save it as a **text** file, and **Save** the file to a location you can remember.
4. In the **Patient Statement Data Selection** window, leave all entries blank except enter the **Date From Range** 02/01/2014 to 02/28/2014. Leave the **Statement Total Range** as is. Click **OK**.
5. Statements for all patients who have had charges for the month or who have a balance will be displayed on the screen. (Patients with balances previously in the software will also print.) Review the contents of the file to make sure the desired statements are included in the file. Send the file to your instructor.

ACTIVITY 11-4 PATIENT DAY SHEET REPORT

To print day sheets summarizing the monthly charges per patient, do the following:

1. On the Medisoft main menu, click **Reports>Day Sheets>Patient Day Sheet.**
2. Specify **Export the report to a file** and click **Start.**
3. Name the file **yourlastname daysheet,** save it as an **rtf** (rich text format) file and **save** the file, to a location you can remember.
4. In the **Search** window, check **show all values** for all fields except enter the **Date From Range 02/01/2014 to 02/28/2014.** Click **OK.**
5. A daysheet summarizing all transactions during February 2014 will be generated. Review the contents of the file to make sure the desired statements are included in the file. Send the file in to your instructor.

ACTIVITY 11-5 PATIENT RECEIPT

To print a patient receipt for an encounter with a provider, do the following:

1. On the **Medisoft** main menu, click **Activities> Transaction entry.** Open the bill for Anthony Peters's visit on 2/3/2014 with Timothy Marks. If necessary, click the drop-down arrow in the **Case** box, click the case with the description **WOR00 020314** to display the charges for the visit.
2. Click **Print Receipt** near the bottom of the window. (Make sure Transaction window is maximized in order to view **Print Receipt** option.) Click **Walkout receipt (All Transactions)>OK.**
3. Click **Export the report to a file>Start.** Name the file **yourlastname receipt,** save it as a **text** document, and click **Save** the file to a location you can remember.
4. In the **Date From Range** enter the date of the encounter **02/03/2014 to 02/03/2014.** Click **OK.**
5. A receipt for the encounter will be generated. Review the contents of the file to make sure the desired receipt is included in the file. Send the file to your instructor.

ACTIVITY 11-6 ESTATE CLAIMS

In your local newspaper, search for an example of a legal notice of estate claims similar to the one shown in Figure 11-6. Determine what the legal requirements are in your state for collecting a debt from an estate.

ACTIVITY 11-7 COLLECTION LETTERS

Draft a collection letter to Matthew Stein, chart number STEMA000. His address is 123 Prairie Parkway, Harvester, AZ 85000. Matthew Stein was mentioned in this chapter. He has an account balance of $1000. His accounts receivable balance is as follows: (Current (0-30 days old): $0. Balance 31-60 days old: $100. Balance 61-90 days old: $50. Balance more than 90 days old: $850.) This is the first collection letter that will be sent to him. Follow the guidelines for collection printed in this chapter, as well as the guidelines for proper letter format given in Chapter 6.

Prepare a letter and an envelope using word processing software.

ACTIVITY 11-8 MEDICAL OFFICE SCENARIOS

Consider the following situations. What is the appropriate response to the situation given?

1. A patient calls the office and asks how much a physical examination costs. What do you say?
2. A patient's account has a balance of $500 that is 120 days past due. No payment has ever been made toward the balance. Reminders and letters to the patient have produced no response. You must now phone the patient to attempt collection. What do you say?

ACTIVITY 11-9 SUPERBILLS

Obtain a copy of a superbill from a medical office in your area. Discuss the following questions:

1. What information is included on the superbill?
2. Is the term *superbill* used by the medical office from which you obtained the form?
3. How does this form compare with the superbills shown in Figure 11-1?

DISCUSSION

The following topics can be used for class discussion or for individual student essay.

DISCUSSION 11-1

Explain why complete documentation regarding a patient's encounter is critical to the billing process.

DISCUSSION 11-2

Is a patient's medical billing information as confidential as his or her medical record? Why?

DISCUSSION 11-3

Identify methods of tracking a guarantor who has moved and left no forwarding address.

Bibliography

The Access Project: *Borrowing to Stay Healthy: How Credit Card Debt Is Related to Medical Expenses*. http://www.accessproject.org/adobe/borrowing_to_stay_healthy_release.pdf. Accessed August 30, 2012.

Centers for Disease Control and Prevention: *Financial Burden of Medical Care: Early Release of Estimates From the National Health Interview Survey*. http://www.cdc.gov/nchs/data/nhis/earlyrelease/financial_burden_of_medical_care_032012.pdf. Accessed September 11, 2012.

Consumer Credit Counseling Service: *Dealing With Medical Debt*. http://www.cccsatl.org. Accessed November 25, 2007.

Families USA: Medical Debt: *What States are Doing to Protect Consumers*. http://www.familiesusa.org/assets/pdfs/medical-debt-state-protections.pdf. Accessed September 11, 2012.

Federal Trade Commission: *The Fair Debt Collection Practices Act*. http://www.ftc.gov/os/statutes/fdcpa/fdcpact.shtm. Accessed August 30, 2012.

Fish-Parcham C, Wu C: National Consumer Law Center: Helping Older Americans Cope with Medical Debt, a presentation dated March 14, 2012. http://www.nclc.org/images/pdf/conferences_and_webinars/webinar_trainings/presentations/2011-2012/helping_older_americans_cope_with_medical_deb_webinar.pdf. Accessed October 24, 2013.

The United States Department of Justice: *Title VII: Equal Credit Opportunity Act*. http://www.justice.gov/crt/about/hce/documents/ecoafulltext_5-1-06.php. Accessed August 30, 2012.

CHAPTER 12 Health Insurance and Health Benefits Programs

LEARNING OUTCOMES

On successful completion of this chapter, the student will be able to

1. Apply health insurance and benefits terminology.
2. Explain the components of the CMS-1500 form.
3. Describe the insurance claims process.
4. Explain the components of an Explanation of Benefits (EOB) statement.
5. Identify reasons claims are denied.
6. Explain managed care policies.
7. Explain Medicare eligibility and coverage.
8. Explain Medicaid eligibility and coverage.
9. Explain TRICARE/CHAMPVA eligibility and coverage.
10. Explain Workers' Compensation eligibility and coverage.
11. Explain group insurance coverage.
12. Explain Blue Cross/Blue Shield coverage.
13. Explain short-term and long-term disability coverage.
14. Explain legal and ethical issues related to health insurance.
15. Utilize medical practice management software to generate insurance claims.

COMMISSION ON ACCREDITATION OF ALLIED HEALTH EDUCATION PROGRAMS (CAAHEP) CORE CURRICULUM FOR MEDICAL ASSISTANTS

- Use office hardware and software to maintain office systems
- Use Internet to access information related to the medical office
- Utilize computerized office billing systems
- Identify types of insurance plans
- Identify models of managed care
- Discuss workers' compensation as it applies to patients
- Describe how guidelines are used in processing an insurance claim
- Compare processes for filing insurance claims both manually and electronically
- Describe guidelines for third-party claims
- Complete insurance claim forms
- Describe the implications of HIPAA for the medical assistant in various medical settings
- Respond to issues of confidentiality
- Apply third-party guidelines
- Identify and respond to issues of confidentiality
- Perform within legal and ethical boundaries
- Use computer software to maintain office systems

ACCREDITING BUREAU OF HEALTH EDUCATION SCHOOLS (ABHES) COMPETENCIES FOR MEDICAL ASSISTING

Graduates

- Prepare and submit insurance claims
- Apply computer application skills using a variety of different electronic programs including both practice management software and EMR software
- Apply third-party guidelines
- Obtain managed care referrals and precertification
- Apply electronic technology

VOCABULARY

Advance Beneficiary Notice (ABN)
beneficiary
birthday rule
capitation
Children's Health Insurance Program (CHIP)
Civilian Health and Medical Program of the Department of Veterans Affairs (CHAMPVA)
claim
coinsurance
Consolidated Omnibus Budget Reconciliation Act (COBRA)
coordination of benefits (COB)
copayment
deductible
dual-eligibles
edits
electronic data interchange (EDI)
explanation of benefits (EOB)
fee-for-service
group insurance
group number
health maintenance organization (HMO)
independent practice association (IPA)
insurance contract
insured
insurer
limiting charge

VOCABULARY—cont'd

managed care
Medicaid
Medicare
Medicare Administrative Contractor (MAC)
participating provider (PAR)
policy
policyholder
preauthorization
preferred provider organization (PPO)
premium
referral
sponsor
subscriber
TRICARE
usual, customary, and reasonable (UCR) fee
Workers' Compensation

Health insurance regulations change frequently and are updated continually. A medical administrative assistant should obtain insurance claim processing information directly from a specific insurance plan. This chapter is intended to serve as a guide to the types of issues that may arise when one is assisting patients with health insurance questions and claims processing. Information received directly from insurance plans is definitive in describing the insurance plan's processes and benefits.

Today, many patients who are seeking health care have some type of coverage that will pay a portion or even all of their health care costs. Approximately 84% of patients seeking medical care are covered by some type of insurance. For these patients, preparation of a billing statement that summarizes charges is not sufficient; many individuals will need insurance claims filed to receive those benefits. Medical office personnel spend many hours filing and collecting health insurance benefits as a customer service for their patients. Knowledge of medical insurance procedures is an integral part of the patient billing process, and claims for health insurance benefits must be filed accurately and promptly to allow patients to collect their benefits and health facilities to be paid in a timely manner.

Insurance Terminology

When studying the various types of health insurance coverage and benefits, a medical administrative assistant must have a firm grasp of the specific language used in the health insurance industry. Several terms are used on a daily basis in working with insurance claims.

An **insurance contract** or **policy** is an agreement between an **insurer** (an insurance company) and an individual or a group of individuals. A policy specifies what types of health care treatment are covered, as well as the amounts that are payable.

The payment required for insurance coverage is known as a **premium.** A premium may be paid by an employer or an individual, or perhaps both may share the payment of the premium. Premiums may be paid on a monthly basis, or the parties may agree to another arrangement. In exchange for a paid premium, an insurance company agrees to provide insurance coverage pursuant to the terms of the contract or policy.

The terms **policyholder, insured,** and **subscriber** are synonymous and refer to the individual who holds the insurance policy. For instance, if one of the two working parents in a family of four has an insurance policy through an employer, that parent is known as the policyholder (or insured or subscriber). A **beneficiary** is any individual, such as the subscriber's spouse or dependent, who qualifies for benefits under that subscriber's policy.

In addition to paying any required premium, a policyholder sometimes may have to pay an additional cost, known as a **copayment,** for health care services. A copayment may have to be paid by a patient (or insured) each time the patient has a visit with a health care provider. A copayment is a set amount (e.g., $20, $30) that must be paid by a patient or policyholder for each encounter, regardless of the cost of the visit.

Consider the following examples for two patients covered by health insurance: (1) Patient A's policy requires a $20 copayment. The patient sees a physician for a sore throat and a strep screen for a total visit cost of $64. The patient will pay a $20 copayment for the encounter with the physician. (2) Patient B's policy also requires a $20 copayment. The patient sees a physician for a cardiology workup and diagnostic tests totaling more than $1500. Patient B will pay a $20 copayment for the entire visit.

The copayment does not change according to the amount charged for a visit. Copayments help hold down costs for the insurer because a portion of every visit must be paid by the patient or the insured, and the patient may think twice about seeing a physician for minor ailments. Copayments usually only apply to visits with the physician and do not apply to services such as laboratory and radiology tests.

A **coinsurance** clause in an insurance contract greatly affects the amount the patient may have to pay for treatment. Coinsurance is a percentage of the claim required to be paid by the patient. In the previous example, if both patients A and B had a 20% coinsurance clause, patient B would pay far more for the visit than would patient A. This is because the total amount for patient B's visit is significantly higher than patient A's total amount. Health insurance policies may require payments of copayments, coinsurance, or both.

Usually, when an insured patient receives services from a health care provider, a medical office files a **claim** on behalf of the patient to collect benefits from the patient's insurance company. A claim refers to any request to an insurance company or government program for benefits on behalf of the insured. Most medical offices will file claims for their patients because it is more likely that claims will be filed and benefits will be received if this service is provided by a medical office. If this process were left up to patients and the insured, it is likely that many claims would not be made, and payments for services would be delayed. Medical billing personnel really become experts in filing insurance claims.

A **deductible** also affects the amount a patient must ultimately pay for medical services. A deductible is a specific amount that a patient must pay for health care services per year before any insurance benefits will be paid. Deductibles are amounts that are larger than copayments, for example, \$100, \$200, or \$500. A policy may set a maximum deductible per patient, as well as for an entire family.

For example, a policy's deductible may be \$200 per family member or \$500 for the entire family per year. If the policy covers a family of three, the first \$200 of services for family member 1 and family member 2 will be applied toward the deductible. Only the first \$100 of expenses for family member 3 will be applied toward the deductible because the maximum family deductible would be met. Likewise, if family member 1 incurred \$50 more in expenses, those expenses would not be applied toward the deductible because the \$200 limit would have already been met for the year. Once the entire family reaches the \$500 deductible, the deductible will be met for that year.

Deductibles usually are applicable for charges from January 1 to December 31 of each year. Also, deductibles apply only to services that are covered under the terms of the insurance policy. Services not covered under an insurance policy are paid solely by the patient (or guarantor) and do not apply toward any deductible. Often deductibles do not apply to some services that are fully covered by insurance, such as routine physicals or eye examinations. In the case of covered examinations, the examinations would be paid regardless of whether or not the deductible is paid.

Coverages can vary greatly among different policies and from company to company, and it is quite common for an insurance policy to change its own coverage amounts from year to year. This can make it quite challenging for patients to understand which benefits they are entitled to each year. To help patients understand their insurance policies and associated coverage, it is very important for an assistant to have a thorough understanding of the terminology used pertaining to health insurance. In addition to the definitions provided in this text, many insurance plans and government programs have information available online including definitions of the terms used for insurance claims processing.

Centers for Medicare and Medicaid Services

The Centers for Medicare and Medicaid Services (CMS), part of the U.S. Department of Health and Human Services (DHHS), is an agency of the federal government. CMS manages the Medicare, Medicaid, and Children's Health Insurance Program (CHIP), all of which provide health care benefits to over 100 million people, and spends more than \$819 billion per year on those benefits. CMS's mission is "to ensure effective, up-to-date health care coverage and to promote quality care for beneficiaries." Their responsibilities include the following:

- Overseeing the operations of state agencies and contractors that carry out the functions of CMS
- Evaluating the quality of health care services
- Studying the effectiveness of matters related to health care services
- Setting policy for payment for health care services

CMS-1500 Claim Form

Most medical office claims are filed on a standard claim form called the CMS-1500 (Fig. 12-1). In the 1960s, the CMS-1500 was developed originally for the purpose of standardizing the submission of claims sent in for payment of government benefits. It was gradually adopted for use by other insurance companies. In 2006, the National Uniform Claim Committee (NUCC) released a revision of the CMS-1500, which was required to be used as of July 2, 2007, and is still in use today. Although CMS and many other providers prefer that electronic claims are filed, there are provisions for CMS-1500 paper claims processing for providers who are exempt from electronic claims processing.

The use of this standard form has helped streamline claims submissions for medical offices and claims processing for insurance companies. Table 12-1 lists CMS guidelines for step-by-step completion of the CMS-1500 for Medicare claims. Other insurance programs and private insurance companies such as Blue Cross/Blue Shield usually have their own specific requirements for completion of the CMS-1500.

HIPAA Hint

If the U.S. Department of Health and Human Services (DHHS) is conducting a review of a provider's billing practices, the provider is allowed to disclose protected health information to DHHS.

The Insurance Claim Process

Remember that the most critical step of the insurance claim process takes place before a patient even sees the physician. Preparation for an insurance claim begins at the moment a patient registers for an appointment with a physician, at which time a medical administrative assistant obtains current insurance information from the patient and records the information for later use when processing the patient's insurance claim. This information can be obtained directly from the patient's insurance card (Fig. 12-2). This card identifies the insurance company's name and address, the policyholder, the policy number, the group number, and information on how to contact the insurance company and where to file claims.

1500

HEALTH INSURANCE CLAIM FORM

FHP HEALTH PLAN
4576 E. W. POWER RD.
MESA AZ 85208

PICA | PICA

1. MEDICARE (Medicare #) MEDICAID (Medicaid #) TRICARE CHAMPUS (Sponsor's SSN) CHAMPVA (VA File #) GROUP HEALTH PLAN (SSN or ID) FECA BLK LUNG (SSN) OTHER (ID)

1a. INSURED'S I.D. NUMBER (FOR PROGRAM IN ITEM 1): 78-555-263

2. PATIENT'S NAME (Last Name, First Name, Middle Initial): DOE, JOHN, C

3. PATIENT'S BIRTH DATE MM DD YY SEX: 07 03 1972 M [X] F [ ]

4. INSURED'S NAME (Last Name, First Name, Middle Initial)

5. PATIENT'S ADDRESS (No., Street): 222 EAST JANE STREET

6. PATIENT RELATIONSHIP TO INSURED: Self [X] Spouse [ ] Child [ ] Other [ ]

7. INSURED'S ADDRESS (No., Street)

CITY: MESA STATE: AZ

8. PATIENT STATUS: Single [ ] Married [ ] Other [ ]; Employed [ ] Full-Time Student [ ] Part-Time Student [ ]

CITY STATE

ZIP CODE: 85213 TELEPHONE (Include Area Code): (010)9999999

ZIP CODE TELEPHONE (INCLUDE AREA CODE) ( )

9. OTHER INSURED'S NAME (Last Name, First Name, Middle Initial)

10. IS PATIENT'S CONDITION RELATED TO:

11. INSURED'S POLICY GROUP OR FECA NUMBER: NONE

a. OTHER INSURED'S POLICY OR GROUP NUMBER

a. EMPLOYMENT? (CURRENT OR PREVIOUS) [ ] YES [X] NO

a. INSURED'S DATE OF BIRTH MM DD YY SEX M [ ] F [ ]

b. OTHER INSURED'S DATE OF BIRTH MM DD YY SEX M [ ] F [ ]

b. AUTO ACCIDENT? PLACE (State) [ ] YES [X] NO

b. EMPLOYER'S NAME OR SCHOOL NAME

c. EMPLOYER'S NAME OR SCHOOL NAME

c. OTHER ACCIDENT? [ ] YES [X] NO

c. INSURANCE PLAN NAME OR PROGRAM NAME

d. INSURANCE PLAN NAME OR PROGRAM NAME

10d. RESERVED FOR LOCAL USE

d. IS THERE ANOTHER HEALTH BENEFIT PLAN? [ ] YES [ ] NO *If yes, return to and complete item 9 a-d.*

READ BACK OF FORM BEFORE COMPLETING AND SIGNING THIS FORM.

12. PATIENT'S OR AUTHORIZED PERSON'S SIGNATURE. I authorize the release of any medical or other information necessary to process this claim. I also request payment of government benefits either to myself or to the party who accepts assignment below.

SIGNED DATE

13. INSURED'S OR AUTHORIZED PERSON'S SIGNATURE. I authorize payment of medical benefits to the undersigned physician or supplier for services described below.

SIGNED

14. DATE OF CURRENT: ILLNESS (First symptom) OR INJURY (Accident) OR PREGNANCY(LMP) MM DD YY

15. IF PATIENT HAS HAD SAME OR SIMILAR ILLNESS GIVE FIRST DATE MM DD YY

16. DATES PATIENT UNABLE TO WORK IN CURRENT OCCUPATION FROM MM DD YY TO MM DD YY

17. NAME OF REFERRING PHYSICIAN OR OTHER SOURCE 17a. 17b. NPI

18. HOSPITALIZATION DATES RELATED TO CURRENT SERVICES FROM MM DD YY TO MM DD YY

19. RESERVED FOR LOCAL USE

20. OUTSIDE LAB? $ CHARGES [ ] YES [X] NO

21. DIAGNOSIS OR NATURE OF ILLNESS OR INJURY (RELATE ITEMS 1,2,3 OR 4 TO ITEM 24E BY LINE)

1. 487 . 1   2. ___ . __   3. ___ . __   4. ___ . __

22. MEDICAID RESUBMISSION CODE ORIGINAL REF. NO.

23. PRIOR AUTHORIZATION NUMBER

24. A. DATE(S) OF SERVICE From MM DD YY	To MM DD YY	B. Place of Service	C. EMG	D. PROCEDURES, SERVICES, OR SUPPLIES (Explain Unusual Circumstances) CPT/HCPCS	MODIFIER	E. DIAGNOSIS POINTER	F. $ CHARGES	G. DAYS OR UNITS	H. EPSDT Family Plan	I. ID QUAL.	J. RENDERING PROVIDER ID. #
02042014	02042014	11		99213		1	60 00	1		NPI	
02042014	02042014	11		71020		1	53 00	1		NPI	
										NPI	
										NPI	
										NPI	
										NPI	

25. FEDERAL TAX I.D. NUMBER SSN EIN [ ] [ ]

26. PATIENT'S ACCOUNT NO.: DOEJO000 76

27. ACCEPT ASSIGNMENT? (For govt. claims, see back) [ ] YES [X] NO

28. TOTAL CHARGE: $ 113.00

29. AMOUNT PAID: $

30. BALANCE DUE: 113.00

31. SIGNATURE OF PHYSICIAN OR SUPPLIER INCLUDING DEGREES OR CREDENTIALS (I certify that the statements on the reverse apply to this bill and are made a part thereof.)

SIGNED DATE 01/02/13

32. SERVICE FACILITY LOCATION INFORMATION a. NPI b.

33. BILLING PROVIDER INFO & PH # (012)5550000
TIMOTHY I MARKS PA
1234 MAIN AVE
FARMINGTON AZ 85000
a. NPI b.

NUCC Instruction Manual available at: www.nucc.org

PLEASE PRINT OR TYPE

Figure 12-1 The CMS-1500 insurance claim form can be used to file paper claims for government and private insurance plans. (From the National Uniform Claim Committee. www.nucc.org.)

TABLE 12-1

Guidelines for Filing Insurance Claims*

Carrier Block	Carrier Information
Located at top of form	Enter name and address of the payer to whom the claim is addressed. 1st line—Name 2nd line—First line of address 3rd line—Second line of address (if necessary) 4th line—City State ZIP
Item Number	**Patient Information**
†1	Check the box that pertains to the insurance plan for the claim that is being filed. *Blue Cross/Blue Shield*—Check the group health plan box. *TRICARE*—Enter name of military sponsor. *Workers' Compensation*—Use patient's social security number (SSN).
†1a	Enter the insured's policy identification (ID) number. This usually (but not always) is the insured's SSN. *Workers' Compensation*—Enter the claim number.
†2	Enter the patient's last name, first name, and middle initial as shown on insurance card.
†3	Enter the patient's birth date using eight digits (MM/DD/YYYY), and identify patient's sex (M or F).
†4	Enter the name of the insured. If the same as item 2, enter **SAME.** *Workers' Compensation*—Enter name of patient's employer. *Workers' Compensation*—Enter name of patient's employer. *Third-Party Liability Claims*—Enter name of insured.
†5	Enter the patient's address and telephone number as identified on the form.
†6	Identify the relationship of the patient to the insured.
†7	If 4 is completed, enter the insured's address and telephone number. If this information is the same as item 5, enter the word SAME.
†8	Check the patient's marital status and employment and student status as they apply. Only one box per line may be checked.
†9	If the patient is covered by a secondary insurance policy, enter the policyholder's name on the secondary policy. If the information is the same, enter SAME.
†9a	Enter policy number of secondary payer. *Medicare*—If Medicare is secondary, enter patient's ID number. *Medigap*—Enter **MEDIGAP, MGP,** or **MGAP** followed by the Medigap policy number.
†9b	Enter the birth date (MM/DD/YYYY) and sex (M or F) of the secondary policyholder.
†9c	If a secondary policy is from an employer, enter the employer's name. If the patient is a student but is also employed, enter the patient's school name. *Medicaid*—Leave blank. *Medicare*—Leave blank. *Medigap*—Enter claims processing address from patient's Medigap card.
†9d	Enter the name of the secondary insurance plan. *Medigap*—Enter the nine-digit payer ID of the Medigap insurer. If the payer ID is not available, enter the Medigap plan name.
†10a-c	Check the appropriate boxes "yes" or "no" as to whether this claim is a result of an employment, auto, or other accident. Yes or no must be checked for each question.
†10d	If the patient is covered by Medicaid, enter **MCD** followed by the patient's Medicaid number.
†11	List the insured's group number in this box. If there is no group number, enter the insured's policy number. *Medicare*—If Medicare is the primary insurance, enter **NONE** and go to item 12. *Workers' Compensation*—Enter policy or group number of employer's Workers' Compensation plan.
†11a	Enter the insured's birth date (MM/DD/YYYY) and identify the insured's sex (M or F) if insured is not the patient.
†11b	Enter insured's employer's name, if policy was issued through the employer. *Medicare*—Leave blank. *Workers' Compensation*—Leave blank.
†11c	Enter the plan name.
†11d	Enter "yes" when a secondary insurance will be billed, then complete box 9 in its entirety. Enter "no" if no other plans. *Workers' Compensation*—Enter "no".

Continued

TABLE 12-1

Guidelines for Filing Insurance Claims—cont'd

Item Number	Patient Information
†12	The patient or authorized representative must sign and date this section of the form to authorize release of medical information to process the claim. This item also authorizes payment of Medicare benefits to the health care facility that accepts assignment. The notation "signature on file" (SOF) may be entered in this blank if the patient has signed a previous authorization and that authorization is kept on file at the facility. Otherwise, leave blank.
†13	The patient's signature or the notation of signature on file in this blank authorizes a health care facility to receive payments of insurance benefits from the patient's insurance company.
Item Number	**Provider or Supplier Information**
†14	Enter an eight-digit date of current illness, injury, or pregnancy. This field is required for treatment related to injury or pregnancy. Date of injury (DOI) must be entered if patient was injured.
†15	Usually not required by most insurance plans.
†16	*Workers' Compensation*—If patient is employed and is unable to work because of a work-related injury, enter the dates the patient is unable to work.
†17	Enter the name of referring physician if applicable. Managed care plans—This field may be required if an authorization is required.
†17a	Enter other ID number of the provider reported in 17.
†17b	Enter the National Provider Identifier (NPI) of the provider listed in 17.
†18	Enter eight-digit date if medical services done pertain to a hospitalization.
†19	Reserved for local use.
†20	If outside laboratory tests were performed, the laboratory will bill the physician and the physician will bill insurance. If so, "yes" must be checked. *Medicare*—If "yes" is checked, enter purchase price under charges and complete information in item 32.
†21	Identify the ICD-9 codes related to the patient's diagnosis(es). Primary and secondary codes should be listed under item 1 and item 2, respectively. *Medicare*—If "yes" is checked in block 10 a, b, or c, an E code describing the injury is required.
†22	*Medicaid*—Enter resubmission code and original reference number.
†23	If applicable, enter a prior authorization number.
†24	Up to six different items may be billed per claim. When a number of identical services are performed, enter on one line and enter number of days or units in 24g.
†24a	Enter eight-digit dates of service. If only one date of service applies, enter the date only in the "From" blank. When "from" and "to" dates are used, enter the number of days or units in 24g.
†24b	Enter the place of service code (see Box 12-1).
†24c	May be required by some insurance plans, not required by Medicare. Use of a type of service code recognized by the insurance plan may provide further explanation of a procedure and may help prevent a claim denial.
†24d	Identify the procedure codes using the HCFA Common Procedure Coding System (HCPCS).
†24e	Reference the diagnosis code (1, 2, 3, or 4) in item 21 that applies to each procedure listed. Up to 4 numbers may be entered.
†24f	Enter the charge for each procedure.
†24g	Enter the number of times the procedure was performed or delivered. Some supplies list the quantity of supply delivered.
†24h	*Medicaid*—This field is used if services are provided under EPSDT (Early Periodic Screening and Diagnostic Testing), a Medicaid program.
†24i	Mark this field (usually an X is used) if service provided was an emergency.
†24j-k	J—Check if coordination of benefits (COB) applies. K—Enter UPIN (unique physician identification number) of physician (if group practice).
†25	Enter the Employer Identification number (EIN—federal tax ID) or the SSN of the provider.
†26	Enter the patient's account number assigned by the provider.
†27	*Medicare and TRICARE*—Check the appropriate box to identify whether the provider accepts assignment for Medicare benefits. If "yes" is entered, the provider agrees to accept payment from payer along with any copayment and deductible as payment in full.
†28	Enter the total of charges listed in 24f, lines 1 through 6.
†29	Enter the amount paid by the patient on charges related to this claim.
†30	Subtract line 29 from line 28. *Medicare*—This field may be left blank.

TABLE 12-1

Guidelines for Filing Insurance Claims—cont'd

Item Number	Provider or Supplier Information
†31	Enter the signature of the provider and the date the form was signed. Electronic signatures are acceptable.
†32	If services were provided in a place other than the patient's home or the physician's office, identify the location where the services were performed.
32a	Enter the NPI of the facility (if listed in 32).
32b	Enter the code for the other ID number followed by the ID number.
†33	Enter the provider's billing name, address, and telephone number along with the NPI if the provider is not a member of a group practice.
†33a	Enter the NPI of the provider in 33.
†33b	Enter the code for the other ID number followed by the ID number.

*When completing the CMS-1500 form, follow these basic instructions if no specific instructions are available from the insurance plan. Special instructions for certain insurance plans are included where applicable.

†A denotes that the item number *must* be completed. More detailed instructions are available from the National Uniform Claim Committee at www.nucc.org.

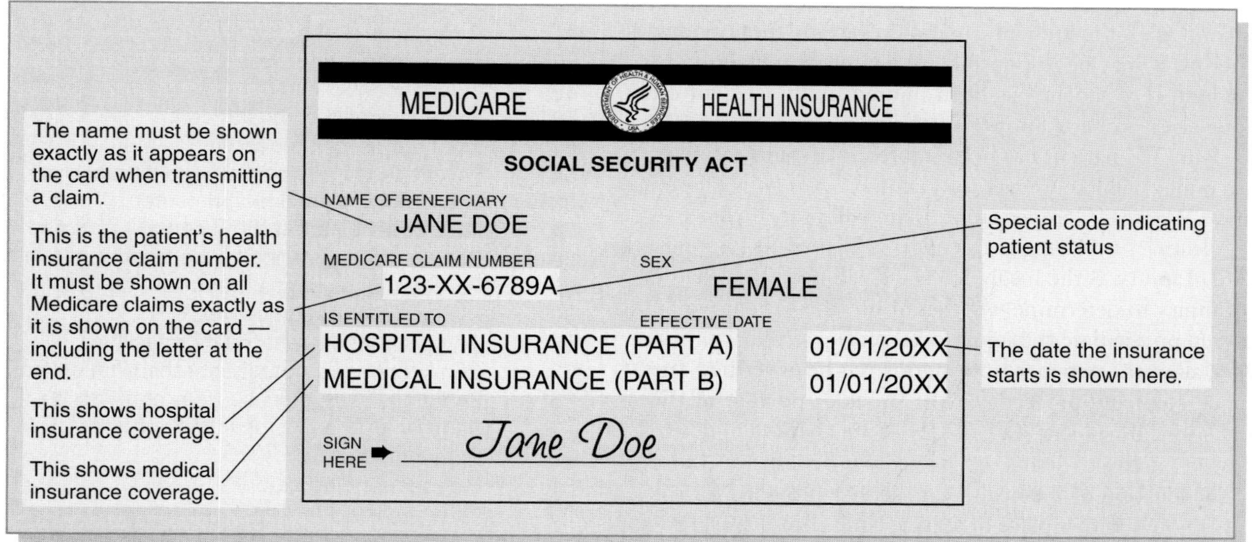

Figure 12-2 Information needed for processing insurance claims can be found on a patient's insurance card. (From Centers for Medicare and Medicaid Services: *Medicare and You.* CMS Publication 10050. Washington, DC: U.S. Department of Health and Human Services; 2008.)

A **group number** appears on many different insurance cards and is used to identify a group of people who all have the same insurance plan and related benefits. An example of a group would be employees who all work for the same company. The policy number identifies individual policyholders within that group.

The medical administrative assistant who registers the patient records all information from the insurance card needed to submit the claim. This information usually is recorded in a computer database used for patient billing but could also be written directly on the superbill. The information collected is the information that will be used to process a future insurance claim unless the patient reports an insurance change to the office. At this point, the patient is ready to see the provider, and the superbill is generated according to the procedures given in Chapter 11.

After the superbill has been completed and entered into the billing system, a claim (Procedure 12-1) is created and sent to the patient's insurance company. Some claims are printed on the CMS-1500 form and mailed to the insurance company. Today, however, many facilities that process large numbers of insurance claims submit them electronically using computerized systems. These systems can keep the facility from using excessive stacks of paper and can speed the actual processing and payment of claims.

Once the insurance company receives the claim, the patient's information on the claim is checked. The patient's name is checked with the company's database to ensure that the person is entitled to benefits from one of the insurance company's plans. The policy number and the group number also are verified to establish whether insurance coverage is available for that patient.

If the patient reports being injured in any type of accident, the insurance company may have to refer the claim back to the

PROCEDURE 12-1

Complete an Insurance Claim Using the CMS-1500

Materials Needed

- Billing and insurance information for a patient
- Computer software or typewriter to complete form
- CMS-1500 claim form

1. Obtain the billing information for the claim.
2. Code the procedures and diagnoses for the claim.*
3. Obtain the patient's insurance information for the claim.*
4. Complete the CMS-1500 claim form following the guidelines established by the insurance plan.*

**Denotes a crucial step in the procedure. The student must complete this step satisfactorily in order to complete the procedure satisfactorily.*

patient and ask for further information regarding the accident. Another party may be responsible for payments pertaining to an accident. If a patient has been injured in an accident on someone else's property, property liability coverage may apply to the claim. If a patient has been injured in an auto accident, an auto policy will likely cover the claim. If a patient is injured at work, a Workers' Compensation claim will probably have to be filed. In cases involving accidents, it is important to obtain the date of injury as the insurance plans will need to have the date of injury to determine whether or not the patient would be covered on the date the injury occurred.

Once all of the patient's information has been verified, the insurance company proceeds to the provider portion of the claim. Date of illness and date of service are checked to determine whether the patient was covered for benefits on those dates. The location of the health care service provided for the patient is noted with a place of service code (Box 12-1). Procedure codes are verified to determine whether those procedures are covered under the policy benefits. Diagnosis codes are also verified to determine whether the diagnosis is covered under the policy. The diagnosis and procedure codes then are matched with each other to reveal whether the procedure is related to or was appropriate treatment for the diagnosis—in other words, does the diagnosis fit the procedure? Example: If the patient had a tonsillectomy, the diagnosis should pertain to the throat. The patient's sex is also checked to make sure the procedure and diagnosis would be appropriate treatment for the patient. Example: A hysterectomy would not be performed on a male patient. If the patient is covered under a managed care policy that may restrict the providers that the patient is allowed to use, the provider name is checked against a list of authorized providers.

Once it has been determined that benefits should be provided for the health care services provided, the next step is for the insurer to determine the **usual, customary, and reasonable (UCR) fee** for those services. The UCR fee is the average amount charged by local physicians for services performed.

BOX 12-1

Place of Service Codes*

Code	Place of Service
03	School
04	Homeless shelter
11	Provider's office
12	Home
13	Assisted living facility
14	Group home
15	Mobile unit
20	Urgent care facility
21	Inpatient hospital
22	Outpatient hospital
23	Emergency room—hospital
24	Ambulatory surgical center
25	Birthing center
26	Military treatment center
31	Skilled nursing facility
32	Nursing facility
33	Custodial care facility
34	Hospice
41	Ambulance—land
42	Ambulance—air or water
49	Independent clinic
50	Federally qualified health center
51	Inpatient psychiatric facility
52	Psychiatric facility partial hospitalization
53	Community mental health center
54	Intermediate care facility/mentally retarded
55	Residential substance abuse treatment facility
56	Psychiatric residential treatment center
60	Mass immunization center
61	Comprehensive rehabilitation facility
62	Comprehensive outpatient rehabilitation facility
65	End-stage renal disease treatment facility
71	State or local public health clinic
72	Rural health clinic
81	Independent laboratory
99	Other unlisted facility

*A complete description of the place of service codes is available on the Centers for Medicare and Medicaid Services website.

Insurers keep track of fees charged within a certain geographic area and average those fees to arrive at the UCR fee. Companies then may not pay any amounts greater than the UCR fee. If the provider charges more than the UCR fee, a UCR reduction will appear on the patient's explanation of benefits, which is defined later in this chapter.

Next, any deductible that applies to the patient and any copayment due at the time of the visit are subtracted from the total bill. If the patient has a coinsurance clause in the policy, the coinsurance is subtracted from the remaining amount of the bill. Coinsurance is usually a percentage of the total *approved* charges (after the deductible is subtracted) for which the insured is responsible. For further illustration of how copayment, deductible, and coinsurance could be applied to a patient's charges, refer to Box 12-2.

BOX 12-2

Insurance Charges

Lisa Stein visits Dr. Mallard for an office visit and routine laboratory tests. She incurs charges for health care of $200.00. Her private insurance company approves of the charges. She pays a $10 copayment for each visit, has a $100 deductible that has not yet been met this year, and has a 20% coinsurance clause in her insurance contract. The amount her insurance will pay for the visit is as follows:

Total approved charges*	$200.00
Copayment	–$10.00
	$190.00
Deductible	–$100.00
	90.00
20% coinsurance	–$40.00
Amount insurance company pays:	$50.00

*If the charges for Lisa's visit were not all approved by the insurer, and a usual, customary, and reasonable fee reduction was taken, the patient may be charged for the reduction, or the medical office may write off the reduction.

For each claim submission, the insurance company prepares an **explanation of benefits (EOB)** (Fig. 12-3) that explains what benefits will be paid, to whom they will be paid, and what (if any) subtractions have been made from the claim. Even if the claim is rejected, the reason for the rejection is listed on the EOB.

If the insurance plan will pay benefits on the claim, the plan writes a check for the benefit amount either to the patient or to the health care provider, or payments may be transferred electronically to the provider. The insurance benefits can be sent directly to the medical office if the patient has agreed to assign benefits to the facility. The assignment of benefits, which causes insurance payments to be sent directly to the health care provider, must be authorized by the patient (or guardian). A signed assignment of benefits must be kept on file in the medical office. An example of an authorization to release medical information and to assign benefits can be found on the bottom of the patient registration form as pictured in Figure 8-2.

Many government programs provide by law a release of information and assignment of benefits (the patient does not have to sign a release and an assignment), and paid benefits are sent directly to the health care facility.

For a procedure and diagnosis to be identified and a claim form submitted to nongovernment programs, a release of information for insurance purposes must be signed by the patient or guardian. This release also allows a copy of the patient's medical record pertaining to the visit to be sent to the insurance company if the insurance company requests more information to process the claim. Whenever an assistant releases information to an insurance company regarding a claim, great care must be taken to release only the information that pertains to the claim and nothing else.

Whether or not benefits are paid on a claim, a copy of the EOB is always sent to the medical office, so the office is aware of what has been paid and what has not been paid. A copy of the EOB is also sent to the insured to inform the insured of the processing of the claim.

When a health care facility receives a payment from the insurance carrier, this payment is applied to the charges that are being paid. This is an important step in the billing process, which allows the patient to be aware of how much money is left to pay for a visit.

Electronic Claims Processing

The federal government and many insurers prefer that claims for insurance benefits are filed electronically using an **electronic data interchange (EDI)**. Providers who file electronic claims must obtain software from vendors or from CMS contractors or may contract with a billing service to file electronic claims. Electronic claims must pass a series of **edits,** which screen the claims and evaluate compliance with Health Insurance Portability and Accountability Act (HIPAA) standards and the accuracy of the claims.

Filing claims electronically has several advantages. Not only are payments received earlier, but mailing costs are virtually eliminated. Software for claims filing is often available for free from CMS contractors. By filing claims electronically, providers often are able to correct claims errors online for more expedient processing and can even look up claim status online.

Paper Processing of CMS-1500

Optical character recognition (OCR) equipment is often used to read a paper copy of a CMS-1500. If a claims processor uses OCR equipment, providers must use CMS-1500 claim forms that are printed in a specific type of red ink. The ink is specialized and cannot be duplicated by a color PC printer. Scannable red CMS-1500 forms must be ordered from the U.S. Government Printing Office, from a printing company, or from a local Medicare claims processor.

OCR scanning equipment requires that special procedures be followed to allow the scanner to read the claim. When completing claim forms, a medical administrative assistant must

- Key the information on the claim using a computer printer or typewriter
- Align the form properly; information must appear in the correct position on the form
- Use only uppercase (CAPITAL) letters
- Use only an original red-ink-on-white-paper Form CMS-1500 claim form
- Use dark ink
- Not print, hand-write, or stamp any extraneous data on the form
- Not staple, clip, or tape anything to the Form CMS-1500 claim form
- Remove pin-fed edges at side perforations
- Use only lift-off correction tape to make corrections
- Place all necessary documentation in the envelope with the Form CMS-1500 claim form
- Not use italics or script

EXPLANATION OF BENEFITS

HEALTHY INSURANCE
1452 West Lake Road
Harvester, MN 55555
010-555-5555

THIS IS NOT AN INVOICE. This document explains the processing of charges submitted by your health care provider to this insurance plan. If you have questions regarding this claim, please contact 010-555-5551 from 8:00 to 5:00 Monday through Friday.

Claim Number	01 - 003 753 865
Date Received	9-11-2001
Date Processed	9-18-2001

Participating Provider	Horizons Healthcare Center
Date of Service	8-14-2001
Description of Service	Office visit, diagnostic laboratory
Provider Charges	$82.50
Usual, Customary, Reasonable Reduction	–12.50
Total Allowed Charges	$70.00
Co-payment	–10.00
Deductible	– 0.00
20% Co-insurance	–14.00
Charges Paid by Insurance Plan	$46.00
Amount You Owe to the Provider	$24.00

If you feel this explanation of benefits is in error, you may appeal this claim. Information on how to appeal is located in your insurance contract or at the number listed above.

Subscriber Information:

Policy number: 123xx6791

Christian B. Olson
1452 Pleasant View Road
Harvester, MN 55555

Figure 12-3 An Explanation of Benefits (EOB) lists the details on how an insurance claim was paid.

- Not use dollar signs, decimals, or punctuation
- Use 10- or 12-pitch (pica) characters and standard dot matrix fonts
- Not include titles (e.g., Dr., Mr., Mrs., Rev., M.D.) as part of the beneficiary's name
- Enter all information on the same horizontal plane within the designated field
- Follow the correct Health Insurance Claim Number (HICN) format. No hyphens or dashes should be used. The alpha prefix or suffix is part of the HICN and should not be omitted. Be especially careful with spouses who have a similar HICN with a different alpha prefix or suffix
- Ensure data are in the appropriate field and do not overlap into other fields
- Use an individual's name in the provider signature field, not a facility or practice name

Even though the majority of today's claims are done electronically, it is important for an assistant to understand requirements for paper processing of claims just in case that is necessary to file a claim.

Coordination of Benefits

If the patient has two or more insurance policies, the insurance plan that receives the claim will have to determine which policy is the primary insurance policy for the patient. The primary insurance is the insurance plan that is first responsible for payment of any benefits.

If an individual has two or more insurance policies that provide coverage for a service, **coordination of benefits (COB)** will take place. Coordination of benefits determines which policy will pay what on a claim and is done so that a health expense is not paid for more than once.

BOX 12-3

Determining the Primary Insurance Carrier

If an individual is covered by two or more policies, the policies will likely pay in the following order:

1. Workers' Compensation
2. Any applicable liability insurance (e.g., property insurance, auto insurance, usually for claims related to accident)
3. Employer-sponsored group insurance or patient's individual policy
4. Medicare
5. TRICARE and CHAMPVA
6. Medigap supplemental insurance
7. Medicaid

Following is how COB works: If a patient's encounter costing $400 is covered by two insurance plans and the first plan pays $320 of the charges, the second plan will pay only a maximum of $80. Both plans' combined benefits will not exceed the total charges.

Most insurance plans have COB provisions within their policies. If there were no coordination of benefits, people might actually profit from seeing a health care provider because each plan would pay the full amount that they would cover. To determine what type of plan should be listed as primary when coverage exists from two or more companies, refer to Box 12-3 for a listing of the priority of insurance coverages.

Coordination of benefits will take place whenever a patient is covered by two different types of insurance plans. Here is another COB example: Suppose a family of four (father, mother, two children) has two policies that provide health care coverage obtained through their employers. The father has a policy through his employer and the mother through her employer. In this case, the father's policy is always the father's primary policy; the mother's policy is his secondary policy. The opposite is true for the mother. Her policy is her primary policy, and the father's policy is her secondary policy. An employee is normally covered by his or her policy first.

How is it determined which policy covers the dependents first? Dependents are covered by the policy of the parent who has a birthday closest to the beginning of the year. This is known as the **birthday rule.** When this rule is implemented, the year of the policyholder's birth is disregarded. For instance, if, in the family previously mentioned, the father's birthday is 10-19-63 and the mother's is 4-4-64, the mother's policy would cover the dependents first even though she is younger. For further explanation of this concept, see the scenario in Box 12-4.

BOX 12-4

Birthday Rule

Martin and Lisa Stein have two children, ages 14 and 12. Martin has an insurance policy (A) through his employer that provides family coverage. Lisa has a policy (B) through her employer that also provides family coverage. Martin's birthday is 10-19-63, and Lisa's birthday is 4-4-64. The primary and secondary policies for the family are as follows:

	Primary Policy	Secondary Policy
Martin	A	B
Lisa	B	A
Dependents	B	A

Using the birthday rule to determine which policy covers the dependents first, B would cover the dependents first because Lisa's birthday (4-4) occurs before Martin's birthday (10-19) during the year. Even though Martin is older than Lisa, the year is disregarded when the policy for primary coverage is determined.

Troubleshooting Claims

It is extremely important for every step of the claims preparation process to be done carefully and without mistakes. When a mistake occurs anywhere during the process, the claim will likely be rejected by the insurance company. Mistakes on insurance claims consist of any information that is missing, incorrect, or incomplete and mistakes can be very costly. Delays in claim processing cost additional time on the part of the office staff to correct and refile the claim. This also slows payments coming into the office, thus reducing the cash flow. Delays and mistakes can also frustrate a patient, possibly even causing the patient to seek health care elsewhere.

When a medical office receives notice of a claim rejection, a medical administrative assistant must review the accuracy of the information on the CMS-1500. The claim rejection will list the reason for the rejection. An error on the upper portion of the claim can be remedied by verifying the information against the data in the patient's file. This information usually can be found in the patient's medical record or financial record. If the patient's address, insurance company, policy number, and group number are verified by an assistant at each appointment (as mentioned in Chapter 8), the possibility of errors in claims will be greatly reduced. A misspelling or incorrect information entered on the form (e.g., a group number listed as a policy number) can cause the claim to be rejected. If the data in the patient's medical record do not agree with the information on the claim form, a medical administrative assistant may have to contact the patient to check the accuracy of the information. Once the correct information has been obtained, a corrected claim form should be generated and sent to the insurance company for processing.

If the claim has been rejected for reasons related to the information pertaining to the provider information or charges for the visit, that information may also have to be verified against information in the patient's medical record. Dates of service, as well as procedures and diagnoses, can be confirmed with the use of documentation from the patient's visit. A rejection also can occur because information such as an employer identification number or facility billing information has been entered incorrectly.

To reduce the possibility of a Medicare or other insurance claim being rejected, follow these tips recommended by CMS:

- Put the beneficiary's name and Medicare number on each piece of documentation submitted. Always use the beneficiary's name exactly as it appears on the beneficiary's Medicare card.
- Include all applicable NPIs on the claim, including the NPI for the referring provider.
- Indicate the correct address, including a valid ZIP code, where the service was rendered to the beneficiary. Any missing, incomplete, or invalid information in the Service Facility Location Information field will cause the claim to be unprocessable. A post office box address is unacceptable in the field for the location where the service was rendered.
- Include special certification numbers for services such as mammography (FDA number) and clinical laboratory (CLIA number).
- Ensure that the number of units/days and the date of service range are not contradictory.
- Ensure that the number of units/days and the quantity indicated in the procedure code's description are not contradictory.

Timelines for Filing

Insurance claims should be filed as quickly as possible after the patient's visit. This is important to keep cash flowing into the medical practice. Claim processing that is delayed means a decrease in cash coming in to the office. Many offices process all of their insurance claims on a regular (at least monthly) schedule. Also, each insurance plan or government program establishes its own specific deadlines for filing claims. If a policy states that all claims must be filed by the end of the next calendar year, then a claim for services provided on 7-9-14 could be filed no later than 12-31-15. Some insurance plans require that claims are filed no longer than one year after the date of service. It is imperative to know each insurance plan's timelines for filing to avoid losing revenue from any claims that may be filed too late.

Filing an Appeal

Occasionally, a patient will disagree with a decision from an insurance company. Patients may appeal such things as amounts paid on insurance claims or denials for surgical procedures. Each plan or program has provisions under which a patient (or insured) can appeal a decision. Specific appeal forms will likely have to be completed and copies of documents that pertain to the dispute may have to be included with the appeal forms.

There often is a time limit as to when an appeal must be made. An assistant may have to help a patient complete an appeal and may need to obtain documentation from the patient's record and/or from the patient's provider. Claims should be appealed if there is any question as to whether a charge was paid correctly or if a denied service should have been covered. Appeals are successful quite often.

Types of Insurance Plans

Insurance plans are set up in a variety of ways. Common types of plans include fee-for-service, health maintenance organization (HMO), and preferred provider organization (PPO). Each of these types of insurance plans has its own unique characteristics, but many plans use a combination of the more desirable features of each type of insurance in order to attract customers.

A common practice in health care today is to control health care costs through **managed care.** Many of the insurance plans or programs highlighted in this chapter have adopted some type of managed care controls to help curtail health care costs.

The general concept of managed care is that accessibility to health care is managed, or restricted, by the insurance company or the health care provider, or both (thus, *managed* care). Managed care places restrictions on the patient's ability to choose a health care provider.

In the past, patients were essentially free to go to almost any health care provider they wished. Under managed care, a network of primary care physicians and specialists is established, and a patient first consults a primary care provider when seeking medical care. That provider may treat the patient or, if necessary, may refer the patient to a specialist. Sometimes, the patient is required to select a specific primary care provider to help coordinate health care services. A patient may be required to see a physician within the network in order to receive maximum benefits from the insurance plan and may be required to receive a referral from a primary care physician in order to see a specialist.

Before a surgical procedure can be done for a managed care patient, a **preauthorization** *must be obtained* from the insurance plan. Preauthorization is an insurance plan's approval for a health care provider to provide a health care service to a patient. Treatment for emergencies is allowed to be given as needed, and, when the danger has passed, a patient may be required to notify an insurance plan of the emergency treatment.

Fee-for-Service

A **fee-for-service** insurance plan pays fees for each service (after deductible, copayments, or coinsurance) obtained by its insured. When a patient sees a physician for a visit, the insurance company reimburses the physician for the service provided. If the patient does not see a physician during a particular month, the insurance company pays the physician nothing.

Fee-for-service plans often allow patients to choose their own provider for health care services. Patients may go back and forth among various providers. Patients can go to any facility they want, whenever they want. No preapproval may be required when health care services are sought; as mentioned previously, however, some fee-for-service plans have instituted restrictions as found in other types of plans. These restrictions might include limiting patients to a specific network of physicians or requiring approval before a visit to a specialist.

Costs for a fee-for-service plan include payment of a monthly premium for the coverage, and, typically, a deductible per individual or family and a coinsurance. Most fee-for-service plans have a maximum deductible and a maximum out-of-pocket expense that the individual or family may have to pay in a single year for health care.

Health Maintenance Organizations

A **health maintenance organization** (**HMO**) is a prepaid plan that provides all the care a patient may need in exchange for a flat monthly fee or premium. This concept is known as **capitation**. No matter how often a patient uses an HMO's health care services, the monthly fee remains the same. With capitation, the physician collects a monthly fee for every patient in the HMO in exchange for providing all of the patient's health care services. With this type of arrangement, physicians count on some patients who are not using any of their services to compensate for those patients who do use their services.

Unlike a fee-for-service plan, subscribers are not free to see whomever they choose for health care. They must see someone who is a provider listed under the HMO. The only exception to this rule is a case of an emergency or a case in which the HMO cannot provide the care (i.e., the HMO does not have a specialist in a particular area). In an emergency, a patient is almost always allowed to seek care outside the HMO. If a patient is admitted to a hospital that is not in the HMO, the patient will likely be moved to a hospital within the HMO as soon as the patient's condition permits.

The fundamental idea behind HMOs is maintaining good health. An HMO typically includes in its policies coverage for preventive care, such as physical examinations, routine eye examinations, Pap smears, mammograms, immunizations, and other medical services. The reasoning is that patients will schedule themselves for regular checkups, thereby catching a potential problem before it becomes a big problem. For example, if a patient, during a physical examination, discovers that he has high blood pressure, this condition can be treated before it becomes dangerously high and the patient has a stroke. Because the HMO is providing a patient's total health care, it is to the HMO's benefit to treat health problems before they become costly.

To control costs related to health care, HMOs customarily require a patient to choose a physician as his or her primary care physician. This means that the patient must see the specified primary care physician for all care (barring emergencies), and the primary care physician provides for the basic health care needs of the patient. If the patient requires the services of a specialist, a **referral** must be approved by the primary care physician. A referral is the approval from the primary care physician for the patient to receive the services of a specialist. This control measure helps the HMO control costs by eliminating unnecessary visits to specialists.

Providers in HMOs may be located all in the same building, or independent groups of providers in various locations may join in an HMO contract to provide coverage for patients. An independent group of providers is referred to as an **independent practice association (IPA)**. If a patient chooses to see a provider not included in the HMO or IPA, coverage for that visit may be greatly reduced or may even be nonexistent.

HMOs typically require a copayment with each visit to the provider. Copayments for HMO office visits are usually a nominal amount ($20 to $25), while copayments for emergency room visits are frequently somewhat higher ($50 to $100).

Preferred Provider Organizations

A **preferred provider organization** (**PPO**) provides a network of providers or preferred providers who contract with the PPO to provide services at a discount for members of the PPO.

A PPO may require patients to choose a primary care physician or primary care clinic. A primary care clinic choice allows the patient to choose from a group of providers in one clinic location. Patients who choose to see providers outside of a designated primary care clinic will likely receive reduced coverage for health care services.

By requiring patients to select a primary care physician or clinic, the PPO, like the HMO, can control costs related to patients' health care. Patients usually are required to pay a copayment with each office visit. Unlike the HMO, however, which receives only a flat monthly fee for each patient, the PPO operates like a fee-for-service plan. With each patient visit, in conjunction with the copayment given by the patient, the health care provider bills the PPO for each service that is provided.

CHECKPOINT

Which coverage could potentially be more costly for an insurance company to provide: a fee-for-service plan or a managed care plan? Why?

Government Health Insurance Programs

Medicare

The **Medicare** program, the largest health insurance program in the United States, is managed by CMS and is a federal program that provides health care benefits for individuals who are eligible for social security or railroad retirement benefits and

- Are 65 years or older
- Are permanently disabled
- Have end-stage renal disease and are awaiting kidney transplant or are undergoing dialysis, or
- Have amyotrophic lateral sclerosis (ALS, also known as Lou Gehrig's disease)

Medicare was established in 1965 under Title XVIII of the Social Security Act. Medicare was initially designed to provide health care services for the elderly. In 1977, the Health Care Financing Administration, now known as Centers for Medicare and Medicaid Services, was established to oversee both Medicare and Medicaid. In 1997, the Children's Health Insurance Program (CHIP) was created (originally known as the State Children's Health Insurance Program) and added to the CMS's responsibilities.

Medicare Coverage and Enrollment

The Medicare program is composed of several parts, all of which provide health insurance coverage for different types of health care services:

- Part A—Hospital Insurance (HI), which covers inpatient care, skilled nursing facility care, and hospice and home health care
- Part B—Supplemental Medical Insurance (SMI), which covers physician's services, outpatient care, and some preventative care services
- Part C—Medicare Advantage Plans, which provide managed care services to persons enrolled in Parts A and B and sometimes D
- Part D—Prescription Drug Coverage, which provides coverage for some prescription drug costs not covered by Part A or B

Medicare Enrollment

Persons aged 65 or older who are entitled to social security or railroad retirement benefits are automatically enrolled in Medicare A. If an individual has not reached age 65 but is receiving social security benefits or railroad retirement benefits, that person is automatically enrolled in Parts A and B of Medicare. Likewise, if an individual is disabled, he or she will automatically be enrolled in Medicare in their 25th month of disability.

Not everyone is automatically enrolled in Medicare. Individuals who do not fit the examples mentioned need to apply for Medicare. These include individuals who do not currently receive social security or railroad retirement benefits and patients with kidney disease. Persons may go to their local social security office to apply for Medicare.

Part A Coverage

Part A coverage for Medicare provides payment assistance for the following:

- Inpatient care, including care in hospitals and inpatient rehabilitation facilities
- Skilled nursing facility (nursing home) services
- Hospice care
- Home health services

Medicare Part A also provides coverage for hospital services such as semiprivate room charges, meals, regular nursing services, rehabilitation services, drugs, medical supplies, laboratory tests, x-rays, operating and recovery room charges, and intensive care and coronary care services. For services to be covered under Medicare, they must be medically necessary. Medically unnecessary services such as telephone, television, or private-duty nurses in the hospital room are not covered by Medicare.

For Medicare to pay for hospitalization charges, the following criteria must be met:

1. A doctor prescribes inpatient hospital care for an illness or injury.
2. The patient's illness or injury requires care that can be provided only in a hospital.
3. The hospital is approved by Medicare.
4. The hospital's Utilization Review Committee or Peer Review Organization (PRO) did not disapprove the patient's stay.

Medicare also pays for home health care services and necessary medical equipment. There is no deductible for home health services. Home health services are covered if the following conditions are met:

1. The patient requires intermittent skilled nursing care, physical therapy, or speech-language pathology services.
2. The patient is confined to home.
3. The patient's doctor determines that the patient needs home health care and devises a plan for care to be provided in the patient's home.
4. The home health agency participates in Medicare.

Hospice care is also provided to Medicare beneficiaries. Hospice care for the terminally ill is focused on relieving the patient's pain and providing comfort to the patient and family members. Medicare pays most of the charges related to hospice care when the patient meets the following conditions:

1. The patient's doctor or doctors certify that the patient is terminally ill.
2. The patient chooses to receive hospice benefits instead of standard Medicare benefits.
3. The hospice care provider participates in Medicare.

Part A Premiums

For people who qualify, there is no charge for Part A Medicare coverage. Most individuals do not have to pay a premium for Part A coverage because they paid Medicare taxes while working. To qualify, a person (1) must have worked at least 10 years in Medicare-covered employment, (2) must be 65 years old or older, (3) must be disabled and receiving social security or railroad retirement disability benefits for 24 months, or (4) must have kidney failure treated with dialysis or transplantation.

For those who cannot meet the requirements for premium-free Part A, the coverage may still be available if they pay a premium. If a patient worked fewer than 39 quarters of Medicare-covered employment, he or she probably will have to pay a premium for Part A. In 2013, this premium was $441 per month.

Part A Deductible

In 2013, the deductible for Part A coverage was $1184 per benefit period. A benefit period begins when a patient is admitted to a hospital and ends when the patient has been out of the hospital for 60 consecutive days. The deductible applies to the first 60 days of hospitalization. If the patient is hospitalized for longer than 60 days, a coinsurance of $296 applies for each day the patient is hospitalized from the 61st to the 90th day of each benefit period. If the patient is hospitalized for longer than 90 days, a $592 per lifetime reserve day coinsurance applies for each day up to 60 days over a lifetime.

If the patient is placed in a skilled nursing facility, a coinsurance of $148 per day from the 21st to the 100th day of the benefit period applies. If a patient stays in a nursing home longer than 100 days, the patient pays all costs for each day after day 100 in the facility.

TABLE 12-2

Summary of Medicare Deductibles, Coinsurance, and Premiums for the Year 2013

	Medicare Part A	Medicare Part B
Deductible	$1184 per benefit period	$147 per year
Coinsurance	$296 per day for the 61st to 90th day of benefit period; $592 per lifetime reserve after day 90 each benefit period (up to 60 days over a patient's lifetime)	20% of Medicare-approved charges (less deductible)
Premium	None unless individual has fewer than 10 years of Medicare-covered employment	$104.90 per month

BOX 12-5

Examples of Medicare Part B Covered Services (some restrictions may apply)

Abdominal Aortic Aneurysm Screening
Ambulance Services
Ambulatory Surgery Center Fees
Blood
Bone Mass Measurement
Cardiovascular Screenings
Clinical Laboratory Services
Clinical Research Studies
Colorectal Cancer Screenings
Diabetes Screenings
Diabetes Self-Management Training
Diabetes Supplies
Doctor Services
Durable Medical Equipment
Emergency Room Services
Eye Exams
Flu Shots
Foot Exams and Treatment
Glaucoma Tests
Hearing and Balance Exams
Hepatitis B Shots
Home Health Services
Kidney Dialysis Services and Supplies
Mammograms (Screening)
Medical Nutrition Therapy Services
Mental Health Care (Outpatient)
Occupational Therapy
Outpatient Hospital Services
Outpatient Medical and Surgical Services and Supplies
Pap Tests and Pelvic Exams (Includes Clinical Breast Exam)
Physical Therapy
Pneumococcal Shot
Prostate Cancer Screenings
Prosthetic/Orthotic Items
Second Surgical Opinions
Speech-Language Pathology Services
Transplants

A summary of Medicare deductibles, premiums, and coinsurance amounts for both Part A and Part B is shown in Table 12-2.

Part B Coverage

Medicare Part B provides coverage for a variety of medical expenses, including physician services (both inpatient and outpatient), outpatient hospital services, clinical laboratory tests, medical equipment, ambulance services, influenza vaccines, home health services, and other specified health services and supplies. Of course, for the provider to be paid, services must be medically necessary or must be a covered preventative. For examples of services and items that are covered or noncovered by Medicare, refer to Boxes 12-5 and 12-6.

A patient will have to have Part B if he or she is to have coverage for services provided within a medical office. To determine whether a patient has Part B, simply look for the words "MEDICAL (PART B)" on the patient's Medicare card. A sample of a Medicare card is shown in Figure 12-2. Most people who are eligible choose to enroll in Part B.

BOX 12-6

Examples of Medicare Part B Noncovered Services (some restrictions may apply)

Acupuncture
Cosmetic Surgery
Dental Care and Dentures (With Few Exceptions)
Hearing Aids
Orthopedic Shoes (With Few Exceptions)
Routine Foot Care (e.g., Cutting Corns and Calluses)
Routine Physical Exams Except for the One-Time "Welcome to Medicare" Exam
Screening Lab Tests Except Those Specifically Covered Under Part B

Part B Premium

In 2013, the monthly premium for Medicare Part B was $104.90. Medicare does charge a higher premium for single enrollees with an income over $85,000 and enrollees who were married and filing joint tax returns with income over

TABLE 12-3

Comparison of Medicare Assignment versus Nonassignment

	Physician 1 (accepts assignment) Patient A (has met deductible for year)	Physician 2 (does not accept assignment) Patient B (has met deductible for year)
A. Doctor charges	$250	$250
B. Medicare allows	$200	$200
C. Minus deductible	0	0
D. Subtotal	$200	$200
E. Coinsurance (20% of D)	$40	$40
F. Amount Medicare pays (D and E)	$160	$160
G. Patient pays (C and E)	$40	$40 + (*) = $70

*This amount equals 15% × B, or 15% × (A − B), whichever is lower. If a provider does not accept assignment, the provider is permitted to charge the Medicare-approved amount plus 15%. A provider who does not accept assignment may charge the patient more for services. Federal law prohibits a provider from charging more than 15% over Medicare's approved amount.

$170,000. If an eligible individual fails to enroll in Medicare Part B within the initial enrollment period in which the individual is eligible, a penalty may be assessed if the individual decides to enroll at a later date. A 10% surcharge may be added to the Part B premium for every year in which an eligible individual fails to enroll. If a patient waited for 2 years to enroll, a penalty of 20% could be added to the cost of the yearly premium. A penalty may not be assessed if an individual or an individual's spouse is working and has group health insurance.

Part B Deductible and Coinsurance

The deductible for Medicare Part B in 2013 was $147 per year. A coinsurance also applies to Medicare Part B claims. The coinsurance is 20% of the Medicare-approved amount (less deductible) for a service. See Table 12-3 for examples of how coinsurance is calculated.

Medicare Advantage Plans (Part C)

Medicare also provides health care coverage in the form of HMOs and PPOs. Advantage plans cover both Part A and Part B but may provide additional coverage for services not normally covered by Medicare such as vision, hearing, dental, or preventative services.

If a patient has an Advantage plan, the patient will be required to seek medical services from providers who are associated with the plan. Also, plans may have different deductibles, copayments, or coinsurance amounts for services.

Medicare Part D

Part D provides coverage for prescription drugs. Patients are required to pay a special premium for Part D coverage. Similar to Part B, if the patient should wait to purchase Part D coverage, a penalty may be applied to the patient's premium. These plans are provided by private insurance companies, and plans can vary greatly as far as costs and drugs covered. Deductibles, copayments and coinsurance may apply before benefits are paid for Part D coverage.

Processing of Medicare Claims

To facilitate the processing of Medicare claims, the federal government has elected to contract for claims processing services. A **Medicare Administrative Contractor (MAC)** is a company that has contracted with Medicare to process claims for Medicare. After a claim is processed, the MAC sends the patient a Medicare Summary Notice (MSN) (Fig. 12-4), Medicare's version of an EOB, detailing what Medicare will pay and what the patient must pay in relation to the claim. The contractor handles all questions regarding the benefits listed on the claim.

Medicare Administrative Contractors are responsible for determining costs and reimbursement amounts, maintaining records, establishing controls, safeguarding against fraud and abuse or excess use, making payments to providers for services, and assisting providers and beneficiaries when needed.

Medicare Assignment

Physicians and other health care providers who accept Medicare assignment agree to accept the amount that Medicare approves for services as payment in full. These providers who accept assignment are known as **participating providers (PARs)**. If a patient sees a PAR, the patient will not have to pay more than the deductible and 20% coinsurance. A participating provider is not allowed to charge the patient any more than Medicare's approved amount. Accepting Medicare assignment means that the patient will pay less. For an example of how participating providers and assignment affect the amount a patient owes for health care, see Table 12-3.

If a provider does not accept assignment, the provider is allowed to charge a patient more than the Medicare-approved amount for services. However, the provider may not charge more than 15% over the Medicare-approved amount. This higher amount is known as the **limiting charge.** However, the limiting charge may apply only to certain services and may not apply to some supplies and medical equipment.

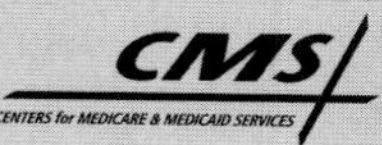

Medicare Summary Notice

Page 1 of 2

July 1, 2006

BENEFICIARY NAME
STREET ADDRESS
CITY, STATE ZIP CODE

CUSTOMER SERVICE INFORMATION

Your Medicare Number: 111-11-1111A

If you have questions, write or call:
Medicare (#12345)
555 Medicare Blvd., Suite 200
Medicare Building
Medicare, US XXXXX-XXXX

Call: 1-800-MEDICARE (1-800-633-4227)
Ask for Doctor Services
TTY for Hearing Impaired: 1-877-486-2048

BE INFORMED: Beware of telemarketers offering free or discounted medicare items or services.

This is a summary of claims processed from 05/10/2006 through 08/10/2006.

PART B MEDICAL INSURANCE – ASSIGNED CLAIMS

Dates of Service	Services Provided	Amount Charged	Medicare Approved	Medicare Paid Provider	You May Be Billed	See Notes Section
Claim Number: 12435-84956-84556						
Paul Jones, M.D., 123 West Street, Jacksonville, FL 33231-0024						a
Referred by: Scott Wilson, M.D.						
04/19/06	1 Influenza immunization (90724)	$5.00	$3.88	$3.88	$0.00	b
04/19/06	1 Admin. flu vac (G0008)	5.00	3.43	3.43	0.00	b
	Claim Total	**$10.00**	**$7.31**	**$7.31**	**$0.00**	
Claim Number: 12435-84956-84557						
ABC Ambulance, P.O. Box 2149, Jacksonville, FL 33231						a
04/25/06	1 Ambulance, base rate (A0020)	$289.00	$249.78	$199.82	$49.96	
04/25/06	1 Ambulance, per mile (A0021)	21.00	16.96	13.57	3.39	
	Claim Total	**$310.00**	**$266.74**	**$213.39**	**$53.35**	

PART B MEDICAL INSURANCE – UNASSIGNED CLAIMS

Dates of Service	Services Provided	Amount Charged	Medicare Approved	Medicare Paid You	You May Be Billed	See Notes Section
Claim Number: 12435-84956-84558						
William Newman, M.D., 362 North Street Jacksonville, FL 33231-0024						a
03/10/06	1 Office/Outpatient Visit, ES (99213)	$47.00	$33.93	$27.15	$39.02	c

THIS IS NOT A BILL – Keep this notice for your records.

Figure 12-4 A Medicare Summary Notice (MSN) is created for inpatient or outpatient claims and is sent from Medicare to a beneficiary to explain coverage provided for a claim.

Continued

Your Medicare Number: 111-11-1111A

Notes Section:

a This information is being sent to your private insurer. They will review it to see if additional benefits can be paid. Send any questions regarding your supplemental benefits to them.

b This service is paid at 100% of the Medicare approved amount.

c Your doctor did not accept assignment for this service. Under Federal law, your doctor cannot charge more than $39.02. If you have already paid more than this amount, you are entitled to a refund from the provider.

Deductible Information:

You have met the Part B deductible for 2006.

General Information:

You have the right to make a request in writing for an itemized statement which details each Medicare item or service which you have received from your physician, hospital, or any other health supplier or health professional. Please contact them directly, in writing, if you would like an itemized statement.

Compare the services you receive with those that appear on your Medicare Summary Notice. If you have questions, call your doctor or provider. If you feel further investigation is needed due to possible fraud and abuse, call the phone number in the Customer Service Information Box.

Appeals Information – Part B

If you disagree with any claims decisions on this notice, your appeal must be received by **November 1, 2006**. Follow the instructions below:

1) Circle the item(s) you disagree with and explain why you disagree.

2) Send this notice, or a copy, to the address in the "Customer Service Information" box on Page 1. (You may also send any additional information you may have about your appeal.)

3) Sign here ______________________________ Phone number ______________________

Revised 08/06

* obtained from
http://www.medicare.gov/publications/pubs/pdf/SummaryNoticeB.pdf 12-17-07

Figure 12-4, cont'd

***(A)* Notifier(s):**
***(B)* Patient Name:** ***(C)* Identification Number:**

Advance Beneficiary Notice of Noncoverage (ABN)

NOTE: If Medicare doesn't pay for *(D)*______________ below, you may have to pay.

Medicare does not pay for everything, even some care that you or your health care provider have good reason to think you need. We expect Medicare may not pay for the *(D)*_____________ below.

*(D)*______________	***(E)* Reason Medicare May Not Pay:**	***(F)* Estimated Cost:**

What you need to do now:

- Read this notice, so you can make an informed decision about your care.
- Ask us any questions that you may have after you finish reading.
- Choose an option below about whether to receive the *(D)*____________listed above.

  Note: If you choose Option 1 or 2, we may help you to use any other insurance that you might have, but Medicare cannot require us to do this.

***(G)* Options:** **Check only one box. We cannot choose a box for you.**

☐ **OPTION 1.** I want the *(D)*__________ listed above. You may ask to be paid now, but I also want Medicare billed for an official decision on payment, which is sent to me on a Medicare Summary Notice (MSN). I understand that if Medicare doesn't pay, I am responsible for payment, but **I can appeal to Medicare** by following the directions on the MSN. If Medicare does pay, you will refund any payments I made to you, less co-pays or deductibles.

☐ **OPTION 2.** I want the *(D)*__________ listed above, but do not bill Medicare. You may ask to be paid now as I am responsible for payment. **I cannot appeal if Medicare is not billed.**

☐ **OPTION 3.** I don't want the *(D)*__________listed above. I understand with this choice I am **not** responsible for payment, and **I cannot appeal to see if Medicare would pay.**

***(H)* Additional Information:**

This notice gives our opinion, not an official Medicare decision. If you have other questions on this notice or Medicare billing, call **1-800-MEDICARE** (1-800-633-4227/**TTY**: 1-877-486-2048).

Signing below means that you have received and understand this notice. You also receive a copy.

***(I)* Signature:**	***(J)* Date:**

According to the Paperwork Reduction Act of 1995, no persons are required to respond to a collection of information unless it displays a valid OMB control number. The valid OMB control number for this information collection is 0938-0566. The time required to complete this information collection is estimated to average 7 minutes per response, including the time to review instructions, search existing data resources, gather the data needed, and complete and review the information collection. If you have comments concerning the accuracy of the time estimate or suggestions for improving this form, please write to: CMS, 7500 Security Boulevard, Attn: PRA Reports Clearance Officer, Baltimore, Maryland 21244-1850.

Form CMS-R-131 (03/08) Form Approved OMB No. 0938-0566

Figure 12-5 An Advance Beneficiary Notice (ABN) should be signed by a patient if the patient is to receive a service or an item that Medicare may not cover. (From U.S. Department of Health and Human Services, Centers for Medicare and Medicaid Services.)

Advance Beneficiary Notice

An **Advance Beneficiary Notice (ABN)** (Fig. 12-5) is a Medicare document that states that Medicare does not provide coverage for certain services. An assistant should ask a patient to sign an ABN if the patient is receiving a service that may not be covered by Medicare. The purpose of an ABN is to inform the patient of Medicare's possible denial of coverage and to protect the patient from incurring an unexpected health care expense. A record of a patient's signed ABN must be retained by the medical office. A checkmark in Option 1 of the ABN also preserves the patient's right to appeal a Medicare denial.

Medicare Statistics

In 2010, Medicare coverage provided health insurance coverage to 95% of the aged population in the United States. Hospital coverage (Part A) was provided to over 47 million people, covering more than $244 billion in benefits. Part B coverage (covering physician services and other medical expenses) was provided to 44 million people and covered more than $209 billion in benefits.

In addition to providing coverage to 95% of the nation's aged population, Medicare also provides health insurance coverage to many disabled persons. Medicare is a major source of health insurance benefits, and a thorough understanding of Medicare's requirements and processes will ensure that claims are filed expediently and correctly.

Medigap

Because Medicare does not completely cover all costs related to medical care, private companies offer insurance policies referred to as *Medigap* policies that will help cover the costs that Medicare does not cover. Medigap policies may cover Medicare deductibles and coinsurance or services not covered by Medicare, or both. Thus, a Medigap policy "bridges the gap," more or less, between what Medicare allows and what Medicare pays.

Twelve basic Medigap plans offer a variety of benefits. Plans are identified with the letters A through L, and all plans with a specific letter must offer the same coverage. For example, a C plan at one insurance company will offer the same coverage as a C plan at another insurance company. This allows Medicare patients to shop and compare plans because the only difference in a C plan among companies will be the cost.

A 6-month open-enrollment period for Medigap usually begins when a Medicare B recipient reaches age 65. If an eligible enrollee purchases a policy during an open enrollment period, the enrollee cannot be charged higher premiums because of poor health.

Medicaid

The **Medicaid** program became law in 1965 with the passage of Title XIX of the Social Security Act. Medicaid, or medical assistance, was created to ensure adequate medical coverage for individuals in need.

A health care program funded by both federal and state dollars, Medicaid covered nearly 57 million people in 2012. The federal government establishes minimal coverages for Medicaid but allows each state to set income guidelines, determine additional coverages, establish reimbursement rates, and administer its own program. Because of the wide latitude given to state governments, Medicaid coverage can vary greatly among states.

Medicaid Eligibility

Medicaid provides coverage for many individuals who otherwise would likely go without medical care. To receive federal funds for a Medicaid program, a state must provide coverage to specific groups of individuals, some of whom are members of low-income families with children, supplemental security income (SSI) recipients, infants born to Medicaid-eligible pregnant women, children younger than age 6, and pregnant women whose income is below 133% of the federal poverty level. A low income is not the only test for Medicaid eligibility. A patient's assets also are taken into account.

States also have the option of adding coverage for specific groups. Many states provide Medicaid benefits for individuals who are medically needy. A medically needy individual may have an income that is greater than the Medicaid limits but may have sizable or catastrophic medical expenses.

Persons who wish to obtain information about eligibility for Medicaid and to apply for Medicaid benefits in their state should contact their local Medicaid agency. If in doubt as to whether or not they may be able to obtain coverage under Medicaid, patients would be encouraged to contact their local Medicaid office and submit an application for Medicaid assistance. Information on the location of local offices is available on the CMS website.

Medicaid Coverage

As was mentioned previously, to receive federal funds for Medicaid, all states must provide the following basic health care services:

- Inpatient and outpatient hospital services
- Physician services
- Nursing facility services for individuals aged 21 and older
- Medical and surgical dental services
- Home health care for persons eligible for nursing facility services
- Family planning services and supplies
- Rural health clinic services
- Laboratory and x-ray services
- Pediatric and family nurse practitioner services
- Federally qualified health center services
- Nurse-midwife services
- Early and periodic screening, diagnosis, and treatment (EPSDT) services for individuals younger than age 21
- Prenatal care
- Vaccinations for children

Each state may then decide what other types of coverage that state will provide for each Medicaid beneficiary. Additional provided services may include the following:

- Vision services, including eyeglasses
- Nursing facility services for persons younger than age 21
- Intermediate care/nursing facility services
- Prescribed medications
- Tuberculosis-related services for persons with tuberculosis
- Prosthetic devices
- Dental services

In some instances, a state may determine that a beneficiary is overusing Medicaid services. Because patients very often do not have to pay to receive Medicaid coverage, the possibility exists that a patient may see a health care provider when it is not necessary. In this situation, a state may place the patient in a Medicaid restriction program, which may restrict the patient to a certain primary care physician and a certain pharmacy. Patients may even be required to contact a nurse by phone before seeing a physician. If the patient doesn't follow the requirements set up by the restriction program, benefits will not be paid. A restriction program is essentially similar to a managed care plan in that patients are required to use specific providers for coordination of their health care treatment.

Some states use the term *lock-in* to describe this type of restriction. A patient may be locked in because the patient has overused or abused Medicaid services. A patient who has seen multiple doctors and has received multiple prescriptions may be restricted to one pharmacy so the patient's medications can be managed better. Patients who have this type of Medicaid restriction may see a physician other than their designated physician only in cases of emergency.

Medicaid Payments

Medicaid benefits are paid directly to the health care provider. Any provider who accepts Medicaid patients and requests reimbursement for Medicaid services is required to accept payment for Medicaid-approved amounts as payments in full. This includes the portion Medicaid pays as well as any copayment or deductible paid by the patient. Some states may have small copayments or deductibles for which the patient is responsible. These amounts cannot be charged for family planning or emergency services. Also, certain Medicaid beneficiaries—pregnant women, children, and some hospital or nursing home patients—are exempt from these copayment or deductible amounts. Besides collecting amounts for copayments or deductibles, a provider is not allowed to bill a patient for any excess charges for a Medicaid-covered service. For example, if a provider normally charges $50 for a particular service and Medicaid only covers $35, the provider may not bill the patient the $15 difference between their charge and the Medicaid-approved amount.

Many elderly patients are covered by both Medicare and Medicaid. Patients with this type of coverage are known as **dual-eligibles**. In the case of benefits for health services received for these patients, as well as for patients with other coverages, Medicaid is always the secondary payer, or the "payer of last resort." All other health insurance benefits must be exhausted before Medicaid will pay benefits.

When serving a Medicaid patient, an assistant should be sure to not use the term "welfare" when referring to Medicaid. This term conjures up such a negative image in the mind of most individuals that it is best never to use the term in the medical office.

Children's Health Insurance Program (CHIP)

To address the needs of uninsured children, the **Children's Health Insurance Program (CHIP),** formerly known as the State Children's Health Insurance Program, was created to help provide health insurance to uninsured children. As part of the Balanced Budget Act of 1997, CHIP was created similarly to Medicaid: state and federal dollars support the program, and each individual state administers its own program.

The program was created to provide insurance to children who did not qualify for Medicaid because their families earned too much money. CHIP covers children whose families earn 200% below the federal poverty level or 50% above the state's Medicaid eligibility limit.

A state's CHIP can be designed in one of three ways:

1. CHIP funds can be used to expand Medicaid coverage to previously unqualified children.
2. A separate CHIP program can be created.
3. The state can create a combination of the two previous options.

States can require that individuals pay some of the costs for services provided under CHIP; however, states cannot impose cost sharing for immunizations or preventative services, and cost sharing cannot exceed 5% of the family's income.

TRICARE

Formerly known as CHAMPUS (Civilian Health and Medical Program of the Uniformed Services), **TRICARE** is a health care benefit program for active duty service members, retired military personnel and their families, survivors, and some former spouses. TRICARE uses the services of military health care providers and facilities and supplements the military health care system with civilian providers and facilities.

TRICARE provides coverage for 9.7 million eligible beneficiaries. All TRICARE recipients must be registered in TRICARE's Defense Enrollment Eligibility Reporting System (DEERS). TRICARE offers several different health plans—TRICARE Prime, TRICARE Extra, TRICARE Standard, and TRICARE for Life—and two dental plans as well.

The plan with the most enrollees, TRICARE Prime provides health care coverage for active-duty and retired military personnel and their families who wish to enroll in the plan. TRICARE Prime operates much as an HMO operates. Preventive care such as physical examinations, Pap smears, mammograms, and prostate screening are provided for enrollees. Care provided to TRICARE Prime enrollees is usually given at military hospitals and clinics.

TRICARE Extra operates much as a PPO operates. Individuals are able to seek health care from a civilian provider in a network of providers. No enrollment is required with TRICARE Extra. Eligible individuals can choose a network provider and must pay a share of the costs of health care.

TRICARE Standard provides care for family members who wish to use civilian health care providers. Similar to TRICARE Extra, there is no enrollment required in TRICARE Standard; of the TRICARE options, this option is often the most expensive, however. This is because an eligible individual may choose any health care provider and is not limited to a specific network of providers. Individuals who choose TRICARE Standard have an annual deductible and also pay a percentage of charges over allowed rates. Health care providers who do not accept assignment of TRICARE benefits may charge patients any extra amounts over allowed rates.

CHAMPVA

In 1973, the Veterans Health Care Expansion Act created a health insurance benefits program that provided health care coverage for dependents of veterans who have a total, permanent service-connected disability, survivors of veterans who died because of a service-connected disability or who at the time of death were totally disabled from a service-connected condition, and survivors of persons who died in the line of duty. This program is known as the **Civilian Health and Medical Program of the Department of Veterans Affairs CHAMPVA**. The program is separate from TRICARE. Individuals are eligible for CHAMPVA provided they are not eligible for TRICARE. The military member on whom TRICARE or CHAMPVA eligibility is based is known as a **sponsor**, and individuals who receive insurance benefits are known as beneficiaries. CHAMPVA covers health care services and supplies that are medically or psychologically necessary.

Workers' Compensation

Workers' Compensation (Workers' Comp) programs cover employees who suffer from work-related injuries, diseases, illnesses, or even death. Each state is responsible for structuring its own Workers' Compensation system. Depending on this structure, employers may be able to provide Workers' Comp insurance in the following ways: (1) state-funded program, (2) self-insured program, (3) private insurance coverage, or (4) a combination of any of the three.

Workers' Compensation insurance provides medical treatment benefits for workers with job-related conditions and pays a portion of wages lost to an employee who is unable to work because of a work-related condition. Death and burial benefits also are available to help cover some of the expenses incurred and income lost as the result of a work-related death. If a worker is permanently injured and unable to perform their current job, vocational rehabilitation may be available to retrain the injured worker for work in another type of employment. Restrictions on Workers' Compensation coverage may apply if a worker was negligent.

Occurrences that may be covered under Workers' Compensation include the following:

- An employee who is setting up a display falls off a ladder and breaks an arm
- A nurse assistant lifts a patient and herniates a disk
- A health care worker experiences a needle stick and must undergo testing for the human immunodeficiency virus
- A medical transcriptionist suffers from pain due to carpal tunnel syndrome
- A fast food employee sustains third-degree burns from a hot grease spill
- A sales manager is killed in a car accident while en route to a work-related meeting
- A factory worker incurs permanent hearing loss due to excessive noise

When a worker is injured, it is important for the worker to complete a first report of injury to document the circumstances of the injury. Time limitations usually exist as to when the report must be completed and when the employer must be notified of a work-related injury. Limitations can range from a few days to almost a month. Requirements for filing an injury report vary from state to state. Information on current reporting guidelines should be obtained from the state. A provider who treats a patient with a work-related injury that requires extended treatment are periodically required to provide a report to the state on the patient's condition.

Premiums for Workers' Compensation insurance are paid by the employer and are determined by the number of employees and by the type of work performed by the business. The more risky the work, the more costly is the premium.

Some states have consultative services available to employers who wish to reduce their Workers' Compensation claims. These services counsel employers and employees on accident prevention and workplace safety and may include inspection services.

HIPAA Hint

A provider is not required to obtain an authorization to disclose protected health information if the provider is determining eligibility for or conducting enrollment in certain government benefit programs.

Private Health Insurance

Many private insurance companies throughout the United States offer health insurance coverage in exchange for a premium. Many individuals get health insurance through their employer. This type of health insurance is called **group insurance.** Group insurance is usually the cheapest way for an individual to obtain insurance because, in many instances, the employer helps pay all or a portion of the cost of the insurance. Although individuals can purchase a health insurance policy on their own, a large number of policies are sold through group insurance plans provided by employers.

Insurance Coverage

The types of benefits provided by most insurance companies are divided into two main categories: basic and major medical. Basic coverage generally pays for charges related to hospitalization, such as hospital room, treatment, procedures, medications, diagnostic tests, and supplies necessary to the hospitalization. Major medical coverage typically covers those types of services provided outside the hospital, such as office visits and prescription medications.

Blue Cross/Blue Shield

The Blue Cross/Blue Shield Association (BCBSA) is a national association composed of independently owned and operated Blue Cross/Blue Shield plans. The BCBSA provides business support and sets quality standards that individual plans must meet. These plans, in order to use the BCBS name, must apply for a license to offer health insurance within a predefined geographic area. For large employers that span a several-state area or the entire country, the Association helps coordinate the insurance coverage available to those groups.

The BCBS group originated from two separate insurance plans: Blue Cross, which provided hospital coverage, and Blue Shield, which provided coverage for physician services. Most corporations today operate as a combined BCBS organization.

Every individual BCBS plan is managed by a board of directors whose membership consists of a majority of public members (individuals not employed in a health care organization). Approximately one of every four Americans is insured by a BCBS plan.

When a group of physicians agrees to join a BCBS organization and provide services for the organization, it is known as a participating provider (PAR). Similar to Medicare, this means that the physician agrees to a payment amount established by the plan. The amount paid will likely be determined by the usual, customary, and reasonable (UCR) fee, which is an amount usually charged for a particular service.

Just as in the Medicare example given earlier, the designation of PAR means a cost savings to the patient. If a provider is a PAR, the provider agrees to accept the payment made by the insurance company (plus any deductible, coinsurance, and copayment) as payment in full for services rendered. In other words, if a physician charges $100 for a service and the UCR is $75, the difference of $25 is discounted off the patient's bill.

Disability Insurance

Disability insurance provides partial income replacement for individuals if they become unable to work. Disability insurance does not cover the cost of medical care but instead provides benefit payments to policyholders who lose income because of an incapacity to work.

Coverage may be paid for or purchased from an individual's employer. Disability insurance policies are also available from private insurance companies on an individual basis. Disability coverage can be purchased for loss of income on a short-term or long-term basis.

A medical office becomes involved with disability insurance if a patient tries to collect benefits from a disability insurance policy. It is normally required that a physician complete a form that details the extent of the patient's disability. No standardized report form is used for this process. Each patient will have to provide the office with the specific form required for the patient's insurance plan.

Long-term Care Insurance

Nursing home costs can easily exceed $5000 to $7000 per month. Nursing home insurance helps cover the costs of nursing home care. Coverage for nursing home care usually is not provided by health insurance, and Medicare provides little coverage for nursing home care. Nursing home insurance helps fill the gap left by other insurance programs.

Nursing home care can quickly exhaust an elderly couple's lifetime savings. In 1988, Congress enacted spousal impoverishment legislation designed to protect a nursing home resident's spouse from losing needed financial resources.

When an individual is placed in a nursing home and is expected to stay for at least 30 days, the couple may apply for Medicaid. An assessment of the couple's assets is conducted, and exemptions for home, household goods, automobile, and burial funds are established. The amount remaining after the exemptions and any state maximums is considered to be available for care of the resident. This legislation helps protect a healthy spouse from having to spend all the couple's resources on nursing home care with little or nothing left to pay the spouse's own living expenses.

Insurance Resources

The study of health insurance is quite vast, and many excellent references are available for the medical administrative assistant who requires a more extensive review of the subject. *The Insurance Handbook for the Medical Office,* by Marilyn T. Fordney, provides a very detailed look at the complexities of the health insurance industry. In addition to federal and state regulations, most health insurance programs provide online information on their specific guidelines for processing of insurance claims.

Many excellent Internet sources are available to provide access to up-to-date information about industry requirements. The federal government's CMS website contains a wealth of information related to Medicaid, Medicare, and government regulations pertaining to health care insurance (Table 12-4). Within the Medicaid portion of the site, information on state Medicaid agencies and programs is available. Additional Internet resources are found in the bibliography section of this chapter.

Current Topics in Health Insurance

Insurance Fraud and Abuse

Health care insurance programs face a tremendous problem in trying to combat fraud and abuse related to health insurance benefits. Fraud can be defined as an intentional act committed by an individual who knows the act to be false or deceptive in order to receive a benefit for himself or someone else. Abuse in billing may be more difficult to identify. An example of abuse would be ordering and billing for a test that may not be necessary. It may be difficult to prove that a test was not necessary.

Insurance fraud and abuse is estimated to cost American taxpayers billions of dollars each year. The federal government continues efforts to reduce fraud and abuse and in turn to reduce the huge amounts of money that are lost each year. Federal and state agencies often work together in a cooperative effort to expose and combat this problem.

Committing insurance fraud and abuse is a willful and conscious act. Following are some examples of the acts that perpetrators intentionally carry out to take advantage of insurance programs:

- Billing for office visits that never occurred
- Billing for procedures never done
- Billing used items as new
- Billing for unnecessary tests
- Paying kickbacks for referrals
- Inflating charges for procedures
- Falsifying credentials
- Misrepresenting a patient's diagnosis for greater payment of benefits

CMS issues fraud alerts that identify schemes used to defraud Medicare. Information is available on the CMS website. Providers and/or employees who suspect fraudulent billing practices should report the suspected perpetrator to the state insurance commissioner's office or other appropriate agency.

TABLE 12-4

CMS Regional Offices

Region	Address and Telephone Number	States Covered
I. Boston Regional Office	John F. Kennedy Federal Building Room 2325 Boston, MA 02203-0003 617-565-1188	Connecticut Maine Massachusetts Hampshire New Rhode Island Vermont
II. New York Regional Office	26 Federal Plaza 38th Floor New York, NY 10278-0063 212-264-3657	New Jersey New York Puerto Rico Virgin Islands
III. Philadelphia Regional Office	The Public Ledger Building 150 South Independence Mall West Suite 216 Philadelphia, PA 19106 215-861-4140	District of Columbia Delaware Maryland Pennsylvania Virginia West Virginia
IV. Atlanta Regional Office	Atlanta Federal Center 61 Forsyth Street, S.W., Suite 4T20 Atlanta, GA 30303-8909 404-562-7500	Alabama North Carolina South Carolina Florida Georgia Kentucky Mississippi Tennessee
V. Chicago Regional Office	233 North Michigan Avenue Suite 600 Chicago, IL 60601 312-886-6432	Illinois Indiana Michigan Minnesota Ohio Wisconsin
VI. Dallas Regional Office	1301 Young Street, Suite 714 Dallas, TX 75202 214-767-6423	Arkansas Louisiana New Mexico Oklahoma Texas
VII. Kansas City Regional Office	Richard Bolling Federal Building 601 East 12 Street, Room 235 Kansas City, MO 64106-2808 816-426-5233	Iowa Kansas Missouri Nebraska
VIII. Denver Regional Office	Colorado State Bank Building 1600 Broadway Suite 700 Denver, CO 80202 303-844-2111	Colorado Montana North Dakota South Dakota Utah Wyoming

TABLE 12-4

CMS Regional Offices—cont'd

Region	Address and Telephone Number	States Covered
IX. San Francisco Regional Office	75 Hawthorne St, Suite 408 San Francisco, CA 94105 415-744-3501	American Samoa Arizona California Commonwealth of Northern Marianas Islands Guam Hawaii Nevada
X. Seattle Regional Office	2201 Sixth Avenue, Suite 911 Seattle, WA 98121-2500 206-615-2306	Alaska Idaho Oregon Washington

As was mentioned in the previous chapter, identity theft is another large problem in health care. Individuals may steal someone's identity with or without the person's knowledge. Patients may receive services under someone else's name and insurance. It is illegal for an individual to use someone else's identity to obtain health care services. To reduce the possibility of this occurrence, many health care facilities are now requiring government-issued photo identification, and many organizations are also requiring photos of patients as part of their registration data.

Confidentiality

As with many activities in the medical office, insurance claims processing involves dealing with sensitive medical information. A patient's insurance claim contains information about dates of treatment, diagnoses, procedures, and providers; this information is confidential and cannot be given or sent to any party unless the patient has authorized release of the information. Telephone inquiries from insurance companies must be scrutinized carefully. In general, it is best to handle these inquiries by asking the insurance company for the patient's name, the insured's name, and the reason for the inquiry, and by taking a message regarding the inquiry. The patient's record then can be checked for a release of information, and the information can be mailed directly to the insurance company if the release has been done.

COBRA

Federal law established in 1985 known as **COBRA (Consolidated Omnibus Budget Reconciliation Act of 1985)** requires that an employee be allowed to continue health insurance coverage if the employee is laid off, or if the employee leaves the job. This continuation of health insurance is provided for a specific length of time. A drawback is that the employee probably will have to pay the entire premium. COBRA also applies if an individual divorces, and a former spouse was covered.

Insurance Industry Statistics

Not all Americans are covered by health insurance. In 2010, 16.3% of the U.S. population, or 49.9 million people, did not have health insurance coverage. Of all those who had health insurance in 2006, 55.3% had employer-sponsored health insurance, 14.5% were covered by Medicare, 15.9% by Medicaid (some individuals were covered by both Medicare and Medicaid), and 4.2% by military health care.

Although some individuals are not covered by an insurance plan, most individuals are covered by some type of plan. Filing of insurance claims is an important responsibility in the medical office, as the financial health of the office is largely dependent on accurate filing and prompt payment of claims. In order to provide timely and informed customer service in the medical office, the medical administrative assistant must be knowledgeable about health insurance regulations and procedures.

SUMMARY

The insurance claims process is an important customer service function that is provided by a medical administrative assistant for the patients of the medical office. In smaller offices, an assistant may be responsible for the entire claims process. In larger offices, a separate billing and insurance department may be responsible for filing insurance claims. Whatever the setup of the medical office, assistants must know the claims process so they can assist patients with insurance claim filing and related questions.

Federal and state governments establish regulations that the insurance industry is required to follow. Insurance plans also establish guidelines that providers are required to follow. An assistant should consult CMS or the insurance plan for the most current information on insurance requirements and claims processing.

YOU ARE THE MEDICAL ADMINSITRATIVE ASSISTANT

You have received an EOB that states that an incorrect policy number was listed on a claim form. What do you do?

REVIEW EXERCISES

Exercise 12-1 True or False

Read each statement, and determine whether the statement is true or false. Record the answer in the blank provided. T = true; F = false.

_______ 1. When an individual is employed, insurance premiums are always paid by the employer.

_______ 2. Copayments help hold down insurance costs for an insurance plan.

_______ 3. Health insurance policies identify what types of treatments are covered by the policy.

_______ 4. The greater the charges for an office visit, the greater is the patient's copayment.

_______ 5. Services that are fully covered by insurance such as yearly physical examinations do not apply to an insurance deductible.

_______ 6. Health insurance policies may have a maximum deductible amount that a family will have to pay in a year.

_______ 7. To draw special attention to new information on a CMS-1500 claim form, the information should be printed in italics.

_______ 8. Assignment of benefits means that the health care provider must accept what the insurance company allows as payment in full for services provided.

_______ 9. A release of information for insurance purposes is necessary to send information to a patient's insurance company.

_______ 10. An MSN is essentially the same type of form as an EOB.

_______ 11. With a fee-for-service insurance plan, an insurance company pays a health provider only if services are performed.

_______ 12. With an HMO, a health care provider is paid a fee to provide all health care for a patient.

_______ 13. Medicare provides health care coverage for some individuals who are younger than 65 years.

_______ 14. Medicare Advantage offers managed care plans for Medicare Part A and Part B.

_______ 15. Medicare is administered by each state, so patient benefits vary from state to state.

_______ 16. Premiums may be charged for Parts A and B of Medicare.

_______ 17. Medicare Part A covers hospital charges.

_______ 18. Hospice care and home health care are provided by Medicare as long as certain conditions are met.

_______ 19. It is the responsibility of the Medicare Administrative Contractor to monitor Medicare claims for fraud and abuse.

_______ 20. Persons with a large income may be eligible to receive Medicaid benefits if they are medically needy.

_______ 21. Because each state determines Medicaid eligibility and additional benefits, Medicaid coverage can vary widely from state to state.

_______ 22. Each state is free to decide what coverage will be provided under Medicaid.

_______ 23. If Medicaid does not cover all of a physician's charges, a physician may bill the patient for the remainder of the charges.

_______ 24. Workers' Compensation covers a worker's injuries that occur on the job.

_______ 25. The first report of injury for a Workers' Compensation claim must be made within 1 year of the injury.

_______ 26. Employees are responsible for paying their own Workers' Compensation premiums.

_______ 27. Major medical covers catastrophic medical expenses resulting from hospitalization.

_______ 28. Patient registration is a critical part of the insurance claim process.

________29. Physicians must personally sign every CMS-1500 claim form before it is sent to the insurance company.

________30. Vocational rehabilitation sometimes is provided by Workers' Compensation for an injured worker.

________31. Premiums are charged for Medicare Part D coverage.

________32. Medicare edits analyze the accuracy of Medicare electronic claims.

________33. Software often is costly for electronic claims processing; therefore, few medical offices file electronic claims.

________34. A patient can appeal an insurance company's decision at any time.

________35. A patient with an income of $200,000 per year probably will have to pay more for Medicare Part B coverage.

________36. The Medicare limiting charge applies to participating providers.

________37. An ABN should be signed by every Medicare patient who receives services in a medical office.

________38. Patients in restriction programs will have limited access to health care services.

________39. Providers who treat patients for work-related conditions may be required to complete periodic reports on the patient's condition.

Exercise 12-2 Insurance Terminology

Match each term in the list with its definition. Record the answer in the blank provided. Each answer is used only once.

(a) Assignment
(b) Beneficiary
(c) Birthday rule
(d) Claim
(e) Coinsurance
(f) Coordination of benefits
(g) Copayment
(h) Deductible
(i) Explanation of benefits
(j) Insured, policyholder, subscriber
(k) Insurance contract, policy
(l) Managed care
(m) Medicare Administrative Contractor
(n) Participating provider
(o) Preauthorization
(p) Premium
(q) Referral
(r) Usual, customary, reasonable fee
(s) Workers' Compensation

________ 1. Agreement between an insurance company and an individual (or group of individuals) in which the insurance company agrees to provide insurance coverage in exchange for a premium

________ 2. A type of insurance that provides benefits for employees who are injured on the job

________ 3. Request to an insurance company to receive insurance benefits

________ 4. An individual who holds an insurance policy

________ 5. An insurance plan's approval for a patient to receive a health care procedure from a health care provider

________ 6. An individual who qualifies for benefits under a subscriber's policy

________ 7. An insurance company that processes Medicare Part B claims

________ 8. Dependents are covered by the policy of the parent who has a birthday closest to the beginning of the year

________ 9. A set amount that must be paid by a patient for each encounter with a physician

________10. Accessibility to health care is controlled by the insurance company or the health care provider

________11. A percentage of a claim is paid by the patient

_______12. Monetary payment paid for insurance coverage

_______13. A specific amount a patient must pay for health care services per year before insurance benefits are paid

_______14. An agreement to accept the amount that Medicare approves for services as payment in full

_______15. An insurance clause that ensures health expenses are not paid for more than once

_______16. Providers who accept assignment

_______17. Approval from a primary care physician for a patient to receive services from a specialist

_______18. Describes what insurance benefits will be paid and what subtractions have been made from an insurance claim

_______19. The average amount charged by local physicians for health care services

Exercise 12-3 Chapter Concepts

Read each statement or question, and choose the answer that best completes the statement or question. Record the answer in the blank provided. Each answer is used only once.

_______1. Which of the following does not belong?
(a) Insured
(b) Policyholder
(c) Beneficiary
(d) Subscriber

_______2. Which of the following is false about preparing a CMS-1500 for processing by OCR equipment?
(a) Forms must be printed in a special type of red ink.
(b) Information should be entered by a computer or typewriter and should be entirely in capital letters.
(c) A scannable font such as Pica 12 should be used.
(d) Punctuation should be used where needed when information is entered on the form.

_______3. A family of six (father, mother, four children) has two insurance policies covering all family members. Each parent has full family coverage through his or her employer. Which policy will cover the children?
(a) The policy that was in effect first
(b) The father's policy
(c) The mother's policy
(d) The policy of the parent whose birthday occurs first in the year
(e) The policy of the parent who was born first

_______4. An insurance claim has been rejected by the insurance company. All of the following might be done to resubmit the claim except
(a) Check the patient's medical record to determine whether the procedure and the diagnosis were correct.
(b) Verify the insurance information by calling the patient.
(c) Confirm the insurance information by checking the office's computer database.
(d) Notify the patient that he or she will have to resubmit the claim.

_______5. All of the following are true about Medicare except
(a) Patients must be 65 years old to receive Medicare.
(b) Medicare Part B covers physician services provided in a clinic setting.
(c) CMS oversees Medicare.
(d) Patients with kidney transplants are eligible for Medicare.

_______6. The 2013 deductible for Medicare Part B is
(a) $104.90 per year
(b) $147 per year
(c) $1184 per year
(d) There is no deductible.

_______7. If a patient is covered under Medicare and Medicaid for an office visit, which insurance is primary?
(a) Medicare
(b) Medicaid

_______8. Medicaid is a health benefits program that is administered by the
(a) Federal government
(b) State government
(c) City government
(d) Centers for Medicare and Medicaid Services

_______9. Which group is covered under Medicare?
(a) People who have retired from their jobs
(b) People who cannot afford health insurance and have children
(c) People 65 and older who are retired and receive social security or railroad retirement benefits
(d) People who are partially disabled

_______10. The proper format for entering a date on a CMS-1500 is
(a) 03 08 1983
(b) 03-08-83
(c) March 8, 1983
(d) 83 03 08

_______ 11. A patient's encounter with a physician included 10 different procedures that must be billed for the visit. How many claim forms are required to be completed for the encounter?
(a) One
(b) Two
(c) Five
(d) Ten

_______ 12. The proper format for entering a patient's name on a CMS-1500 is
(a) Shepard, Alice R.
(b) SHEPARD, ALICE R.
(c) Alice R. Shepard
(d) ALICE R SHEPARD
(e) SHEPARD ALICE R

_______ 13. A child is covered under both parents' group insurance policies. The father's birthdate is 5-12-62, and the mother's birthdate is 3-14-61. Which policy is primary for the child?
(a) Father
(b) Mother
(c) Neither

_______ 14. A patient is injured while at work. Identify the policy that likely provides primary coverage.
(a) Liability policy
(b) Long-term care policy
(c) Group insurance policy
(d) Workers' Compensation
(e) Medicaid

_______ 15. If a patient has Medicare and Medigap, which plan will provide the primary insurance coverage for the patient?
(a) Medicare
(b) Medigap
(c) Whichever plan provides the most benefits

_______ 16. The portion of each bill that a Medicare B patient must pay is
(a) $0
(b) $20
(c) 20%
(d) $147

_______ 17. All of the following are true about Medicaid except
(a) State and federal funds are used to fund Medicaid.
(b) Each state must provide certain minimum coverage for all Medicaid recipients.
(c) If Medicaid cannot pay a patient's entire bill, a physician can bill the patient for the remainder of the bill.
(d) Copayments may be required for some Medicaid services.

_______ 18. If a patient is injured and unable to work, which box on the CMS-1500 should be completed?
(a) Box 18
(b) Box 14
(c) Box 16
(d) b and c only
(e) All of the above

_______ 19. The procedure code for services provided to a patient is located in which box on the CMS-1500?
(a) Box 21
(b) Box 23
(c) Box 24D
(d) Box 24C

_______ 20. Which box on the CMS-1500 identifies how many times a procedure was performed for a patient?
(a) Box 24C
(b) Box 24G
(c) Box 24J
(d) Box 24F

Exercise 12-4 Life Cycle of an Insurance Claim

Read the following steps in the insurance claim process, and number the steps in the order in which they occur. Record the number in the blank provided.

_______ The superbill is generated.

_______ The CMS form is completed and sent to the insurance plan.

_______ The insurance plan determines the UCR fees.

_______ The superbill is completed.

_______ Any insurance payment received by a health care provider is applied to the appropriate charges on the patient's account.

_______ The patient's information on CMS-1500 is verified by the insurance company.

_______ The EOB is prepared, and any copayment, deductible, or coinsurance is subtracted.

_______ The provider's information on CMS-1500 is verified by the insurance company.

_______ The patient's insurance information is obtained at registration.

_______ If the insurance plan owes benefits, a check is prepared for either the patient or the health care provider.

_______ A copy of the EOB is sent to the patient and the provider. Any check for payment of benefits is also sent.

Exercise 12-5 Medicare Computations

Read the following scenarios and determine the amounts requested in each scenario. Happy Valley Medical Center accepts assignment for all Medicare patients. Record your answers in the blanks provided. Use rates for the year 2013 when calculating amounts.

1. Linda Larson has Medicare Part B coverage. She sees Dr. Lee for an office visit and laboratory tests pertaining to diabetes. Ms. Larson has already met her deductible this year. The charges for the visit and tests are $325, of which Medicare allows only $300. Identify the following amounts:
   _______ (a) Amount discounted from Ms. Larson's charges
   _______ (b) Amount Medicare pays
   _______ (c) Amount Ms. Larson pays

2. Abner Wright has Medicare Part B coverage. He sees Dr. Hinckle for an office visit and diagnostic tests pertaining to arthritis. He has already met his deductible for the year. The charges for the visit and tests are $800, of which Medicare allows only $684. Identify the following amounts:
   _______ (a) Amount discounted from Mr. Wright's charges
   _______ (b) Amount Medicare pays
   _______ (c) Amount Mr. Wright pays

3. Martha Maye has Medicare Part B coverage. She sees Dr. Mallard for an office visit and diagnostic tests pertaining to influenza. She has not met her deductible for the year. The charges for the visit and tests are $250, of which Medicare allows only $225. Identify the following amounts:
   _______ (a) Amount discounted from Ms. Maye's charges
   _______ (b) Amount Medicare pays
   _______ (c) Amount Ms. Maye pays

4. Martha Maye has Medicare Part B coverage. She sees Dr. Mallard again for an additional office visit and tests pertaining to influenza. She has now met her deductible for the year. The charges for the visit and tests are $330, of which Medicare allows only $286. Identify the following amounts:
   _______ (a) Amount discounted from Ms. Maye's charges
   _______ (b) Amount Medicare pays
   _______ (c) Amount Ms. Maye pays

5. Marge Armstrong has a urinary tract infection and sees Dr. Lee for an office visit and diagnostic tests. She has already met her Medicare Part B deductible for the year. The charges for the visit and tests are $126, of which Medicare allows only $84. Identify the following amounts:
   _______ (a) Amount discounted from Ms. Armstrong's charges
   _______ (b) Amount Medicare pays
   _______ (c) Amount Ms. Armstrong pays

6. Amy Gordon has been having blackouts and sees Dr. Mallard for an office visit and numerous tests. Her Medicare Part B deductible has not been met for the year. The charges for the visit and tests are $1232, of which Medicare allows $998. Identify the following amounts:
   _______ (a) Amount discounted from Ms. Gordon's charges
   _______ (b) Amount Medicare pays
   _______ (c) Amount Ms. Gordon pays

7. Arthur Hunter sees Dr. Lee for an office visit and diagnostic tests pertaining to cellulitis. He has paid $50 toward his Medicare Part B deductible for the year. The charges for the visit and tests are $400, of which Medicare allows only $350. Identify the following amounts:
   _______ (a) Amount discounted from Mr. Hunter's charges
   _______ (b) Amount Medicare pays
   _______ (c) Amount Mr. Hunter pays

8. Charles Webster sees Dr. Hinckle for an office visit and diagnostic tests pertaining to bladder problems. He has Medicare Part A and has not paid any deductible this year. The charges for the visit and tests are $200. Identify the following amounts:
   _______ (a) Amount discounted from Mr. Webster's charges
   _______ (b) Amount Medicare pays
   _______ (c) Amount Mr. Webster pays

9. Mr. Webster (as mentioned in question 8) is found to have a kidney infection and is hospitalized at Happy Valley Hospital for 5 days. The charges for his hospital stay total $5317, of which Medicare allows $4645. Mr. Webster has not been hospitalized at all for the past year. Identify the following amounts:
   _______ (a) Amount discounted from Mr. Webster's charges
   _______ (b) Amount Medicare pays
   _______ (c) Amount Mr. Webster pays

Exercise 12-6 Other Insurance Computations

Read the following scenarios, and determine the amounts requested in each scenario. Happy Valley Medical Group accepts assignment for all BCBS patients. Coinsurance is based on the UCR fee. Record your answers in the blanks provided.

1. Susan Miller has BCBS coverage and sees Dr. Mallard for an ankle fracture. The total charges for the initial treatment of the fracture are $863, of which BCBS has a UCR reduction of $92. Ms. Miller has not yet paid her $200 deductible for the year. She has no copayment required for the visit and has a 20% coinsurance in her contract. Identify the following amounts:
   _______ (a) Amount discounted from Ms. Miller's charges
   _______ (b) Amount BCBS pays
   _______ (c) Amount Ms. Miller pays
2. Rayanne Roberts has BCBS coverage and sees Dr. Lee for a foreign body in her eye. Total charges for the office visit and slit lamp examination are $162. BCBS allows all charges, and Ms. Roberts has met her deductible for the year. She has a $10 copayment for each visit and a 20% coinsurance clause in her contract. Identify the following amounts:
   _______ (a) Amount discounted from Ms. Roberts' charges
   _______ (b) Amount BCBS pays
   _______ (c) Amount Ms. Roberts pays
3. Nan Johnson has Medicaid coverage. She sees Dr. Lee for an office visit regarding otalgia. Ms. Johnson has no deductible requirement but has a $3 copayment for each office visit. No coinsurance applies. The charges for the visit are $48, of which Medicaid allows only $36. Identify the following amounts:
   _______ (a) Amount discounted from Ms. Johnson's charges
   _______ (b) Amount Medicaid pays
   _______ (c) Amount Ms. Johnson pays
4. Henry Sherman has Priced Right insurance coverage. He sees Dr. Hinckle for an office visit and laboratory tests pertaining to gout. Horizons Healthcare does not accept assignment for Priced Right insurance and will bill the patient for any UCR reduction taken by the insurance company. Mr. Sherman has already met his deductible this year. The charges for the visit and tests are $164, of which Priced Right insurance allows only $124. A $10 copayment is paid by Mr. Sherman for his visit, and no coinsurance applies. Identify the following amounts:
   _______ (a) Amount discounted from Mr. Sherman's charges
   _______ (b) Amount Priced Right pays
   _______ (c) Amount Mr. Sherman pays
5. Kaye Evenson has Medicaid coverage and is a restricted patient at another clinic. She sees Dr. Lee for an office visit that is not urgent. Medicaid does not provide coverage. Ms. Evenson has no deductible requirement but has a $3 copayment for each office visit. The charges for the visit are $48. Identify the following amounts:
   _______ (a) Amount discounted from Ms. Evenson's charges
   _______ (b) Amount Medicaid pays
   _______ (c) Amount Ms. Evenson pays

Exercise 12-7 CMS-1500 Claim Form

Look at the CMS-1500 as pictured in Figure 12-1, and identify the box number where the following information would be located.

_______ Patient's name
_______ Insured's name
_______ Primary insurance name
_______ Secondary insurance name
_______ Primary insurance policy number
_______ Date patient was seen by physician
_______ Patient's diagnosis(es)
_______ Procedure(s) done for patient
_______ Physician who provided services
_______ Location where services were provided

ACTIVITIES

ACTIVITY 12-1 SET DEFAULT FOR INSURANCE CLAIM PROCESSING

Using Medisoft, set the default billing method for insurance claims. Most claims are filed electronically, but for the purposes of this practice version of Medisoft, claims will need to be set for **paper** processing.

1. On the Medisoft main menu, click **Lists>Insurance>Carriers.**
2. Double-click on **Blue Cross Blue Shield 231. Options and Codes** tab. Set the **Default Billing Method 1** to **Paper.** Click **Save.**
3. Repeat the actions in #2 for **Blue Cross Blue Shield 225** and remaining insurance companies.

ACTIVITY 12-2 CREATE INSURANCE CLAIMS WITH MEDISOFT

Using Medisoft, create insurance claims for the following patients. (To complete this exercise, billing activity 11-2 must be completed.)

1. On the Medisoft main menu, click **Activities>Claim Management**.

2. Click **Create Claims**. Specify the **Range of Transaction Dates** as **02/03/2014 to 02/04/2014.** Leave remaining fields blank.
3. Click **Create**. Claims will be added to the **Claims Management** window.
4. Click **Print/Send** near the bottom of the claim management window. Specify **Paper Claim>OK**. Click **Laser CMS (Primary) W/Form.** Click **OK.**
5. Click **Export the report to a file>Start**.
6. Name the file **yourlastname claims.** Save as a **text document.** Click **Save.**
7. In the **Date Created Range** enter **today's date** if you created the claims today. Enter today's date in both date boxes. If you did not create the claims today, check the **Date Created Column** in the **Claim Management** window. The claims you created will be in the last group of claims on the list. Use the date in the **Date Created Column.**
8. Click OK.

If you wish to reprint claims after you complete this exercise, you must highlight the claims you wish to print and then choose the **Reprint Claims** option near the bottom of the Claim Management window.

ACTIVITY 12-3 CLAIM FILING GUIDELINES

Obtain guidelines for submitting claims from your local BCBS office, another commercial health insurance company, your local Medicaid office, or all three.

ACTIVITY 12-4 RELEASE OF INFORMATION EXPLANATION

Explain to a patient the purpose of the release of information statement in Figure 8-2.

ACTIVITY 12-5 CMS-1500 CLAIM FORM

Compare a completed CMS-1500 claim form with the instructions provided in Table 12-1. Are the computerized forms consistent with the instructions in the table? If not, are any differences significant enough to affect the processing of a claim?

ACTIVITY 12-6 MEDICARE FACTS

Locate a summary of Medicare Part A, B, and D costs for patients for the current year at the CMS website. The information should include amounts that a patient must pay for Medicare-covered services. For example, what part of a home health care service must a patient pay? (In 2013, a patient paid $0 for home health care services but paid 20% of the Medicare-approved amount for durable medical equipment.)

ACTIVITY 12-7 INSURANCE TERMINOLOGY

Locate an online glossary of insurance terminology.

ACTIVITY 12-8 MEDICAID BENEFITS

Determine what services are covered and not covered by Medicaid in your state.

ACTIVITY 12-9 MEDIGAP PLANS

Identify the services covered under Medigap A-L plans.

ACTIVITY 12-10 WORKERS' COMPENSATION REQUIREMENTS

Identify your state requirements for employers, health care providers, and injured employees in working with patients covered by Workers' Compensation claims.

DISCUSSION

The following topic can be used for class discussion or for individual student essay.

DISCUSSION 12-1

A health care provider agrees to accept Medicare assignment. Is this beneficial for patients? Why or why not?

Bibliography

Assistant Secretary for Planning and Evaluation, U.S. Department of Health and Human Services: Overview of the Uninsured in the United States: A Summary of the 2011 Current Population Survey. aspe.hhs.gov. Accessed October 1, 2012.

Centers for Medicare and Medicaid Services: Advance Beneficiary Notice. www.cms.gov. Accessed October 7, 2012.

Centers for Medicare and Medicaid Services: Brief Summaries of Medicare and Medicaid. www.cms.gov. Accessed 3-24-12.

Centers for Medicare and Medicaid Services: Form CMS-1500 at a Glance. www.cms.gov. Accessed October 7, 2012.

Centers for Medicare and Medicaid Services: Medicare Costs at a Glance. www.cms.gov. Accessed October 7, 2012.

Fordney MT: *Insurance Handbook for the Medical Office*, ed 10, St. Louis, MO, 2008, WB Saunders.

Fordney MT, French LL, Follis JJ: *Administrative Medical Assisting*, ed 5, Clifton Park, NY, 2004, Delmar.

National Uniform Claim Committee: 1500 Health Insurance Claim Form Reference Instruction Manual, July 2012. www.nucc.org. Accessed October 7, 2012.

Newby C: *From Patient to Payment: Insurance Procedures for the Medical Office*, ed 4, New York, NY, 2005, Glencoe McGraw-Hill.

Office of Civil Rights: U.S. Summary of the HIPAA Privacy Rule, Department of Health and Human Services. http://www.hhs.gov/ocr/privacy/hipaa/understanding/summary/privacysummary.pdf, last revised May 2003. Accessed October 7, 2012.

TRICARE. Media Center: www.tricare.mil. Accessed October 7, 2012.

U.S. Department of Veterans' Affairs: *Frequently Asked Questions*. www.va.gov. Accessed October 7, 2012.

CHAPTER 13 Business Operations of the Medical Office

LEARNING OUTCOMES

On successful completion of this chapter, the student will be able to

1. Identify types of ownership of medical facilities.
2. Explain the function of The Joint Commission and the purpose of accreditation.
3. Examine facility safety, the Occupational Safety and Health Administration (OSHA), and OSHA requirements.
4. Explain ergonomics and recognize its importance.
5. Define the function of the Clinical Laboratory Improvement Amendments.
6. Explain managing office supplies.
7. Explain effective methods of interoffice communication.
8. Determine planning considerations for meetings.
9. Explain coordination of travel arrangements.

COMMISSION ON ACCREDITATION OF ALLIED HEALTH EDUCATION PROGRAMS (CAAHEP) CORE CURRICULUM FOR MEDICAL ASSISTANTS

- Use Internet to access information related to the medical office.
- Describe personal protective equipment.
- Describe the importance of Materials Safety Data Sheets (MSDS) in a health care setting.

VOCABULARY

agenda
corporation
ergonomics
Material Safety Data Sheet (MSDS)
minutes
musculoskeletal disorders (MSDs)
Occupational Safety and Health Administration (OSHA)
partnership
sole proprietorship
universal precautions

Medical practices vary widely in size and scope of practice, and an office manager is responsible for various activities in the office. The assistant's role in office management is determined by the arrangement and needs of the organization. This chapter examines the fundamental considerations of organizing and operating a medical practice. An understanding of the organizational makeup of the medical office and functions that support the operation of the medical office is necessary to help a medical administrative assistant develop a "big picture" of an organization—how it works and what supportive functions are necessary to keep an office running smoothly.

Organizational Structure of the Medical Office

Types of Ownership

Medical practices can be structured in various ways to accommodate the physicians who are practicing within the organization. Medical practices may be incorporated, with the physicians as shareholders of the corporation. A **corporation** is a recognized separate entity that operates independently of its employees and stockholders. Health care systems that consist of a medical practice and a hospital may choose to operate as a for-profit or as a nonprofit corporation. Organizing as a corporation is advantageous because the organizational structure stays intact and does not have to be reorganized as physicians come and go from the organization. Also, individual physicians may be protected from actions attributed to the corporation.

Some independent physicians choose not to incorporate and instead operate a practice as a **sole proprietorship.** A sole proprietor assumes all liabilities for the practice and receives all of the income for the practice. With this type of business arrangement, a physician makes all business decisions and could be on call 24 hours a day. This business arrangement means that a physician assumes personal liability for the actions of the practice. A sole proprietor physician may risk losing personal assets in a suit against the practice. Sole proprietorships were much more common in the earlier part of this century and have been declining with the advent of group practices operating as corporations.

Two or more physicians who do not wish to incorporate may choose to form a **partnership.** Partner physicians share all income and expenses of a practice. A disadvantage of a partnership is that one partner may be found liable for the actions of another partner. An advantage of working in a partnership or working for a corporation is that the partnership or corporation can purchase equipment that might otherwise be too expensive for a sole proprietor to purchase.

Financial Interests of Physicians

In today's medical community, it is common for physicians to have part or full ownership of health-related businesses such as pharmacies, home health agencies, laboratories, nursing homes, or other medically related services. Although such ownership is legal, the ethical standards of the American Medical Association state that a physician's financial interest in a company should not influence the physician's decision making, and that a physician should never place personal financial interest above a patient's best interest. It is a patient's prerogative to choose where prescriptions and other medical products and services will be purchased.

This ethical standard is evident in the everyday practice of physicians. Consider the following example: When a physician decides that a prescription is necessary to treat a patient, the physician either writes the prescription and gives it to the patient or electronically sends the prescription to a pharmacy. When a written prescription is given to a patient, the patient may fill the prescription wherever he or she chooses. If a physician electronically sends a prescription to a pharmacy, the physician asks the patient which pharmacy should be contacted. A physician does not automatically select a pharmacy of the physician's choice; the physician lets the patient decide where the prescription will be purchased.

Many practices make a point of notifying patients of a physician's financial interest in a health-related business that may be connected to the medical office. A notice may be legally required to be posted in the office to inform patients of a physician's ownership in the equipment or business.

Organizational Hierarchy

Depending on the nature of the medical office, the size of the office staff can vary from just a few people to hundreds and, in the case of large facilities, even thousands.

When the hierarchy of a medical organization is established, employees usually are divided into groups according to the nature of their work, that is, the clinical staff, consisting of registered nurses, licensed practical nurses, certified nurse assistants, and clinical medical assistants, usually report to the same superior because their job duties are somewhat similar. Supervisors have work experience related to the group that they supervise. A registered nurse, not an accountant, is a logical choice to manage the nursing staff. An accountant would be a logical choice to manage the business office, however.

Of course, if the organization consists of only 5 to 10 employees, it may not be necessary, or even possible, to hire a professional to manage each group in the office. In this case, key personnel may be assigned duties within the office. Professional services then can be contracted on an as-needed or a regular basis.

Following is an example of how the contracting of certain professional services might work: A key person of the office staff (e.g., a medical administrative assistant) may collect financial information, such as charges and payments to patients' accounts and payroll information. Monthly totals are tabulated by the assistant and are given to an outside accounting firm that maintains the accounts of the office and files necessary government reports such as those required for payroll.

Large corporate practices typically are managed by a board of directors. The board may be elected by the shareholders of the corporation and may consist of staff physicians, retired physicians, community leaders, and key people of the organization. The board then elects a chairperson from the group to conduct board meetings. These meetings consist of reports from key personnel within the organization and any matters that require the attention of the board. Examples of key personnel of an organization include chief of medical staff, chief financial officer, human resources director, and facilities manager.

It is important for everyone to know the hierarchy of the medical organization in which they are employed and to understand the importance of the organizational hierarchy. An organizational hierarchy is developed to establish a chain of command for accountability and decision making. If a question or concern about the procedures of the medical office arises, an assistant should communicate with the individual who is most directly responsible for the procedure in question.

Consider the following situation: An assistant has a question regarding a physician's wishes for scheduling patients for physical examinations. Depending on the hierarchy of the organization, the situation could be handled in one of two ways: (1) If the assistant is a supervisor in charge of the registration and appointment services for a larger medical practice, the assistant probably talks directly with the physician to determine the appropriate method for scheduling patients. The assistant then communicates the decision of the physician to the rest of the registration and appointment staff. (2) If the assistant is a member of the registration and appointment services staff and has another assistant as an immediate supervisor, the staff assistant speaks with the supervisor, and the supervisor, in turn, speaks with the physician, if necessary. The supervisor then returns to the assistant and the rest of the staff and reports the physician's decision.

An assistant should not go above an immediate supervisor unless the situation is urgent and following the chain of command would cause a delay in handling the situation, or injury or harm could come to someone. Another possible reason for not following the chain of command is when the problem is with the supervisor. In such cases, the assistant may have to use personal judgment as to what action is appropriate. If possible, a supervisor should be given an opportunity to correct any situations for which the supervisor may be responsible. Circumventing an immediate supervisor may provoke some unnecessarily tense situations in the medical office. If possible, always try to resolve a problem by speaking directly with the supervisor first.

Health Care–Related Organizations

The Joint Commission

A key component in the operation of a medical facility is accreditation by a recognized accreditation agency. Health care organizations all across the country participate in various types of accreditation processes. Some health care organizations are reviewed by outside accreditation agencies and some by respective state government organizations. States have licensing authority over health care organizations but may accept other accreditation in lieu of inspection by a state agency.

The Joint Commission is an independent national organization that reviews the practices of many types of health care organizations, such as hospitals, home health agencies, mental health providers, ambulatory care facilities, laboratories, and nursing homes. The Joint Commission reviews a health care facility's operations and determines whether the services the facility provides and the organization's business practices meet predetermined quality standards of The Joint Commission.

Accreditation may or may not be voluntary. Accreditation is often necessary to conduct business as a health care organization. Many states require that health care organizations be accredited by a recognized organization to obtain and maintain a license to do business in the state. Accreditation by the commission also may satisfy Medicare certification requirements.

The accreditation process requires a health care facility to conduct a careful study of its organizational practices and document the practices in a written response. This study process, sometimes referred to as a self-study, requires the organization to conduct an in-depth review of all procedures and policies used in the everyday operation of the health care facility. Procedures and policies are reviewed in the self-study, along with documented evidence of how those procedures and processes are carried out within the organization.

The self-study process is often an eye-opening experience for the organization because it examines what is and is not working within the organization. After the self-study has been completed, an investigative team consisting of industry experts conducts an on-site visit, known as an on-site survey, to verify that the organization is indeed meeting the standards as established by The Joint Commission. At the end of the on-site visit, the team reports its recommendation on accreditation to the organization and files a report with The Joint Commission, which then determines whether to grant the accreditation recommendations of the on-site team. If the health care facility wishes to appeal an unfavorable decision of The Joint Commission, it is allowed to do so. More information on The Joint Commission is available on its website.

Occupational Safety and Health Administration

In addition to accreditation from a nationally recognized agency, safe work practices and a safe work environment are essential to the success of a medical practice. The management team of the medical practice must effectively and continually communicate to all employees the importance of safety in the workplace. A single incident caused by an unsafe environment or unsafe practices can ruin an otherwise successful practice. The management team as well as all employees of the organization should stress workplace safety and should expect everyone to ensure a safe workplace.

Setting standards to ensure safe workplaces is the chief responsibility of the **Occupational Safety and Health Administration** (OSHA, pronounced "o-sha"). OSHA was created by the Occupational Safety and Health Act of 1970 and applies to all employers and employees, with the exception of self-employed persons, farms on which only family members are employed, worksites (e.g., mining, nuclear energy) that are covered by other federal statutes, and employees of certain identified state and local governments.

OSHA carries out its responsibility by setting workplace standards and conducting workplace inspections to ensure that standards are being met. Employers are responsible for knowing the standards that apply to their workplace, eliminating any hazardous conditions, and making sure employees comply with applicable standards.

OSHA establishes standards that impose basic requirements for ensuring a safe workplace. The Personal Protective Equipment Standard requires that employers provide employees with personal protective equipment necessary to do their job. This equipment must be provided at no cost to the employee. Examples of protective equipment in a medical office include latex gloves, splashguards for eyes, and other protective coverings that may be necessary for performing a task in the office.

Employee Injury

If an employee injury occurs, OSHA Form 301 Injury and Illness Incident Report (Fig. 13-1) is used to report the incident and describe in detail the injury or illness that has occurred. An insurance or Workers' Compensation form may be substituted for Form 301 if it provides the same type of information. Form 301 contains information about the name and location of the employer; the name, address, age, sex, and occupation of the injured or ill employee; information about the incident that caused the employee's injury or illness; circumstances of the injury or illness itself; and information regarding the treating physician and hospital (if the employee was hospitalized). OSHA forms must be kept a minimum of 5 years after the end of the calendar year in which the incident occurred. For instance, a report for an incident that occurred on July 9, 2011, would have to be kept until December 31, 2016.

On Form 300 Log of Work-Related Injuries and Illnesses (Fig. 13-2), an employer is also required to keep a log of work-related injuries and illnesses that require the attention of a physician or other health care personnel. Injuries that result in days off work, job transfer or restricted work, loss of consciousness, or medical attention beyond first aid are required to be reported on Form 300.

Because of the sensitive nature of the information included on OSHA forms, all information contained within the forms should be treated as confidential and should be protected as much as possible when the information is used for occupational safety and health purposes. An employee's personal medical record is always considered confidential, and an employee must give specific written consent for anyone to view the records. Employers are not entitled to a copy of an employee's medical record without the employee's permission.

If a work-related death occurs, or if three or more employees require hospitalization because of a work-related accident, the employer is required to contact the nearest OSHA office within 8 hours of the accident. This time requirement is

OSHA's Form 301
Injury and Illness Incident Report

Attention: This form contains information relating to employee health and must be used in a manner that protects the confidentiality of employees to the extent possible while the information is being used for occupational safety and health purposes.

U.S. Department of Labor
Occupational Safety and Health Administration

Form approved OMB no. 1218-176

This *Injury and Illness Incident Report* is one of the first forms you must fill out when a recordable work-related injury or illness has occurred. Together with the *Log of Work-Related Injuries and Illnesses* and the accompanying *Summary*, these forms help the employer and OSHA develop a picture of the extent and severity of work-related incidents.

Within 7 calendar days after you receive information that a recordable work-related injury or illness has occurred, you must fill out this form or an equivalent. Some state workers' compensation, insurance, or other reports may be acceptable substitutes. To be considered an equivalent form, any substitute must contain all the information asked for on this form.

According to Public Law 91-596 and 29 CFR 1904, OSHA's recordkeeping rule, you must keep this form on file for 5 years following the year to which it pertains.

If you need additional copies of this form, you may photocopy and use as many as you need.

Completed by ______

Title ______

Phone (___)___-______ Date ___/___/___

Information about the employee

1) Full name

2) Street ______

City ______ State ___ ZIP ______

3) Date of birth ___/___/___

4) Date hired ___/___/___

5) ☐ Male
☐ Female

Information about the physician or other health care professional

6) Name of physician or other health care professional

______

7) If treatment was given away from the worksite, where was it given?

Facility ______

Street ______

City ______ State ___ ZIP ______

8) Was employee treated in an emergency room?
☐ Yes
☐ No

9) Was employee hospitalized overnight as an in-patient?
☐ Yes
☐ No

Information about the case

10) Case number from the *Log* ______ *(Transfer the case number from the Log after you record the case)*

11) Date of injury or illness ___/___/___

12) Time employee began work ______ AM / PM

13) Time of event ______ AM / PM ☐ Check if time cannot be determined

14) **What was the employee doing just before the incident occurred?** Describe the activity, as well as the tools, equipment, or material the employee was using. Be specific. *Examples*: "climbing a ladder while carrying roofing materials"; spraying chlorine from hand sprayer"; "daily computer key-entry."

15) **What happened?** Tell us how the injury occurred. *Examples:* "When ladder slipped on wet floor, worker fell 20 feet"; "Worker was sprayed with chlorine when gasket broke during replacement"; "Worker developed soreness in wrist over time."

16) **What was the injury or illness?** Tell us the part of the body that was affected and how it was affected; be more specific than "hurt", "pain," or "sore". *Examples:* "strained back"; "chemical burn, hand"; "carpal tunnel syndrome."

17) **What object or substance directly harmed the employee?** *Examples*: "concrete floor"; "chlorine"; "radial arm saw." *If this question does not apply to the incident, leave it blank.*

18) **If the employee died, when did death occur?**
Date of death ___/___/___

Public reporting burden for this collection of information is estimated to average 22 minutes per response, including time for reviewing instructions, searching existing data sources, gathering and maintaining the data needed, and completing and reviewing the collection of information. Persons are not required to respond to the collection of information unless it displalys a current valid OMB control number. If you have any comments about this estimate or any other aspects of this data collection, including suggestions for reducing this burden contact: US Department of Labor, OSHA Office of Statistics, Room N-3644, 200 Constitution Avenue, NW, Washingon, DC 20210. Do not send the completed forms to this office.

Figure 13-1 Occupational Safety and Health Administration Form 301 documents the circumstances of an individual employee injury. (From Occupational Safety and Health Administration, U.S. Department of Labor. www.osha.gov. Accessed December 26, 2007.)

OSHA's Form 300

Log of Work-Related Injuries and Illnesses

Attention: This form contains information relating to employee health and must be used in a manner that protects the confidentiality of employees to the extent possible while the information is being used for occupational safety and health purposes.

Year 20

U.S. Department of Labor
Occupational Safety and Health Administration

Form approved OMB no. 1218-0176

You must record information about every work-related death and about every work-related injury or illness that involves loss of consciousness, restricted work activity or job transfer, days away from work, or medical treatment beyond first aid. You must also record significant work-related injuries and illnesses that are diagnosed by a physician or licensed health care professional. You must also record work-related injuries and illnesses that meet any of the specific recording criteria listed in 29 CFR Part 1904.8 through 1904.12. Feel free to use two lines for a single case if you need to. You must complete an Injury and Illness Incident Report (OSHA Form 301) or equivalent form for each injury or illness recorded on this form. If you're not sure whether a case is recordable, call your local OSHA office for help.

Establishment name

City   State

Identify the person		Describe the case				Classify the case										
						Using these four categories, check ONLY the most serious result for each case:				Enter the number of days the injured or ill worker was:		Check the "Injury" column or choose one type of illness: (M)				
(A) Case no.	(B) Employee's name	(C) Job title (e.g., *Welder*)	(D) Date of injury or onset of illness	(E) Where the event occurred (*e.g., Loading dock north end*)	(F) Describe injury or illness, parts of body affected, and object/substance that directly injured or made person ill (*e.g., Second degree burns on right forearm from acetylene torch*)	(G) Death	(H) Days away from work	Remained at work: (I) Job transfer or restriction	Remained at work: (J) Other record-able cases	(K) On job transfer or restriction	(L) Away from work	(1) Injury	(2) Skin disorder	(3) Respiratory condition	(4) Poisoning	(5) All other illnesses
			/ month/day			☐	☐	☐	☐	days	days	☐	☐	☐	☐	☐
			/ month/day			☐	☐	☐	☐	days	days	☐	☐	☐	☐	☐
			/ month/day			☐	☐	☐	☐	days	days	☐	☐	☐	☐	☐
			/ month/day			☐	☐	☐	☐	days	days	☐	☐	☐	☐	☐
			/ month/day			☐	☐	☐	☐	days	days	☐	☐	☐	☐	☐
			/ month/day			☐	☐	☐	☐	days	days	☐	☐	☐	☐	☐
			/ month/day			☐	☐	☐	☐	days	days	☐	☐	☐	☐	☐
			/ month/day			☐	☐	☐	☐	days	days	☐	☐	☐	☐	☐
			/ month/day			☐	☐	☐	☐	days	days	☐	☐	☐	☐	☐
			/ month/day			☐	☐	☐	☐	days	days	☐	☐	☐	☐	☐
			/ month/day			☐	☐	☐	☐	days	days	☐	☐	☐	☐	☐
			/ month/day			☐	☐	☐	☐	days	days	☐	☐	☐	☐	☐
			/ month/day			☐	☐	☐	☐	days	days	☐	☐	☐	☐	☐
					Page totals ➤	___	___	___	___	___	___	Injury (1)	Skin disorder (2)	Respiratory condition (3)	Poisoning (4)	All other illnesses (5)

Be sure to transfer these totals to the Summary page (Form 300A) before you post it.

Public reporting burden for this collection of information is estimated to average 14 minutes per response, including time to review the instructions, search and gather the data needed, and complete and review the collection of information. Persons are not required to respond to the collection of information unless it displays a currently valid OMB control number. If you have any comments about these estimates or any other aspects of this data collection, contact: US Department of Labor, OSHA Office of Statistics, Room N-3644, 200 Constitution Avenue, NW, Washington, DC 20210. Do not send the completed forms to this office.

Page ___ of ___

Figure 13-2 Employers are required to keep a Form 300, Log of Work-Related Injuries and Illnesses. Injuries that require medical attention beyond basic first aid, cause loss of consciousness, or result in days missed from work or restricted work activity must be recorded in the log. (From Occupational Safety and Health Administration, U.S. Department of Labor. www.osha.gov. Accessed November 18, 2011.)

necessary in case an investigation of an accident is needed to ensure that workplace standards were being met at the time of the accident.

Employers found in violation of OSHA standards are subject to a fine for each offense, and if an employer knows of a serious violation and does not attempt to correct it, the violation may be punishable by a fine and incarceration.

Ergonomics

A very common type of work-related injury occurs when work done by an employee is done incorrectly or is done under improper conditions. If a job task is not suited to an employee, that employee may sustain a work injury because of job conditions.

If a task does not match the physical capacity of an employee, a musculoskeletal injury is likely to result. A **musculoskeletal disorder (MSD)** is an injury or disorder of the muscles, nerves, tendons, ligaments, and joints and does not include injury resulting from trips or falls. MSDs are likely to occur in employees who use repetitive motions throughout the day, lift heavy objects, or perform a task in an awkward position. An example of a common MSD is carpal tunnel syndrome. Office personnel who perform repetitive motions as part of their job are especially susceptible to MSDs.

The largest work-related type of injury, MSDs make up one third of all work-related injuries as reported to the Bureau of Labor Statistics every year. In 2010, MSDs accounted for 29% of days spent away from work. Some employees may become permanently disabled because of an MSD and may not even be able to perform simple tasks like combing hair or picking up a child.

An improperly designed workstation (e.g., a chair that is nonadjustable, a desk that is too high) that causes a worker to perform a task in an unnatural position may lead to injury. Often, something as simple as an adjustable chair can prevent a work-related injury. The concept of **ergonomics** involves fitting the work to the worker. Results of OSHA studies reveal that ergonomics programs for injury prevention help reduce injuries in the workplace. Studies by the National Research Council/National Academy of Sciences have demonstrated a direct, positive correlation between ergonomics education and a reduction in work-related musculoskeletal disorders (Fig. 13-3).

Because of the large number of work-related disorders, all employees of the medical office should be educated about the hazards that may cause a work-related injury. To reduce the chance of injury, an employer should monitor the following situations:

- Proper lifting techniques should be used to avoid back injury.
- Computer workstations should be set at an appropriate ergonomic height for the employee. Computer keyboards should be at a comfortable height to relieve pressure on shoulders and upper back, and monitors should be at eye level and should have a nonglare screen.
- Employees who work at computer stations or at other tasks for long periods should take frequent breaks to relax muscles in use.

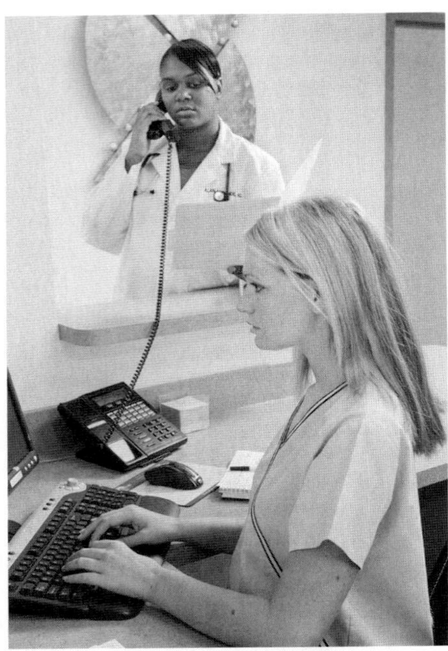

Figure 13-3 Proper attention to ergonomics reduces the chances of a work-related injury. (From Young AP. *Kinn's The Administrative Medical Assistant.* 7th ed. St. Louis, MO: Saunders Elsevier; 2011, Figure 4-1.)

- Appropriate lighting should be available for the task at hand.
- Proper ventilation should be ensured throughout the building. Air cleaning services should be regularly employed to clean ductwork and remove dust and other foreign particles that accumulate in air systems. Improper or dirty ventilation systems can cause employee illness.

Employee Rights Under the Occupational Safety and Health Act

The Occupational Safety and Health Act protects employee rights on the job. Employees have the right to complain to OSHA about safety and health conditions in their workplace and to have their identities kept confidential. Employees are allowed to participate in workplace inspections and may challenge the time OSHA allows for the employer to comply with any violations. Also, if an employee feels that he or she has been discriminated against, the employee must notify OSHA within 30 days of the time the employee became aware of the discrimination.

CHECKPOINT

A medical office employee trips and falls over some boxes in the medical records room. One of the staff physicians examines the employee, obtains radiographs of the employee's wrist, and determines that the radiographs are negative and that the employee has sustained only a wrist sprain. Because the worker is already employed by the clinic, these services are performed at no charge. Should anything else be done by the employee?

Material Safety Data Sheets

All products that are potentially hazardous to a person's health must be appropriately labeled, and the facility must keep information on file documenting the contents of the products and actions that should be taken if an employee has improper exposure to the products. Employees also must be educated about what should be done if they come into contact with a hazardous substance.

Product information is recorded on a **Material Safety Data Sheet (MSDS)** (Fig. 13-4). An MSDS details the ingredients of a product, as well as first aid measures that should be taken in case of wrongful exposure to the product (e.g., a product splashes the eye). All facilities with hazardous substances are required to have an MSDS on file for every hazardous substance. MSDSs usually are included with shipments of substances.

MATERIAL SAFETY DATA SHEET (MSDS)

Date of Issue: 4/28/04 | Date of Revision: 8/8/07

SECTION 1 IDENTIFICATION

GENERIC NAME: Glutaraldehyde	INFORMATION TELEPHONE NUMBER: 1 (800) 733-8690
BRAND NAME: Aldecide	EMERGENCY TELEPHONE NUMBER: 1 (800) 331-0766
MANUFACTURER'S NAME: Brennan Corporation	
MFG. ADDRESS: P.O. Box 93	
CITY: Camden STATE: NJ ZIP: 08106	

SECTION 2 COMPOSITION OF INGREDIENTS

CAS NUMBER	CHEMICAL NAME OF INGREDIENTS	PERCENT	PEL	TLV
111-30-8	Glutaraldehyde	2.5	0.2 ppm	0.2 ppm
7732-18-5	Water	97.4	None	None
7632-00-0	Sodium Nitrite	<1	None	None

SECTION 3 PHYSICAL AND CHEMICAL PROPERTIES

BOILING POINT: 212° F	SPECIFIC GRAVITY (H_2O = 1): 1.004
VAPOR PRESSURE (mm Hg): 0.20 at 20° C	VAPOR DENSITY (AIR = 1): 1.1
ODOR: Sharp odor	pH: 7.5-8.5
SOLUBILITY IN WATER: Complete (100%)	MELTING POINT: n/a
APPEARANCE: Bluish-green liquid	FREEZING POINT: 32° F
EVAPORATION RATE: 0.98 (Water = 1)	ODOR THRESHOLD: 0.04 ppm

SECTION 4 FIRE AND EXPLOSION HAZARD DATA

FLASH POINT: Not flammable (aqueous solution)		NFPA Rating:
FLAMMABILITY LIMITS:	LEL: n/a	Health: 2
EXTINGUISHING MEDIA: n/a (aqueous solution)		Flammability: 0
SPECIAL FIRE FIGHTING PROCEDURES: n/a		Reactivity: 0
UNUSUAL FIRE/EXPL HAZARDS: None		

SECTION 5 REACTIVITY DATA

STABILITY: Stable under recommended storage conditions.

CONDITIONS TO AVOID: Avoid direct sunlight and temperatures above 104° F (40° C).

INCOMPATIBILITY (MATERIAL TO AVOID): Strong acids and alkalines will neutralize active ingredient.

HAZARDOUS DECOMPOSITION BYPRODUCTS: None

HAZARDOUS POLYMERIZATION: Will not occur

Figure 13-4 A Material Safety Data Sheet identifies the chemical makeup of a hazardous substance and suggests remedies that should be used in case of exposure. (From Bonewit-West K. *Clinical Procedures for Medical Assistants.* 5th ed. Philadelphia, PA: WB Saunders; 2000, pp. 161–163.)

Continued

MATERIAL SAFETY DATA SHEET			PAGE 2
SECTION 6 HEALTH HAZARD DATA			
ROUTE OF ENTRY: SKIN: yes	EYES: yes	INHALATION: yes	INGESTION: yes
SIGNS AND SYMPTOMS OF OVEREXPOSURE: SKIN: Moderate irritation. May aggravate existing dermatitis. EYES: Serious eye irritant. May cause irreversible damage which could permanently impair vision. INHALATION: Vapors may be severely irritating and cause stinging sensations in the eyes, nose, throat, and lungs. May aggravate pre-existing asthma. INGESTION: May cause irritation or chemical burns of the mouth, throat, esophagus, and stomach. May cause vomiting, diarrhea, epigastric distress, headache, dizziness, faintness, mental confusion, and general systemic illness.			
CARCINOGENICITY DATA: NTP: No	AIRC: No	OSHA: No	
SECTION 7 EMERGENCY FIRST AID PROCEDURES			
SKIN: Wash skin with soap and water for 15 minutes. If skin redness or irritation persists, seek medical attention. Remove contaminated clothing and wash before reuse.			
EYES: Immediately flush with water for 15 minutes. Seek medical attention.			
INHALATION: Remove to fresh air. If irritation persists, seek medical attention.			
INGESTION: Do not induce vomiting. Seek medical attention immediately. Call a physician or Poison Control Center.			
SECTION 8 PRECAUTIONS FOR SAFE HANDLING AND USE			
SPILL PROCEDURES: Ventilate area, wear protective gloves and eye gear. Wipe with sponge, mop, or towel. Flush with large quantities of water. Collect liquid and discard it.			
WASTE DISPOSAL METHOD: Container must be triple rinsed and disposed of in accordance with federal, state, and/or local regulations. Used solution should be flushed thoroughly with water into sewage disposal system in accordance with federal, state, and/or local regulations.			
PRECAUTIONS IN HANDLING AND STORAGE: Store in a cool, dry place (59-86° F) away from direct sunlight or sources of intense heat. Keep container tightly closed when not in use.			
SECTION 9 CONTROL MEASURES			
VENTILATION: Ensure adequate ventilation to maintain recommended exposed limit.			
RESPIRATORY PROTECTION: None normally required for routine use.			
SKIN PROTECTION: Wear chemical resistant protective gloves. Butyl rubber, nitrile rubber, polyethylene, or double-gloved latex.			
EYE PROTECTION: Safety goggles or safety glasses			
WORK/HYGIENE PRACTICES: Prompt rinsing of hands after contact. Handle in accordance with good personal hygiene and safety practices. These practices include avoiding unnecessary exposure.			

Figure 13-4, cont'd

OSHA Information

Information on OSHA standards is published in the *Federal Register*, which is available in many public libraries. Additional information about OSHA standards and regulations is also available on the federal government's OSHA website.

Bloodborne Pathogens and Standard Precautions

In 1991, OSHA established the Occupational Exposure to Bloodborne Pathogens Standard. This standard is designed to protect health care workers from pathogens that may be distributed by means of blood and other bodily fluids and applies to all employees who have occupational exposure to these potentially infectious materials. Bloodborne pathogens are microorganisms that are present in bodily fluids and cause infection in humans. The following infections may be transmitted through exposure to bodily fluids:

- Hepatitis A, B, and C
- Human immunodeficiency virus (HIV)
- Staphylococcal and streptococcal infections
- Pneumonia
- Tuberculosis
- Blood infections
- Chickenpox
- Measles

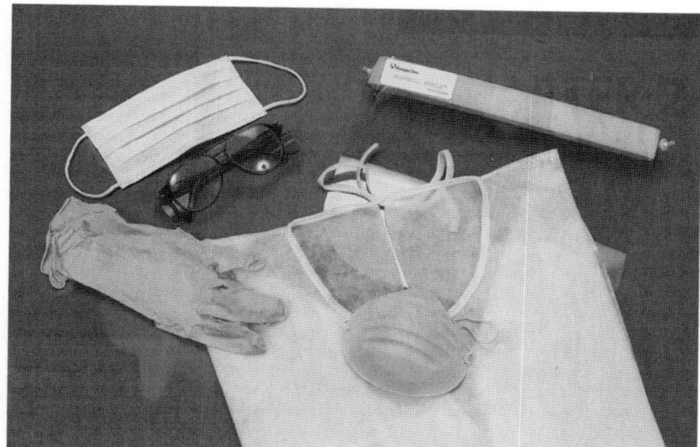

Figure 13-5 All employees are provided with the protective equipment necessary to perform their jobs within the medical office.

- Urinary tract infections
- Syphilis
- Herpes

The most common way that an employee may come into contact with a bloodborne pathogen is by needlestick; however, a hazardous substance could be splashed on an employee or could enter an opening in an employee's skin. All employees who handle a specimen of blood or other bodily fluids should exercise **universal precautions.** The term "universal precautions" refers to the treatment of all human blood and certain bodily fluids as potentially infectious for pathogens such as the HIV virus or hepatitis virus. Whether an office employee knows the patient is not important. Every medical office employee—or anyone —who comes into contact with any bodily fluids at any time should treat every bodily fluid as potentially infectious. Examples of bodily fluids included in this standard are human blood; semen; vaginal secretions; cerebrospinal, synovial, pleural, pericardial, peritoneal, and amniotic fluid; any body fluid contaminated with blood or saliva in dental procedures; and unfixed human tissues or organs (other than intact skin).

When a medical administrative assistant comes into contact with any type of potentially infectious bodily fluid, precautions should be taken. For instance, if a patient drips blood from a laceration on the registration desk, the assistant should consult the physician's written instructions for cleaning and disinfecting the area. These instructions should be on hand at all times and likely will include using an approved disinfectant and using appropriate equipment, such as wearing gloves during decontamination of the area (Fig. 13-5).

Any employee who is potentially contaminated with a bloodborne pathogen should complete an incident report (OSHA or Workers' Compensation, or both) immediately after the incident occurs. Employers are required to inform employees as to procedures that should be followed if an employee experiences an exposure incident. Employers also must provide free medical evaluation and treatment to any employee who has an exposure incident.

Hazard Communication Standard

This standard is frequently referred to as the "Right to Know." The standard specifies that employees have a right to know about hazards in their workplace. It requires that a written communication program should disseminate information about hazards, that a list of hazardous chemicals and associated MSDS sheets should be maintained, and that employees should receive training about hazards within the workplace. Employees receive training as new employees, and training is provided to all employees on an annual basis.

Clinical Laboratory Improvement Amendments Program

Health care laboratory facilities must undergo inspection in order to conduct laboratory tests. All laboratory testing (with the exception of research testing) is regulated by the Clinical Laboratory Improvement Amendments (CLIA) as passed by the U.S. Congress in 1988. CLIA was enacted to ensure that quality standards are followed in clinical laboratory testing. All health care facilities that conduct laboratory testing on specimens from human beings for the purpose of providing diagnosis or treatment require CLIA certification. Laboratories may be exempt from CLIA certification if the laboratory has been inspected and accredited by an approved agency, or if it is located in a CLIA-exempt state (in which case the state inspects the laboratory).

Other Office Support Responsibilities

It will be the assistant's duty to perform some supportive functions that are necessary to keep the office running smoothly. Depending on the nature of the practice, an assistant may have to perform a variety of supportive functions to avoid interruption of services.

Office Supplies

It is often an assistant's responsibility to maintain a stock of office supplies needed to complete the tasks of the front office. A well-equipped medical office should have a 6-month stock of office supplies on hand. Items such as pens, pencils, note pads, computer supplies, appointment reminders, and office forms are used daily, and an adequate supply must be available.

A quick inventory of supplies should be done once a month to monitor the supply stock and to order any items that may be needed within 6 months. A log of inventory and supply orders can be kept to monitor the frequency of ordering. To determine the average monthly usage of a supply, the log can be reviewed when supplies are ordered. Maintaining a 6-month supply of materials should minimize the amount of ordering that is necessary but will not overstock the supply cabinet. Of course, the quantity of office supplies that can be stocked will depend on the amount of storage space available. A larger supply generally saves money because larger quantities usually can be purchased at a discount.

Ordering insufficient quantities of supplies (e.g., a 1-month supply of computer ink) to save money will actually cost the practice money in the long run because the item will have to be reordered constantly. Frequent reordering requires a great deal of time that might be better spent elsewhere in the office. The stock of office supplies should be replenished to minimize the frequency of reordering, with the shelf life of the supply kept in mind. Supply orders that may last years should be avoided because some items may become unusable or may become outdated.

Supply Scams

The office supply business has had some unscrupulous business practices associated with the industry. An assistant should be aware of office supply scams. One of the practices that sometimes is used is to send the office a document that looks like an invoice but is really an offer to order some merchandise. An assistant, on looking at the document, may believe that it is an invoice and may authorize a check to be written for the supplies. Because many people work in an office, an assistant may believe that someone else ordered the merchandise. To avoid this situation, all invoices should be reviewed carefully, and it should be determined whether the material was ordered legitimately. Whenever supplies are received, they should be counted and checked with the packing slip. The packing slip then can be attached to the invoice to verify that all merchandise was received.

Another scam is a solicitation over the telephone in which an office receives a call to verify the make of the office copier and the number of copies that are tallied on the machine. The caller then says that the office's address will have to be verified and requests an authorization to ship copier supplies. An assistant may inadvertently say yes (thinking someone else originally ordered the supplies), and soon a large order of supplies—along with an invoice—arrives.

To avoid falling victim to such a scam when purchasing office supplies, an assistant should conduct business only with reputable local businesses or with nationally recognized office supply companies. Keeping the practice's business with well-known suppliers may save a few surprises down the road.

Office Meetings and Communications

Communication between the physicians of the practice and the office staff is critical to the success of the organization. The larger the office staff, the more difficult it may be to communicate information to everyone in the office. Depending on the type of information that must be disseminated, interoffice memos or meetings are effective ways of keeping communication open in the office.

A meeting should be called when

- Input from the office staff may be necessary to solve a situation
- A matter is crucial to the practice, and office staff may need an opportunity to ask questions
- The supervisor must be sure that information is clearly understood

If information merely needs to be circulated, an interoffice memo or e-mail should suffice to communicate that information.

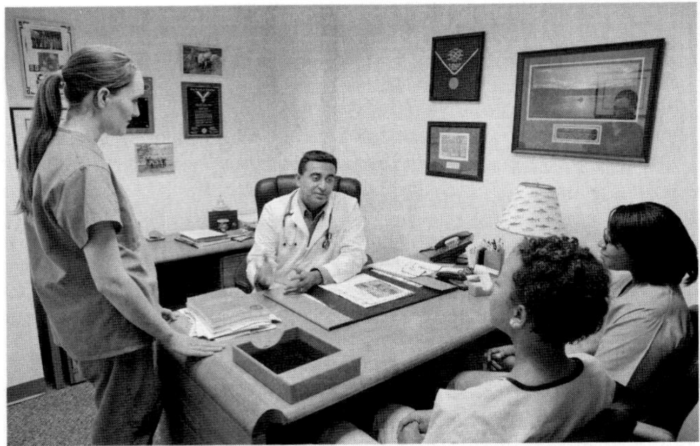

Figure 13-6 A staff meeting provides an excellent opportunity to communicate important information about the practice. (From Young. *Kinn's The Administrative Medical Assistant*. 7th ed. St. Louis, MO: Saunders Elsevier; 2011, Figure 25-1.)

Interoffice Memo

Many times it is necessary to inform the office staff of simple changes in policy and procedure. Whenever possible, simple changes should be disseminated by interoffice memo (see Fig. 6-14) instead of at an employee meeting.

Memos are advantageous because everyone gets a written copy of the information, and a memo serves as documentation of the information that was communicated. Memos can be sent expediently via e-mail, by leaving the memo in an employee mailbox, or by posting the information in a prominent place in the office. Distribution of routine information can be done quickly, the assistant does not have to find a convenient time to schedule a meeting, and employees are not required to sit through a meeting. An interoffice memo can be cost-effective because many medical offices pay employees to attend office meetings.

Memos do have some disadvantages, however. The author of the memo must be sure that everyone who needs the memo sees a copy of it. If the subject is complicated, a memo would be discouraged because the information may be misunderstood. Complicated subjects usually are better communicated in person to give employees a chance to ask questions for clarification.

Office Meetings

Meetings are an effective way to communicate detailed, complex, or easily misunderstood information (Fig. 13-6). Office meetings should be held on a regular basis to give employees a chance to get together to discuss concerns relevant to the practice. However, a meeting should be productive and time well spent. A meeting should not be called if there is nothing of substance to discuss. Meetings are not effective if they simply become an "oral memo." The office management must decide if information should be disseminated via memo or meeting.

Meetings offer several advantages. Important information can be given, and office management can ask for feedback or check for understanding of the information during the meeting time. At meetings, employees usually have a chance

Happy Valley Medical Group
Monthly Staff Meeting
Agenda for July 11, 20xx 8:00 a.m.
Room C12

1. Office cleaning services
2. Training for new phone system
3. Annual Family Practice Conference, October 24–25, 2001, Minneapolis, MN
4. Expansion planned for 2002–2003
5. Other

Figure 13-7 An agenda identifies the topics to be covered in a meeting.

to work together to solve a problem or, sometimes, to get to know one another better.

Meetings also have disadvantages. It is often difficult to find a convenient time for a meeting. If all employees are not present at the meeting, the information will not be received by everyone. If the practice pays employees to attend meetings, a meeting may be costly.

In planning a meeting, an **agenda** (Fig. 13-7) is prepared to inform participants about the subject matter of the meeting and to serve as a plan for the person who is conducting the meeting. An agenda should be distributed to meeting participants ahead of the meeting time to give participants a chance to prepare for or to research agenda items before the meeting. As was mentioned previously, a meeting should be productive, and any information that can be communicated by means of a memo should not be included in a meeting. Participants must feel as though a meeting has been worthwhile and has accomplished something. Otherwise, participants may be tempted to skip future meetings.

Depending on the size of the medical practice, an office meeting may include all staff or may be conducted for specific employees of the practice (e.g., nursing or office staff). It sometimes is very helpful if all departments can attend because more often than not, the items discussed may have some significance to other members of the office staff. All meetings should be conducted in a well-organized manner, with sufficient time allotted for discussion of important agenda items. The individual who is conducting the meeting should allow attendees to ask questions and to offer feedback if necessary (Procedure 13-1).

A recorder should be appointed to write down the **minutes** (Fig. 13-8) of the meeting. Minutes are a summary of the information disseminated and discussion that occurred during the meeting. After the meeting, minutes should be produced in written form and distributed to all persons attending the meeting or to those with an interest in the minutes. The minutes serve as a written archive of information given in the meeting and should be kept in a specific location in the office for future reference (Procedure 13-2).

PROCEDURE 13-1
Prepare an Agenda

Materials Needed
- Information about the meeting
- Computer

1. Identify the meeting date, time, and place.
2. Identify the agenda items to be discussed and the order of discussion.
3. List the agenda items in order of discussion.
4. Proofread the agenda for typos and grammatical errors.
5. Print a copy of the agenda.*
6. Make the required number of copies of the agenda, and distribute them to designated individuals.

**Denotes crucial step in procedure. Student must complete this step satisfactorily in order to complete the procedure satisfactorily.*

PROCEDURE 13-2
Prepare Minutes of a Meeting

Materials Needed
- Meeting agenda
- Attendance at the meeting
- Laptop computer or paper and pencil

1. Identify the meeting date, time, and place.
2. Obtain a copy of the agenda.
3. Attend the meeting and list those present at the meeting.
4. During the meeting, take notes regarding the meeting discussion. Record these minutes in chronological order.
5. Prepare the minutes using the format provided in this chapter.
6. Proofread the minutes for typos and grammatical errors.*
7. Print a copy of the minutes.
8. Make the required number of copies of the minutes, and distribute them to designated individuals.

**Denotes crucial step in procedure. The student must complete this step satisfactorily in order to complete the procedure satisfactorily.*

Other Meetings

Occasionally, an assistant may have to host meetings for outside groups. The practice may host patient education seminars or profession-related workshops for employees or outside groups or may conduct meetings for other business purposes.

Happy Valley Medical Group
Minutes of Monthly Staff Meeting
July 11, 20xx 8:00 a.m.
Room C12

Staff members present: Patrick Scott, Rae Smith, Margaret Gordon, Robert Dorland, Jackie Sears, Amy Dixon, Connie Michaels, Taylor Hudson, Dr. O'Brian, Dr. Marks, Dr. Sanchez

Office cleaning services–So Bright Cleaning Services has been contracted to provide cleaning services for the office starting on August 1, 2001. Office staff is asked to communicate any services that are not satisfactory to Taylor, the office manager, and she will speak with the supervisor of the cleaning crew.

Training for new phone system–A new telephone system was recently purchased and will be installed the last week in September. The system has several new features and the company is providing free training immediately after installation. It is important that all employees attend. Anyone requesting vacation days is asked to reconsider as this training cannot be repeated.

Annual Family Practice Conference, October 26–27, 2001, Minneapolis, MN–The conference will be held on the date noted above. The office would like to pay for at least 4 staff members to attend and bring back information to share with the rest of the staff. Conference brochures were distributed and Patrick, Amy, and Connie will attend. There is room for one more, so if anyone is interested, contact Taylor immediately.

Expansion planned for 2002–2003–The clinic physicians have just finished meeting with architects regarding the addition of office space. HMC is expecting to add a physician in each of the following areas: OB-GYN, orthopedics, and dermatology. The architects will be distributing surveys to all employees regarding uses and needs for space within the office. When the survey is received, please complete it and return to Taylor ASAP.

No other business was discussed.

CM

Prepared by Connie Michaels

Figure 13-8 Minutes of a meeting provide a written record of what transpired during the meeting.

Whatever the reason for a meeting, an assistant usually is responsible for any arrangements. Several items must be considered when meetings are scheduled. These include the following.

Size of Room. Obviously, the number of people expected to attend the meeting will influence where the meeting will be held. The assistant must approximate the number of attendees in order to secure an adequate meeting room. Facilities should provide adequate, comfortable seating within view of the speaker. Also, the assistant must determine whether the attendees will be seated all the time, or whether additional room will be necessary for the participants to stand or move around.

Number of Meeting Attendees. Certainly, the number of people affects many of the considerations for the meeting. Room size, refreshments, and the need for printed materials will be influenced by the number of attendees. Often, when one is planning refreshments for a large group (more than 10 people), it is a good idea to ask participants to reply via an RSVP. This will help avoid overspending for any of the meeting's requirements.

If some of the attendees of the meeting will be coming in from out of town, it may be necessary to secure hotel rooms for these people as well. Attendees may also need transportation if they are arriving by air.

Equipment Needed. The speaker may need an overhead screen or computer setup. Considerations as simple as where outlets are located to plug in equipment must be taken into account. Depending on the speaker's preferences, a speaker's podium may be needed. If the room is large, an audience microphone may be needed so that audience members can ask the speaker questions.

Refreshments. As was mentioned previously, an RSVP will help the assistant plan for an expected number of people. The assistant must consult with the physician and other necessary personnel to determine what type of refreshments are desired for the meeting. Depending on the meeting needs, catering services are an excellent resource for planning. They offer many suggestions and can provide an appropriate quantity of refreshments for the expected number of participants. If money is an issue, many grocery vendors provide affordable box lunches, fruit trays, and bakery goods with paper goods at no extra charge to the customer. This requires the assistant to be more involved in the planning, however. When planning for refreshments, an assistant should not forget to include all the extras, such as plates, napkins, silverware, and sugar and cream for coffee.

Notification of Participants. Once the meeting date has been determined, participants should be invited to attend. Depending on the size of the facility reserved, the meeting may be limited to a specific number of participants. The meeting notice should include date, time, location, topic, and RSVP information (if applicable). If participants are coming from another location or are new to the area, they may have to be given directions as to the meeting's location.

Not all meetings require every item mentioned on the list, but the list gives the essential requirements that must be taken into consideration when one is planning an event. Depending on the nature of the meeting, the assistant may have to adjust plans as needed to conduct a successful meeting.

Travel Planning

From time to time, the physician or some of the office staff may have to travel to attend a conference or another event away from the office. Very often, the cost of professional conferences is covered by the practice. It may be the responsibility of the assistant to make travel arrangements for the office staff.

Perhaps the easiest way to make travel arrangements is to have someone who is an expert do the work. Travel agents can make all reservations needed for a trip, such as air travel, rental cars, and hotel accommodations. Very often, even dinner arrangements and recreational outings can be scheduled in advance. Travel agents may or may not charge for their services, but agents usually are aware of the best fares available for travel and accommodations. Even if a rate may be slightly higher with use of a travel agent, the service may be well worth the money to save the assistant some time in the office.

If an assistant does take the time to do the travel planning, many airlines, rental agencies, and hotel chains have information available on the Internet and toll-free telephone numbers for inquiries about arrangements. Usually, no charge is required for reservations made over the Internet, although time spent researching fares and accommodations might be better spent on other tasks in the office.

Once the travel plans have been set, it is important for the assistant to prepare an itinerary for the trip (Fig. 13-9). An itinerary is a complete schedule of the trip from beginning to end and should include the following information:

- Dates and times of arrivals and departures
- Name of airline or train service
- Hotel accommodations
- Rental car
- Confirmation numbers for travel and hotel
- Telephone numbers for airline, hotel, and rental agency, and any other necessary numbers
- Schedule of events

Once the itinerary has been prepared, two copies should be given to the individual who is traveling (one for the traveler and one for spouse or family members), and a copy should be retained at the office. The office copy will enable the practice to easily locate the traveler if necessary (Procedure 13-3).

PROCEDURE 13-3

Prepare a Travel Itinerary

Materials Needed

- Information regarding travel plans
- Computer

1. Obtain information on air or ground transportation. Identify the name of the transportation provider, departure and arrival locations, and travel confirmation numbers.
2. Obtain information on hotel accommodations. Identify the name, address, telephone number, and confirmation numbers.
3. Obtain information on any meetings, conferences, or other activities that will be attended. Identify the name, address, and telephone numbers of contacts when possible.
4. Prepare an itinerary that lists in chronological order all the information obtained.*
5. Distribute two copies of the itinerary to the traveler (one for the traveler and one for the traveler's family), and retain one copy for the office.

**Denotes crucial step in procedure. Student must complete this step satisfactorily in order to complete the procedure satisfactorily.*

SUMMARY

Many of the topics discussed in this chapter are "behind-the-scenes" functions that are necessary for the office to operate efficiently. Many individuals in the office may not realize the importance of each of these topics until a situation arises to bring the topic to their attention. Even then, it may be difficult for some individuals to understand why some things are done the way they are—because of legal issues or other considerations. A complete understanding of the operations of the medical office enables a medical administrative assistant to understand why things are done a certain way and aids the assistant in providing optimal support to the physician and the medical practice.

YOU ARE THE MEDICAL ADMINISTRATIVE ASSISTANT

You are the office supervisor in a medical office. The staff physicians have just informed you that the office will be extending its office hours from 9 AM to 6 PM Monday through Friday to 9 AM to 8 PM Monday through Friday and 9 AM to 3 PM on Saturday. This change will affect the hours that the current medical administrative assistants will be scheduled to work, and an additional assistant will be hired. What would be the best way to communicate this change to current employees?

Travel Itinerary for Dr. Timothy I. Marks
National Medical Conference
Newark, NJ
November 9–11, 20xx

November 9, 20xx

Depart:	**1:01 p.m.**	E-ticket #384029476SLK Fairair Airlines Flight #6510–Coach Farmington National Airport Farmington, ND
Arrive:	**4:44 p.m.**	Newark International Airport Newark, NJ
Rental Car:		Confirmation #XTD383501 Reliable Rent-a-Car Rental agency will have directions to hotel.
Hotel:		Parkside Inn, 1751 Lake Street, Newark, NJ Phone 000-555-1111 1 room with king-size bed Confirmation # GH40892
7:00–9:00		Early conference registration and social hour Eagle Room, Parkside Inn

November 10, 20xx

8:00–9:00	Continental breakfast Eagle Room, Parkside Inn
9:00–5:00	Conference agenda
5:00–6:00	Social hour Meadow Terrace, Parkside Inn
6:00–9:00	Dinner Plains Room, Parkside Inn

November 11, 20xx

8:00–9:00		Continental breakfast Eagle Room, Parkside Inn
9:00–3:00		Conference agenda
3:30		Leave for airport
Depart:	**6:30 p.m.**	Fairair Airlines Flight #648–Coach Newark International Airport Newark, NJ
Arrive:	**8:48 p.m.**	Farmington National Airport Farmington, ND

Figure 13-9 A travel itinerary summarizes important information regarding an individual's travel arrangements.

REVIEW EXERCISES

Exercise 13-1 True or False

Read each statement, and determine whether the statement is true or false. Record the answer in the blank provided. T = true; F = false.

_____ 1. It is against the law for physicians to own pharmacies associated with the medical office.

_____ 2. A physician may select the pharmacy that will fill a patient's prescription.

_____ 3. A board of directors is usually responsible for overall management of a large health care corporation.

_____ 4. An assistant does not have to be concerned about the chain of command in any situation.

_____ 5. Joint Commission accreditation is required for all medical offices.

_____ 6. Accreditation by independent accrediting organizations may fulfill licensing requirements in some states.

_____ 7. The Joint Commission establishes standards that health care organizations are required to meet in order to receive accreditation.

_____ 8. Circumventing the chain of command may be necessary if a problem exists with a direct supervisor.

_____ 9. OSHA conducts workplace inspections to determine whether a safe work environment exists.

_____ 10. Employees can be required to purchase their own safety equipment for work.

_____ 11. An employer with an unsafe workplace may be fined by OSHA.

_____ 12. A work-related injury may develop over time, depending on the work environment.

_____ 13. Carpal tunnel syndrome sometimes can be a work-related injury.

_____ 14. The identity of an employee who files a complaint with OSHA cannot be kept confidential.

_____ 15. Because a medical administrative assistant does not draw blood, there is no reason for the assistant to be concerned about bloodborne pathogens.

_____ 16. A 6-month stock of every office supply should always be on hand.

_____ 17. CLIA certification is required for facilities that conduct laboratory tests.

_____ 18. An interoffice memo is an effective way to communicate easily understood information instead of convening a meeting.

_____ 19. E-mail can be used to circulate an office memo quickly.

_____ 20. Complicated topics regarding the medical office are better explained in a memo than at a meeting.

_____ 21. A meeting agenda informs the staff about what the meeting will cover.

_____ 22. Meeting minutes should be retained in the office for future reference.

_____ 23. Some travel agents charge for services.

_____ 24. An itinerary details what transpired at a meeting.

_____ 25. A work-related injury is a matter of public record, and all documents related to the injury are open to the public.

_____ 26. "Right-to-Know" training gives employees training regarding hazardous substances in the workplace.

Exercise 13-2 Chapter Concepts

Read each statement or question, and choose the answer that best completes the statement or question. Record the answer in the blank provided.

_____ 1. An inventory of office supplies should be done
(a) Daily
(b) Weekly
(c) Monthly
(d) Yearly

_____ 2. The type of organizational structure in which two physicians share expenses and income is a
(a) Sole proprietorship
(b) Corporation
(c) Partnership

_____ 3. An organization in which ownership consists of stockholders or shareholders is a
(a) Sole proprietorship
(b) Corporation
(c) Partnership

_____ 4. An organization in which structure does not have to be reorganized as physicians come and go from the organization is a
(a) Sole proprietorship
(b) Corporation
(c) Partnership

_____ 5. A physician makes all decisions regarding operation of a medical office in a
(a) Sole proprietorship
(b) Corporation
(c) Partnership

_____ 6. To avoid work-related injury, a worker should do all of the following except
(a) Have appropriate lighting for the task
(b) Use proper lifting techniques
(c) Use personal funds to purchase necessary protective equipment
(d) Use an adjustable chair when working at a desk

_____ 7. Which of the following is false regarding ordering supplies for a medical office?
(a) Frequent ordering saves time in the long run.
(b) Buying supplies from regular local suppliers reduces the risk of falling victim to a scam.
(c) It is usually an assistant's responsibility to order office supplies.
(d) Supply inventory should be done on a regular basis to determine how frequently a supply is used.

_____ 8. Which of the following is false regarding office meetings?
(a) Meetings can give a supervisor the chance to check for understanding of an important topic.
(b) Meetings help keep communication open in the medical office.
(c) Meetings should be held only to discuss a crucial situation.
(d) Meetings provide a good opportunity for staff members to ask questions.

_____ 9. When hosting a meeting, an assistant will need to do all of the following except
(a) Verify the number of persons attending
(b) Prepare the minutes before the meeting
(c) Invite necessary participants
(d) Determine what refreshments should be ordered

_____ 10. When making travel arrangements for members of the office staff, an assistant may expect to do all of the following except
(a) Prepare an itinerary
(b) Search for travel arrangements on the Internet
(c) Obtain confirmation numbers for travel arrangements
(d) Pay cash for arrangements made with a travel agent

ACTIVITIES

ACTIVITY 13-1 THE JOINT COMMISSION

Research The Joint Commission on the Internet at www.jointcommission.org.

ACTIVITY 13-2 OSHA COMPLIANCE

Research OSHA compliance for medical and dental offices on the Internet.

ACTIVITY 13-3 ERGONOMICS

Research ergonomics on the Internet.

ACTIVITY 13-4 ERGONOMICS FOR A COMPUTER WORKSTATION

Research specifications of a safe workstation for a computer-related position.

ACTIVITY 13-5 MUSCULOSKELETAL DISORDERS

Research musculoskeletal disorders that may affect workers in a health care organization.

ACTIVITY 13-6 MATERIAL SAFETY DATA SHEETS

Identify the following information from the MSDS pictured in Figure 13-4.

(a) Product name
(b) Manufacturer
(c) Is the product flammable?
(d) What may happen if the product is swallowed?
(e) First aid required for exposure to skin

ACTIVITY 13-7 MEETING AGENDA

Prepare a meeting agenda for the following:

- An all-staff meeting will be held next Monday at 8 AM in the staff lounge. The following will be presented:
- Change in employee parking areas
- Holiday hours for the office
- Employment openings
- Medicare workshop on the first Tuesday of next month

ACTIVITY 13-8 MINUTES

Attend a meeting of a local group and prepare minutes of that meeting following the format given in this chapter.

DISCUSSION

The following topic can be used for class discussion or for individual student essay.

DISCUSSION 13-1

Three employees of a medical office with 20 employees have had persistent allergy problems over the past year. The employees have asked the employer to conduct an inspection of the ventilation systems in the building. Is this the responsibility of the employer?

Bibliography

Pathogens Bloodborne: http://www.osha.gov/SLTC/bloodbornepathogens/index.html/gen_guidance.html. Accessed November 18, 2011.

Bureau of Labor Statistics: Safety and Health Statistics. *Nonfatal Occupational Injuries and Illnesses Requiring Days Away From Work*. http://www.bls.gov. Accessed November 18, 2011.

Centers for Medicare and Medicaid Services: *Clinical Laboratory Amendments*. http://www.cms.hhs.gov/clia/. Accessed November 18, 2011.

Occupational Safety and Health Administration: The Occupational Safety and Health Act of 1970. www.osha.gov. Accessed November 18, 2011.

Office of Civil Rights Office of Civil Rights: Summary of the HIPAA Privacy Rule, U.S. Department of Health and Human Services, last revised May 2003. http://www.hhs.gov/ocr/privacysummary.pdf. Accessed November 18, 2011.

The Joint Commission on Accreditation of Healthcare Organizations: http://www.jointcommission.org/. Accessed November 18, 2011.

CHAPTER 14 Financial Management

LEARNING OUTCOMES

On successful completion of this chapter, the student will be able to

1. Demonstrate accounts receivable procedures and associated banking practices.
2. Explain the use of change funds.
3. Demonstrate use of petty cash funds.
4. Demonstrate accounts payable procedures and associated banking practices.
5. Describe bookkeeping and accounting procedures and financial record retention.
6. Utilize medical practice management software for bookkeeping and accounting purposes.

COMMISSION ON ACCREDITATION OF ALLIED HEALTH EDUCATION PROGRAMS (CAAHEP) CORE CURRICULUM FOR MEDICAL ASSISTANTS

- Use office hardware and software to maintain office systems.
- Use the Internet to access information related to the medical office.
- Explain basic bookkeeping computations.
- Differentiate between bookkeeping and accounting.
- Describe banking procedures.
- Differentiate between accounts payable and accounts receivable.
- Describe common periodic financial reports.
- Prepare a bank deposit.
- Use computerized office billing systems.
- Describe the implications of HIPAA for the medical assistant in various medical settings.

ACCREDITING BUREAU OF HEALTH EDUCATION SCHOOLS (ABHES) COMPETENCIES FOR MEDICAL ASSISTING

Graduates

- Prepare and reconcile a bank statement and deposit record.
- Perform accounts payable procedures.
- Perform accounts receivable procedures.
- Establish and maintain a petty cash fund.
- Use manual or computerized bookkeeping systems.

VOCABULARY

accounting
accounts payable
accounts receivable
assets
balance sheet
bookkeeping
capital
cash flow statement
change fund
income statement
liabilities
nonsufficient funds or (NSF) check
purchase order (PO)
reconciling
restrictive endorsement
vendor

Bookkeeping and Accounting Procedures in a Medical Office

The past 20 years have brought about tremendous change in the financial operations of a medical office. Although computers were used in billing 30 years ago, the incorporation of computer systems throughout the office has made billing functions more streamlined in the office. Today, even very small offices usually use some type of computer software that tracks the financial transactions of the business.

No matter what the size of the practice, professional accounting services should always be retained by a medical practice. Large practices usually employ accountants to oversee all financial operations of the practice, and smaller practices typically hire accountants on a consultant (contractual) basis to work with the financial information that is provided by a medical administrative assistant. The law pertaining to taxes and other parts of the financial operations of a medical practice is so complex that physicians are wise to use experts to oversee this part of a practice.

Although an assistant may not be solely responsible for the bookkeeping and accounting procedures, it is important for an assistant to understand his or her part in the financial transactions of a practice. **Bookkeeping** refers to the recording of business transactions, whereas **accounting** involves developing reports from those financial transactions and analyzing those reports. Periodic financial reports are prepared to reveal the financial condition of a medical practice.

Financial Reports

Computerizing the financial transactions of a medical office saves a tremendous amount of time in keeping track of the practice's finances. Imagine what it might be like to gather the total of outstanding balances on patients' accounts if the accounts were kept manually. The balance of every account would have to be entered into a calculator. This would take a substantial amount of time. With the use of a computer program, a few buttons are clicked and a report with the entire balance of patients' accounts can be generated.

Computer programs allow many different types of reports to be generated to give a picture of the financial health of the office. Reports usually can be run periodically that will give the practice any information that is desired, such as the numbers of particular procedures done within a specified period, the number of patients treated with a particular diagnosis, and the number of patients served on a particular day or during a month or year. Such reports (Fig. 14-1) are helpful in planning. For example, if several people with a particular diagnosis are treated monthly by a practice, it may be prudent to buy new or additional equipment to treat those patients. Likewise, if few patients are treated, it may be prudent to make arrangements for patients to receive treatment elsewhere.

An **income statement**, also called a profit and loss statement, identifies profit earned during a specific period of time. Income statements are often done monthly. Income received over a particular period less expenses paid during that period demonstrates either a profit or a loss for the period.

A **balance sheet** reveals a practice's financial condition. Income statements may look good or bad for a particular period, but a balance sheet shows the true financial health of a practice. A balance sheet lists the amounts of assets, liabilities, and owners' equity in the practice. **Assets** are items of value, such as bank accounts, furniture, or equipment, whereas **liabilities** are debts (**accounts payable**) or something that is owed by the practice, and **capital** consists of the investments of the owners of the practice. When a balance sheet is prepared, the following equation is always true: ASSETS = LIABILITIES + CAPITAL. Two practices might have similar quantities of assets, but if one practice has a far greater number of liabilities, the practice with fewer liabilities may be more financially healthy.

A **cash flow statement** gives a picture of the cash transactions of a practice. The cash balance at the beginning of the month, cash received during the month, cash disbursed during the month, and the ending cash balance are identified.

Although most offices have computerized their financial recordkeeping, a fundamental understanding of the financial operations of a medical office helps an assistant understand how occurrences in the office can have an impact on an office's finances. For example, if charges are not entered for patients, **accounts receivable** will get behind because insurance claims and statements are not generated. Such activity will have a great impact on the financial picture of the practice because accounts receivable for that month may be greatly reduced and this will be reflected on the monthly income statement. Although the practice may have generated lots of revenue in a particular month, if the claims are not filed and patients are not billed, the practice's finances may look bleak.

Accounts Receivable

Chapter 11 conveys how accounts receivable balances can be determined with the use of a computerized medical practice accounting system such as Medisoft. Such a system can provide totals of patients' charges and payments for a period of time, whether this might be a day, a week, or even a month. Every medical practice uses some method of tracking charges and payments for the accounts receivable of the office. In a smaller office, a physician may expect a medical administrative assistant to handle the accounts receivable and to report a balance of accounts to a bookkeeper or an accountant at the end of the month.

In larger offices with many physicians, a separate billing department is typically responsible for managing the accounts receivable for the practice. Billing staff may be assigned to handle specific patient accounts or specific functions within the billing department, such as patient payments, insurance payments, and charges from certain areas of the practice. Because of the various procedures followed for different types of insurance plans or government benefit programs, some practices might assign specific personnel to handle payments for each plan. For instance, one individual could be responsible for Medicare accounts, another for Medicaid, another for Blue Cross/Blue Shield, and so on.

Given the complexity of the financial management of businesses today, a medical administrative assistant usually plays a supporting role in the financial management of the practice. It is often an assistant's responsibility to collect data and then to report the data to a financial expert who is employed by the office or is hired as an outside consultant to the office.

Receiving Payments on Account

Every medical office needs some cash on hand to conduct the daily business of the practice. A **change fund** of approximately $100 to $200 should be sufficient for most medical practices and is necessary to have on hand for those patients who pay their charges on the day the charges are incurred. Some patients prefer to pay their bill immediately after their visit, and it is necessary to have cash on hand to make change. Also, some offices require that patients outside the immediate vicinity of the office pay for their visit on the day they are seen. A practice may require that all patients who live out of state pay their bill immediately after the visit. This requirement may be instituted to prevent future problems in collecting a bill from a patient who lives far away. In addition to receiving payments made with cash or check, an office may allow patients to pay their bill using a major credit card, and an assistant may be required to process the payment by using the card.

When a patient makes a payment in person, the payment should be entered immediately in the computer system and a receipt printed as proof of payment by the patient (Fig. 14-2 and Procedure 14-1). The following items should be identified on a receipt:

- Amount of the payment
- Who made the payment
- How the payment was made (check, cash, credit card)
- Account number on which to apply the payment
- Date of the payment
- Description of where the payment should be applied

Happy Valley Medical Group

Insurance Analysis

December 28, 20YY

Insurance Carrier	--Claims-- #	%	--Charges-- Amount	%	--Payments*-- Amount	%
AET00 Aetna						
Primary	1	12.5	396.00	28.2	0.00	0.0
Secondary	1	25.0	150.00	23.4	0.00	0.0
Copay Payments					-10.00	
Data Filters:					Outstanding Balance:	$546.00
BLU00 Blue Cross Blue Shield 231						
Primary	1	12.5	105.00	7.5	-84.00	17.9
Secondary	2	50.0	395.00	61.7	-82.40	100.0
					Outstanding Balance:	$60.00
BLU01 Blue Cross Blue Shield 225						
Secondary	1	25.0	95.00	14.8	0.00	0.0
Tertiary	1	100.0	335.00	100.0	-20.60	100.0
					Outstanding Balance:	$95.00
CIG00 Cigna						
Primary	2	25.0	155.00	11.0	-48.00	10.2
Copay Payments					-10.00	
					Outstanding Balance:	$95.00
FHP00 FHP Health Plan						
Primary	1	12.5	335.00	23.8	-162.00	34.5
					Outstanding Balance:	$0.00
MED00 Medicaid						
Primary	1	12.5	160.00	11.4	-56.00	11.9
Copay Payments					-10.00	
					Outstanding Balance:	$0.00
MED01 Medicare						
Primary	2	25.0	255.00	18.1	-119.00	25.4
					Outstanding Balance:	$105.00

	Primary	Secondary	Tertiary
Total Charges:	$1,406.00	$640.00	$335.00
Total Number of Claims:	8	4	1
Average Charge/Claim:	$175.75	$160.00	$335.00

Figure 14-1 Financial reports can be used to analyze different aspects of a practice's business.

All of these items must appear on a receipt if one is to have enough information to process or track (or both) the payment internally. A copy of the receipt (usually electronic) should always be retained by the practice because a receipt provides documentation that a payment should be entered into a computer system. Payments should be entered as soon as possible to keep account totals up to date. Payment may be processed where the payment is received, or payments may be forwarded to a central office for processing.

When a check is received, it should be endorsed immediately with a **restrictive endorsement** on the reverse of the check. A restrictive endorsement, as shown in Figure 14-3, includes the wording "For deposit only" and allows the check to be deposited only in the account of Happy Valley Medical Group. If a check were lost or stolen, a check with a restrictive endorsement could not be cashed by anyone else. A check should always be stamped with an endorsement as soon as it is received. It is not enough to sign or stamp the name of the party to whom the check was written, such as "Happy Valley Medical Group," because such an endorsement entitles whoever has the check to cash it.

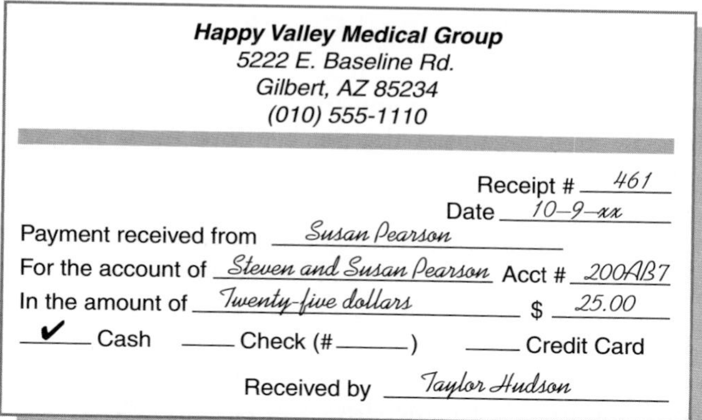
Happy Valley Medical Group
5222 E. Baseline Rd.
Gilbert, AZ 85234
(010) 555-1110

Receipt # 461
Date 10-9-xx
Payment received from Susan Pearson
For the account of Steven and Susan Pearson Acct # 200AB7
In the amount of Twenty-five dollars $ 25.00
✔ Cash ___ Check (#___) ___ Credit Card
Received by Taylor Hudson

Figure 14-2 A receipt should be issued whenever a patient pays for services while in the office.

PROCEDURE 14-1

Prepare a Receipt for a Payment Received

Materials Needed

- Receipts
- Payments received
- Pen

1. Using the receipts in number order, enter the date on which the payment is received.
2. Enter the name of the payee.
3. Specify the method of payment (check or cash).
4. Enter the amount of the payment both numerically and descriptively in the spaces provided.*
5. Identify the account to which the payment should be applied.*
6. Enter the account balances if known.
7. Sign the receipt.*

**Denotes crucial step in procedure. Student must complete this step satisfactorily in order to complete the procedure satisfactorily.*

CHECKPOINT

1. At the end of many workdays, your coworkers comment that there is "too much to be done" to get ready for patients the next day, and that the receipts of the day should be handled when the office atmosphere is less hectic—maybe at the end of the week or the next week. What is your response?
2. One of the assistants in the office proposes that receipts should no longer be written for payments received in person in the office, citing that patients who send checks in the mail do not get a receipt. What is your response?

Preparing a Bank Deposit

At the end of the day, the cash and checks received are totaled, and a deposit slip is prepared to accompany the checks to the bank. Deposits to a practice's bank account should be made daily to ensure that there is only a minimum amount of cash on hand when the office is closed (Fig. 14-4). Before a check is deposited, the check must be logged in a receipts journal or must be entered into a computer system to ensure that the guarantor's account is properly credited. The checks and the deposit slip should each be totaled to verify the amount that will be deposited into the practice's account (Procedure 14-2).

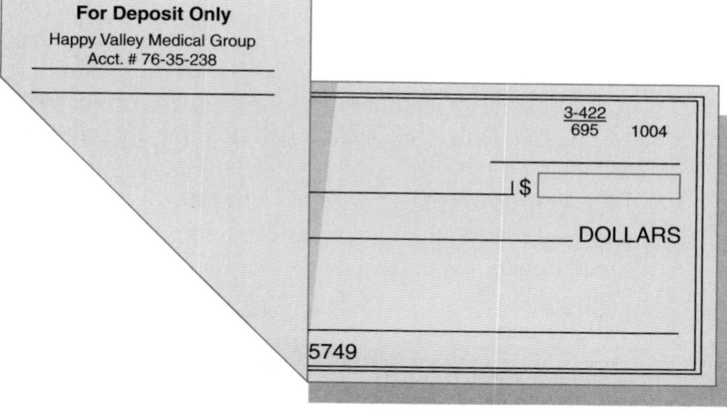

Figure 14-3 A restrictive endorsement can be used to limit where a check is deposited. (Modified from Chester GA. *Modern Medical Assisting*. Philadelphia, PA: WB Saunders; 1998, p. 146.)

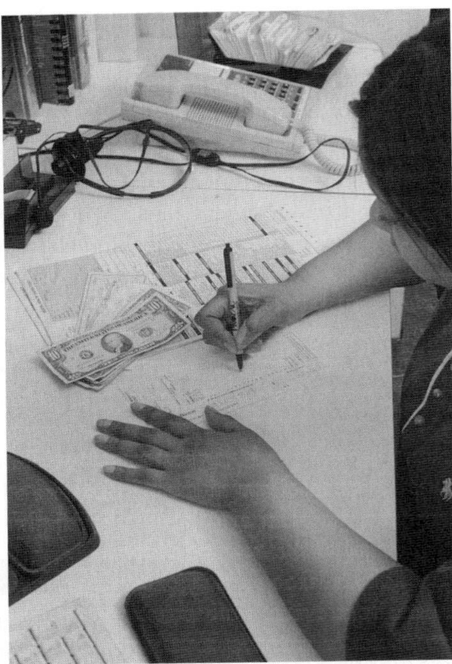

Figure 14-4 Deposits should be made daily to an office's bank account.

PROCEDURE 14-2

Prepare a Bank Deposit

Materials Needed

- Checks and currency to be deposited
- Deposit slip
- Pen

1. Enter the date of the deposit on the deposit slip.
2. Count the currency to be deposited. Enter the amount after "Currency" on the deposit slip.
3. Count the coins to be deposited. Enter the amount after "Coins" on the deposit slip.
4. Individually write the amount of each check to be deposited in the "Checks" portion of the deposit slip.
5. Calculate the total of currency, coin, and checks to be deposited, and enter the amount under "Total."
6. Verify that the deposit is correct by adding currency, coin, and the amount of each check.*
7. Record the deposit in the check register.

**Denotes crucial step in procedure. Student must complete this step satisfactorily in order to complete the procedure satisfactorily.*

Refunding Overpayment of a Patient's Account

If a guarantor has a credit, or a negative balance, on account, the amount may be refunded to the guarantor. A negative balance can result when a patient pays for a service and an insurance company pays for the same service. Alternatively, an unexpected discount might have been applied to the account.

When money must be refunded to a guarantor, a check is written in the amount of the credit balance. The check is issued from the practice's account to the guarantor and is posted as a charge to the guarantor's account. This procedure should bring the account to zero. If patients on the guarantor's account are seen in the office frequently, a note may be included with the account statement that the credit balance will be applied to any future balances instead of a check written for the credit balance.

Processing Returned Checks

Occasionally, a check may be received from a patient or other payer for which there are **nonsufficient funds** in the payer's checking account to pay the check. When the office presents the check to the bank for payment, the payer's bank may refuse to pay the check, will return the check to the office, and will identify that there are nonsufficient funds to pay the check. This is also known as an **NSF check**.

When a check for a patient is deposited, the amount of the check is subtracted from the patient's balance. If a practice is unable to receive payment for a check, an assistant can call to notify the patient that the check was returned. The returned check then should be listed as a charge to the patient's account, and the explanation should be something similar to "NSF check."

A check may be returned because a payer's account has been closed. This should be handled in the same way as an NSF check: The payer should be notified and the amount charged back to the patient's account.

If a check has been returned to the office as an NSF check, an attempt can be made to deposit the check again. It is possible that funds may later be available to cover the check. If a check is successfully deposited the second time around, there will be no need to notify the patient of the difficulty, and no NSF adjustments will have to be made to the patient's account.

If an NSF check is not paid by the bank, the amount of the check that was subtracted when the check was recorded will need to be added back to the patient's account.

Petty Cash

From time to time, small amounts of cash are needed to purchase incidental items for use in a medical office. These types of expenses (often $10 or less) generally are too small to require that a check be written to pay for the items, and they should instead be paid for with cash. The purpose of a petty cash fund is to enable the staff to purchase items of small value quickly and easily.

Physicians should communicate to their staff what types of expenses are allowed to be paid out of the petty cash fund. Following are examples of various types of expenses that may be covered by petty cash:

- Refreshments for an office meeting or a special office visitor
- Inexpensive office supplies (usually costing less than $10 to $20)
- Batteries for a physician's digital recorder
- Coffee for the employee lounge or reception area
- Small donations
- Postage due
- Parking fees
- Any other approved item costing $20 or less

Petty Cash Log

date	description	amount	balance
10-1-0x	*balance*		$100.00
10-1-0x	*AA batteries*	$4.59	$95.41
10-4-0x	*postage due*	0.35	$95.06
10-4-0x	*parking*	$6	$89.06
10-8-0x	*staples*	$2.26	$86.80
10-15-0x	*cleaning supplies*	$10.72	$76.08
10-16-0x	*refreshments for staff meeting*	$16.83	$59.25

Figure 14-5 A petty cash log should be maintained to track disbursements and deposits into the fund.

PROCEDURE 14-3

Maintain a Petty Cash Fund

Materials Needed

- Petty cash record
- Receipts for expenditures
- Pen/pencil

1. A cash fund of a predetermined amount, possibly $100, is placed in a secure location in a locked, zippered bank bag.
2. When an approved purchase must be made, cash is removed from the bag that will cover the purchase, and an employee makes the purchase.
3. When the employee returns, a receipt for the item and change (if any) is placed in the bag. The receipt and change should total the amount that was removed to make the purchase.
4. The item purchased is written in a petty cash log (see Fig. 14-5).*
5. When the fund becomes depleted, the expenses from the petty cash log are totaled, and the log and receipts are kept as proof of expenses. A check is then written to "Petty Cash" for the amount of the expenses.
6. The check is cashed by the employee responsible for the fund, and the fund is replenished by placing the check proceeds in the bank bag. A new log sheet is started.
7. After the fund has been replenished, the cash in the bank bag should equal the original amount of the petty cash fund.*

**Denotes crucial step in procedure. Student must complete this step satisfactorily in order to complete the procedure satisfactorily.*

The petty cash fund is separate from the change fund that the medical office uses to process patient payments. The petty cash fund should be kept in a location separate from the change fund or in a separate container to distinguish it from the change fund so that funds are not mixed. One individual should be responsible for disbursing cash from the petty cash fund, receiving the receipt and any change for items purchased, and maintaining the petty cash log (Fig. 14-5). This individual should also be responsible for reconciling the fund when the fund is replenished (Procedure 14-3). At any time, the amount of the fund can be checked by adding all receipts obtained since the last time the fund was replenished to any remaining cash. This amount should equal the original amount of the fund.

Accounts Payable

The accounts payable functions of a practice include payment for items purchased for use by the practice and expenses incurred by the practice. When an invoice or a bill is received for payment, the invoice may be due immediately or at a specified time. If the invoice is not due immediately, it may be filed in a folder designated for payment at a later date.

Purchase Orders

Supplies, equipment, and other items purchased for use in the medical office frequently are ordered with the use of a purchase order (Fig. 14-6). A **purchase order (PO)** is a request to purchase merchandise from an identified supplier. A PO specifies certain items to be purchased, as well as the quantity and price of the items.

A PO can be originated by anyone in an organization as long as that individual has the authority to purchase items. After a PO is written, it can be mailed or faxed to the **vendor** (business or supplier from which merchandise is being purchased), or someone from the office may take the PO directly to the vendor when the merchandise is picked up.

A PO signifies to a vendor that purchase of the identified merchandise has been authorized for the items listed on the order. POs are also signed by someone in the medical office. Using a PO gives a vendor the assurance that when a bill is sent for the purchased items, the bill will be paid.

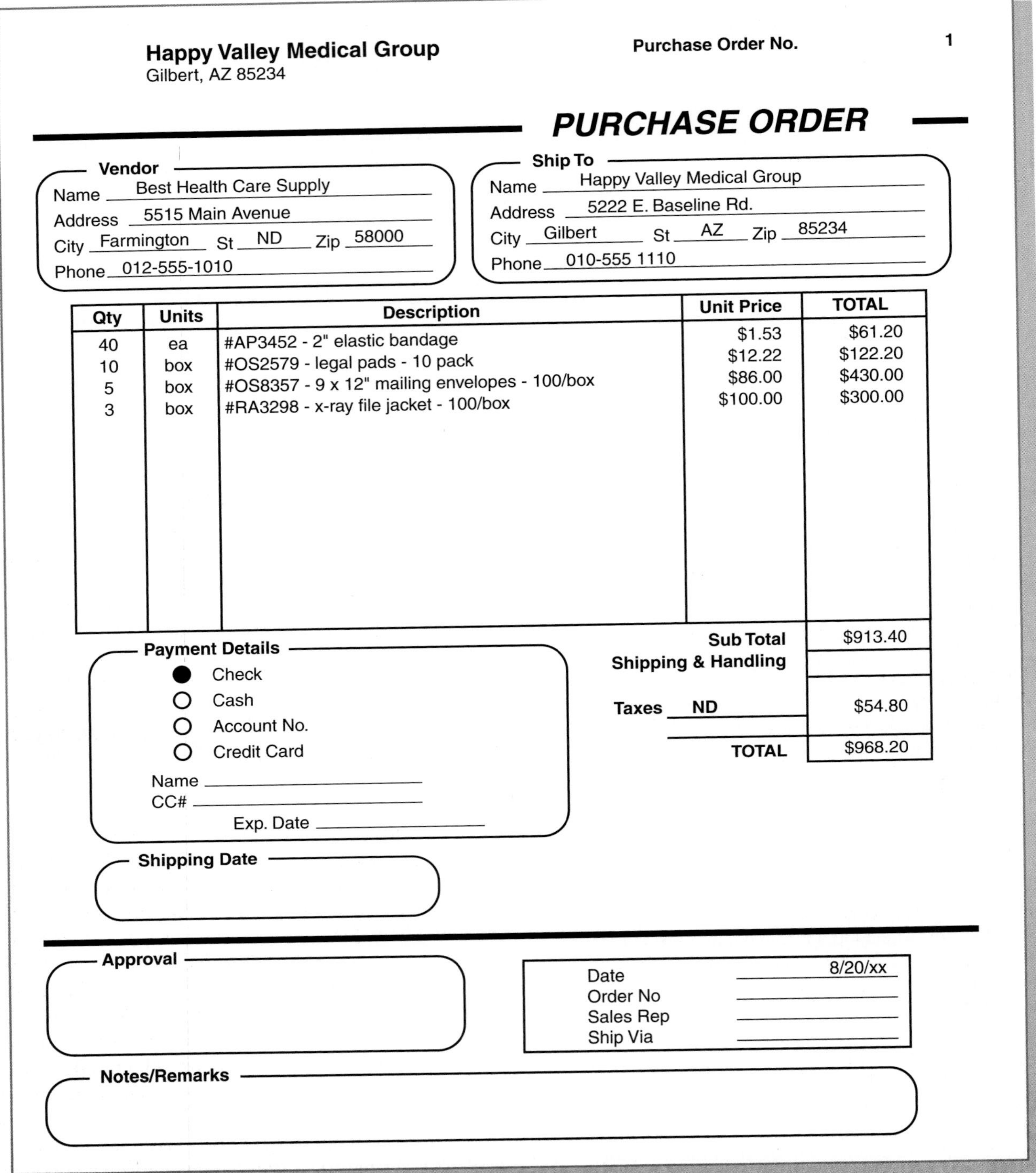

Happy Valley Medical Group
Gilbert, AZ 85234

Purchase Order No. 1

PURCHASE ORDER

Vendor
Name Best Health Care Supply
Address 5515 Main Avenue
City Farmington St ND Zip 58000
Phone 012-555-1010

Ship To
Name Happy Valley Medical Group
Address 5222 E. Baseline Rd.
City Gilbert St AZ Zip 85234
Phone 010-555 1110

Qty	Units	Description	Unit Price	TOTAL
40	ea	#AP3452 - 2" elastic bandage	$1.53	$61.20
10	box	#OS2579 - legal pads - 10 pack	$12.22	$122.20
5	box	#OS8357 - 9 x 12" mailing envelopes - 100/box	$86.00	$430.00
3	box	#RA3298 - x-ray file jacket - 100/box	$100.00	$300.00

Sub Total	$913.40
Shipping & Handling	
Taxes ND	$54.80
TOTAL	$968.20

Payment Details
● Check
○ Cash
○ Account No.
○ Credit Card
Name
CC#
Exp. Date

Shipping Date

Approval

Date 8/20/xx
Order No
Sales Rep
Ship Via

Notes/Remarks

Figure 14-6 A purchase order is used to authorize purchases from a vendor.

Banking Procedures for Accounts Payable

If a medical administrative assistant is responsible for processing payments to pay bills that the practice has incurred, payments can be made by entering them into a computer system and by laser printing checks. With this method, the computer will account for all information that should be kept as a record of the transactions. Payments also can be made by writing checks by hand; however, this method is far more time consuming than is use of a computer-based system.

Writing checks and authorizing payment are considerable responsibilities. Great care should be taken to make certain that the charges are truly owed by the practice. Many different

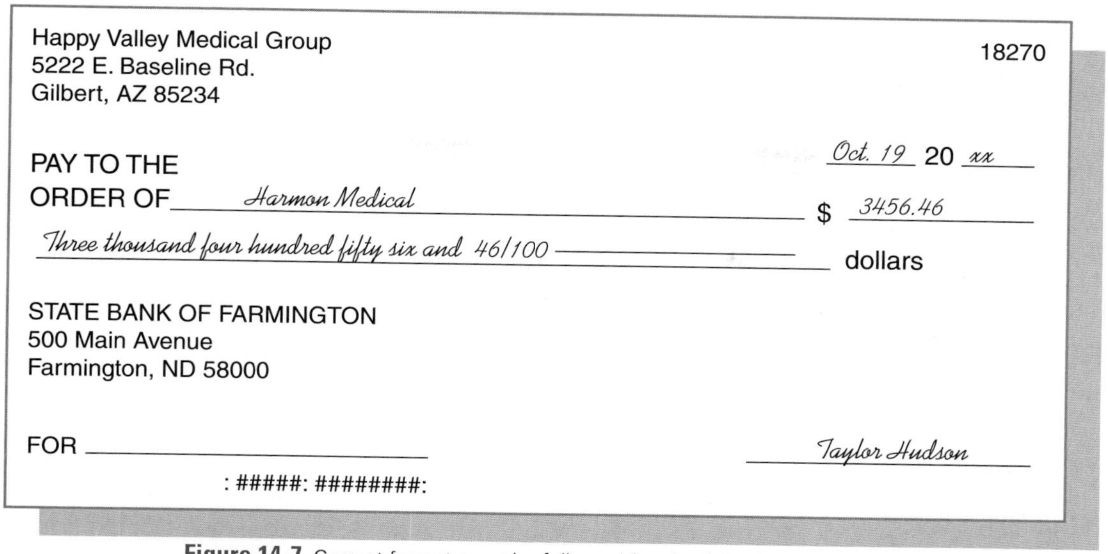

Happy Valley Medical Group
5222 E. Baseline Rd.
Gilbert, AZ 85234

18270

Oct. 19 20 xx

PAY TO THE
ORDER OF Harmon Medical $ 3456.46

Three thousand four hundred fifty six and 46/100 dollars

STATE BANK OF FARMINGTON
500 Main Avenue
Farmington, ND 58000

FOR

Taylor Hudson

: #####: ########:

Figure 14-7 Correct format must be followed for checks written on account.

PROCEDURE 14-4

Write a Check for Payment of an Invoice

Materials Needed

- Check register with checks
- Invoices to be paid
- Pen

1. Complete the check stub, subtracting the amount of the check from the current balance on the account.
2. Complete the check using a pen. Use checks in numerical order.*
3. Enter the current date on the check.
4. On the "PAY TO THE ORDER OF" line, enter the payee's name.*
5. Enter the amount of the check numerically in the blank provided after the "$." Begin entering the amount immediately after the "$" to prevent anything from being added to the check amount.*
6. Enter the amount of the check in words on the line below the "PAY TO THE ORDER OF" line. If the entire line is not used, use dashes or a solid line to cross out the remainder of the line.*
7. The check is signed by an individual who has been authorized to sign checks for the account. The check can then be placed in a window envelope for mailing to the payee if necessary.*

**Denotes crucial step in procedure. Student must complete this step satisfactorily in order to complete the procedure satisfactorily.*

types of check-writing systems are available for handwritten checks or computer-generated checks. Regardless of what type of check-writing system is used, the following features should be included on each check:

- Payer of check is identified.
- Check is listed in numerical order so all checks can be accounted for.
- Date the check was written is listed.
- Amount of the check is subtracted from the account balance.
- Amount of the check is assigned to an account for accounting purposes.

When writing a check, an assistant should be careful to write legibly. There should never be a question as to what was written on the check. If a mistake is made, the check should be voided. Information should not be crossed out. No information on the check should be erasable. Information regarding the amount of the check should not be alterable in any way (Fig. 14-7 and Procedure 14-4).

Reconciling the Bank Account

If maintaining the check register is the responsibility of an assistant, the account will have to be reconciled each month to ensure that no clerical errors have been made when checks were entered. Each month, the bank sends to the office a statement of account (Fig. 14-8) that lists the checks, the deposits, and other charges that have been incurred by the account, as well as any bank charges applied to the account.

When the monthly statement arrives, it has to be **reconciled** with the office's check register (Procedure 14-5). This is necessary to ensure that the checkbook balance and the bank balance are in agreement. Again, the responsibility of maintaining the checkbook for a practice is an important one, and the account should never go unreconciled any month. One mistake in the check register might lead to embarrassment when checks have to be returned to payers.

Business Record Retention

In the course of business in the medical office, many important documents are received. Insurance policies for property liability and malpractice insurance should be retained by the practice until the statutes of limitations have expired for any potential liability. In the case of malpractice policies for physicians who treat children, remember that the statute of limitations may not begin until the patient is 18 years of age.

State Bank of Farmington
500 Main Avenue
Farmington, ND 58000
012-555-5000

Statement of Account for:
Happy Valley Medical Group
5222 E. Baseline Rd.
Gilbert, AZ 85234

Date: 11-30-xx
Account number: 76-375-238

Previous Balance:	5,012.45
Deposits/credits:	10,347.78
Checks/debits:	9,385.13
Service charges:	0.00
Ending Balance:	5,975.10

Deposits:

Date	Amount
11-5	2,305.46
11-8	456.38
11-9	235.90
11-15	4038.98
11-21	2972.00
11-28	339.06

Checks drawn on account:

Check No.	Date	Amount	Check No.	Date	Amount
18275	11-1	493.47	18285	11-16	890.56
18276	11-2	50.00	18286	11-16	1500.00
18277	11-2	37.50	18288*	11-19	234.34
18278	11-6	395.00	18289	11-21	470.00
18279	11-5	500.00	18290	11-21	3310.00
18280	11-9	40.00	18291	11-26	500.00
18281	11-8	120.00	18292	11-28	39.46
18282	11-8	324.52	18294*	11-29	109.78
18283	11-9	35.50			
18284	11-14	335.00			

Figure 14-8 A bank sends a monthly statement to identify checks, deposits, and other charges made to an account.

PROCEDURE 14-5

Reconcile a Bank Statement

Materials Needed

- Current month's bank statement
- Record of checks drawn or check register
- Calculator
- Pen/pencil

1. All checks that have been paid by the bank should be checked on the record of checks drawn or the check register.
2. Any charges applied to the account by the bank should be listed on the record/register and subtracted from the balance.
3. Any interest deposits from the bank should be listed on the record/register and added to the balance.
4. Take the ending monthly balance on the account and do the following:*
   (a) Add any deposits made by the practice that are not included on the statement.
   (b) Subtract any checks written by the practice that have not been paid by the bank.
   (c) The total should then equal the ending balance in the record. If the total does not equal the balance in the record, you should look for errors in addition and subtraction when figuring the ending balance, as well as any other errors that may be present in the record/register.

**Denotes crucial step in procedure. Student must complete this step satisfactorily in order to complete the procedure satisfactorily.*

All office documents related to the business practices of the office should be retained until all statutes of limitations have expired. The statute of limitations varies from state to state, and an assistant should verify the statute of limitations for the state in which the medical office does business. Financial records must be retained until they are no longer needed according to the applicable statute of limitations.

HIPAA Hint

A health care entity must keep records for privacy practices, complaints, and other items the Privacy Rule requires to be kept, for 6 years after the last effective date of the record.

SUMMARY

The size of the practice and the scope of the responsibilities of the medical administrative assistant dictate whether an assistant is responsible for handling the financial operations of the practice. As was mentioned previously, in many large offices today, professionals may be hired or contracted by the practice to perform many of the financial functions of the practice. Whether an assistant has a small or a large role, an understanding of the financial operations of the practice will give an assistant a greater appreciation for how office activities affect the financial health of the office.

REVIEW EXERCISES

Exercise 14-1 True or False

Read each statement, and determine whether the statement is true or false. Record the answer in the blank provided. T = true; F = false.

_______ 1. A change fund is used to pay for small expenditures such as supplies used in the office.

_______ 2. It is best if several people are responsible for the petty cash fund; this reduces the chance that mistakes will be made in handling the fund.

_______ 3. Reports generated from a computer billing system provide detail on the financial health of the practice.

_______ 4. It is common for a medical administrative assistant to have the sole responsibility of managing the financial operations of a medical practice.

_______ 5. A medical practice must be ready to accept cash, checks, or credit cards for payment of patients' account balances.

_______ 6. Because medical charges are billed directly to insurance companies, a medical office has no need to have cash on hand.

_______ 7. A receipt provides proof of payment on a patient's account.

_______ 8. A restrictive endorsement limits where a check can be deposited.

_______ 9. A negative balance on a patient's account is an amount that is owed to the practice.

_______10. NSF and returned checks should be subtracted from a patient's account balance.

_______11. All business records should be kept for a period of 5 years.

_______12. If a bank refuses to pay a check, this is known as a restrictive endorsement.

_______13. Reconciling a checking account ensures that the check register agrees with the bank's balance on a checking account.

_______14. Once a checking account has been reconciled and the check register agrees with the bank statement, the bank statement can be shredded.

_______15. A credit balance on an account may be applied to future charges on an account.

_______16. Patients who live outside the vicinity of a medical practice may be expected to pay their bill on the date of an office visit because it may be difficult to collect a bill if it goes unpaid at a later date.

Exercise 14-2 Chapter Concepts

Read the following statements or questions, and choose the answer that best completes each statement or question. Record the answer in the blank provided.

_______ 1. Identifies profit earned over a period of time.
(a) Transaction journal
(b) Check register
(c) Income statement
(d) Balance sheet

_______ 2. Identifies the amounts of assets, liabilities, and owners' equity in a medical practice.
(a) Cash flow statement
(b) Balance sheet
(c) Check register
(d) Accounts payable

_______ 3. Which of the following is false about a petty cash account?
(a) Petty cash is used to purchase small items for use in a medical office.
(b) Receipts should be kept for petty cash expenditures.
(c) A petty cash fund is different from a change fund.
(d) Petty cash is normally used to cover expenditures of more than $100.

_______ 4. All of the following are true about writing checks except
(a) Some practices may use computer-generated checks.
(b) Checks should be used in numerical order.
(c) When the amount is entered on a check, care should be taken to eliminate the possibility that the amount may be altered.
(d) Mistakes on a check can be crossed out with a single line and corrected with red ink.

_______ 5. All of the following can be found on a purchase order except
(a) Name of vendor
(b) Listing of items purchased
(c) Balance of the account to which the purchase will be charged
(d) Name of person authorizing the purchase

_______ 6. Accounts payable is an example of
(a) An asset
(b) A liability
(c) Owners' equity

_______ 7. Cash is an example of
(a) An asset
(b) A liability
(c) Owners' equity

_______ 8. Deposits to a practice's bank account should be made
(a) When there is time
(b) Weekly
(c) Daily
(d) After each check is received

_______ 9. Which of the following is not included on a receipt?
(a) Date of the patient's visit
(b) Name of the person who made the payment
(c) Method of payment
(d) Name of person who received the payment

_______10. All of the following are true about bookkeeping and accounting in a medical office except
(a) An assistant can expect to play a supporting role in the financial management of a practice.
(b) Computer systems can provide in a matter of seconds important financial data needed for planning.
(c) An assistant should expect to be responsible for analyzing financial reports to plan for future expansion of a practice.
(d) Office documents should be retained until applicable statutes of limitations have expired.

ACTIVITIES

ACTIVITY 14-1 PATIENT PAYMENTS

Using Medisoft, record the following payments on account by completing the following:

1. At the Medisoft main menu, click **Activities>Enter Deposits/Payments.**
2. In the **Deposit List** window, list the deposit date as 02/28/2014. Click **New.**
3. Enter the information from the table in the following fields in the **Deposits: New** window.
   a. **Payer type**: Identify whether the payment is from a patient or an insurance company.
   b. **Method**: Identify the form of payment (check, cash, credit card, electronic). If a check, enter the check number in the field.
   c. **Payment Amount**: Enter total amount of payment.
   d. **Chart # or Insurance**: Identify who or what company made the payment.
   e. Leave other fields as is.
   f. Click **Save.**
   g. Highlight the deposit you just entered on the **Deposit List.** Click **Apply.**
   h. Uncheck the box **Show Remainder Only.**
   i. Enter the amount paid by the patient or insurance company in the **payment** field. Press **tab.** The payment will show as a negative number.
   j. Click **Save Payments/Adjustments.**
   k. In the **Create Statements** window, click **Cancel.** When asked **Do you want to print the last created statement for this patient?,** click **No.**
   l. Click **Close.**
4. Enter the next deposit following the instructions in #3. When done entering and applying payments, click **Close.**

Note: At any time during this process, lines can be deleted to wipe out any mistakes.

Payor type	Payment Method	Amount	Payer name	Payment Information
Patient	Check #3247	$20	Deanne Olson OLSDE000	Apply to 2/4/2014 visit
Insurance	Check #126583	$80	BCBS225	$50 Sammy Catera 2/4/14 $30 Suzy Jones 2/3/14
Insurance	Check #47536	$40	Cigna	$40 Lindsey Nielsen
Patient	Check #4328	$20	Michael Youngblood YOUMI000	Apply to 2/3/2014 visit
Patient	Cash	$10	Anthony Zimmerman ZIMAN000	Apply 2/3/2014

ACTIVITY 14-2 FINANCIAL REPORTS

Open Medisoft. Complete the following to print the identified reports, and explain how the reports could be used in financial planning for the office.

Practice Analysis

1. Click **Reports>Analysis Reports>Practice Analysis.**
2. Click **Print>Start or Preview>Start.** In the **Search** window, all options should have **Show All Values** checked.
3. After reviewing the report, explain how the report could be used in financial planning in the office.

Patient Aging

1. Click **Reports>Aging Reports>Patient Aging.**
2. Click **Print>Start** or **Preview>Start.** In the **Search** window, all options should have **Show All Values** checked.
3. After reviewing the report, explain how the report could be used in financial planning in the office.

Patient Ledger

1. Click **Reports>Patient Ledger.**
2. Click **Print>Start** or **Preview>Start.** In the **Search** window, all options should have **Show All Values** checked.
3. After reviewing the report, explain how the report could be used in financial planning in the office.

Patients by Diagnosis

1. Click **Reports>Standard Patient Lists>Patients by Diagnosis.**
2. Click **Print>Start** or **Preview>Start.** In the **Search** window, **Show All Values** should be checked.
3. After reviewing the report, explain how the report could be used in financial planning in the office.

ACTIVITY 14-3 PREPARE DEPOSIT SLIP

Following Procedure 14-2, prepare the deposit slip below for the checks listed in Activity 14-1.

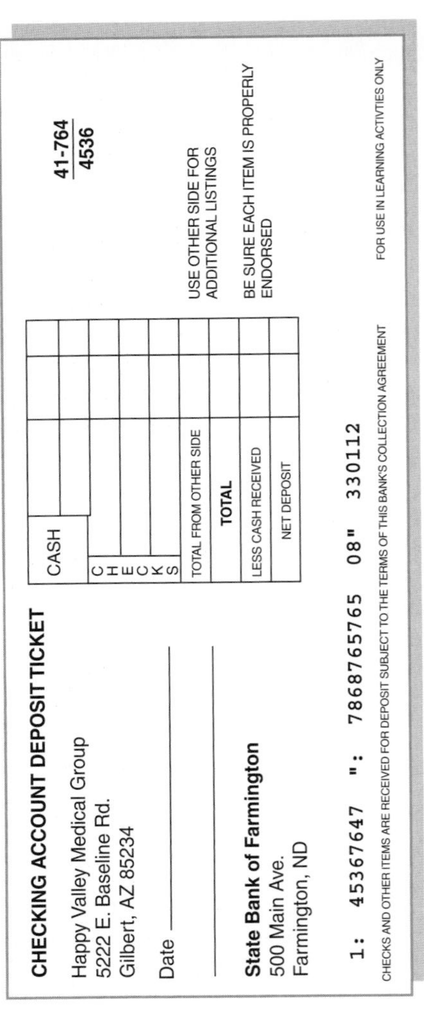

CHECKING ACCOUNT DEPOSIT TICKET

Happy Valley Medical Group
5222 E. Baseline Rd.
Gilbert, AZ 85234

Date ________

State Bank of Farmington
500 Main Ave.
Farmington, ND

1: 45367647 ": 7868765765 08" 330112

CHECKS AND OTHER ITEMS ARE RECEIVED FOR DEPOSIT SUBJECT TO THE TERMS OF THIS BANK'S COLLECTION AGREEMENT

CASH	
CHECKS	
TOTAL FROM OTHER SIDE	
TOTAL	
LESS CASH RECEIVED	
NET DEPOSIT	

USE OTHER SIDE FOR ADDITIONAL LISTINGS

BE SURE EACH ITEM IS PROPERLY ENDORSED

41-764/4536

FOR USE IN LEARNING ACTIVTIES ONLY

DEPOSIT TICKET

FOR CLEAR COPY, PRESS FIRMLY WITH BALL POINT PEN.

State Bank of Farmington
500 Main Ave.
Farmington, ND 58000

DATE ________

	DOLLARS	CENTS
CURRENCY		
COIN		
LIST EACH CHECK		
1.		
2.		
3.		
4.		
5.		
6.		
7.		
8.		
9.		
10.		
11.		
12.		
13.		
14.		
15.		
16.		
17.		
18.		
19.		
20.		
PLEASE ENTER TOTAL		

TOTAL DEPOSIT

DEPOSITS MAY NOT BE AVAILABLE FOR IMMEDIATE WITHDRAWAL

PLEASE BE SURE ALL ITEMS ARE PROPERLY ENDORSED

TOTAL ITEMS

50-17/223 0107

1: 45890277": 6334792445 08" 6221

CHECKS AND OTHER ITEMS ARE RECEIVED FOR DEPOSIT SUBJECT TO THE PROVISIONS OF THE UNIFORM COMMERCIAL CODE OR ANY APPLICABLE COLLECTION AGREEMENT

ACTIVITY 14-4 PURCHASE ORDER

Using the purchase order in Figure 14-6, identify the following:
Vendor: ____________________
Date of PO: ____________________
How many different items are going to be purchased: ____________________
Total amount of PO: ____________________

ACTIVITY 14-5 BACK ACCOUNT RECONCILIATION

Reconcile a bank account using the check register and form below and the statement pictured in Figure 14-8.

Ending balance per statement $____________

Plus deposits not included on statement + ____________

Subtotal $____________

Minus outstanding checks – ____________

Total $____________

Check Register

Number	Date	Description	Payment/debit	Ref	Deposit/credit	Balance
						9703.63
18270	10/19/02	Harmon Medical	3465.46	X		6238.17
18271	10/22/02	Acme Rental	789.00	X		5449.17
18272	10/22/02	Custodial Suppliers	46.72	X		5402.45
18273	10/24/02	Taylor Hudson	50.00	X		5352.45
18274	10/24/02	Bob Smith	340.00	X		5012.45
18275	10/25/02	Timothy Marks	493.47			4518.98
18276	10/25/02	GM Supply	50.00			4468.98
18277	10/30/02	Hearty Bakery	37.50			4431.48
18278	10/31/02	Palm Tree Inn	395.00			4036.48
18279	11/1/02	Lincoln Mutual	500.00			3536.48
	11/5/02	deposit			2305.46	5841.94
18280	11/5/02	BAP Printing	40.00			5801.94
18281	11/5/02	NT Phone Services	120.00			5681.94
18282	11/5/02	Custodial Suppliers	324.52			5357.42
18283	11/5/02	Office Suppliers Inc	35.50			5321.92
18284	11/6/02	Electric Co-op	335.00			4986.92
18285	11/7/02	Harmon Medical	890.56			4096.36
	11/8/02	deposit			456.38	4552.74
	11/9/02	deposit			235.90	4788.64
18286	11/12/02	TMI Leasing	1500.00			3288.64
18287	11/12/02	Mary Sanchez	573.00			2715.64
	11/15/02	deposit			4038.98	6754.62
18288	11/15/02	French Pharmaceuticals	234.34			6520.28
18289	11/15/02	Goodwin Oil	470.00			6050.28
18290	11/17/02	Payroll Account	3310.00			2740.28
18291	11/19/02	GM Supply	500.00			2240.28
18292	11/20/02	Hearty Bakery	39.46			2200.82
	11/21/02	deposit			2972.00	5172.82
18293	11/23/02	BAP Printing	100.00			5072.82
18294	11/23/02	ABC plumbing	109.78			4963.04
	11/28/02	deposit			339.06	5302.10
18295	11/28/02	Furniture Outlet Inc	50.00			5252.10
	11/29/02	deposit			585.00	5837.10
18296	11/29/02	Federated Delivery	23.00			5814.10
18297	11/29/02	Vision Security Services	420.00			5394.10
18298	11/29/02	United Supply	34.00			5360.10
18299	11/29/02	U S Postmaster	375.00			4985.10
18300	11/29/02	Custodial Suppliers	180.50			4804.60
X = check received						

ACTIVITY 14-6 PETTY CASH LOG

Using the petty cash log pictured below, enter the following transactions to the log using Procedure 14-3 as a guide.

Petty Cash Log

Date	Description	Amount	Balance

10-17-YY spent $3.52 for pens for the front office
10-19-YY paid $1.21 for postage due
10-23-YY purchased coffee and filters for employee lounge—$6.73
10-24-YY purchased new surge protector for computer—$9.95
10-26-YY paid $15.00 for cab fare for visiting physician
On 10-26-YY, a check was written to replenish the petty cash fund to the original amount of $100. The amount of the check was $_____ _____ _____ _____.

Optional: Design a spreadsheet that would keep track of expenditures from a petty cash account. Enter the amounts identified in Figure 14-5, and add the expenses identified in Activity 14-6. The spreadsheet should automatically calculate the fund balance. Print two copies of the spreadsheet—one showing the amounts and the other showing the formulas used to calculate the amounts.

ACTIVITY 14-7 CHECK PREPARATION

Following Procedure 14-4, prepare check #18300 as listed in the check register in Activity 14-7.

Happy Valley Medical Group
5222 E. Baseline Rd.
Gilbert, AZ 85234

18300

_______ 20 _____

PAY TO THE
ORDER OF______________________________ $ __________

______________________________________ dollars

STATE BANK OF FARMINGTON
500 Main Avenue
Farmington, ND 58000

FOR ____________________ ____________________

: #####: ########:

DISCUSSIONS

The following topics can be used for class discussion or for individual student essay.

DISCUSSION 14-1

Explain why it is important that the services of a financial professional, such as an accountant, be used to monitor the financial operations of a medical practice.

DISCUSSION 14-2

Explain how financial software can aid in financial planning for a medical practice.

Bibliography

U.S. Department of Health and Human Services Office of Civil Rights: Summary of the HIPAA Privacy Rule. Last revised May 2003 http://www.hhs.gov/ocr/privacysummary.pdf. Accessed November 18, 2011.

CHAPTER 15 Human Resource Management

LEARNING OUTCOMES

On completing this chapter, the student will be able to

1. Describe a management style that can help create an efficient yet effective office environment for patients.
2. Explain components of the employee selection process.
3. Explain policy and procedure manuals.
4. Prepare payroll.
5. Identify components of employee records.
6. Identify essentials of employee discipline and termination.
7. Describe employee health issues.
8. Describe labor laws and legal issues related to human resources.

COMMISSION ON ACCREDITATION OF ALLIED HEALTH EDUCATION PROGRAMS (CAAHEP) CORE CURRICULUM FOR MEDICAL ASSISTANTS

- Use office hardware and software to maintain office systems.
- Use Internet to access information related to the medical office.
- Describe the implications of HIPAA for the medical assistant in various medical settings.
- List and discuss legal and illegal interview questions.

VOCABULARY

employee compensation record
employer identification number (EIN)
empower
human resources
job description
participatory management
performance review
policy manual
probationary period
procedure manual
sexual harassment

Perhaps the most vital component in the operation of any organization is the people who are employed by or who represent the organization—the **human resources** of the organization. All staff members of a medical office are vital to a practice's success. No practice would function efficiently or effectively without all groups working together, complementing one another's efforts. Creating a harmonious work environment in which all employees truly value and support each other is perhaps the greatest challenge for many managers, but such an environment promotes the growth and stability of the practice.

In this chapter, components of human resource management are introduced along with fundamental legal topics pertinent to human resource management. Even if an assistant is not employed as a manager, knowledge of human resource management can help an assistant recognize the various human resource components that enter into creating an optimal work environment in which all staff members work together to provide optimal service for all patients.

Participatory Management Style

The atmosphere of the medical office is influenced by variables such as the size of the office staff, the facility itself, what types of patients are served, and the management style that is inherent in the operation of the office. Physicians and associated staff who manage the day-to-day operations of the office significantly influence the atmosphere of the office by the type of management style they use (Fig. 15-1). Management style is an integral part of a practice's success.

A common trend in management of employees today is to **empower** all employees to become involved in how they contribute to the overall goals or mission of an organization. In a medical office, a typical mission statement would likely include a declaration about supporting one another as a team in providing the finest quality health care and service to all patients. A mission statement might appear as the following:

> The mission of Horizons Health Partners is to provide an atmosphere of caring and compassion for all patients while offering state-of-the-art health care services. This is accomplished through the selection, hiring, and training of the best-qualified staff available.

Mission statements are important in that they give an overall direction for the office staff. Consider the mission statement and primary value of Mayo Clinic identified on mayoclinic.org. The Mayo mission is brief but to the point: "To inspire hope and contribute to health and well-being by providing the best care to every patient through

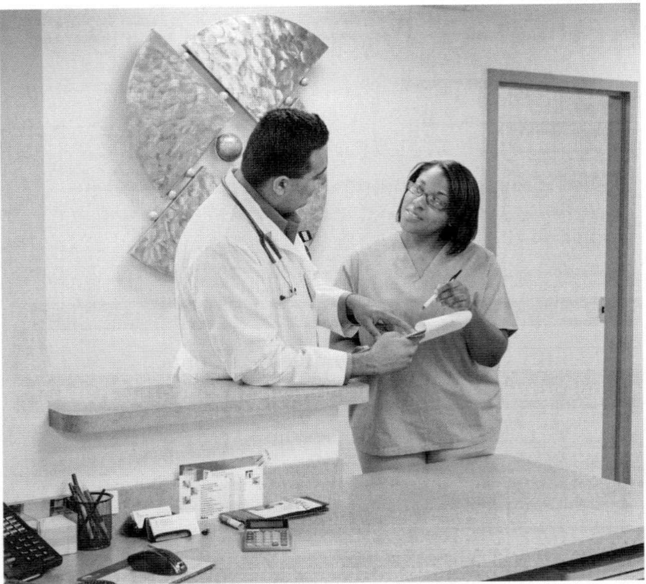

Figure 15-1 Management style greatly influences the environment of the medical office. (From Young AP: *Kinn's The Administrative Medical Assistant*, ed7, St. Louis, Saunders, 2011.)

BOX 15-1

Characteristics of a Participatory Management Style

A manager
- Communicates openly and honestly
- Is team oriented
- Encourages employees to grow
- Presents clear guidelines to let employees know what is expected of them
- Recognizes quality work; gives staff credit and positive feedback
- Informs employees about what is expected of them
- Does not have hidden agendas
- Delegates work
- Welcomes new ideas or suggestions from staff
- Does not micromanage or make every decision
- Is a mentor, role model, and leader

integrated clinical practice, education and research." The primary value of Mayo Clinic is "The needs of the patient come first."

In the book *Management Lessons From Mayo Clinic*, authors Leonard Berry and Kent Seltman present how the employees of this leading health care organization have been living out that mission for longer than 100 years. All employees contribute to the mission of the Mayo Clinic. The input of staff members across the organization is gathered for organizational planning involving finances, staffing, and strategic planning. All employees plan, organize, and perform their work to match the mission of the organization.

When empowerment is applied to a medical practice, all employees are given some degree of responsibility in achieving the mission within their area of expertise. To demonstrate how employees are empowered in a medical office, consider the following example.

All office staff members can be given authority to organize and coordinate their work to meet the mission of the practice and to support the other work groups in the practice. Each work group or department within the practice can collaborate within the group to meet staffing needs from the start to the end of the day. As long as the group meets its work goals, management may leave it up to the group to decide how the work will be accomplished. In addition, group managers (or department managers) will work together to ensure that the business operations of the office are working as they should.

In this example, the front office staff will plan their schedule to meet the staffing needs of the physicians and other support staff. Of course, the staffing may have some budget constraints, but in general, the front office staff members in association with management cooperatively make decisions as to how staffing needs will be met. They may work 8-hour days 5 days a week or 10-hour days 4 days a week, depending on which best meets the needs of the practice. The physicians and other management depend on the front office staff to meet the day-to-day scheduling needs of the practice, and they appreciate a smooth flow of operations that allows them to practice medicine and see patients. As long as the front office staff can meet the needs of the physicians, the physicians may leave how that is done up to the front office staff.

Empowerment creates the type of environment that is often appreciated by employees. Many people, when given the chance, welcome the opportunity to decide what type of schedule works best for them. People, in general, appreciate opportunities to be in charge of their surroundings. A few individuals may wish to be told what to do, but in an empowered environment, these individuals will be encouraged to join in the decision making.

The concept of empowerment is present in what is frequently called a **participatory management** style (Box 15-1). This type of style works well in a medical office for the following reasons:
- A medical office is usually a very fast-paced environment, and empowering employees to make decisions allows employees to serve patients quickly and efficiently.
- Empowered employees are typically happy employees, and a medical office with happy employees attracts and retains more patients.
- Employees who have input into the decisions of the medical office are more dedicated to the practice; thus, employee turnover is reduced.

Depending on the size of the organization, the front office staff may consist of one, several, or many assistants. If there are many assistants and a participatory management style is used, the management of the practice must identify individual positions, such as office manager or supervisor, to facilitate communication among the various groups of the organization and to define the delegation of duties and tasks. As both a supervisor and coordinator of office operations, the manager serves as a communication link among physicians, the front office staff, and other groups within the organization. When performing job duties, the office manager gathers input from the front office staff, yet he or she is ultimately responsible for making and implementing decisions that are consistent with the mission and goals of the organization.

Empowerment is a newer trend and may not reflect the management style present in some offices around the country. Some offices may still have management that is dictated from the top down. Some physicians or office managers may wish to make most of the decisions that affect their practice. If this is the case, an assistant must respect the wishes of the office's management. An assistant should always work for the good of the patients and the organization.

The Employment Process

Posting an Open Position

Suppose there is an opening in the office, and people in the office are commenting that the "right" person is needed to fill the position. What constitutes the "right" person? Of course, it is the person with the qualifications—education, experience, and personal qualities—to fill the position.

When listing the necessary qualifications for a position, it is important to include only those items that are related to and necessary to perform the job. A **job description** identifies what a person employed in a particular position will be required to do in that position (Fig. 15-2). A job description usually also identifies who supervises the position and the wage range for the position. The job description serves as the basis for the qualifications identified in an advertisement for a position.

Happy Valley Medical Group
Job Description

Position title: Medical Administrative Assistant
Reports to: Office Manager
Payroll rate: 10.36–14.32/hour

Responsibilities:

- maintain appointment schedule
- release medical records
- process telephone calls
- transcribe medical dictation
- maintain patient's registration/insurance information
- process patient billing
- prepare insurance claims

Revised: July 2001

Figure 15-2 A job description identifies the responsibilities of a position.

Generally, objective criteria, or those items that can be measured, should be listed as qualifications for a position. Examples of these include a certain level of education (e.g., diploma, associate's degree, bachelor's degree), a certain type of skill or knowledge (e.g., typing, knowledge of medical terminology, billing and coding, proficiency using certain types of computer software), or a certain number of years of experience in a similar position in a medical office.

Subjective criteria, or soft skills, can be qualifications for a position, but these skills are often difficult to measure. Soft skills are related to a person's attitude or behavior and include such attributes as motivation and enthusiasm, enjoying working with people, or being a team player.

When each candidate is interviewed, the objective and subjective criteria listed for the position must be applied equally to all applicants. For instance, when an opening for a medical administrative assistant is advertised, objective criteria might include computer skills at a certain level, such as typing 45 words per minute, knowledge of a particular computer software, medical administrative assistant education or experience in a medical office, or any combination of these. The ability to lift 100 pounds or run a marathon would not fulfill the qualifications necessary to perform the job and obviously could not be considered during the selection process, but all applicants could be evaluated for typing speed.

Once the qualifications for a position have been determined, the position is advertised (Fig. 15-3) or published in a variety of sources. Many health care employers advertise employment openings on their own website. This is perhaps the most common method for advertising openings as it can be easily controlled by the employer. Openings can also be listed with state employment services, school placement services, employment agencies, newspapers, and even professional publications. Job postings should list deadlines by which résumés or applications should be submitted for consideration.

When the deadline for the position has passed, the résumés that have been submitted for consideration are reviewed. The committee or interviewer should establish a list of evaluation criteria necessary for the position and should assign points to each of the criteria. After all résumés are received, copies of each are reviewed by committee members, and points are assigned for each candidate's qualifications. Point assignments are totaled and reviewed by the committee. Candidates with the greatest number of points are invited to come to the office for an interview (Procedure 15-1).

Help Wanted – Health

Medical Administrative Assistant

Full-time opening in our family practice clinic working 8-5 Monday through Friday. Position requires excellent communication skills, medical transcription proficiency and knowledge of medical office procedures such as appointment scheduling, registration, billing, coding, and insurance. Applicants must possess a working knowledge of XYZ Office software.

Interested applicants should apply in person to Human Resources at Horizons Medical Center, 123 Main Ave, Farmington, ND 58000.

Figure 15-3 Employment openings in a medical office are advertised in a variety of locations.

PROCEDURE 15-1

Select Candidates for Interviewing

Materials Needed

- Résumés or job applications
- Selection criteria
- Pen or pencil

1. If possible, form a committee that will be involved in all aspects of the selection process. Using the committee selection process helps eliminate potential biases and future conflicts. (Sometimes this is not possible, and the applicants will be interviewed by only one individual.) However, there should always be more than one interview. A second interview ensures proper selection of the most qualified candidate.
2. The committee or interviewer should establish a list of criteria necessary for the position and should assign points to each of those criteria.
3. After all résumés have been received, give copies of each résumé to each member of the committee.
4. Résumés are evaluated by each member, and points are assigned for each candidate's qualifications.*
5. Point assignments are totaled and reviewed by the committee. The candidates with the greatest number of points are invited for an interview.

**Denotes crucial step in procedure. Student must complete this step satisfactorily in order to complete the procedure satisfactorily.*

If at all possible, a committee should be formed that will be involved in all aspects of the selection process. Using the committee selection process helps eliminate potential biases and future conflicts. Sometimes this is not possible, and the applicants are interviewed by only one individual. Whether a committee or an individual does the interviewing, there should always be more than one interview. A second interview ensures proper selection of the most qualified candidate because it allows the interviewer to determine whether the preferred candidate is presenting a consistent appearance.

The Interview

After the résumés have been reviewed and candidates selected for interviewing, appropriate questions must be selected for the interviews. It is of the utmost importance that the questions relate to the position itself and to the person's qualifications for the position. Questions regarding marital status or whether or not the candidate owns a home or has a car to drive to work cannot be asked. Questions cannot be asked about a person's family or plans to have a family, nor can questions be asked about a person's age, race, or religion. Such questions could bring a lawsuit for discrimination.

All applicants should be asked the same questions to allow each applicant the same interview opportunities and to ensure that equal opportunity standards are being followed. Female applicants cannot be asked additional questions that may appear related to their gender, such as "Will you be able to make daycare arrangements for your children?" Instead of asking "Will children make it difficult to get to work at a certain hour?" ask the applicant whether he or she will be able to work the designated hours for the job, and if there is flexibility in case office hours change or unexpected needs arise. Employers are allowed to ask such questions as "Will you be able to work flexible hours?" (if needed for the job) or "Will you have any problems getting to work?" All applicants, regardless of gender, race, age, or religion, must receive equal opportunity to respond to all questions and must not be discriminated against. Most interview questions should be focused on the applicant's ability to perform job requirements.

Questions for the interview should be prepared, and a separate copy of the questions should be available for every interview. The interviewer can then refer to the sheet during the interview. Some interviewers choose to rate each candidate's answer on a scale, such as from 1 to 5, with 1 being "poor or no answer" and 5 being an "excellent answer." At the end of all interviews, the interviewer can add up the total points for each applicant. The applicant with the highest score should be the best candidate for the position (Fig. 15-4).

When possible, the top two or three candidates should be chosen for the position. References listed by each candidate are then checked. During a reference check, the previous employer is asked questions about when the applicant worked with the organization and what type of work was performed, as well as other questions related to the applicant's position, such as about production and attendance. Concerns about giving references are identified later in this chapter, and those concerns may influence the responses obtained during a reference check.

If the references support the selection of a top candidate, the interviewer should contact the top candidate and offer the position to that candidate. If the top candidate declines the offer (for whatever reason), the interviewer can offer the position to

INTERVIEW EVALUATION AND REFERENCE INVESTIGATION FORM, MEDICAL or DENTAL OFFICE

SUMMARY OF EVALUATION	
POINTS FROM APPLICATION AND INTERVIEW	
POINTS FROM REFERENCES	
TOTAL POINTS	
OVERALL IMPRESSION	

NAME OF APPLICANT	DATE

RATING: GOOD - 2 POINTS
FAIR - 1 POINT
POOR - 0 POINTS

POSITION APPLIED FOR:

FROM APPLICATION FOR POSITION, GAUGE APPLICANT IN FOLLOWING AREAS	GOOD	FAIR	POOR
APPLICATION SECTION REFERENCE			
1. STABILITY (REMAINED IN ONE PLACE OF RESIDENCE AND ONE JOB FOR A REASONABLE LENGTH OF TIME)?			
2. HEALTH?			
3. THE PROPER EDUCATIONAL BACKGROUND TO FILL THE POSITION?			
4. LEGIBLE HANDWRITING?			
5. AN EMPLOYMENT HISTORY THAT POINTS TOWARD DEPENDABILITY?			
6. LIMITATION ON WORKING HOURS?			
7. THE PROPER EXPERIENCE AND / OR SKILLS TO FILL THE POSITION?			
8. SALARY REQUIREMENT COMMENSURATE WITH POSITION?			
FROM THE PERSONAL INTERVIEW - (SHOULD BE SPECIFIC QUALITIES - OBJECTIVE)			
9. SUFFICIENT CAPABILITY TO HANDLE ANY SITUATION THAT MAY ARISE WHEN ALONE IN OFFICE?			
10. AN APPROPRIATE ATTITUDE TOWARD WORK?			
11. AN APPROPRIATE VOICE, DICTION, GRAMMAR?			
12. POISE?			
13. SELF CONFIDENCE (NOT OVER-CONFIDENCE)?			
14. TACT?			
15. SUFFICIENT MATURITY FOR JOB?			
16. AN ABILITY TO EXPRESS ONESELF WELL?			
17. AN INITIATIVE OR INTEREST IN LEARNING?			
18. ABILITY TO WORK WITH OTHERS IN OFFICE?			
19. APPROPRIATE APPEARANCE (NEAT, CLEAN; SUITABLE TO BUSINESS)			
20. ENERGY, VITALITY, AND PERCEIVED ABILITY TO HANDLE PRESSURE OF POSITION?			
21. EAGERNESS TO OBTAIN THE POSITION IN QUESTION?			
COLUMNAR TOTALS			
	GRAND TOTAL		

DIRECTIONS FOR USE OF FORM:
1. Look over your ratings. A zero score on any one VITAL question should automatically eliminate applicant. Add up the total rating points and enter in the SUMMARY OF EVALUATION BLOCK in the upper right-hand corner of this page.
2. After finishing all interviews, choose the "best bets" and check their references using the reverse side of this form.
3. Enter, as above, the results of your reference check and then your overall impression. (E - Excellent, G - Good, F - Fair, P - Poor)

ORDER # **72-120** • BIBBERO SYSTEMS, INC. • PETALUMA, CA.
TO REORDER CALL TOLL FREE: (800) BIBBERO (800-242-2376) OR FAX (800) 242-9330 M FG IN U.S.A.

(PLEASE TURN OVER)

Figure 15-4 An interview form helps management to objectively identify the best candidates for an office position. (Form courtesy of Bibbero Systems, Inc., Petaluma, California, 800-242-2376; fax, 800-242-9330; www.bibbero.com.)

Continued

NOTES:

REFERENCE INVESTIGATION			
1. OFFICE CONTACTED	PHONE: ( )	DATE	
PERSON CONTACTED			
HOW LONG HAVE YOU KNOWN THIS PERSON ?			
BETWEEN WHAT DATES WAS THIS PERSON EMPLOYED BY YOU?	FROM	TO	
WHAT TYPE OF WORK DID THIS PERSON DO FOR YOU?	TITLE OF POSITION:	SATISFACTORILY?	
WAS THIS PERSON CONSISTENTLY COOPERATIVE?	WHAT WERE SHORTCOMINGS?		
DID THIS PERSON GET ALONG WELL WITH OTHERS?			
WAS THIS PERSON TRUSTWORTHY / DEPENDABLE?		ATTENDANCE RECORD:	
WHY DID THIS PERSON LEAVE YOUR EMPLOY?		SALARY LEVEL:	
WOULD YOU REHIRE THIS PERSON?			
NOTES:			
		RATING:	
2. OFFICE CONTACTED	PHONE: ( )	DATE	
PERSON CONTACTED			
HOW LONG HAVE YOU KNOWN THIS PERSON ?			
BETWEEN WHAT DATES WAS THIS PERSON EMPLOYED BY YOU?	FROM	TO	
WHAT TYPE OF WORK DID THIS PERSON DO FOR YOU?	TITLE OF POSITION:	SATISFACTORILY?	
WAS THIS PERSON CONSISTENTLY COOPERATIVE?	WHAT WERE SHORTCOMINGS?		
DID THIS PERSON GET ALONG WELL WITH OTHERS?			
WAS THIS PERSON TRUSTWORTHY / DEPENDABLE?		ATTENDANCE RECORD:	
WHY DID THIS PERSON LEAVE YOUR EMPLOY?		SALARY LEVEL:	
WOULD YOU REHIRE THIS PERSON?			
NOTES:			
		RATING:	
3. OFFICE CONTACTED	PHONE: ( )	DATE	
PERSON CONTACTED			
HOW LONG HAVE YOU KNOWN THIS PERSON ?			
BETWEEN WHAT DATES WAS THIS PERSON EMPLOYED BY YOU?	FROM	TO	
WHAT TYPE OF WORK DID THIS PERSON DO FOR YOU?	TITLE OF POSITION:	SATISFACTORILY?	
WAS THIS PERSON CONSISTENTLY COOPERATIVE?	WHAT WERE SHORTCOMINGS?		
DID THIS PERSON GET ALONG WELL WITH OTHERS?			
WAS THIS PERSON TRUSTWORTHY / DEPENDABLE?		ATTENDANCE RECORD:	
WHY DID THIS PERSON LEAVE YOUR EMPLOY?		SALARY LEVEL:	
WOULD YOU REHIRE THIS PERSON?			
NOTES:			
		RATING:	

INTERVIEWER ____________________ DATE: ________________

Figure 15-4, cont'd

BOX 15-2

Sample of Policy Manual Components

The following topics usually are found in a policy manual or employee handbook. This list is not inclusive:

- Payroll periods
- Performance reviews
- Work schedule
- Overtime
- Dress code
- Absence from work
- Sick leave
- Maternity/paternity leave
- Vacation leave
- Holiday pay
- Religious holidays
- Bereavement leave
- Jury/legal leave
- Military leave
- Educational leave
- Health insurance
- Dental insurance
- Life insurance
- Retirement plans
- Work-related injuries and OSHA requirements
- Confidentiality
- Employee reprimand
- Employee dismissal

the next best qualified candidate, provided that candidate's references are favorable. After the position has been accepted, the interviewer should notify all remaining candidates by telephone or mail to thank them for applying and to inform them that someone else has been selected for the position. Notification of all applicants helps the practice maintain a positive public image.

CHECKPOINT

1. You are responsible for hiring an additional medical assistant to work in the office. A physician in the practice has asked you to find an older woman whose children are grown so that she will be able to stay late if necessary. How do you reply?
2. You are working for a pediatric practice. When hiring, the pediatricians have asked you to screen for an assistant who likes children. Would this be acceptable in an interview?

Hiring a New Employee

When a new employee is hired, a few items must be taken care of immediately. An employer is required to verify that each employee is eligible for employment in the United States. Form I-9, Employment Eligibility Verification, must be completed; eligibility may be confirmed by phoning the U.S. Citizenship and Immigration Services office.

Every new employee is asked to complete a W-4 form. In addition, new hires are reported to a designated state office that tracks new hires. Some states will accept a copy of the employee's completed W-4 in lieu of any other reporting. More on the W-4 appears later in this chapter.

Employee Training and Probationary Period

Once an employee is selected, orientation and training sessions are arranged to familiarize the employee with the specific expectations and operations of the office. Even if an employee has received formal education in medical administrative assisting, each office has specific procedures that are required when the business operations of the office are performed. A training period allows the new employee to become familiar with office procedures specific to that office. During this period, it is most beneficial if a new employee works alongside other members of the staff in addition to a senior employee. The senior employee may serve as a mentor, guiding the new employee in the philosophy, policies, and procedures of the organization. In addition, working alongside other employees helps the new employee acclimate as a team member.

New employees are usually subject to a **probationary period,** which is a specific length of time such as 90 days or 6 months in which the employee is working under a temporary employment arrangement. This is a "no strings attached" type of arrangement; shortly before the end of the probationary period, the employer meets with the employee and decides whether the employment arrangement should continue, and the employee evaluates whether or not to stay in the position permanently. This period gives both the employee and the employer a chance to measure performance and observe whether the employer/employee arrangement is compatible.

HIPAA Hint

A health care provider is required to train all workforce members (paid and unpaid) on its privacy policy and procedures.

Policy Manuals

When an employee is newly hired, one of the first documents the employee receives is a **policy manual** detailing the practice's policies on various human resource–related topics.

Policy manuals, or employee handbooks, contain information on matters such as vacation, sick leave, personal leave, holidays, retirement plans, dress codes, and confidentiality (Box 15-2). Basically, anything an employee would want to

BOX 15-3

Sample Dress Code for Office Staff

1. Clothing must be clean and pressed.
2. A name tag must be worn at all times while on duty.
3. Hosiery must be worn at all times.
4. Hair should be neat and trimmed.
5. Perfume or cologne is not allowed because patients and other employees may be sensitive.
6. Tennis shoes may be worn only with uniforms.
7. Use of cosmetics and jewelry should be conservative.
8. Crop top, tank top, backless, or low-cut apparel is not acceptable.
9. Shorts of any kind are not allowed.
10. Jeans of any color are not allowed.

Employees in violation of the dress code will be asked to leave and to remedy the situation on their own time.

know about working in an organization should be included in the policy manual. The manual may apply to all employees in the organization or just to a specific group of employees. In large organizations, it is common to have a separate policy manual for professional staff such as physicians and executive staff. Because professional staff may be under a contractual arrangement with the organization, different standards may be established as a condition of their employment.

The items included in a policy manual detail the organization's guidelines or rules on certain behaviors or actions. A sample policy regarding sick leave might appear as follows:

Employees shall be granted 40 hours of sick leave on the day employment begins. For every 80 hours worked, the employee shall earn an additional 4 hours of sick leave. Employees may accumulate sick leave to a maximum of 800 hours.

Sick leave may be used for personal illness or injury; illness or injury of an employee's dependent, spouse, or parent; or medical or dental appointments of the employee or the employee's dependent, spouse, or parent. Sick leave used for medical and dental appointments may be used in 1-hour increments. Sick leave used for other reasons is used in half-day increments. Sick leave may be used in accordance with the Family and Medical Leave Act.

A dress code is often developed to ensure that standards of professional dress are established and followed. Dress codes may vary for different positions within an organization. Office staff may have a certain dress code, and the clinical staff may have another. An example of a dress code for office staff is included in Box 15-3.

Procedure Manuals

What is the standard procedure for business activities in the medical office? Just as this text details procedures on how the medical administrative assistant would accomplish a given task, a medical office's **procedure manual** gives specific instructions and guidelines for procedures used in that medical office. It provides step-by-step information on how to complete a specific task. Having established procedures ensures consistency in completion of tasks because each employee can follow the same steps every time a procedure is completed.

A procedure manual can be developed with input from all staff members and can be available to the staff in both written and electronic form. The manual should explain approved established procedures and should have the capacity to add new procedures as they are incorporated into the office activities. A procedure manual is an important reference for both new and established employees.

Payroll

Payroll is a major responsibility of individuals responsible for human resource management. Processing of payroll can be quite an involved process. There are many components in payroll processing: gathering required documents for payroll

PROCEDURE 15-2

Prepare Payroll

Materials Needed

- Time cards and records (as in Fig. 15-6 or a similar form)
- Tax tables or percentages
- Calculator

1. Calculate wages earned by multiplying hours worked by hourly rate. If the employee has worked overtime, the overtime hours worked will be multiplied by 1.5 times the employee's hourly rate.*
2. Enter the total wages earned for the period in the gross salary column.*
3. Enter Social Security and Medicare taxes in the FICA column.*
4. Determine the amount of federal tax to be withheld by referring to the employee's wages and withholding allowance amounts. (Refer to the employee's Form W-4 to obtain his or her marital status and withholding allowances. Include any additional amount the employee wishes to have withheld.) Enter the federal income tax withheld amount in the FWT column.*
5. Determine the amount of state tax to be withheld by referring to the employee's wages and withholding allowance amounts. Enter the state tax in the SWT column.*
6. Enter any other deductions on the payroll record.*
7. To figure the employee's net salary, subtract the total deductions from the employee's gross earnings.*
8. Prepare payroll checks by listing all payroll amounts in the check summary.*

**Denotes crucial step in procedure. Student must complete this step satisfactorily in order to complete the procedure satisfactorily.*

processing (e.g., time sheets, records of absence); maintaining salary and withholding information for each employee; calculating the amount due each pay period; and depositing, reporting, and paying payroll taxes and other withholding amounts (Procedure 15-2).

Each practice determines the intervals in which payroll processing will be done. Employees may be paid on a weekly, biweekly, bimonthly, or monthly basis.

Computerized software can be used to calculate payroll and generate payroll checks. This type of software tracks all employee data related to payroll and can calculate payroll information automatically. Such software can quickly generate reports needed for payroll reporting. Some small offices choose to hire an outside expert such as payroll services to process payroll and associated payroll reports necessary for government filing.

Complete information on employer tax requirements is available in Publication 15 (Circular E), Employer's Tax Guide, which is available from the Internal Revenue Service (IRS). This guide provides information on what time of the year required forms should be filed and taxes deposited.

Timekeeping

Depending on the employment arrangements of the medical office staff, time cards (Fig. 15-5) may be used to account for the hours a staff member works. The time card is inserted into a time clock and is imprinted with the correct time and date.

In the example pictured in Figure 15-5, the employee either punches a time clock or writes in the time next to the corresponding date of the month. The reverse of the card contains boxes for the 8th to the 15th or the 24th to the 31st of the month. This type of card works well for a 2-week or bimonthly pay period. The employee or supervisor totals the hours worked for each day and enters the total in the left-hand column of the card. At the end of the week, the total hours worked for that week are written on the time card. The time card then serves to document the hours worked when payroll is calculated.

Many larger organizations now track employee hours electronically. Computer software is now readily available to electronically track employee time-in and time-out. Employees may be issued an employee ID card or name badge with a magnetic strip. The employee swipes the badge through an electronic time clock that will record when the employee enters and leaves the office.

Employees also may sign in to a computer system with a special log-in. Some systems even have the ability to require an employee's fingerprint for sign-in to the system.

Computerized time-keeping software enables management to easily track hours for each employee. Reports can be generated within seconds that would enable management to monitor absenteeism, vacation hours, and other information that may be desired. These systems also greatly reduce the possibility that employees may log in for each other.

Smaller practices with few employees may decide to forgo the use of a time clock altogether. Practices in which the same people work every day, all day long, may decide not to use a time clock to track hours. When a time clock is not used, work hours may be written by the employee on a time sheet (Fig. 15-6), or the employee may be paid a salary.

NAME Dale, Julia — Apr 1 20XX

Hours	Date		Time
	16	IN	
		OUT	
		IN	
		OUT	
8	(1) 17	IN	8:00
		OUT	12:00
		IN	1:00
		OUT	5:00
8.5	(2) 18	IN	8:00
		OUT	12:00
		IN	12:30
		OUT	5:00
8.5	(3) 19	IN	7:45
		OUT	12:00
		IN	12:45
		OUT	5:00
8.5	(4) 20	IN	8:00
		OUT	12:30
		IN	1:00
		OUT	5:00
8.25	(5) 21	IN	8:00
		OUT	12:00
		IN	1:00
		OUT	5:15
	6-22	IN	
		OUT	
		IN	
		OUT	
(41.75)	7-23	IN	
		OUT	
		IN	
		OUT	

ORDER #72-113 • BIBBERO SYSTEMS, INC. • PETALUMA, CA.
TO REORDER CALL TOLL FREE: (800) BIBBERO (800-242-2376) OR FAX (800) 242-9330 M FG IN U.S.A.

Figure 15-5 Time cards are used to document an employee's hours worked. (Form courtesy of Bibbero Systems, Inc., Petaluma, California, 800-242-2376; fax, 800-242-9330; www.bibbero.com.)

Employee Compensation Record

At the end of each payroll period, every employee is paid wages earned during that period. Employees may be paid

Happy Valley Medical Group TIME SHEET

1234 Main Ave
Gilbert AZ 85234
800.333.4747 Fax 012.555.0001

Employee Name: ____________ Title: ____________

Employee Number: ____________ Status: ____________

Department: ____________ Supervisor: ____________

Date	Start Time	End Time	Regular Hours	Overtime Hours	Total Hours
		WEEKLY TOTALS:			

Employee Signature: ____________ Date: ____________

Supervisor Signature: ____________ Date: ____________

Figure 15-6 A time sheet may be used to record an employee's hours worked.

an hourly wage or a salary. With an hourly wage, the employee's hourly rate is multiplied by the number of hours worked in the pay period. Overtime hours, usually those hours worked in excess of 8 hours per day or 40 hours per week, usually are paid at 1.5 times the hourly rate.

A salaried employee is paid a specific amount each pay period. Salaried employees usually are not paid overtime and normally are not required to punch a time clock.

The **employee compensation record** (Fig. 15-7) keeps the payroll data for each individual employee. Amounts paid and deducted from each check, as well as year-to-date totals, are available on this record. At the end of the year, this record provides documentation that can be used in preparing a W-2 form for the employee.

Payroll Deductions

Many deductions are subtracted from an employee's paycheck. Some deductions are mandatory; some are optional. Federal and state income taxes and Social Security and Medicare taxes are mandatory (with very few exceptions). Optional deductions may include premiums for health or dental insurance (or both), retirement contributions, and even deductions for medical or child care expenses (see Fig. 15-7).

Some employers offer pre-tax plans for employees who have medical or child care expenses. Pre-tax plans can save money for an employee. With a pre-tax arrangement, health and dental insurance premiums, child care, and other medical expenses may be deducted from the gross salary. For medical and child care expenses, employees enroll in a pre-tax plan and specify the amount they want subtracted from each paycheck (throughout the year) for those expenses. Taxes then are computed on the amount left after the pre-tax deductions. To be reimbursed for the amounts withheld from each paycheck, the employee must submit a written request or claim with receipts for the expenses to a plan administrator. A separate check for the claim is then written from the plan to the employee.

Premiums for health, dental, and life insurance may be completely or partially the employee's responsibility. Employees may have the option to make retirement contributions, in addition to what their employer may provide. These deductions should be detailed on the employee's paycheck (Fig. 15-8) and listed on the employee's compensation record.

Occasionally, an employee may have court-ordered deductions subtracted from each paycheck. This practice is known as garnishing wages and is not optional for an employee. Wages may be garnished for child support payments to ensure that the money is given to a child.

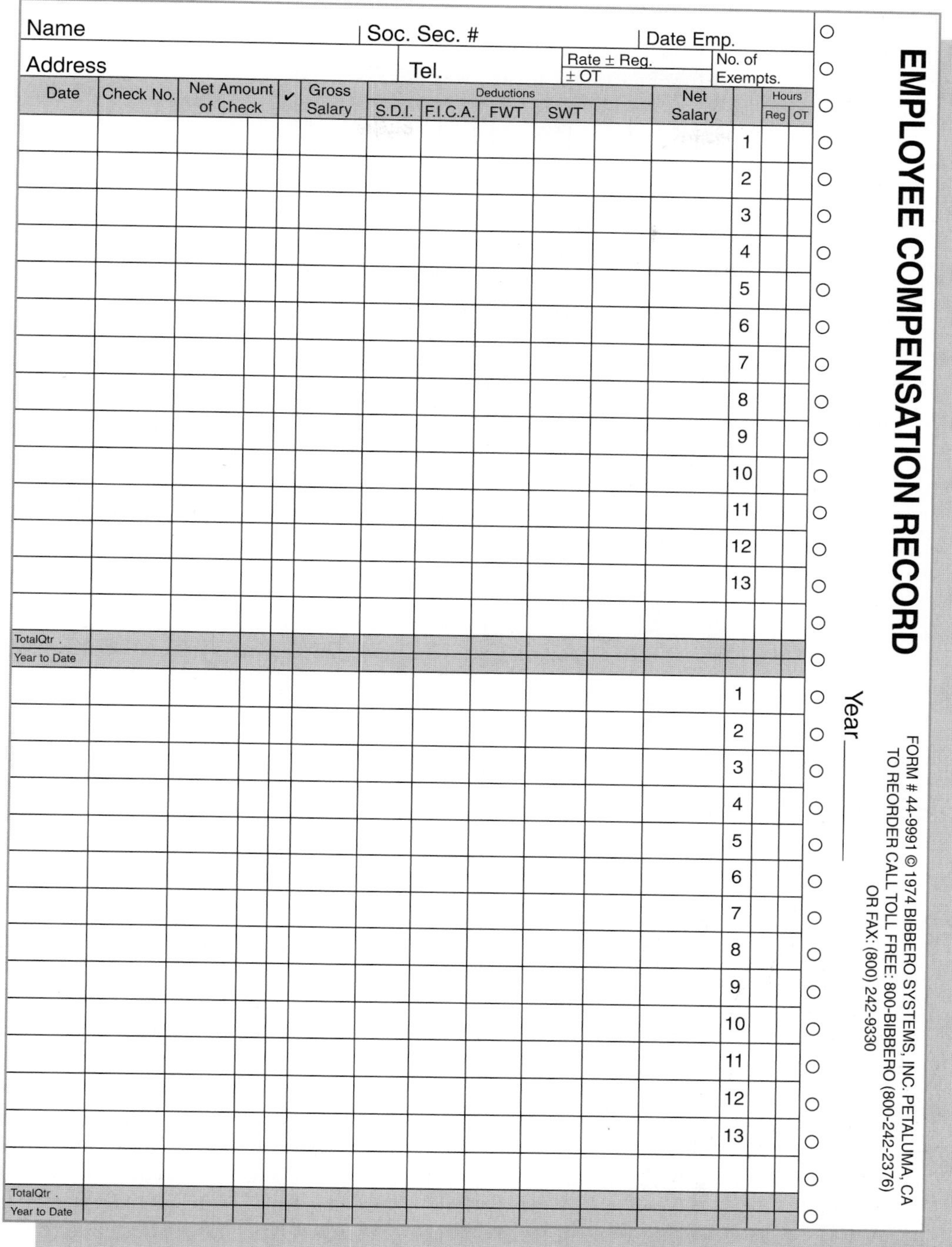

EMPLOYEE COMPENSATION RECORD

Year ______

FORM # 44-9991 © 1974 BIBBERO SYSTEMS, INC. PETALUMA, CA
TO REORDER CALL TOLL FREE: 800-BIBBERO (800-242-2376)
OR FAX: (800) 242-9330

Name | Soc. Sec. # | Date Emp.

Address | Tel. | Rate ± Reg. ± OT | No. of Exempts.

Date	Check No.	Net Amount of Check	✔	Gross Salary	Deductions S.D.I.	F.I.C.A.	FWT	SWT		Net Salary		Hours Reg	OT
											1		
											2		
											3		
											4		
											5		
											6		
											7		
											8		
											9		
											10		
											11		
											12		
											13		
TotalQtr .													
Year to Date													
											1		
											2		
											3		
											4		
											5		
											6		
											7		
											8		
											9		
											10		
											11		
											12		
											13		
TotalQtr .													
Year to Date													

Figure 15-7 A compensation record tracks an employee's earnings. (Form courtesy of Bibbero Systems, Inc., Petaluma, California, 800-242-2376; fax, 800-242-9330; www.bibbero.com.)

Payroll Taxes

Employers must withhold federal income tax, state income tax (if any), Social Security tax, and Medicare tax from employee paychecks. There are few exceptions to this requirement. Under special circumstances, some people may be exempt from federal income tax withholding. Otherwise, employers are required to withhold taxes and must pay taxes for all employees of an organization. An individual is deemed to be an employee if the employer controls what work will be done and how it will be done.

Federal Income Tax. All wages paid to employees are subject to federal income tax. Wages may take the form of cash or other compensation, such as daycare assistance, stock options, bonuses, or educational assistance. The amount of tax on wages earned is determined by the amount of wages the employee earned during that specific payroll period and the information the employee has provided on the W-4 form. The tax due is calculated by using the tax table applicable to the length of the payroll period. Tables for single or married individuals in a biweekly payroll are

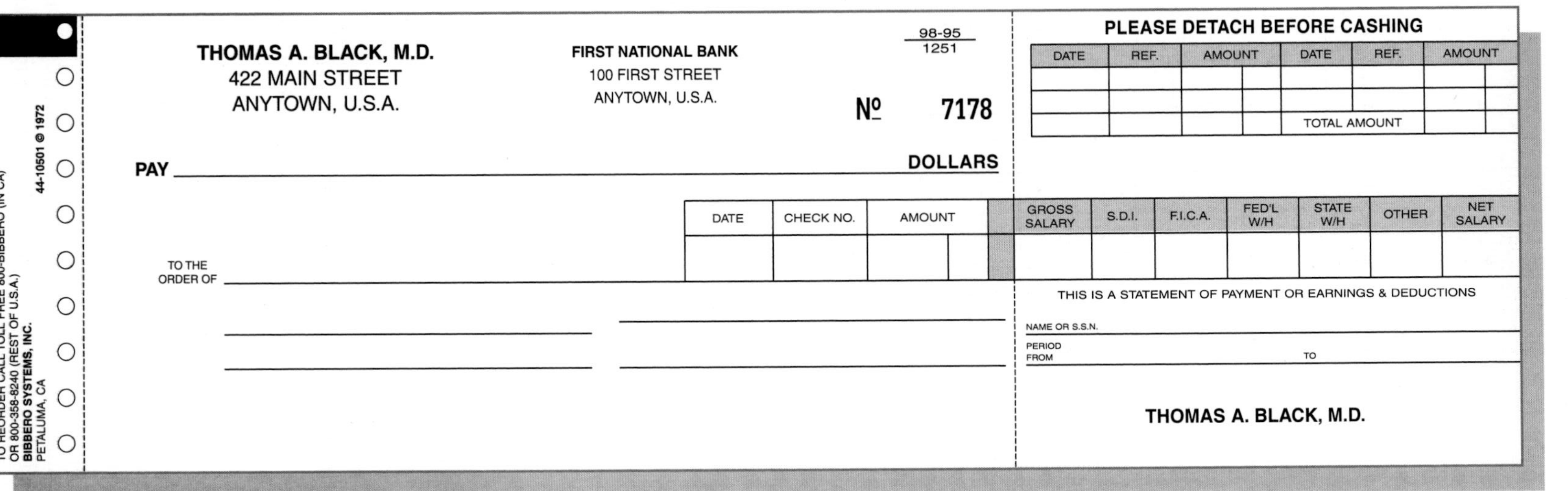

TO REORDER CALL TOLL FREE 800-BIBBERO (IN CA)
OR 800-358-8240 (REST OF U.S.A.)
BIBBERO SYSTEMS, INC.
PETALUMA, CA
44-10501 © 1972

THOMAS A. BLACK, M.D.
422 MAIN STREET
ANYTOWN, U.S.A.

FIRST NATIONAL BANK
100 FIRST STREET
ANYTOWN, U.S.A.

98-95
1251

№ 7178

PAY ______ DOLLARS

TO THE ORDER OF ______

DATE	CHECK NO.	AMOUNT

PLEASE DETACH BEFORE CASHING

DATE	REF.	AMOUNT	DATE	REF.	AMOUNT
			TOTAL AMOUNT		

GROSS SALARY	S.D.I.	F.I.C.A.	FED'L W/H	STATE W/H	OTHER	NET SALARY

THIS IS A STATEMENT OF PAYMENT OR EARNINGS & DEDUCTIONS

NAME OR S.S.N. ______

PERIOD FROM ______ TO ______

THOMAS A. BLACK, M.D.

Figure 15-8 Every payroll check identifies the earnings and deductions for an employee. (Form courtesy of Bibbero Systems, Inc., Petaluma, California, 800-242-2376; fax, 800-242-9330; www.bibbero.com.)

SINGLE Persons—**BIWEEKLY** Payroll Period
(For Wages Paid in 2007)

If the wages are –		And the number of withholding allowances claimed is—										
At least	But less than	0	1	2	3	4	5	6	7	8	9	10
		The amount of income tax to be withheld is—										
600	620	62	42	25	12	0	0	0	0	0	0	0
620	640	65	45	27	14	1	0	0	0	0	0	0
640	660	68	48	29	16	3	0	0	0	0	0	0
660	680	71	51	32	18	5	0	0	0	0	0	0
680	700	74	54	35	20	7	0	0	0	0	0	0
700	720	77	57	38	22	9	0	0	0	0	0	0
720	740	80	60	41	24	11	0	0	0	0	0	0
740	760	83	63	44	26	13	0	0	0	0	0	0
760	780	86	66	47	28	15	1	0	0	0	0	0
780	800	89	69	50	30	17	3	0	0	0	0	0

A

MARRIED Persons—**BIWEEKLY** Payroll Period
(For Wages Paid in 2008)

If the wages are –		And the number of withholding allowances claimed is—										
At least	But less than	0	1	2	3	4	5	6	7	8	9	10
		The amount of income tax to be withheld is—										
780	800	48	35	21	8	0	0	0	0	0	0	0
800	820	50	37	23	10	0	0	0	0	0	0	0
820	840	52	39	25	12	0	0	0	0	0	0	0
840	860	54	41	27	14	0	0	0	0	0	0	0
860	880	56	43	29	16	2	0	0	0	0	0	0
880	900	58	45	31	18	4	0	0	0	0	0	0
900	920	60	47	33	20	6	0	0	0	0	0	0
920	940	63	49	35	22	8	0	0	0	0	0	0
940	960	66	51	37	24	10	0	0	0	0	0	0
960	980	69	53	39	26	12	0	0	0	0	0	0

B

Figure 15-9 Sample of tax tables for a biweekly payroll. **A**, Single persons. **B**, Married persons. (From U.S. Department of Treasury, Internal Revenue Service, Washington, DC, 2008.)

shown in Figure 15-9. If an employer's payroll period is every 2 weeks, the employer uses the tax table for a biweekly payroll period, looking up the amount of wages earned and the number of exemptions listed. Even if an employee does not work the entire payroll period, the employer should use the table for the established length of the payroll period. Current tax tables in their entirety are available on the website of the IRS.

Form W-4. All new employees should be asked to complete a form W-4 (Fig. 15-10) when they begin work. The W-4 identifies the employee's name, address, Social Security number, marital status, and the number of exemptions that he or she wishes to take for tax purposes. A personal allowances worksheet is available at the top of form W-4 to help the employee determine the number of exemptions that should be claimed. The more exemptions an employee claims, the less tax will be withheld from the employee's paycheck.

Employees should take only those exemptions to which they are entitled, or they may be underwithheld and owe significant tax at the end of the year. If an employee is grossly underwithheld, a penalty may be assessed to the employee for failure to pay enough tax. Employees may wish to claim fewer exemptions than those to which they are entitled to ensure that they have enough tax withheld throughout the year. If an employee believes he or she will owe significant tax at the end of the year, the employee may authorize additional tax to be withheld, as listed on line 6 of form W-4.

If an employee wishes to change the amount of tax withholding, the employee is required to complete a new form W-4. The new W-4 does not take effect until the date the employee lists on the form.

A form W-4 must be signed by an employee in order to be valid. The language on a form W-4 may not be altered by an employee. If an employee fails to turn in a form W-4, if the form is altered, or if it is otherwise not completed correctly, taxes will be withheld as though the employee were single with no dependents—this would be withholding at the highest rate possible.

FICA Tax. The Federal Insurance Contributions Act (FICA) includes provisions for Social Security tax and Medicare tax. Employees must pay these taxes, and an employer must match an employee's contribution. Tax rates and wages limits are identified in Figure 15-11. Using the

Form W-4 (2013)

Purpose. Complete Form W-4 so that your employer can withhold the correct federal income tax from your pay. Consider completing a new Form W-4 each year and when your personal or financial situation changes.

Exemption from withholding. If you are exempt, complete **only** lines 1, 2, 3, 4, and 7 and sign the form to validate it. Your exemption for 2013 expires February 17, 2014. See Pub. 505, Tax Withholding and Estimated Tax.

Note. If another person can claim you as a dependent on his or her tax return, you cannot claim exemption from withholding if your income exceeds $1,000 and includes more than $350 of unearned income (for example, interest and dividends).

Basic instructions. If you are not exempt, complete the **Personal Allowances Worksheet** below. The worksheets on page 2 further adjust your withholding allowances based on itemized deductions, certain credits, adjustments to income, or two-earners/multiple jobs situations.

Complete all worksheets that apply. However, you may claim fewer (or zero) allowances. For regular wages, withholding must be based on allowances you claimed and may not be a flat amount or percentage of wages.

Head of household. Generally, you can claim head of household filing status on your tax return only if you are unmarried and pay more than 50% of the costs of keeping up a home for yourself and your dependent(s) or other qualifying individuals. See Pub. 501, Exemptions, Standard Deduction, and Filing Information, for information.

Tax credits. You can take projected tax credits into account in figuring your allowable number of withholding allowances. Credits for child or dependent care expenses and the child tax credit may be claimed using the **Personal Allowances Worksheet** below. See Pub. 505 for information on converting your other credits into withholding allowances.

Nonwage income. If you have a large amount of nonwage income, such as interest or dividends, consider making estimated tax payments using Form 1040-ES, Estimated Tax for Individuals. Otherwise, you may owe additional tax. If you have pension or annuity income, see Pub. 505 to find out if you should adjust your withholding on Form W-4 or W-4P.

Two earners or multiple jobs. If you have a working spouse or more than one job, figure the total number of allowances you are entitled to claim on all jobs using worksheets from only one Form W-4. Your withholding usually will be most accurate when all allowances are claimed on the Form W-4 for the highest paying job and zero allowances are claimed on the others. See Pub. 505 for details.

Nonresident alien. If you are a nonresident alien, see Notice 1392, Supplemental Form W-4 Instructions for Nonresident Aliens, before completing this form.

Check your withholding. After your Form W-4 takes effect, use Pub. 505 to see how the amount you are having withheld compares to your projected total tax for 2013. See Pub. 505, especially if your earnings exceed $130,000 (Single) or $180,000 (Married).

Future developments. Information about any future developments affecting Form W-4 (such as legislation enacted after we release it) will be posted at *www.irs.gov/w4*.

Personal Allowances Worksheet (Keep for your records.)

A Enter "1" for **yourself** if no one else can claim you as a dependent . . . . . **A** ______

B Enter "1" if:
- You are single and have only one job; or
- You are married, have only one job, and your spouse does not work; or
- Your wages from a second job or your spouse's wages (the total of both) are $1,500 or less.

. . . **B** ______

C Enter "1" for your **spouse.** But, you may choose to enter "-0-" if you are married and have either a working spouse or more than one job. (Entering "-0-" may help you avoid having too little tax withheld.) . . . . . **C** ______

D Enter number of **dependents** (other than your spouse or yourself) you will claim on your tax return . . . . . **D** ______

E Enter "1" if you will file as **head of household** on your tax return (see conditions under **Head of household** above) . . **E** ______

F Enter "1" if you have at least $1,900 of **child or dependent care expenses** for which you plan to claim a credit . . . **F** ______
(**Note.** Do **not** include child support payments. See Pub. 503, Child and Dependent Care Expenses, for details.)

G **Child Tax Credit** (including additional child tax credit). See Pub. 972, Child Tax Credit, for more information.
- If your total income will be less than $65,000 ($95,000 if married), enter "2" for each eligible child; then **less** "1" if you have three to six eligible children or **less** "2" if you have seven or more eligible children.
- If your total income will be between $65,000 and $84,000 ($95,000 and $119,000 if married), enter "1" for each eligible child . . . **G** ______

H Add lines A through G and enter total here. (**Note.** This may be different from the number of exemptions you claim on your tax return.) ▶ **H** ______

For accuracy, **complete all worksheets that apply.**
- If you plan to **itemize** or **claim adjustments to income** and want to reduce your withholding, see the **Deductions and Adjustments Worksheet** on page 2.
- If you are **single and have more than one job** or are **married and you and your spouse both work** and the combined earnings from all jobs exceed $40,000 ($10,000 if married), see the **Two-Earners/Multiple Jobs Worksheet** on page 2 to avoid having too little tax withheld.
- If **neither** of the above situations applies, **stop here** and enter the number from line H on line 5 of Form W-4 below.

Separate here and give Form W-4 to your employer. Keep the top part for your records.

Form **W-4** Department of the Treasury Internal Revenue Service

Employee's Withholding Allowance Certificate

▶ **Whether you are entitled to claim a certain number of allowances or exemption from withholding is subject to review by the IRS. Your employer may be required to send a copy of this form to the IRS.**

OMB No. 1545-0074 **2013**

1 Your first name and middle initial	Last name	2 **Your social security number**
Home address (number and street or rural route)	3 ☐ Single ☐ Married ☐ Married, but withhold at higher Single rate. **Note.** If married, but legally separated, or spouse is a nonresident alien, check the "Single" box.	
City or town, state, and ZIP code	4 **If your last name differs from that shown on your social security card, check here. You must call 1-800-772-1213 for a replacement card.** ▶ ☐	

5 Total number of allowances you are claiming (from line **H** above **or** from the applicable worksheet on page 2) **5** ______

6 Additional amount, if any, you want withheld from each paycheck . . . . . **6** $ ______

7 I claim exemption from withholding for 2013, and I certify that I meet **both** of the following conditions for exemption.
- Last year I had a right to a refund of **all** federal income tax withheld because I had **no** tax liability, **and**
- This year I expect a refund of **all** federal income tax withheld because I expect to have **no** tax liability.

If you meet both conditions, write "Exempt" here . . . . . ▶ **7** ______

Under penalties of perjury, I declare that I have examined this certificate and, to the best of my knowledge and belief, it is true, correct, and complete.

Employee's signature
(This form is not valid unless you sign it.) ▶ **Date** ▶

8 Employer's name and address (Employer: Complete lines 8 and 10 only if sending to the IRS.)	9 Office code (optional)	10 Employer identification number (EIN)

For Privacy Act and Paperwork Reduction Act Notice, see page 2. Cat. No. 10220Q Form **W-4** (2013)

Figure 15-10 Form W-4 identifies an employee's exemptions for tax purposes. (From U.S. Department of the Treasury, Internal Revenue Service, Washington, DC, 2013.)

Form W-4 (2013) Page 2

Deductions and Adjustments Worksheet

Note. Use this worksheet *only* if you plan to itemize deductions or claim certain credits or adjustments to income.

1 Enter an estimate of your 2013 itemized deductions. These include qualifying home mortgage interest, charitable contributions, state and local taxes, medical expenses in excess of 10% (7.5% if either you or your spouse was born before January 2, 1949) of your income, and miscellaneous deductions. For 2013, you may have to reduce your itemized deductions if your income is over $300,000 and you are married filing jointly or are a qualifying widow(er); $275,000 if you are head of household; $250,000 if you are single and not head of household or a qualifying widow(er); or $150,000 if you are married filing separately. See Pub. 505 for details . . . **1** $

2 Enter: { $12,200 if married filing jointly or qualifying widow(er); $8,950 if head of household; $6,100 if single or married filing separately } . . . **2** $

3 **Subtract** line 2 from line 1. If zero or less, enter "-0-" . . . **3** $

4 Enter an estimate of your 2013 adjustments to income and any additional standard deduction (see Pub. 505) **4** $

5 **Add** lines 3 and 4 and enter the total. (Include any amount for credits from the *Converting Credits to Withholding Allowances for 2013 Form W-4* worksheet in Pub. 505.) . . . **5** $

6 Enter an estimate of your 2013 nonwage income (such as dividends or interest) . . . **6** $

7 **Subtract** line 6 from line 5. If zero or less, enter "-0-" . . . **7** $

8 **Divide** the amount on line 7 by $3,900 and enter the result here. Drop any fraction . . . **8**

9 Enter the number from the **Personal Allowances Worksheet,** line H, page 1 . . . **9**

10 **Add** lines 8 and 9 and enter the total here. If you plan to use the **Two-Earners/Multiple Jobs Worksheet,** also enter this total on line 1 below. Otherwise, **stop here** and enter this total on Form W-4, line 5, page 1 **10**

Two-Earners/Multiple Jobs Worksheet (See *Two earners or multiple jobs* on page 1.)

Note. Use this worksheet *only* if the instructions under line H on page 1 direct you here.

1 Enter the number from line H, page 1 (or from line 10 above if you used the **Deductions and Adjustments Worksheet**) **1**

2 Find the number in **Table 1** below that applies to the **LOWEST** paying job and enter it here. **However,** if you are married filing jointly and wages from the highest paying job are $65,000 or less, do not enter more than "3" . . . **2**

3 If line 1 is **more than or equal to** line 2, subtract line 2 from line 1. Enter the result here (if zero, enter "-0-") and on Form W-4, line 5, page 1. **Do not** use the rest of this worksheet . . . **3**

Note. If line 1 is **less than** line 2, enter "-0-" on Form W-4, line 5, page 1. Complete lines 4 through 9 below to figure the additional withholding amount necessary to avoid a year-end tax bill.

4 Enter the number from line 2 of this worksheet . . . **4**

5 Enter the number from line 1 of this worksheet . . . **5**

6 **Subtract** line 5 from line 4 . . . **6**

7 Find the amount in **Table 2** below that applies to the **HIGHEST** paying job and enter it here . . . **7** $

8 **Multiply** line 7 by line 6 and enter the result here. This is the additional annual withholding needed . . **8** $

9 Divide line 8 by the number of pay periods remaining in 2013. For example, divide by 25 if you are paid every two weeks and you complete this form on a date in January when there are 25 pay periods remaining in 2013. Enter the result here and on Form W-4, line 6, page 1. This is the additional amount to be withheld from each paycheck **9** $

Table 1

Married Filing Jointly		All Others	
If wages from **LOWEST** paying job are—	Enter on line 2 above	If wages from **LOWEST** paying job are—	Enter on line 2 above
$0 - $5,000	0	$0 - $8,000	0
5,001 - 13,000	1	8,001 - 16,000	1
13,001 - 24,000	2	16,001 - 25,000	2
24,001 - 26,000	3	25,001 - 30,000	3
26,001 - 30,000	4	30,001 - 40,000	4
30,001 - 42,000	5	40,001 - 50,000	5
42,001 - 48,000	6	50,001 - 70,000	6
48,001 - 55,000	7	70,001 - 80,000	7
55,001 - 65,000	8	80,001 - 95,000	8
65,001 - 75,000	9	95,001 - 120,000	9
75,001 - 85,000	10	120,001 and over	10
85,001 - 97,000	11		
97,001 - 110,000	12		
110,001 - 120,000	13		
120,001 - 135,000	14		
135,001 and over	15		

Table 2

Married Filing Jointly		All Others	
If wages from **HIGHEST** paying job are—	Enter on line 7 above	If wages from **HIGHEST** paying job are—	Enter on line 7 above
$0 - $72,000	$590	$0 - $37,000	$590
72,001 - 130,000	980	37,001 - 80,000	980
130,001 - 200,000	1,090	80,001 - 175,000	1,090
200,001 - 345,000	1,290	175,001 - 385,000	1,290
345,001 - 385,000	1,370	385,001 and over	1,540
385,001 and over	1,540		

Privacy Act and Paperwork Reduction Act Notice. We ask for the information on this form to carry out the Internal Revenue laws of the United States. Internal Revenue Code sections 3402(f)(2) and 6109 and their regulations require you to provide this information; your employer uses it to determine your federal income tax withholding. Failure to provide a properly completed form will result in your being treated as a single person who claims no withholding allowances; providing fraudulent information may subject you to penalties. Routine uses of this information include giving it to the Department of Justice for civil and criminal litigation; to cities, states, the District of Columbia, and U.S. commonwealths and possessions for use in administering their tax laws; and to the Department of Health and Human Services for use in the National Directory of New Hires. We may also disclose this information to other countries under a tax treaty, to federal and state agencies to enforce federal nontax criminal laws, or to federal law enforcement and intelligence agencies to combat terrorism.

You are not required to provide the information requested on a form that is subject to the Paperwork Reduction Act unless the form displays a valid OMB control number. Books or records relating to a form or its instructions must be retained as long as their contents may become material in the administration of any Internal Revenue law. Generally, tax returns and return information are confidential, as required by Code section 6103.

The average time and expenses required to complete and file this form will vary depending on individual circumstances. For estimated averages, see the instructions for your income tax return.

If you have suggestions for making this form simpler, we would be happy to hear from you. See the instructions for your income tax return.

Figure 15-10, cont'd

Social Security and Medicare tax limits and rates

Type of tax	Wage base limit	Employee rate	Employer rate
Social Security	$113,700	6.2% of wages	6.2% of wages
Medicare	No wage limit; all wages are subject to Medicare tax	1.45% of wages	1.45% of wages

Figure 15-11 The 2013 Social Security and Medicare tax limits and rates. (From U.S. Department of the Treasury, Internal Revenue Service, Washington, DC, 2012.)

amounts shown in Figure 15-11, employees who earn more than $113,700 in 2013 would not have Social Security tax withheld on any earned amounts greater than $113,700, although Medicare tax would still be owed on all wages earned for that calendar year.

State Income Tax. Depending on the state in which the employee works or resides, state income tax may also be required to be withheld from an employee's wages. Employees who reside in a different state from the one in which they work may have to file an exemption from tax in the employer's state. Depending on arrangements made between neighboring states, employers may be able to withhold taxes from other states for employees who reside out of state. A few states do not have any state income tax.

Tax Reports and Deposits. All employers are required to file tax reports to the government and to make deposits for payroll taxes withheld. Each employer is assigned a unique **employer identification number (EIN)** to use when reporting employment taxes or when giving tax statements to employees. An EIN is a nine-digit number (00-0000000) issued by the IRS. This number is used to identify the tax account of the employer. The EIN should be used on all documents sent to the IRS or the Social Security Administration.

Employers are required to deposit the employee's and employer's portions of income tax, Social Security, and Medicare tax either monthly or biweekly. The deposit schedule is determined by the amount of taxes previously reported by the employer in a four-quarter look-back period. Employers are required to deposit all of the taxes owed on or before the deposit due date. Deposits can be made by using electronic deposit via the Electronic Federal Tax Payment System or by means of deposit coupons.

Form 941, Employer's Quarterly Federal Tax Return (Fig. 15-12), and Form 941-V are used when taxes owed are reported and deposited. All employers (with few exceptions) are required to file Form 941. Employers should file only one Form 941 per quarter and should include only one quarter (3 months' worth) of wages on a return. Employers who fail to pay all of the tax due will face a penalty.

Federal Unemployment Tax. Employees who lose their jobs are often paid unemployment compensation that is funded in part by the federal unemployment tax (FUTA). Employers, not employees, pay FUTA tax. Generally, employers are required to pay FUTA tax if they pay more than $1500 in wages to nonfarm or nonhousehold employees. Beginning July 1, 2011, the FUTA tax rate was 6.0% of the first $7000 in wages paid to each employee during the year. In some states, the employer may also be required to pay state unemployment tax. Certain types of employees may be exempt from this tax. FUTA tax is calculated quarterly, and, depending on the amount owed, deposits may be due quarterly. FUTA tax is reported on Form 940 (Fig. 15-13) or 940-EZ.

Depending on state requirements, the employer may be required to pay taxes to a state unemployment fund. Employers should check with individual state agencies to determine what state unemployment taxes may be due.

Form W-2. Employers are required to report each employee's name, Social Security number (SSN), wages earned, and taxes paid each year. An employee's earnings from the previous year's are reported in January on a W-2 form. The W-2 form is a federal form that summarizes the employee's payroll record for the year (Fig. 15-14). W-2 information can be electronically filed with the IRS. Employers should ask for the employee's Social Security card, and the name of the employee should be entered on the W-2 exactly as it appears on the card. If the name on the card is not the same as the employee's current name (as in cases of marriage or divorce), the employee should be instructed to obtain a new card from the Social Security Administration. If an employer wishes to verify an employee's SSN as listed on a W-2, up to 50 names may be verified by calling the local Social Security office.

Human Resource Records

Individual files should be kept for every employee of an organization and that file should contain only information that is objective and well substantiated. Items such as the employee's application, résumé, form W-4, records of employee evaluations, letters of commendation, and any written reprimands may be kept in the employee's human resource file. Subjective information and items that are not substantiated do not belong in an employee's file.

Form **941 for 2013: Employer's QUARTERLY Federal Tax Return** 950113
(Rev. January 2013) Department of the Treasury — Internal Revenue Service OMB No. 1545-0029

Employer identification number (EIN) [ ][ ] – [ ][ ][ ][ ][ ][ ][ ]

Name *(not your trade name)* [ ]

Trade name *(if any)* [ ]

Address [ ]
Number Street Suite or room number
[ ]
City State ZIP code

Report for this Quarter of 2013
(Check one.)

- ☐ **1:** January, February, March
- ☐ **2:** April, May, June
- ☐ **3:** July, August, September
- ☐ **4:** October, November, December

Instructions and prior year forms are available at *www.irs.gov/form941*.

Read the separate instructions before you complete Form 941. Type or print within the boxes.

Part 1: Answer these questions for this quarter.

		Column 1		Column 2		
1	**Number of employees who received wages, tips, or other compensation for the pay period including:** ***Mar. 12*** **(Quarter 1),** ***June 12*** **(Quarter 2),** ***Sept. 12*** **(Quarter 3), or** ***Dec. 12*** **(Quarter 4)**				1	
2	**Wages, tips, and other compensation**				2	.
3	**Income tax withheld from wages, tips, and other compensation**				3	.
4	**If no wages, tips, and other compensation are subject to social security or Medicare tax**					☐ **Check and go to line 6.**
5a	**Taxable social security wages** . .	.	× .124 =	.		
5b	**Taxable social security tips** . . .	.	× .124 =	.		
5c	**Taxable Medicare wages & tips** . .	.	× .029 =	.		
5d	**Taxable wages & tips subject to Additional Medicare Tax withholding**	.	× .009 =	.		
5e	**Add Column 2 from lines 5a, 5b, 5c, and 5d**				5e	.
5f	**Section 3121(q) Notice and Demand—Tax due on unreported tips** (see instructions) . .				5f	.
6	**Total taxes before adjustments** (add lines 3, 5e, and 5f)				6	.
7	**Current quarter's adjustment for fractions of cents**				7	.
8	**Current quarter's adjustment for sick pay**				8	.
9	**Current quarter's adjustments for tips and group-term life insurance**				9	.
10	**Total taxes after adjustments.** Combine lines 6 through 9				10	.
11	**Total deposits for this quarter, including overpayment applied from a prior quarter and overpayment applied from Form 941-X or Form 944-X filed in the current quarter** . . .				11	.
12a	**COBRA premium assistance payments** (see instructions)				12a	.
12b	**Number of individuals provided COBRA premium assistance** . .					
13	**Add lines 11 and 12a**				13	.
14	**Balance due.** If line 10 is more than line 13, enter the difference and see instructions . . .				14	.
15	**Overpayment.** If line 13 is more than line 10, enter the difference	.				Check one: ☐ Apply to next return. ☐ Send a refund.

► **You MUST complete both pages of Form 941 and SIGN it.** Next ➡

For Privacy Act and Paperwork Reduction Act Notice, see the back of the Payment Voucher. Cat. No. 17001Z Form **941** (Rev. 1-2013)

Figure 15-12 Form 941, Employer's Quarterly Federal Tax Return, is used to report taxes owed. (From U.S. Department of the Treasury, Internal Revenue Service, Washington, DC, 2013.)

Continued

950213

Name *(not your trade name)* | **Employer identification number (EIN)**

Part 2: Tell us about your deposit schedule and tax liability for this quarter.

If you are unsure about whether you are a monthly schedule depositor or a semiweekly schedule depositor, see Pub. 15 (Circular E), section 11.

16 Check one: ☐ **Line 10 on this return is less than $2,500 or line 10 on the return for the prior quarter was less than $2,500, and you did not incur a $100,000 next-day deposit obligation during the current quarter.** If line 10 for the prior quarter was less than $2,500 but line 10 on this return is $100,000 or more, you must provide a record of your federal tax liability. If you are a monthly schedule depositor, complete the deposit schedule below; if you are a semiweekly schedule depositor, attach Schedule B (Form 941). Go to Part 3.

☐ **You were a monthly schedule depositor for the entire quarter.** Enter your tax liability for each month and total liability for the quarter, then go to Part 3.

Tax liability: Month 1 ______ .

Month 2 ______ .

Month 3 ______ .

Total liability for quarter ______ . **Total must equal line 10.**

☐ **You were a semiweekly schedule depositor for any part of this quarter.** Complete Schedule B (Form 941), Report of Tax Liability for Semiweekly Schedule Depositors, and attach it to Form 941.

Part 3: Tell us about your business. If a question does NOT apply to your business, leave it blank.

17 If your business has closed or you stopped paying wages . . . . ☐ Check here, and

enter the final date you paid wages ___ / ___ / ___ .

18 If you are a seasonal employer and you do not have to file a return for every quarter of the year . . ☐ Check here.

Part 4: May we speak with your third-party designee?

Do you want to allow an employee, a paid tax preparer, or another person to discuss this return with the IRS? See the instructions for details.

☐ Yes. Designee's name and phone number ______ ______

Select a 5-digit Personal Identification Number (PIN) to use when talking to the IRS. ☐☐☐☐☐

☐ No.

Part 5: Sign here. You MUST complete both pages of Form 941 and SIGN it.

Under penalties of perjury, I declare that I have examined this return, including accompanying schedules and statements, and to the best of my knowledge and belief, it is true, correct, and complete. Declaration of preparer (other than taxpayer) is based on all information of which preparer has any knowledge.

X Sign your name here ______

Print your name here ______

Print your title here ______

Date ___ / ___ / ___

Best daytime phone ______

Paid Preparer Use Only Check if you are self-employed . . . ☐

Preparer's name		PTIN	
Preparer's signature		Date	/ /
Firm's name (or yours if self-employed)		EIN	
Address		Phone	
City	State	ZIP code	

Page **2** Form **941** (Rev. 1-2013)

Figure 15-12, cont'd

Form 941-V, Payment Voucher

Purpose of Form

Complete Form 941-V, Payment Voucher, if you are making a payment with Form 941, Employer's QUARTERLY Federal Tax Return. We will use the completed voucher to credit your payment more promptly and accurately, and to improve our service to you.

Making Payments With Form 941

To avoid a penalty, make your payment with Form 941 **only if:**

- Your total taxes after adjustments for either the current quarter or the preceding quarter (Form 941, line 10) are less than $2,500, you did not incur a $100,000 next-day deposit obligation during the current quarter, and you are paying in full with a timely filed return, or
- You are a monthly schedule depositor making a payment in accordance with the Accuracy of Deposits Rule. See section 11 of Pub. 15 (Circular E), Employer's Tax Guide, for details. In this case, the amount of your payment may be $2,500 or more.

Otherwise, you must make deposits by electronic funds transfer. See section 11 of Pub. 15 (Circular E) for deposit instructions. Do not use Form 941-V to make federal tax deposits.

Caution. *Use Form 941-V when making any payment with Form 941. However, if you pay an amount with Form 941 that should have been deposited, you may be subject to a penalty. See* Deposit Penalties *in section 11 of Pub. 15 (Circular E).*

Specific Instructions

Box 1—Employer identification number (EIN). If you do not have an EIN, you may apply for one online. Go to IRS.gov and click on the *Apply for an EIN Online* link under "Tools." You may also apply for an EIN by calling 1-800-829-4933, or you can fax or mail Form SS-4, Application for Employer Identification Number, to the IRS. If you have not received your EIN by the due date of Form 941, write "Applied For" and the date you applied in this entry space.

Box 2—Amount paid. Enter the amount paid with Form 941.

Box 3—Tax period. Darken the circle identifying the quarter for which the payment is made. Darken only one circle.

Box 4—Name and address. Enter your name and address as shown on Form 941.

- Enclose your check or money order made payable to the "United States Treasury." Be sure to enter your EIN, "Form 941," and the tax period on your check or money order. Do not send cash. Do not staple Form 941-V or your payment to Form 941 (or to each other).
- Detach Form 941-V and send it with your payment and Form 941 to the address in the Instructions for Form 941.

Note. You must also complete the entity information above Part 1 on Form 941.

▼ Detach Here and Mail With Your Payment and Form 941. ▼

Form **941-V** Department of the Treasury Internal Revenue Service	**Payment Voucher** ► Do not staple this voucher or your payment to Form 941.		OMB No. 1545-0029 **2013**
1 Enter your employer identification number (EIN).	**2** **Enter the amount of your payment.** ► Make your check or money order payable to **"United States Treasury"**	Dollars	Cents
3 Tax Period	**4** Enter your business name (individual name if sole proprietor).		
○ 1st Quarter ○ 3rd Quarter	Enter your address.		
○ 2nd Quarter ○ 4th Quarter	Enter your city, state, and ZIP code.		

Figure 15-12, cont'd

Form **940 for 2012: Employer's Annual Federal Unemployment (FUTA) Tax Return** 850112

Department of the Treasury — Internal Revenue Service OMB No. 1545-0028

Employer identification number (EIN) ☐☐ – ☐☐☐☐☐☐☐

Name *(not your trade name)*

Trade name *(if any)*

Address

Number Street Suite or room number

City State ZIP code

Type of Return
(Check all that apply.)

☐ **a.** Amended

☐ **b.** Successor employer

☐ **c.** No payments to employees in 2012

☐ **d.** Final: Business closed or stopped paying wages

Instructions and prior-year forms are available at *www.irs.gov/form940.*

Read the separate instructions before you complete this form. Please type or print within the boxes.

Part 1: Tell us about your return. If any line does NOT apply, leave it blank.

1a **If you had to pay state unemployment tax in one state only, enter the state abbreviation** . 1a ☐☐

1b **If you had to pay state unemployment tax in more than one state, you are a multi-state employer** . . . . . 1b ☐ Check here. Complete Schedule A (Form 940).

2 **If you paid wages in a state that is subject to CREDIT REDUCTION** . . . . . 2 ☐ Check here. Complete Schedule A (Form 940).

Part 2: Determine your FUTA tax before adjustments for 2012. If any line does NOT apply, leave it blank.

3 **Total payments to all employees** . . . . . 3 ______ .

4 **Payments exempt from FUTA tax** . . . . . 4 ______ .

Check all that apply: 4a ☐ Fringe benefits 4c ☐ Retirement/Pension 4e ☐ Other
4b ☐ Group-term life insurance 4d ☐ Dependent care

5 **Total of payments made to each employee in excess of $7,000** . . . . . 5 ______ .

6 **Subtotal** (line 4 + line 5 = line 6) . . . . . 6 ______ .

7 **Total taxable FUTA wages** (line 3 – line 6 = line 7) (see instructions) . . . . . 7 ______ .

8 **FUTA tax before adjustments** (line 7 x .006 = line 8) . . . . . 8 ______ .

Part 3: Determine your adjustments. If any line does NOT apply, leave it blank.

9 **If ALL of the taxable FUTA wages you paid were excluded from state unemployment tax, multiply line 7 by .054** (line 7 × .054 = line 9). Go to line 12 . . . . . 9 ______ .

10 **If SOME of the taxable FUTA wages you paid were excluded from state unemployment tax, OR you paid ANY state unemployment tax late** (after the due date for filing Form 940), complete the worksheet in the instructions. Enter the amount from line 7 of the worksheet . . 10 ______ .

11 **If credit reduction applies,** enter the total from Schedule A (Form 940) . . . . . 11 ______ .

Part 4: Determine your FUTA tax and balance due or overpayment for 2012. If any line does NOT apply, leave it blank.

12 **Total FUTA tax after adjustments** (lines 8 + 9 + 10 + 11 = line 12) . . . . . 12 ______ .

13 **FUTA tax deposited for the year, including any overpayment applied from a prior year** . 13 ______ .

14 **Balance due** (If line 12 is more than line 13, enter the excess on line 14.)
- If line 14 is more than $500, you must deposit your tax.
- If line 14 is $500 or less, you may pay with this return. (see instructions) . . . . . 14 ______ .

15 **Overpayment** (If line 13 is more than line 12, enter the excess on line 15 and check a box below.) . . . . . 15 ______ .

► You **MUST** complete both pages of this form and **SIGN** it. Check one: ☐ Apply to next return. ☐ Send a refund.

Next ►

For Privacy Act and Paperwork Reduction Act Notice, see the back of Form 940-V, Payment Voucher. Cat. No. 11234O Form **940** (2012)

Figure 15-13 Federal Form 940 is used to report federal unemployment tax. (From U.S. Department of the Treasury, Internal Revenue Service, Washington, DC, 2013.)

850212

Name (*not your trade name*) | Employer identification number (EIN)

Part 5: Report your FUTA tax liability by quarter only if line 12 is more than $500. If not, go to Part 6.

16 Report the amount of your FUTA tax liability for each quarter; do NOT enter the amount you deposited. If you had no liability for a quarter, leave the line blank.

16a 1st quarter (January 1 – March 31) . . . . **16a** ________ .

16b 2nd quarter (April 1 – June 30) . . . . **16b** ________ .

16c 3rd quarter (July 1 – September 30) . . . . **16c** ________ .

16d 4th quarter (October 1 – December 31) . . . . **16d** ________ .

17 Total tax liability for the year (lines 16a + 16b + 16c + 16d = line 17) **17** ________ . **Total must equal line 12.**

Part 6: May we speak with your third-party designee?

Do you want to allow an employee, a paid tax preparer, or another person to discuss this return with the IRS? See the instructions for details.

☐ **Yes.** Designee's name and phone number ________ ________

Select a 5-digit Personal Identification Number (PIN) to use when talking to IRS ☐☐☐☐☐

☐ **No.**

Part 7: Sign here. You MUST complete both pages of this form and SIGN it.

Under penalties of perjury, I declare that I have examined this return, including accompanying schedules and statements, and to the best of my knowledge and belief, it is true, correct, and complete, and that no part of any payment made to a state unemployment fund claimed as a credit was, or is to be, deducted from the payments made to employees. Declaration of preparer (other than taxpayer) is based on all information of which preparer has any knowledge.

✗ Sign your name here ________

Print your name here ________

Print your title here ________

Date ___ / ___ / ___

Best daytime phone ________

Paid Preparer Use Only

Check if you are self-employed . . . ☐

Preparer's name ________ PTIN ________

Preparer's signature ________ Date ___ / ___ / ___

Firm's name (or yours if self-employed) ________ EIN ________

Address ________ Phone ________

City ________ State ________ ZIP code ________

Page **2** Form **940** (2012)

Figure 15-13, cont'd

Continued

Form 940-V, Payment Voucher

Purpose of Form

Complete Form 940-V, Payment Voucher, if you are making a payment with Form 940, Employer's Annual Federal Unemployment (FUTA) Tax Return. We will use the completed voucher to credit your payment more promptly and accurately, and to improve our service to you.

Making Payments With Form 940

To avoid a penalty, make your payment with your 2012 Form 940 **only if** your FUTA tax for the fourth quarter (plus any undeposited amounts from earlier quarters) is $500 or less. If your total FUTA tax after adjustments (Form 940, line 12) is more than $500, you must make deposits by electronic funds transfer. See *When Must You Deposit Your FUTA Tax?* in the Instructions for Form 940. Also see sections 11 and 14 of Pub. 15 (Circular E), Employer's Tax Guide, for more information about deposits.

Caution. *Use Form 940-V when making any payment with Form 940. However, if you pay an amount with Form 940 that should have been deposited, you may be subject to a penalty. See* Deposit Penalties *in section 11 of Pub. 15 (Circular E).*

Specific Instructions

Box 1—Employer Identification Number (EIN). If you do not have an EIN, you may apply for one online. Go to IRS.gov and click on the *Apply for an EIN Online* link under *Tools*. You may also apply for an EIN by calling 1-800-829-4933, or you can fax or mail Form SS-4, Application for Employer Identification Number. If you have not received your EIN by the due date of Form 940, write "Applied For" and the date you applied in this entry space.

Box 2—Amount paid. Enter the amount paid with Form 940.

Box 3—Name and address. Enter your name and address as shown on Form 940.

- Enclose your check or money order made payable to the "United States Treasury." Be sure to enter your EIN, "Form 940," and "2012" on your check or money order. Do not send cash. Do not staple Form 940-V or your payment to Form 940 (or to each other).

- Detach Form 940-V and send it with your payment and Form 940 to the address provided in the Instructions for Form 940.

Note. You must also complete the entity information above Part 1 on Form 940.

▼ **Detach Here and Mail With Your Payment and Form 940.** ▼

Form **940-V** Department of the Treasury Internal Revenue Service	**Payment Voucher** ► **Do not staple or attach this voucher to your payment.**	OMB No. 1545-0028 **2012**
1 Enter your employer identification number (EIN).	2 **Enter the amount of your payment.** ► Make your check or money order payable to **"United States Treasury"**	Dollars / Cents
	3 Enter your business name (individual name if sole proprietor). Enter your address. Enter your city, state, and ZIP code.	

Figure 15-13, cont'd

a Employee's social security number ###-##-####	OMB No. 1545-0008	Safe, accurate, FAST! Use IRS e-file	Visit the IRS website at *www.irs.gov/efile*.
b Employer identification number (EIN) #######		1 Wages, tips, other compensation 37439.23	2 Federal income tax withheld 4565.72
c Employer's name, address, and ZIP code Happy Valley Medical Group 5222 E Baseline Rd Gilbert AZ 85234		3 Social security wages 37439.23	4 Social security tax withheld 2321.23
		5 Medicare wages and tips 37439.23	6 Medicare tax withheld 542.89
		7 Social security tips	8 Allocated tips
d Control number		9 Advance EIC payment	10 Dependent care benefits
e Employee's first name and initial Last name Suff. Amy G Dixon 1567 Meadow Valley Rd Harvester AZ 85000		11 Nonqualified plans	12a See instructions for box 12 Code
		13 Statutory employee ☐ Retirement plan ☐ Third-party sick pay ☐	12b Code
		14 Other	12c Code
f Employee's address and ZIP code			12d Code

15 State	Employer's state ID number	16 State wages, tips, etc.	17 State income tax	18 Local wages, tips, etc.	19 Local income tax	20 Locality name
AZ	######	37439.23	374.39			

Form **W-2** **Wage and Tax Statement** **2013** Department of the Treasury—Internal Revenue Service

Copy B—To Be Filed With Employee's FEDERAL Tax Return.
This information is being furnished to the Internal Revenue Service.

Figure 15-14 Portion of a W-2 form. (From U.S. Department of the Treasury, Internal Revenue Service, Washington, DC, 2013.)

Employee Evaluation

As mentioned previously, many employees when initially hired serve a probationary period of 3 to 6 months. Within that time, the employee has a chance to become familiar with the procedures of the office. Near the end of the probationary period, a review of the employee's performance is conducted, and the employer ascertains whether the employee should remain permanently.

After the initial review, a **performance review** then should be conducted on a regular basis. No more than 1 year should pass between reviews. A schedule for employee reviews should be included in the organization's policy manual. In addition to receiving feedback on individual performance, an employee usually receives a pay increase based on performance at the time of the review. This evaluation also gives the employee and the employer a chance to set goals for performance in the coming year. The evaluation process provides an employee and an employer the opportunity to offer suggestions and feedback.

All employees should be given a performance review. Reviews should not be conducted only for employees who need to improve job skills. A review gives an employer the chance to notify the employee regarding any behavior that needs correction or modification, and it gives the employer a chance to praise an employee for a job well done.

It is important that performance reviews be objective and honest. Employees should not be given false praise if performance is less than acceptable. Problems may result if a longtime employee is suddenly discharged after receiving exceptional reviews throughout the years. Performance reviews are based on fact, and an employee's file should contain all pertinent factual information about the employee, whether positive or negative, and should accurately reflect the employee's performance on the job.

Essentials of a Performance Review

When an employee performance review is conducted, the evaluation (Fig. 15-15) should be based on objective criteria that can be evidenced by action on the job. On the evaluation form itself, such information as the employee's name, date of hire, and current position with the organization is included.

The employee's direct supervisor then ranks the employee's performance on several criteria, such as quality and quantity of work, judgment, and other items as listed in Figure 15-15. The supervisor should rate the employee objectively, based on the criteria specified, and should be very careful not to include any personal bias. The example in Figure 15-15 allows for detailed assessment of an employee's performance. It allows the employer to address concerns and provides an opportunity to document the employee's plan for personal growth. A performance review may be conducted by more than one reviewer to ensure that no misunderstanding occurs. In some instances, employees who work with an employee may be asked to give feedback on the employee's performance.

PERFORMANCE EVALUATION AND DEVELOPMENT PLAN
(OFFICE AND CLERICAL)

NAME: ____________________ DATE OF EVALUATION: ____________________

DATE OF HIRE: ____________________ DEPARTMENT: ____________________

JOB TITLE: ____________________ SUPERVISOR: ____________________

DATE APPOINTED THIS JOB: ____________________ MANAGER: ____________________

LAST REVIEW DATE: ____________________ LAST REVIEW RATING: ____________________

NEXT REVIEW DATE: ____________________ CURRENT REVIEW RATING: ____________________

PURPOSE

The purpose of this evaluation is to:

1. SET GOALS WITHIN SCOPE OF PRESENT JOB.
2. COMMUNICATE OPENLY ABOUT PERFORMANCE.
3. EVALUATE PAST PERFORMANCE.
4. DISCUSS FUTURE DEVELOPMENT PLANS FOR GROWTH.

INSTRUCTIONS

1. Supervisor to review form prior to completion. If specific items are not applicable they should be left blank.
2. Supervisor and employee to review job description prior to review.
3. In "COMMENTS" section supervisor may indicate which factors should be more heavily weighted in this particular evaluation.
4. Comments should be specific and job-related. All appropriate evaluation factors should be commented on to some degree.

I. POSITION OBJECTIVES AND MAJOR RESPONSIBILITIES. Summarize specific responsibilities of the job.

____

____

____

II. ACCOMPLISHMENTS AND/OR IMPROVEMENTS. What specific accomplishments and/or improvements has employee made since last review with respect to set goals?

____

____

____

PLEASE CONSIDER THE EMPLOYEE'S DEMONSTRATED PERFORMANCE AND MARK THE CIRCLE WHICH MOST CLOSELY DESCRIBES THAT PERFORMANCE.

4 - Performance consistently far exceeds expectations and requirements.
3 - Performance consistently exceeds normal expectations and job requirements.
2 - Performance consistently meets expectations and job requirements
1 - Performance usually meets expectations and minimum job requirements.
0 - Performance does not meet job requirements.

– CONTINUED, NEXT PAGE –

Figure 15-15 A performance review gives an employer and an employee an opportunity to review past performance and to make plans for future growth. (Form courtesy of Bibbero Systems, Inc., Petaluma, California, 800-242-2376; fax, 800-242-9330; www.bibbero.com.)

1. WORK QUALITY: CONSIDER COMPLETENESS, ACCURACY, NEATNESS AND RELIABILITY .

○ 0 ○ 1 ○ 2 ○ 3 ○ 4

2. WORK QUANTITY: CONSIDER ACCEPTABLE LEVEL EXPECTED AND TIME UTILIZATION.

○ 0 ○ 1 ○ 2 ○ 3 ○ 4

3. JUDGMENT: CONSIDER ABILITY TO MAKE WELL-REASONED, SOUND DECISIONS WHICH AFFECT WORK PERFORMANCE.

○ 0 ○ 1 ○ 2 ○ 3 ○ 4

4. INITIATIVE: CONSIDER JOB INTEREST, DEDICATION AND WILLINGNESS TO EXTEND ONESELF TO COMPLETE ASSIGNED TASKS. CONSIDER RESOURCEFULNESS.

○ 0 ○ 1 ○ 2 ○ 3 ○ 4

5. TEAMWORK: CONSIDER WORKING RELATIONSHIPS WITH FELLOW EMPLOYEES AND MANAGEMENT WITHIN THE WORK ENVIRONMENT .

○ 0 ○ 1 ○ 2 ○ 3 ○ 4

6. JOB UNDERSTANDING: CONSIDER KNOWLEDGE OF SPECIFIC JOB FUNCTION

○ 0 ○ 1 ○ 2 ○ 3 ○ 4

– CONTINUED, NEXT PAGE –

Figure 15-15, cont'd

Continued

7. DEPENDABILITY: CONSIDER ATTENDANCE, PUNCTUALITY, IDLE TIME AND RELIANCE THAT CAN BE PLACED ON EMPLOYEE TO PERSEVERE AND CARRY THROUGH TO COMPLETION ALL ASSIGNED TASKS

○ 0 ○ 1 ○ 2 ○ 3 ○ 4

8. COMPLIANCE WITH COMPANY POLICIES: DOES THE EMPLOYEE COMPLY WITH RULES AND REGULATIONS THAT APPLY TO SAFETY, FAIR EMPLOYMENT PRACTICES AND GENERAL ADMINISTRATIVE PROCEDURE.

○ 0 ○ 1 ○ 2 ○ 3 ○ 4

SPECIFIC PERFORMANCE	1	2	3	4	COMMENTS
A. Ability to handle scheduling:					
B. Willingness to work OT when necessary:					
C. Handling of calls and follow-up:					
D. Maintenance of equipment:					
E. Ability to handle patient complaints:					
F. Tact in dealing with patients:					
G. Speed (in specific technical procedures):					
H. Secretarial accuracy:					
I. Professional terminology:					
J. Assisting procedures:					
K. Laboratory techniques:					
L. X-ray techniques:					
M. Physical therapy:					
N. Collections:					
O. Medical Insurance:					
P. Bookkeeping:					

10. PERSONAL	1	2	3	4	COMMENTS
A. Grooming:					
B. Professional conduct:					
C. Energy, enthusiasm:					
D. Ability to handle stress:					

ADDITIONAL COMMENTS: ______________________________

— CONTINUED, NEXT PAGE —

Figure 15-15, cont'd

III. AREAS OF CONCERN: SPECIFY, IF ANY, PROBLEM AREAS:

IV. DEVELOPMENT PLANS: WHAT SPECIFIC ACTION CAN YOU SUGGEST TO HELP THE EMPLOYEE IMPROVE PERFORMANCE? HOW CAN YOU, AS THE SUPERVISOR, HELP?

☐ Promotable with additional training and experience.
☐ Promotable now ☐ Properly placed ☐ Not properly placed.

V. GOAL STATEMENT FOR NEXT REVIEW PERIOD: WITH THE EMPLOYEE, ESTABLISH GOALS WHICH MAY INCLUDE NEW AND BETTER WAYS TO CARRY OUT JOB RESPONSIBILITIES, AS WELL AS PLANS FOR PERSONAL DEVELOPMENT. STATED GOALS SHOULD BE CONSIDERED THE BASIS FOR THE NEXT FORMAL PERFORMANCE EVALUATION.

VI. EMPLOYEE COMMENTS:

I am signing this evaluation form to indicate that my supervisor and I have had a discussion of the above comments and ratings. Signature does not imply agreement.

EMPLOYEE: ____________________ DATE: __________

NAME OF REVIEWER ____________________

SIGNATURE ____________________ DATE: __________

TO REORDER CALL TOLL FREE:
800-BIBBERO /(800 242-2376) OR
FAX: (800) 242-9330 MFG IN U.S.A.

FORM # 72-119 ' 1987 BIBBERO SYSTEMS, INC. PETALUMA, CA

Figure 15-15, cont'd

BOX 15-4

Dealing With Poor Work Performance

When dealing with poor employee performance,

- Choose a private location for the discussion.
- Be calm and professional.
- Approach the employee in a positive manner. Negativity will help create a hostile atmosphere.
- Focus on the performance, not the person. Remain objective.
- Assume that the employee wants to improve performance.
- Allow enough time to discuss the employee's performance.
- Describe what is acceptable performance. Describe the situation as you see it.
- Ask the employee how he or she sees it. Let the employee explain the situation in full without interruption. There are always two sides to a story.
- Keep the discussion on neutral ground.
- Check for understanding. Be sure the employee understands what is acceptable and not acceptable performance.
- Encourage the employee to develop a solution. Employee ownership in the solution goes a long way toward correcting poor performance.
- Try to arrive at a solution that is beneficial to both parties.
- Remember that the goal of the discussion is to improve performance.
- Establish a time to meet again and follow up on the situation.

Employee Discipline or Termination

One of the more difficult situations in office management is dealing with an employee who is performing poorly in the workplace. Most employees do not want to perform poorly, but owing to a variety of personal, work, or educational circumstances, their work may not be adequate.

The first instinct for some managers may be to say to an employee, "Shape up!" A good manager, however, investigates the situation thoroughly. When dealing with an employee problem, a manager must be sure to consider all parties involved and should act in a way that is best for all concerned.

If an employee problem exists, the employee should be notified that there is a problem with job performance and should be given an adequate opportunity to respond to and correct the problem. Tips on dealing with employee problems are shown in Box 15-4. Significant employee problems—ones that could possibly warrant future termination—should be objectively and adequately documented and should be included in the employee's human resource file.

Separation of Employment

If an employee must be discharged, firing should never be a surprise. An employee who is not performing properly should be given sufficient warning that a problem with performance exists. A "paper trail" must be kept to demonstrate that the employee has been notified about poor performance. Well-documented evidence of reprimands and the reasons for reprimands as well as evidence of any suspensions must be included in the employee's file. It is critical to cover issues at the time of release from employment. Failure to do so may invite a discrimination suit against the employer.

If it has been decided that an employee should be discharged, the employer should carefully document the reason for termination. All reasons for termination must have been applied to all employees equally. For example, if an employee was discharged because the employee was late for work five times in a month and other employees were late that many times or more, a lawsuit may ensue because office policy was not consistently applied to all individuals in the office and discrimination has possibly occurred.

A breach of patient confidentiality would likely warrant an immediate termination from employment. The office's policy manual should contain a clear statement about confidentiality and the consequences of violating confidentiality. A confidentiality statement similar to the one shown in Figure 3-2 should be signed by every employee at the time of hire and at each performance review. In very obvious instances of violation, an employee would be terminated immediately and the reasons clearly documented in the employee's file.

HIPAA Hint

A person who knowingly obtains or discloses protected health information in violation of HIPAA faces fines of $50,000 to $250,000 or more and up to 1 to 10 years' imprisonment (depending on the nature of the disclosure). The larger fines and longer incarceration times apply to cases where the person intended to use the information for commercial advantage, personal gain, or malicious harm.

References for Former Employees

When an employee leaves a position under good terms, he or she may request a reference from the office when applying for employment elsewhere. Giving references can be a potentially "sticky" legal situation and must be handled with care.

Many defamation lawsuits have been pursued by former employees who received unfavorable references from former employers. A defamation lawsuit may be initiated and won against an employer who gives detrimental information and does not have records to substantiate the information. Even the simple act of saying a former employee was fired may bring a lawsuit because the employee may have to reveal damaging information about the release from employment.

Because of concern about legal entanglements, employers may decide to give references only for good employees. If a positive recommendation cannot be made, an employer may choose to not comment. An employer should refrain from giving good references for employees who do not deserve them because this can create other problems. Not all employees deserve good references, and by giving everyone a good reference, the employer may lose the respect of peers in the community and may actually support the hiring of a person who is wrong for a position.

A safe approach to handling references is to give only limited information about the employee, such as the dates of employment, salary information, and the type of position held. Such references are unfavorable to employees who have performed well on the job, however, and a quality reference should be given for an employee for work well done.

Some employers choose to give no references directly to other employers after the employee is gone and instead will provide a written reference letter to an employee before the employee leaves. Such references may be addressed "To Whom It May Concern" and are given directly to the employee. The employee may make photocopies of the reference letter to give to prospective employers. The employee is then responsible for disclosure of the information in the letter. If a reference letter is given, a copy of the letter should be filed in the employee's personnel file. This may well be the best approach to take, because the employee controls whether or not information is given to potential employers.

Employee Health

Much time and effort goes into selecting the best candidate for a position in the medical office. Once good employees are selected, the organization should expend every possible effort to keep them. To reduce turnover of employees, the practice should pay particular attention to the work environment and the needs of the people who work there. Frequent turnover is costly to the practice because new employees require training and undergo a period of adjustment when acclimating with the rest of the office staff. Frequent turnover can hurt a practice because inexperienced staff members are not as readily familiar with office procedures and with established patients of the practice.

Creating a healthy work environment is not difficult. First and foremost, management sets the tone for the office atmosphere. A friendly, teamwork-type atmosphere helps to create an enjoyable place to work. Honest and open communication among all employees in the office contributes to a harmonious work environment. A medical office is no place for personal agendas or competitiveness that works against an atmosphere of teamwork. A health care organization requires an atmosphere of teamwork to effectively and efficiently handle all patients served by the physicians and staff.

Occasionally, employees have personal problems that affect their job performance. Oftentimes when an employee is in a difficult situation, the employee's productivity is reduced. It is important to discuss performance with employees and provide support if possible. An employer may choose to refer employees in serious situations to an outside counseling service. Employee assistance programs provide counseling services for employees who are experiencing difficult situations at work or at home. Initial sessions with these types of programs are usually free to the employee. Employers who participate in such programs are aware that such participation goes a long way in heading off future difficulties at work. Happy, satisfied employees generally provide quality customer service. Disgruntled, troubled employees tend to reduce service.

Adapting to Change

It is often said that the only thing one can be sure of is that things will change. Certainly, change is inevitable in the health care industry. Constant advances in technology mean that employees must adapt to new systems, technologies, and procedures in the workplace. Only 25 years ago, for example, many medical offices used very little computer equipment in the front office. Today, changes in the business office of a medical practice have been dramatic, with the addition of computerized systems to support everyday front office functions. New technologies are used by the medical staff as well, and office staff will need to be aware of new services that are available. The future will probably bring many more changes, and the skills learned by the office staff today will have to be continually updated to keep pace with these changes.

Coping with change is a concern in any office, even the medical office. Everyone reacts in his or her own way to change. Some people adapt to change quite well. Others may be very resistant and may find it difficult to cope with change. People may have this difficulty for a variety of reasons.

Job Security

When any noticeable change is made in how an organization accomplishes its work, employees may be concerned that they are no longer needed in the office. A shift in the workload or in the organizational structure may produce anxiety in some employees. The addition of a new technology in the office may lead an employee to believe that he or she will no longer be needed. Most employers take preventive action in assuring employees that layoffs will not occur because of a proposed change. The addition of technology does not have to be a threat in the workplace. In actuality, employee security may be more threatened if changes were not made. An office that fails to keep up with technology may soon find that it will not be able to keep a quality level of service for existing customers and may risk losing them.

Resistance to Change

Employees may resist change simply because the present is comfortable. It is important for the office management to discuss the reasons for change with the office staff. Depending on the management style of the organization, the staff may even be asked to find solutions for addressing a problem. If it fits with the management style in the office, this tactic can help give employees ownership of the solution to a problem. When the staff has participated in a solution, the solution often becomes easier to implement.

New Technology

Sometimes office employees are intimidated by the new technology that may accompany change. When change is necessary, office management should provide the training and support needed to implement new technology. Training sessions on new equipment and offsite workshops provide opportunities for employees to learn new technologies and to network with other professionals.

Whatever the reason for change, the transition will be smoother if employees are made aware of why change is necessary and how it will affect them. Employees often need the assurance that management will provide necessary support to implement change.

Stress Management

Stress can be a serious problem in the workplace. There are good and bad types of stress. Good stress is the deadline that motivates someone to get a job done or an office environment that may be busy with activity. Examples of bad stress are constant deadlines that can almost never be met or being the only assistant available to answer eight incoming phone lines.

Sometimes stress is a result of conditions at work, and sometimes individuals are under stress because of situations in their personal lives. Whatever the case, it is important for the management of the medical office to be aware of employee behaviors that can be signals of bad stress.

- Frequent absenteeism or illness
- Tension at work
- Crying spells
- Acting "out of character," or "spacey," daydreaming
- Poor work quality, frequent mistakes
- Feeling unappreciated or picked on

Employers should be aware of the effects of stress and should take the following measures to reduce or prevent work-related stress:

- Establish reasonable work expectations. Provide adequate staff coverage. Recognize impossible workloads.
- Give employees reasonable break time during the workday. Don't allow employees to frequently skip breaks. Breaks rejuvenate employees.
- Provide a comfortable work environment. The right furniture and equipment are necessary to get the job done. A workstation that is not designed to facilitate completion of office responsibilities will have a negative effect on productivity.
- Solicit employees' input on work-related matters and incorporate input whenever possible.
- Give employees adequate time to complete job tasks.

It is important to help employees deal with stress in their lives. Continual, prolonged stress affects not only the employee, but coworkers as well. Office productivity will be reduced. Working to lessen or prevent employee stress can go a long way toward creating a pleasing environment not only for employees but also for patients. Employees who are satisfied, appreciated, and comfortable in their work environment will convey that feeling to patients of the practice.

Labor Laws and Legal Issues

At the beginning of the 20th century, the world of work was a dangerous and difficult place. Workers had little legal protection in various cases of work-related matters. As more and more people left family farm employment and began to work in an industrial setting, the need for legal protection for workers became more apparent. Throughout the past century, great strides have occurred in developing laws that protect employees in the workplace. Following are a few of the major legislative enactments that affect the workplace today.

Labor Law Enforcement

A federal agency within the U.S. Department of Labor, the Employment Standards Administration (ESA), enforces many laws and regulations pertaining to working conditions. Within the ESA, agencies have been established to enforce specific groups of laws and regulations pertaining to labor. The Wage and Hour Division, a division within the ESA, is responsible for protecting workers against unfair labor practices. The Wage and Hour Division enforces laws regarding minimum wage, overtime, child labor, and the Family and Medical Leave Act (FMLA).

Fair Labor Standards Act

In 1938, the Fair Labor Standards Act (FLSA), which included provisions for minimum wage, overtime pay, and child labor, was passed. Certain groups of individuals are exempt from overtime pay and minimum wage requirements. The FLSA also sets standards for hiring youth workers, such as work time restrictions and separate minimum wage requirements. Currently, the FLSA protects approximately 130 million government and private sector workers throughout the United States.

Family and Medical Leave Act

Promoting family stability is one of the chief purposes of the Family and Medical Leave Act of 1993 (FMLA). The Family and Medical Leave Act applies to all public sector employers and private sector employers who employ 50 or more workers and who are engaged in any activity that affects commerce.

The FMLA allows employees to take up to 12 weeks of leave during any 12-month period for the following reasons:

- Birth and care of an employee's child or placement of an adopted or foster care child with the employee
- Care of an immediate family member (spouse, child, parent) who has a serious health condition
- Care of an employee's own serious health condition

During a leave, the employee is entitled to health insurance benefits that the employee was receiving at the time the leave began. Employees may be required by their employer to take any accrued paid leave, such as sick or vacation pay, while on an FMLA leave; otherwise the leave is unpaid.

When returning to work after taking a leave under the FMLA, employees are entitled to their previous job or a job of equal status. If an employee takes a leave for reasons of personal illness, an employer may require that the employee provide certification from a physician that the employee is able to return to work.

No state law can supersede the FMLA, but if a state law is more beneficial to an employee, the employer must abide by the more beneficial law. The provisions of the FMLA apply to federal, state, and local government employers and private employers who employ more than 50 employees. The specifics of the FMLA are available from the U.S. Department of Labor at the U.S. Department of Justice website at www.dol.gov.

Americans With Disabilities Act

What are an employer's responsibilities in hiring or employing individuals who are disabled? Federal law does provide protection against discrimination toward disabled individuals. Enacted in 1990, the Americans With Disabilities Act (ADA) prohibits discrimination in employment practices that are based on a disability. The ADA also prohibits discrimination in commercial facilities and requires governmental agencies to provide access to programs offered to the public.

This law states that reasonable accommodations must be made for disabled individuals when policies or procedures may be discriminatory. An accommodation is a modification in a structure or process that helps a disabled individual. Included in this legislation are provisions for improving access for disabled individuals to new construction and existing buildings that provide goods and services to the public. New construction accommodations include ramps for individuals who use wheelchairs, automatic door openers, and Braille signage.

In the medical office, the ADA might apply in the following ways: (1) an employee who has a musculoskeletal injury may need a special chair in which to sit while working, (2) a diabetic employee may be given time to monitor blood sugar levels and administer insulin during the workday, or (3) an employee who cannot hear may be given a special hearing device.

The application of ADA requirements is often a gray area. The ADA requires only that an employer make reasonable accommodations; it does not require an employer to make all possible accommodations. The employer must decide what is reasonable and what is not. The U.S. Department of Justice does provide technical assistance with ADA regulations and is responsible for enforcing the regulations. However, the department is very strict when cases are reported regarding an apparent lack of effort to accommodate the disabled.

Sexual Harassment

Fair treatment of everyone in the workplace is an important issue in the workplace today. In the interviewing section of this chapter, we learned that it is unlawful to discriminate against individuals in employment practices.

Another issue that has grabbed many headlines in the past several years is the issue of sexual harassment in the workplace. **Sexual harassment** can be defined as unwelcome sexual behavior or innuendo. Sexual harassment can take the form of threats such as "If you don't give in to me, you'll be out of a job" or other activity that creates a hostile working environment, such as lewd jokes, foul language, inappropriate touching, or sexual comments.

Companies can be, and very often are, held responsible for the actions of their employees. If an individual in a position of authority uses that authority to coerce or intimidate an employee, the office management has a responsibility to protect the worker and must be vigilant in maintaining a work environment free of sexual harassment. A medical office should have established policy on sexual harassment, as well as identified procedures on how to report incidents. Sexual harassment policy should be reviewed, and education about recognizing and dealing with sexual harassment should be presented on an annual basis (at a minimum) for all employees. Employees may be asked to sign a form acknowledging that such behavior is against office policy.

When hearing the term sexual harassment, people often think of women being harassed. Even though most legal cases involve women as the subject of harassment, it is important to note that men can be victims of sexual harassment too and are afforded the same rights as women with regard to this subject.

Sexual harassment has been defined as unwelcome sexual behavior or innuendo, but what really is it? Perpetrators of harassment can be supervisors, coworkers, or subordinates. Sexual harassment may take the form of one of the following examples:

- Giving special treatment to a woman or man who is a sexual partner, even if the relationship is consensual
- Using terms such as "honey" or "babe"
- Telling or displaying jokes of a sexual nature
- Commenting on someone's physical appearance, such as "Nice legs" or "That outfit is sexy"
- Touching, hugging, or bumping against someone
- Whistling or winking suggestively

These are only a few examples of what might constitute sexual harassment. An employee who is feeling harassed should notify the perpetrator that the actions are unwelcome. Comments such as "Stop doing that" or "I find that offensive" communicate displeasure. An employee sometimes is unable to inform the perpetrator that the actions are unwelcome because the employee may fear retaliation from the perpetrator. Even in such a case, harassment has taken place. The employee may go directly to a supervisor, and the employee's supervisor will be expected to address the unwanted behavior.

Once the incident has been reported to the appropriate individual, an investigation of the allegations should be conducted. One incident, if severe enough, is sufficient to bring allegations of harassment. The office should have a well-defined investigative procedure that identifies a specific individual to whom allegations are given. Dealing with situations of harassment requires special training, and specific individuals usually are assigned to investigate such matters.

Workers' Compensation

Much is written in Chapter 13 about matters relating to Workers' Compensation. The Occupational and Safety Health Administration (OSHA) has specific guidelines for mandatory reporting of workplace injuries. When an employee is injured on the job, a report of injury must be completed as required by law. Timelines required for reporting vary from state to state. The state Workers' Compensation office and private Workers' Compensation carriers have specific information on how and when reports must be filed. It is important to acknowledge and properly report injuries or even potential injuries when they are reported to management and management should never discourage employees from seeking medical care or filing reports for work-related injuries.

Information on Employment Matters

The information in this chapter is meant to serve as an introduction to the essentials of human resource management and to provide a basis for inquiry when financial or legal counsel is consulted regarding human resource issues. There is no substitute for prudent planning. Professional counsel is an essential component of planning when managing the human resources of an organization.

Experts in payroll accounting provide a valuable service when meeting the various requirements for processing payroll. The services of an accountant should be available for answers to specific questions and for legal and tax advice about payroll requirements.

Because the area of employment practices has such potential for litigation, a medical practice is wise to retain the services of legal counsel before dealing with employment matters such as contracts, discipline, hiring, firing, and other potentially litigious situations. A few dollars spent on legal counsel will potentially save thousands in future litigation.

Information on employment laws and regulations can be obtained from the federal government on the U.S. Department of Labor and other Internet sites. Popular sites are listed in the Bibliography section of this chapter.

SUMMARY

The human resources of the organization are vital to the longevity and effective operations of an organization. Appropriate management of a practice's human resources can keep a medical office growing and running smoothly. A medical administrative assistant, whether an office manager or a staff member, should be aware of the various human resource issues that may affect employment and compensation of employees. The assistant who is well informed will know how to facilitate a positive employer/employee relationship and can help alleviate any legal entanglements related to employment.

YOU ARE THE MEDICAL ADMINISTRATIVE ASSISTANT

Several of your coworkers comment that they are upset about a recent staff meeting in which they were asked for input regarding a specific situation, but the office manager did not incorporate the input. Is management obligated to incorporate the input? How could this situation be handled? How would you respond to this situation?

REVIEW EXERCISES

Exercise 15-1 True or False

Read each statement, and determine whether the statement is true or false. Record the answer in the blank provided. T = true; F = false.

_______ 1. The participatory management style works well in a fast-paced medical office because it allows employees some decision making without the need to always refer to a supervisor.

_______ 2. A chain of command is still necessary if a participatory management style is used in the medical office.

_______ 3. When applications for a position in the medical office are reviewed, the best candidate from the résumés should be invited for an interview. If the interview goes well, no other candidates will have to be interviewed.

_______ 4. Inappropriate questions by an interviewer can trigger a lawsuit.

_______ 5. Employees are allowed to take as many exemptions as they want in order to reduce taxes.

_______ 6. If a W-4 is not completed by an employee, taxes at the lowest rate possible will be subtracted for the employee.

_______ 7. Social Security tax is withheld on all wages earned during a year.

_______ 8. Some employees may be exempt from federal income tax withholding.

_______ 9. The amount of taxes previously paid by an employer will determine how often the employer must make deposits of taxes that are withheld.

_______ 10. Employers should use an employee's name as it appears on the employee's Social Security card.

_______ 11. Anything that pertains to an employee, whether verified or not, should be included in the employee's file in order to avoid any future lawsuits.

_______ 12. Personal bias is acceptable and is expected on an employee's performance review.

_______ 13. Every employee should receive a performance review regardless of the quality of the employee's work.

_______ 14. Frequent employee turnover can be costly to a medical office.

_______ 15. When asked for a reference, an employer should tell everything about an employee, especially the negative points.

_______ 16. An employer should give a positive job reference for an employee who does not deserve one.

_______ 17. Giving a reference letter to a previous employee is a safe way to give an employment reference.

_______ 18. Because change is so frequent in the workplace, it is expected and easy for employees to handle.

_______ 19. Sexual harassment has not taken place if the perpetrator has not been told.

_______ 20. All allegations of sexual harassment must be investigated.

_______ 21. A medical office may be liable for the actions of an office manager if sexual harassment is alleged.

_______ 22. In some offices, employees may have to sign a form acknowledging their understanding of a sexual harassment policy.

_______ 23. The ADA may require an employer to adapt a work environment for an employee who needs it.

_______ 24. Unemployment tax is paid by the employee and the employer.

_______ 25. Employers must make all accommodations that an employee requests.

Exercise 15-2 Chapter Concepts

Read the statement, and determine the answer that best fits the statement. Record the answer in the blank provided.

_______ 1. Which of the following is a subjective criterion for a job opening?
(a) Experience using word processing and spreadsheet software
(b) Works well under pressure
(c) Medical administrative assistant education
(d) Two years' previous experience working in a medical office

_______ 2. Which of the following is false about a probationary period?
(a) Probationary periods are typically 90 to 180 days.
(b) An employee's performance is measured during a probationary period.
(c) If an employee leaves the job after a probationary period, severance must be paid by the employer.
(d) An employer and an employee meet at the end of a probationary period to determine whether the employment arrangement should continue.

_______ 3. Which of the following keeps a record of what an employee has earned over a year?
(a) Policy manual
(b) Employee compensation record
(c) Payroll tax record
(d) Form W-4

_______ 4. A change in income tax withholding must be reported using
(a) Form W-2
(b) Form W-4
(c) An employee compensation record
(d) A written personal note from the employee

_______ 5. Which of the following is an optional deduction from an employee's paycheck?
(a) State income tax
(b) Medicare tax
(c) Dental insurance premium
(d) Federal income tax
(e) Court-ordered deduction

_______ 6. Which of the following is a form used for reporting and depositing taxes owed to the federal government?
(a) Form 941
(b) Form 940
(c) Form W-2
(d) Form W-4

_______ 7. Which of the following is false when an employee is discharged?
(a) Sufficient warning should be given to the employee that performance is not acceptable.
(b) Reason(s) for termination should be well documented.
(c) Office policies can be applied differently for every employee.
(d) Failure to inform an employee of the reason that the employee is terminated could lead to a lawsuit.

_______ 8. All of the following could lead to work-related stress except
(a) Adequate breaks during the day
(b) Not enough time to complete necessary work
(c) Hectic, tense work environment
(d) No opportunity to give input on office matters

_______ 9. Which of the following is false regarding the FMLA?
(a) The Act applies to both private and public sector employers of more than 50 persons.
(b) Twelve weeks of leave is allowed for each 12-month period.
(c) Leave can be used to care for certain ill family members.
(d) The FMLA does not apply if the company has a sick leave policy that differs from the provisions of the Act.

_______ 10. Which of the following is not a likely example of sexual harassment?
(a) Telling lewd jokes
(b) Shaking hands
(c) Rubbing up against someone
(d) Winking suggestively

_______ 11. Which of the following is an inappropriate question to ask in an interview?
(a) Can you work weekends?
(b) Which religious holidays do you observe?
(c) Are you able to work 12-hour days?
(d) Can you work overtime?

Exercise 15-3 Payroll Calculations

Determine the correct amount for the situation given. Use the information in this chapter and the amounts listed here when figuring tax. Record the correct answer in the blank provided.

_______ 1. An employee earning $12.63 per hour working 40 hours per week using a biweekly pay period would have gross earnings of
(a) $505.20
(b) $1010.40
(c) $1094.60
(d) None of the above

_______ 2. What are the gross monthly earnings of an employee hired at $30,000 per year?
(a) $3000
(b) $2500
(c) $2307.69
(d) None of the above

_______ 3. Assuming that the employee mentioned in question 2 works 40 hours per week, what is the employee's hourly wage?
(a) $23.07
(b) $11.54
(c) $14.42
(d) None of the above

_______ 4. An employee works the following hours in a week: Monday, 6.75 hours; Tuesday, 4.5 hours; Wednesday, 8.25 hours; Thursday, 8 hours; and Friday, 7.75 hours. What are the total hours worked during the week?
(a) 33.75
(b) 35
(c) 35.25

_______ 5. The amount of FUTA withheld from an employee who earned $1000 is
(a) $6.00
(b) $60
(c) $0.60
(d) None

_______ 6. An employee earning $24,000 per year will pay how much in Social Security tax?
(a) $348
(b) $1488
(c) $2184
(d) $2976

ACTIVITIES

ACTIVITY 15-1 PAYROLL PREPARATION

Compute the payroll amounts for a biweekly period using the information in this table. Use information given in the chapter and the amounts listed here when figuring tax. Complete the payroll record. (No employee has met the maximum amount for Social Security tax.) Procedure 15-2 can be used as a guide in completing this exercise.

Payroll Information

Employee Name	Hours Worked	Hourly Rate	Marital Status	Exemptions
Dixon, Amy	80	14.73	M	0
Dorland, Robert	75	13.40	M	2
Gordon, Margaret	48	14.80	S	1
Michaels, Connie	64	16.25	S	0
Scott, Patrick	80	14.02	M	3
Sears, Jackie	80	13.21	M	1

Payroll Record

Employee Name	Gross Earnings	FICA Tax	Federal Withholding Tax	State Income Tax (2% of gross earnings)	Total Deductions	Net Earnings
Dixon, Amy						
Dorland, Robert						
Gordon, Margaret						
Michaels, Connie						
Scott, Patrick						
Sears, Jackie						

ACTIVITY 15-2 FEDERAL INCOME TAX

Using the Internet, locate official government information pertaining to federal income taxes, and identify under which circumstances an individual is exempt from federal income tax.

ACTIVITY 15-3 STATE INCOME TAX

Investigate the state income tax requirements in your state and/or adjoining states in which individuals may reside.

ACTIVITY 15-4 FAMILY AND MEDICAL LEAVE ACT (FMLA)

Research the Family and Medical Leave Act.

ACTIVITY 15-5 STRESS MANAGEMENT

Conduct research on the causes, signs, and symptoms of stress. Locate information on how to alleviate or reduce the effects of stress.

ACTIVITY 15-6 SEXUAL HARASSMENT

Research sexual harassment in the workplace. Locate examples of harassment, as well as strategies for handling harassment situations.

DISCUSSION

The following topics can be used for class discussion or for individual student essay.

DISCUSSION 15-1

You are one of five assistants in the office. One of the assistants seems to have a persistently negative, down attitude. What should you do?

DISCUSSION 15-2

Discuss what causes stress for you and positive or negative ways that you handle it.

DISCUSSION 15-3

Find two or more mission statements from health care organizations in your area. Compare the content of the statements.

Bibliography

Coleman DL: What you must know before you hire or fire an employee, *Phys Manage* volume number:60-70, 1992.

Office of Civil Rights: Summary of the HIPAA Privacy Rule, U.S. Department of Health and Human Services, last revised May 2003. http://www.hhs.gov/ocr/privacy/hipaa/understanding/summary/privacysummary.pdf. Accessed January 15, 2012.

U.S. Internal Revenue Service. www.irs.gov Accessed January 15, 2012.

U.S. Department of Labor. www.dol.gov Accessed January 15, 2012.

U.S. Equal Employment Opportunity Commission. www.eeoc.gov Accessed January 15, 2012.

U.S. Office of Personnel Management, Federal Employees Health Benefits. http://www.opm.gov/insure/index.aspx Accessed January 15, 2012.

Weiss DH: *Fair, Square and Legal: Safe Hiring, Managing, and Firing Practices to Keep You and Your Company Out of Court*, New York, 1991, AMACOM.

State of Minnesota Department of Employee Relations: *Your Health Your Choice*, vol. VIII, Kalamazoo, MI, 1997, Hope Publications.

CHAPTER 16 Job Search Essentials

LEARNING OUTCOMES

On successful completion of this chapter, the student will be able to

1. Prepare a cover letter and résumé.
2. Identify where job openings may be advertised.
3. Complete an application for employment.
4. Identify successful interview techniques.

ACCREDITING BUREAU OF HEALTH EDUCATION SCHOOLS (ABHES) COMPETENCIES FOR MEDICAL ASSISTING

Graduates

- Project a positive attitude.
- Perform the essential requirements for employment such as résumé writing, effective interviewing, dressing professionally, and following up appropriately.

VOCABULARY

clinical
externship
internship
practicum
résumé

Throughout a medical administrative assistant's education, a student studies and hones the skills required for work in a medical office. At some point near the end of his or her formal education, an assistant will need to begin the application for employment process by presenting his or her acquired skills, knowledge, and personal attributes to prospective employers. Following are some fundamental details an assistant should consider when seeking a position in a medical office.

Preparation for Employment

During the course of their education, students in a medical office–related program are exposed to many different subjects. Health science–related courses on anatomy and physiology, medical terminology, and disease conditions, as well as office-related courses such as medical office procedures, procedure and diagnosis coding, medical billing, health insurance, bookkeeping, and computer technology, provide a well-rounded education for anyone who wishes to work as a medical administrative assistant.

As mentioned in Chapter 1, however, an assistant's formal education is just the beginning. Technological advances in health care keep the industry moving at a fast pace. An assistant must learn to adapt to those changes and to implement new procedures in the medical office. Continuing education is necessary to keep pace with those changes. Opportunities for continuing education can be found in evening or weekend classes at a local college, in distance education courses available via the Internet, and in workshops conducted by industry professionals, government agencies, and career development companies.

Throughout education and training, an assistant should work to gain as much exposure as possible to all aspects of the operation of the medical office. Courses in human relations, accounting, and management can enhance an assistant's education and increase his or her employability.

In preparation for employment, focus on your particular skills and interests. Not everyone is suited to the same type of position. Try to match your interests to a position that is well suited to you. By identifying your interests, you will be able to identify special qualities that you can bring to a position.

For example, suppose that you have identified excellent math skills as one of your strengths. Obviously, such skills would be a great asset in a position in which an assistant may be responsible for managing a practice's accounts receivable or accounts payable. Or maybe you speak a foreign language. In many locales, a bilingual assistant can be a tremendous asset when serving as an interpreter for patients.

Applying For a Position

When advertising an open position, medical offices may elect to gather interested applicants in a number of ways. They may choose to do the following:

- Have applicants telephone the medical office to inquire about the position.
- Ask interested applicants to send a résumé to the office or another location.
- Require interested applicants to come to the office to complete an application (Fig. 16-1).

(In answering questions, use extra blank sheet if necessary)

APPLICATION FOR POSITION / Medical or Dental Office
AN EQUAL OPPORTUNITY EMPLOYER

No employee, applicant, or candidate for promotion, training or other advantage shall be discriminated against (or given preference) because of race, color, religion, sex, age, physical handicap, veteran status, or national origin.

Date of Application

PLEASE READ CAREFULLY AND WRITE OR PRINT ANSWERS TO ALL QUESTIONS. DO NOT TYPE.

A. PERSONAL INFORMATION

Name - Last	First	Middle	Social Security No.	Area Code/Phone No. ( )

Present Address: - Street	(Apt #)	City	State	Zip	How Long At This Address?:

Previous Address: - Street	City	State	Zip	Person to notify in case of Emergency or Accident - Name:
From:	To:			Address: Telephone:

B. EMPLOYMENT INFORMATION

For What Position Are You Applying?:	☐ Full-Time ☐ Part-Time ☐ Either	Date Available For Employment?:	Wage/Salary Expectations:
List Hrs./Days You Prefer To Work	List Any Hrs./Days You Are Not Available: (Except for times required for religious practices or observances)		Can You Work Overtime, If Necessary? ☐ Yes ☐ No
Are You Employed Now?: ☐ Yes ☐ No	If So, May We Inquire Of Your Present Employer?: ☐ No ☐ Yes, If Yes: Name Of Employer: Phone Number: ( )		
Have You Ever Been Bonded? ☐ Yes ☐ No	If Required For Position, Are You Bondable? ☐ Yes ☐ No ☐ Uncertain	Have You Applied For A Position With This Office Before? ☐ No ☐ Yes If Yes, When?:	

Referred By / Or Where Did You Learn Of This Job?:

Can You, Upon Employment, Submit Verification Of Your Legal Right To Work In The United States?: ☐ Yes ☐ No
Submit Proof That You Meet Legal Age Requirement For Employment? ☐ Yes ☐ No

Language(s) Applicant Speaks or Writes (If Use Of A Language Other Than English is Relevant To The Job For Which The Applicant Is Applying:

C. EDUCATIONAL HISTORY

Name & Address Of Schools Attended (Include Current)	Dates From	Dates Thru	Highest Grade/Level Completed	Diploma/Degree(s) Obtained/Areas of Study
High School				
College				Degree/Major
Post Graduate				Degree/Major
Other				Course/Diploma/License/ Certificate

Specific Training, Education, Or Experiences Which Will Assist You In The Job For Which You Have Applied.

Future Educational Plans

D. SPECIAL SKILLS

CHECK BELOW THE KINDS OF WORK YOU HAVE DONE:		☐ MEDICAL INSURANCE FORMS	☐ RECEPTIONIST
☐ BLOOD COUNTS	☐ DENTAL ASSISTANT	☐ MEDICAL TERMINOLOGY	☐ TELEPHONES
☐ BOOKKEEPING	☐ DENTAL HYGIENIST	☐ MEDICAL TRANSCRIPTION	☐ TYPING
☐ COLLECTIONS	☐ FILING	☐ NURSING	☐ STENOGRAPHY
☐ COMPOSING LETTERS	☐ INJECTIONS	☐ PHLEBOTOMY (Draw Blood)	☐ URINALYSIS
☐ COMPUTER INPUT	☐ INSTRUMENT STERILIZATION	☐ POSTING	☐ X-RAY
OFFICE EQUIPMENT USED: ☐ COMPUTER	☐ DICTATING EQUIPMENT	☐ WORD PROCESSOR	☐ OTHER:
Other Kinds Of Tasks Performed Or Skills That May Be Applicable To Position:		Typing Speed	Shorthand Speed

ORDER # **72-110** • © 1976 BIBBERO SYSTEMS, INC. • PETALUMA, CA. • (REV. 1/95)
TO REORDER CALL TOLL FREE: (800) BIBBERO (800-242-2376) OR FAX (800) 242-9330 MFG IN U.S.A.

(PLEASE COMPLETE OTHER SIDE)

Figure 16-1 Applicants for an open position in a medical office may be required to complete an employment application. Applications also may be done online at many health care organizations. (Form courtesy of Bibbero Systems, Inc., Petaluma, California, 800-242-2376; fax, 800-242-9330; www.bibbero.com.)

E. EMPLOYMENT RECORD

LIST MOST RECENT EMPLOYMENT FIRST **May We Contact Your Previous Employer(s) For A Reference?** ☐ **Yes** ☐ **No**

1) Employer		Worked Performed. Be Specific:
Address Street City State Zip Code		
Phone Number ( )		
Type of Business	Dates From Mo. Yr. To Mo. Yr.	
Your Position	Hourly Rate/Salary Starting Final	
Supervisor©s Name		
Reason For Leaving		
2) Employer		Worked Performed. Be Specific:
Address Street City State Zip Code		
Phone Number ( )		
Type of Business	Dates From Mo. Yr. To Mo. Yr.	
Your Position	Hourly Rate/Salary Starting Final	
Supervisor©s Name		
Reason For Leaving		
3) Employer		Worked Performed. Be Specific:
Address Street City State Zip Code		
Phone Number ( )		
Type of Business	Dates From Mo. Yr. To Mo. Yr.	
Your Position	Hourly Rate/Salary Starting Final	
Supervisor©s Name		
Reason For Leaving		

F. REFERENCES — FRIENDS / ACQUAINTANCES NON-RELATED

(1) ____________________

Name Address Telephone Number (☐ Work ☐ Home) Occupation Years Acquainted

(1) ____________________

Name Address Telephone Number (☐ Work ☐ Home) Occupation Years Acquainted

Please Feel Free To Add Any Information Which You Feel Will Help Us Consider You For Employment

READ THE FOLLOWING CAREFULLY, THEN SIGN AND DATE THE APPLICATION

"I certify that all answers given by me on this application are true, correct and complete to the best of my knowledge. I acknowledge notice that the information contained in this application is subject to check. I agree that, if hired, my continued employment may be contingent upon the accuracy of that information. If employed, I further agree to comply with Company/Office rules and regulations."

Signature: ____________________ Date: ____________

Figure 16-1, cont'd

Some employers may prefer to use an application; others may prefer to ask for a résumé. Regardless of how the medical office asks applicants to inquire, a well-prepared medical assistant will always bring along a résumé to give to the employer. Even if the medical office asks the assistant to complete an application, the assistant should give a résumé to the employer along with the completed application.

If the office asks an assistant to come to the office to pick up an application, the assistant should always go to the office dressed in attire that is suitable for an interview. "Stopping by" the office in a pair of jeans or the like is not appropriate and would probably create a bad first impression. When going into the office of a possible future employer, an assistant should dress as he or she would for an interview. You never know—the employer might decide to hold an interview right then and there!

Developing a Winning Résumé

As a medical administrative student prepares to enter the workforce, information should be gathered for compiling and producing a **résumé** (Fig. 16-2). A résumé documents an individual's qualifications for a position. It provides a place for the student to highlight his or her education, work experience, personal achievements, strengths, and qualities.

The résumé is sometimes the first contact the student will have with the employer. Because first impressions are so important, much time and effort should go into creating a résumé. Tips for creating a great résumé are listed in Box 16-1.

Quite a collection of information is needed to complete an assistant's résumé. In preparing a résumé, it is a good idea to keep all gathered information in one place that is easy to access. Procedure 16-1 outlines how to prepare a résumé. Following is the basic information included within many résumés.

Taylor J. Reed
272 Meadowlawn Lane
Farmington, ND 58000
(012) 555-7717

Objective To obtain a position as a medical administrative assistant in a family practice clinic.

Education

2006–2008 Best Technical College **Farmington, ND**
- Medical Assisting, AAS.
- Graduated with honors, GPA 3.92

2003–2006 Southside High School **Farmington, ND**
- Diploma
- Member of National Honor Society

Experience

2004–2006 Southside School Bookstore **Farmington, ND**
Sales Clerk
- Worked in school store helping customers and stocking shelves.
- Responsible for totaling daily receipts and making bank deposits.

2006–2008 Green Valley Pharmacy **Farmington, ND**
Sales Associate
- Maintain computerized customer database.
- Responsible for financial transactions (charges and cash payments).
- Performed store opening and closing procedures.
- Worked 30 hours per week while attending college.

Interests Bike riding, team sports, reading, crossword puzzles

References

Mary K. Hanson, Faculty Advisor
Best Technical College
308 Main Ave.
Farmington, ND 58000
(555) 111-7899

Christian Matthew, Store Manager
Green Valley Pharmacy
709 Pine St.
Farmington, ND 58000
(555) 111-3456

Figure 16-2 A professional-looking résumé that identifies an applicant's education and experience is essential when one is applying for a position in a medical office.

BOX 16-1

Tips for a Great Résumé

- List the most important items first on the résumé. For example, if education in a medical office–related program has just been completed and the graduate has no experience working in a medical office, list the education first.
- If possible, keep a résumé to one page; employers may look only at the first page. A résumé should not be longer than two pages.
- Use a font that is easy to read. A résumé is no place to experiment with elaborate font styles.
- Pay attention to format. Use a format that makes the résumé easy to read.
- Use high-quality paper with matching envelopes. Office supply stores carry a wide variety of papers. White or off-white papers look professional; avoid colors, especially vivid ones.
- Make the résumé unique. Incorporate a personal touch, if possible.
- Use a résumé template found in many popular office software packages, or use specific software, to develop a professional-looking résumé. Research approaches to preparing résumés.

PROCEDURE 16-1

Prepare a Résumé

Materials Needed

- Professional résumé paper (white or off-white) and matching envelope
- Computer with word processing software
- Education, work experience, and student portfolio information

1. Choose a format for the résumé. A résumé computer program or a résumé template from a word processing program may be used.
2. List your full name, address, telephone number, and email address at the top of the résumé.
3. Write a career objective specific to the position desired.
4. List your education, with the most recent first.
5. List your work experience, with the most recent first. Any volunteer experience or student internship experience can be listed under "Work experience."
6. List your personal achievements, awards, interests, and/or skills.
7. List your personal references. Instructors and work supervisors are good choices. Friends and relatives should not be listed as personal references. Be sure to ask each reference for permission before listing him or her as a reference.
8. Proofread the résumé for typos or grammatical errors.*
9. Review the résumé to ensure that the format is easy to read. Make any necessary adjustments.
10. Print a copy of the résumé, and retain a copy for yourself.
11. (Optional) If mailing the résumé, print an envelope.

**Denotes crucial step in procedure. Student must complete this step satisfactorily in order to complete the procedure satisfactorily. If possible, have another person read the résumé.*

Heading

Usually located at the very top of a résumé, a heading identifies the applicant. Included in a heading are the applicant's complete legal name (nicknames should not be used), address, telephone number, and email address. Use a professional email address (not partyanimal@mail.com). Be sure to list an email address at which you will receive mail *after* you are out of school. Complete information will enable the employer to contact the applicant in numerous different ways. A bold, larger font should be used to accentuate the assistant's name.

Career Objective

Usually listed first in the body of the résumé, the career objective identifies where the applicant hopes to go with his or her education and experience. It should have some connection with the position for which the assistant is applying.

Education

Generally, the education section should be listed near the top of the résumé before a person's work experience. This is done because most people who have just completed their education will not have any work experience in a medical office. In this case, a person's education is more relevant to the position applied for than the person's work experience.

If an individual should have some type of medical office experience and medical office-related education, the individual should choose to list either education or work experience first depending on which is more relevant to the position being sought. Information regarding an assistant's formal and informal education is listed in the education section. Any and all post-secondary education at a business school, college, or university should be given to the prospective employer. This should include the name of a program and a brief description of specific courses taken during post-secondary training, and identification of any degree awarded or the highest grade completed should be listed in this section. If a student's grade point average (GPA) was good, it should be specifically listed. If the employer requests a transcript of education, the GPA will be included on the transcript; however, a good GPA should be highlighted on the résumé as well.

List all education in reverse chronological order. There is no need to list high school unless the applicant was an honor student or if there was something outstanding to mention about the high school experience. It is assumed students went to high school if they went to college.

List all college experience even if the applicant did not graduate. If special awards (e.g., Dean's List) were received, mention those also.

If an advertisement for a medical office position lists specific requirements, such as medical transcription, an assistant should mention specifically whether he or she has taken courses in that subject. Information can also be included in this section about medical office–related workshops that the assistant has attended.

Work Experience or Work History

After education that may be preferred or even required for a position, employers often want to know the applicant's work history and whether it is related to the position for which the assistant has applied. Work experience is usually listed in reverse chronological order, that is, the most recent experience is listed first and the oldest experience is listed last. Volunteer experience can be listed in this section.

When listing work experience, an assistant should give specific information related to each position, such as:

- Name and address of previous employer
- Dates of employment
- Position held
- Job responsibilities

The assistant may choose to add other information, such as that he or she worked at the job while going to college. Applicants may or may not choose to give the reason for leaving a previously held position. It is not necessary to give a reason for leaving employment.

Applicants should never be embarrassed to list job experience that is entry level or unrelated to the position sought. Listing this previous experience gives applicants the chance to let employers know more about their work history. In the example provided in Figure 16-2, note how the assistant has mentioned specific duties that may enhance his or her ability to work in a medical office.

Achievements, Awards, Interests, or Skills

Students should keep track of achievements, awards, or other personal or professional accomplishments that might interest an employer (e.g., fluency in a language other than English). Membership in professional organizations should also be mentioned. Any personal interests can be listed at the applicant's discretion. If the assistant has any certifications such as certified nursing assistant (CNA), emergency medical technician (EMT), or cardiopulmonary resuscitation (CPR), those should be included on the résumé as well.

References

Some publications recommend that references be listed as "available on request." Why would an applicant make a potential employer work to get references? It is much easier for an employer if the references are included with the résumé. For this reason alone, it is recommended to include references with a résumé. Before listing references on a résumé, an applicant should obtain permission from each reference. This is done as a common courtesy and to alert the person that he or she may be receiving a call regarding a reference.

When listing a reference, be sure to include the name, company or organization, address, phone, and email of the reference, and identify how you know them. Do *not* use a relative or friend as a reference. Even coworkers are not great references because usually they are not in a supervisory position over the applicant. Try to find instructors or previous or current supervisors who would be willing to give a reference.

Cover Letter

With each résumé, a cover letter should be included to introduce the applicant to the interviewer or the interview team. The cover letter highlights some of the best qualifications of the candidate and should get the reader's attention so that the applicant will be called for an interview.

The sample of the cover letter shown in Figure 16-3 identifies the applicant's interest in the position, as well as chief qualifications for the position. The use of a cover letter is a good way to highlight an applicant's major qualifications for a position twice—once in the cover letter and once in the résumé. Procedure 16-2 outlines how to prepare a cover letter.

It is good practice to use the same heading that is on the résumé on the cover letter. A heading on both the résumé and cover letter gives a professional look to both documents.

Finding out about Job Openings

Employment openings for individuals with training as medical administrative assistants occur in a variety of places (see Chapter 1 and Box 16-2).

How do employers advertise for open positions? Positions are "advertised" in a multitude of places. When many people think of looking for a job, one of the first places they think of is the newspaper classified advertising section. It is sometimes said, however, that the best jobs never appear in a newspaper classified section. The newspaper classified ads should never be the sole method of locating a job; in fact, no method listed in this section should be the sole method of locating a position. An assistant should use a combination of sources to locate the employment openings.

Networking

It is often said, "It's not what you know; it's who you know." Although having the right skills or qualifications is necessary to secure employment, information about job openings is often gathered casually from individuals with whom an assistant comes in contact. For instance, someone may mention at

February 14, 20xx

Ms. Taylor Hudson, Office Manager
Horizons Healthcare Center
123 Main Avenue
Farmington, ND 58000

Dear Ms. Hudson:

I have recently completed my education for Medical Administrative Assistant at Best Technical College in Farmington, ND. I am interested in staying in the local area to begin my career in the health care industry. I am applying for a customer service position in your insurance department and am enclosing my résumé.

I am a hard-working, dedicated individual with customer service-related work experience over the past few years. I enjoy working with the public and have a particular interest in work related to the financial aspects of a business.

I would appreciate the opportunity to interview with you and appreciate your consideration of my qualifications for this position. I look forward to hearing from you.

Sincerely,

Taylor J. Reed

Taylor J. Reed

enclosure

Figure 16-3 A cover letter is used to introduce an applicant and is included along with a résumé. A cover letter gives the applicant the opportunity to highlight his or her specific qualifications for the position.

PROCEDURE 16-2

Prepare a Cover Letter

Materials Needed

- Professional résumé paper (white or off-white) and matching envelope
- Computer with word processing software Completed résumé

1. Use a proper format for the letter (see Chapter 6).
2. Address the letter to the individual designated to receive applications.
3. Write the letter to express your interest in a position and identify some of your qualifications and strengths.
4. Close the letter with the appropriate salutation and your full name.
5. Proofread the letter for typos and grammatical errors. If possible, have another person also read the letter.*
6. Print a copy of the letter, and retain a copy for yourself.
7. Sign the letter that will be included with your résumé.*
8. Place the letter appropriately in a business envelope along with the résumé (see Fig. 6-13).
9. (Optional) If you are mailing the cover letter with the résumé, print an envelope.

**Denotes crucial step in procedure. Student must complete this step satisfactorily in order to complete the procedure satisfactorily. If possible, have another person read the cover letter.*

BOX 16-2

Possible Employment Opportunities for a Medical Administrative Assistant

- Large multispecialty clinic
- Private practice
- Hospital
- Nursing home
- Insurance company
- Home health agency
- Hospice
- Dental office
- Law office specializing in medical cases
- Medical school
- Pharmaceutical company
- Chiropractic office

a professional meeting that an opening is becoming available in a physician's office. Assistants may hear the information directly, or the information may be given to them by someone they know. Assistants who are seeking employment should spread the word about the type of position they are looking for and should let people know of their search for employment. An acquaintance or a close friend may be the lead to the ideal position.

Academic Placement Services

Educational institutions often provide assistance in helping their graduates obtain employment. Placement services offered by educational institutions are usually free to a graduate. Sometimes, many of the best jobs are found through an academic placement service. Many employers prefer to list openings with schools that they know provide top-quality training.

Educational placement services allow graduates to receive information on employment listings that are sent to the placement office. The placement service, in turn, sends information about employment listings to the graduate. Schools very often receive notice of job openings that may never appear in the newspaper. For this reason, the graduate may have an advantage over other job seekers who do not have access to a school's placement services.

Students should establish a relationship with their instructors and should let instructors know what type of position they are seeking. Many employers telephone or email instructors directly when looking for new employees.

Professional Employment Services

There are two types of professional employment services: those that charge a fee and those that do not charge a fee. For services that charge a fee, the fee may be paid by the employer or by the employee. A medical administrative assistant with the right job skills should never have to pay a fee to obtain a job.

Many employment agencies assist employers in finding the right people for jobs. Some agencies also place people in temporary positions to assist employers with short-term employment shortages. Sometimes, these temporary positions lead to permanent employment.

Many states have government-run employment agencies (sometimes called Job Service) that provide services to employers looking to hire employees. A large practice may require that all entry level positions be applied for through the state employment service in its city. Services are provided at no cost to the employer, and positions are available at no cost to the employee.

Classified Ads

One of the traditional spots to look for a job is in the classified section of a local newspaper. Sometimes, these ads can bring a flood of applicants to the office, and competition may be tough. Ads may offer little information about the position, such as the job responsibilities or the wages, so the assistant may not be able to discern whether the position is one that he or she would like. The best day for job listings is usually Sunday, but classified ads should be read every day to ensure that all openings are seen. Many newspapers now have classified ads that can be accessed for free over the Internet.

Internet Job Search

The Internet can be a useful tool for recruiting employees. Several large health care institutions have established their own employment listings on their websites. Government agencies and large health care facilities such as the Mayo Clinic post open positions on their specific websites. Assistants who wish to relocate may find the Internet a valuable resource for locating employment in the area desired. Many health care organizations' websites allow interested applicants to fill out online employment applications and to submit résumés online.

Professional Organizations

Students who belong to a professional organization while in school may find out about openings in the organization's newsletter or at membership meetings. Membership in a professional organization provides an excellent opportunity for students to network with people currently employed in the health care profession.

Cold Calls

If an assistant desires employment with a specific medical practice, the assistant should not wait for a position to be advertised. The assistant may choose to apply to an office by sending a résumé and cover letter that expresses interest in working with the organization. The possibility always exists that an opening might be available. Even if there currently is not an opening, many offices keep résumé on file for reference purposes when a position opens.

Internship Opportunities

In preparation for entering the workforce, medical administrative assistants should take advantage of internship experiences that may become available to them (Fig. 16-4).

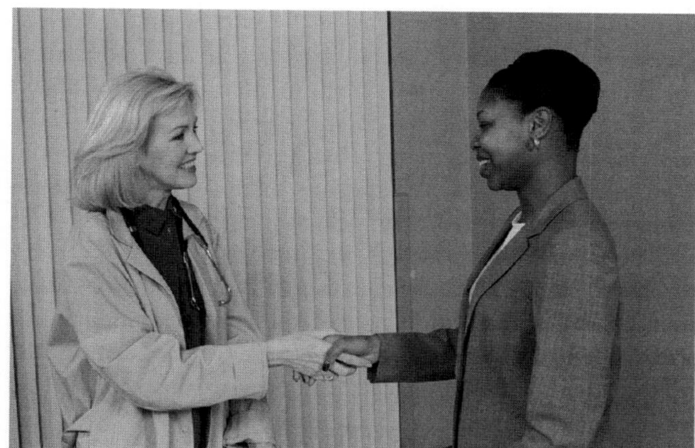

Figure 16-4 An applicant should shake the interviewer's hand both before and after an employment interview. At the end of an interview, the applicant should be sure to thank the interviewer for the interview.

As part of many educational programs, an **internship** can provide an assistant with an opportunity to apply learned skills and behaviors and to experience the work environment of the medical office. In an internship, a student works under the supervision of a medical office employee and receives on-the-job experience in a medical office.

Depending on the arrangements made, an internship experience also may be referred to as an **externship, clinical**, or **practicum**. No matter what it is called, this experience can prove invaluable to the assistant when beginning the job hunt. An internship should be listed on the student's résumé under "Work experience." Often, if the internship experience goes well and the medical office has an opening, the intern may have a good chance of securing employment at the internship site.

An Application for Employment

Sometimes, an application (see Fig. 16-1) is used in the medical office to gain specific information from each applicant. If the office needs specific expertise in a certain area, that area may be specifically listed on the application form. The application shown in Figure 16-1 asks specific questions about when the applicant is available for work. The use of an application form ensures that certain information is asked of each applicant that might not be included in a résumé.

When filling out an application, an assistant should carefully complete all required blanks on the form and should follow all instructions on the form. An employer will look unfavorably upon an assistant who does not complete the application properly or who leaves the application incomplete. Procedure 16-3 outlines how to complete an employment application.

CHECKPOINT

You want to work in a large, well-known facility that is located about 700 miles from your current home. What are some good strategies for locating and applying for a position there?

PROCEDURE 16-3

Complete an Employment Application

Materials Needed

Many employment applications are now available online over the Internet. The same steps would be followed, but the information would be entered electronically.

- Employment application
- Pen

1. Read the instructions on the form, and follow them carefully. Provide the information requested here, in addition to any other information requested on the application.
2. Identify your personal information.
3. List your educational history.
4. List your employment history.
5. List your medical office–related skills.
6. List your personal references.
7. Review the application to make sure it is complete.*
8. Sign and date the application.*
9. Submit the application to the individual designated.

**Denotes crucial step in procedure. Student must complete this step satisfactorily in order to complete the procedure satisfactorily.*

Preparing for a Great Interview

Once the assistant has been selected to be interviewed for a position, he or she should consider many things that are part of a successful interview. Good preparation for an interview can help make it a successful experience.

- Know something about the organization. Research information on company operations. Know where branch offices might be located and what medical specialties they have. Be ready to ask questions about the organization.
- Practice, practice, practice. Rehearse answers out loud to questions that may be asked. Prepare answers to basic questions, such as "Tell me about your education at the technical college" or "What makes you the best person for the job?" Be prepared to answer tough questions, such as "Why are you leaving your present position?" or "What would you do if…?"
- Practice interviewing with a friend. Practicing or role-playing an interview can help relieve the anxiety often present during an interview.
- Arrive on time. Do not be late. Try to arrive 5 to 10 minutes early for the interview but not so early that it may appear you are overanxious.
- Make sure to emphasize strong points. If you have outstanding or exceptional skills in a certain area, do not be afraid to "toot your own horn"—with a certain degree of modesty, of course.
- Dress appropriately. Remember that what is worn to an interview creates a first impression for others. Good grooming is expected. Do not smoke before the interview. A smoke odor on clothing may offend an interviewer. An example of proper interview dress is included in Figure 16-5.

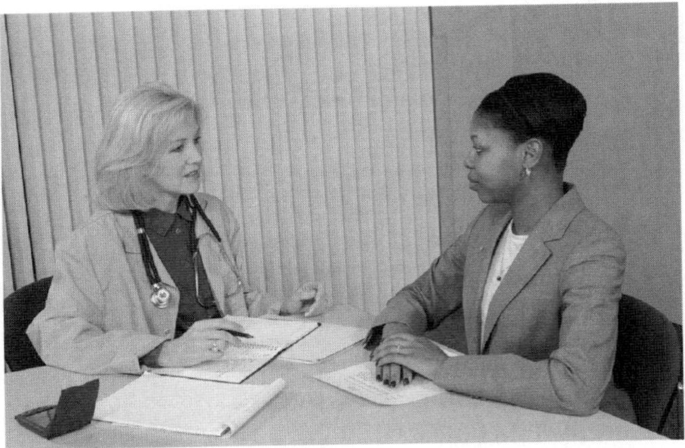

Figure 16-5 During an employment interview, proper posture, eye contact, and professional dress convey genuine interest in a job opening. (From Young AP. *Kinn's The Administrative Medical Assistant.* ed 7, St. Louis, Saunders, 2011.)

- Do not chew gum during the interview.
- Be prepared to ask questions about the position. Be ready with questions about the work hours, responsibilities, opportunities for advancement, and employee benefits. Be careful, though, not to dwell on items that are monetary in nature, as money should not be the focus of your questions or interest in the job.

The Interview

The anticipation of a job interview is often enough to make most people a little nervous. Rest assured, it is okay to be apprehensive—as a matter of fact, it is perfectly normal. It is very important to relax and trust that if you have the right qualifications, appear genuinely interested in working for the practice, and are sincere in your answers to interview questions, you will have a good chance of receiving a job offer.

The interview is an applicant's chance to support the qualifications presented in the résumé and an opportunity to display personal qualities. Some tips for a successful interview are as follows:

- Shake hands with the interviewer at the beginning of the interview. Practice a friendly greeting when preparing for the interview, such as "Good morning, my name is Jane Doe. I'm here for the 11:00 interview" or "Hello, my name is John Doe. It's a pleasure to meet you." Be sure to get the interviewer's name—you will need it later.
- Even if an application is required, give a résumé along with the application, or bring one to the interview.
- Be positive. Do not spend time "bashing" a former employer. Present a positive attitude.
- Shake hands with the interviewer at the end of the interview. Use the person's name and thank him or her for the interview.
- Send a follow-up letter (Fig. 16-6) to thank the interviewer for the interview. Be sure to address the letter to the interviewer personally.

Employee Benefits Packages

An important item of discussion during an interview is the types of benefits available for the position. Because of health care industry forecasts of continued employment growth, employers will likely need to provide incentives to attract and retain employees. Many employers offer substantial benefit packages that provide essential insurance coverage and some "perks" as well.

Individuals who are employed on a full-time basis usually have many benefits paid in full by the employer. Part-time employees in some facilities may have full benefits, but others may receive partial benefits or may have to pay a sum to obtain full benefits.

Not all benefits are available from every organization. Large organizations are able to offer more benefits simply because of their size. Depending on the organization, it may be possible to negotiate some components of a benefit package.

Health Insurance. Health insurance varies widely in the types of incidents covered. Health insurance plans usually cover hospital and clinic charges related to illness or injury, and some plans even provide coverage for preventive care, such as routine physicals and eye examinations. Employers may cover the entire cost of the insurance premium or may require employees to pay a portion of the premium. Many health insurance plans are quite comprehensive and provide many benefits, including reduced costs for prescriptions.

Life Insurance. Many employers provide a basic life insurance benefit that may be a set amount or may be proportionate to the employee's salary. The life insurance benefit is usually provided at no cost to the employee, but occasionally, additional life insurance coverage for the employee or for any member of the employee's immediate family may be available for purchase at the employee's discretion.

Dental Insurance. Dental insurance coverage customarily covers illness or trauma related to the teeth, as well as regular dental checkups. Dental procedures usually are covered, and many dental policies have an orthodontics benefit.

Disability Insurance. Disability insurance covers people who become disabled and are not able to work. Disability insurance is available in two forms: short term and long term. This type of insurance is designed to make up for income that might otherwise be lost if an employee were out of work for a brief or extended time.

Disability insurance is a type of insurance that is different from Workers' Compensation. Workers' Compensation covers injuries that are job related; disability insurance provides coverage for time missed from work because of illness that may not be work related.

Sick Leave. Sick leave benefits provide paid time off when an employee is sick. Some employers allow employees to use sick leave if a family member is sick and needs to be cared for by the employee. Sick leave may be issued in terms of hours or days. It may be awarded at a set time each year or may be accrued during each pay period. Limits sometimes are set by employers on the number of sick leave days or hours an employee may accumulate.

February 21, 20xx

Ms. Taylor Hudson, Office Manager
Horizons Healthcare Center
123 Main Avenue
Farmington, ND 58000

Dear Ms. Hudson:

Thank you for the opportunity to interview yesterday for the customer service position in the insurance department at your facility. I appreciate the time you took to give me a tour of the facility as well as to discuss the responsibilities and expectations for the position.

If you have any additional questions for me, I can be reached after 3:00 weekdays at 555-7717. I look forward to receiving your decision regarding the position.

Sincerely,

Taylor J. Reed

Taylor J. Reed

Figure 16-6 Even though an applicant should personally thank an interviewer at the end of an interview, a follow-up letter also should be sent to thank an interviewer for the opportunity to interview.

Vacation. Almost every health care employer offers some type of paid time off. Similar to sick leave, vacation leave may be accumulated by hours or per day and may be awarded at a specific time of the year or may accrue each pay period. A limit on vacation accumulation is common among employers.

Holidays. Employers in facilities that are not open around the clock usually establish paid holidays. Commonly recognized holidays include religious holidays and many federal holidays.

Paid Time Off. For facilities that are open 24 hours a day, 365 days a year, employers may consolidate vacation pay, holiday pay, and sick leave in one pool for the employee. This pool is often referred to as paid time off (PTO). Employers then allow employees to use the time as they choose, provided that adequate coverage is maintained throughout the facility's vital areas.

Pre-Tax Plans. Employers may offer the chance for employees to set aside from each paycheck a specified amount that is not taxed for eligible expenses. Typical eligible expenses include child care and medical and dental expenses. The money that is set aside is deposited in an account with an outside agency. Participation in a pre-tax plan is totally voluntary. Participants in the plan submit proof of expenses to the plan administrator (an outside company) and are reimbursed for their expenses up to the amount they have set aside.

Retirement. Many employers offer some type of retirement plan. Some plans allow employees to take additional money out of their paychecks to set aside for retirement. The additional money may even be matched by the employer. The thought of a retirement plan when you are just starting out in a career may seem strange, but the sooner an employee participates in a retirement plan, the more time an investment will have to grow.

Education Reimbursement. One of the less common benefits that is sometimes available is an educational reimbursement program provided by the employer. These programs encourage employees to continue their education and keep up with current technologies and trends. Educational reimbursement can pay some or all of the tuition associated with a course for credit. An employer may choose to fund only courses related to the individual's employment or may pay for any educational opportunity in which the employee has an interest. Some employers require proof of successful completion of the course before the tuition is reimbursed. Educational reimbursement can help employees continue their education and can enable employees to earn degrees at little or no cost.

Choosing the Right Position

An assistant who is just right for a position shows that when interacting with patients and coworkers. An assistant should take an honest look at the positions available and should choose the one for which he or she is best suited. For instance, a talkative person may have difficulty in a transcription position that has little to no contact with people during the day, or a person who is relaxed and methodical may have difficulty in a fast-paced urgent care center. An assistant spends a good portion of each day at work, and the type of employment chosen will have an impact on his or her life. That impact will be a good one if an assistant is prepared for and interested in the job he or she chooses.

When a job offer is made, must you give an answer right away? Of course not. Very few employers expect an answer immediately after an offer is made. Very often, an applicant will ask to "sleep on it" and get back to the employer the next day with an answer to the offer. This practice allows the applicant to think about what it would be like to work in that particular office.

How do you tell whether a position is right for you? Basically, you need to be satisfied with your answers to questions such as the following:

- Is the job interesting?
- Does the practice appear to be an enjoyable place to work?
- Are the wages appropriate? (Information on wages in a local area usually can be obtained through state employment offices, school placement offices, or local libraries.)
- Are the benefits satisfactory?
- Does the work schedule meet your expectations?

Once you have asked yourself questions such as these and have given yourself some time to think over a job offer, chances are good that you will make the right decision.

SUMMARY

Now that you have come to the end of this book, you may think that you have read and learned all you need to know to go out and get a job as a medical administrative assistant. However, this book is part of the beginning of your education for working in a medical office. Recall what was mentioned in the very first chapter: In the medical field, learning never ends! Technologies used in health care change almost as quickly as we become aware of them.

Entering the world of work will bring many new challenges and opportunities. Working in a medical office will bring about many opportunities to apply the skills and techniques learned while in school. A career in medical administrative assisting is an exciting, interesting, and worthwhile occupation that a dedicated assistant will find continually rewarding. Best of luck to you in your career ahead!

YOU ARE THE MEDICAL ADMINISTRATIVE ASSISTANT

You are currently working full-time for a small group medical practice and are applying for another position at another local health care facility. What is acceptable to list as contact information in your cover letter?

REVIEW EXERCISES

Exercise 16-1 True or False

Read each statement, and determine whether the statement is true or false. Record the answer in the blank provided. T = true; F = false

_______ 1. When applying for a position in a medical office, an assistant should bring along a résumé even if an employment application is completed.

_______ 2. Information on wages in your local area may be obtained through a state employment office or through other resources.

_______ 3. An applicant should review an application for completeness before handing it in.

_______ 4. On a résumé, it is best to list "Available on request" for personal references to save you the time of asking individuals for permission to list them as personal references.

_______ 5. Mistakes on an application can cost you a chance at an interview.

_______ 6. Medical and life insurance are typical employee benefits provided by employers.

_______ 7. If an employee is injured on the job, he or she must have disability insurance, or compensation will not be received for time missed from work or injuries caused by work.

_______ 8. Retirement plans may allow additional contributions to be made by employees.

_______ 9. Employers may offer medical, dental, and life insurance to their employees at little or no additional cost.

_______ 10. A pre-tax plan allows employees to set aside part of their earnings tax-free to pay for medical and child care expenses.

Exercise 16-2 Chapter Concepts

Read each statement, and choose the answer that best completes the statement. Record the answer in the blank provided.

_______ 1. Which of the following is false about seeking employment in a medical office?

(a) Some offices require an application to be completed.
(b) Courses in computer technology are of little value because technology changes too rapidly.
(c) An applicant's personal strengths and interests should be considered when seeking employment.
(d) Continuing education will be necessary to keep pace with industry changes.

_______ 2. Which of the following is true about a cover letter?

(a) A cover letter contains detailed information regarding an applicant's education and work history.
(b) It is best to address the letter "To Whom It May Concern."
(c) A cover letter allows an applicant to emphasize chief qualifications for a position.
(d) A cover letter is sent separately from a résumé.

_______ 3. Which of the following is true about locating job openings?

(a) Fees are normally charged for using an academic placement service.
(b) Health care job openings are listed only in the Sunday newspaper.
(c) To find a job, an assistant should expect to use a professional employment service and should expect to pay a fee.
(d) Openings in another part of the country may be located using the Internet.

_______ 4. All of the following apply to a student internship EXCEPT

(a) During an internship, a student experiences real-life situations.
(b) A student may be paid while on an internship.
(c) Internships often increase a student's chances of being employed later at the internship site.
(d) Every student who wishes to work in a medical office must complete an internship.

_______ 5. Benefits are an important consideration when accepting employment. Which of the following is false with regard to employee benefits?

(a) An employee may be required to pay part of a health insurance premium.
(b) All employers are required to provide dental insurance for employees.
(c) PTO is an accumulation of vacation, holiday, and sick leave pay.
(d) Employers may limit the amount of vacation time that an employee can accumulate.

_______6. Which of the following is true about employee benefits?
(a) Employers may limit the amount of sick leave that an employee can accumulate.
(b) An education reimbursement benefit means that an employer may pay for some educational courses or programs in which employees enroll.
(c) An employee may be able to purchase additional life insurance coverage for himself or herself.
(d) All are correct.
(e) Only (b) and (c) are correct.

_______7. Which of the following does not belong?
(a) Reference
(b) Internship
(c) Practicum
(d) Clinical
(e) Externship

_______8. Which of the following does not belong on a résumé?
(a) Applicant's interests
(b) Applicant's street address
(c) Applicant's phone number
(d) Applicant's birth date
(e) Applicant's email address

Exercise 16-3 Interview Techniques

Identify whether the following interview techniques are good or bad practice when applying for a position. Record the answer in the blank provided. G = good practice; B = bad practice.

_______ 1. Leave résumé at home until it is requested.

_______ 2. Be prepared to ask questions about the position and the organization.

_______ 3. Establish eye contact with the interviewer.

_______ 4. It is acceptable to chew gum during an interview.

_______ 5. Rehearse answers to potentially difficult questions.

_______ 6. Ask the employer ahead of time for all questions that will be discussed during the interview.

_______ 7. Have a cigarette or an alcoholic drink before the interview to relax.

_______ 8. Arrive on time or slightly late because doctors' offices usually are behind schedule.

_______ 9. Rehearse for the interview with a friend.

_______10. Focus on your needs and wants.

_______11. Shake hands with the interviewer before and after the interview.

_______12. Be interested in the position for which you are interviewing.

_______13. Ask current employees what they do not like about the office atmosphere.

_______14. Ask questions about the work schedule.

_______15. Send a follow-up letter thanking the interviewer for the opportunity to interview.

_______16. Use proper speech during the interview.

_______17. At the end of the interview, thank the interviewer by name.

ACTIVITIES

ACTIVITY 16-1 STUDENT PORTFOLIO

Review the contents of your student portfolio begun in Activity 1-8 and compare with the list here. Identify items that are included and items that should be added.

- Copy of school transcripts
- Record of employment
- Academic awards
- Other achievement awards, personal accomplishments
- Organization membership information
- Committee membership/leadership information
- Certifications or licensures
- Examples of school projects

ACTIVITY 16-2 RÉSUMÉ PREPARATION

Prepare a résumé. Refer to the chapter for the complete list of everything that should be included in a résumé. You may design the résumé yourself or use a template from a word processing program. Follow the guidelines listed in Procedure 16-1.

ACTIVITY 16-3 COVER LETTER

Prepare a cover letter by using a word processing program. Follow the guidelines in Procedure 16-2.

ACTIVITY 16-4 INTERVIEW QUESTIONS

Prepare a list of questions that may be asked by an interviewer. Stay within the guidelines presented in Chapter 15. Then participate in a mock interview, with you acting as the interviewer.

ACTIVITY 16-5 MOCK INTERVIEW

Participate in a mock interview, with another individual acting as the interviewer. Bring a prepared résumé to the interview, and be prepared to answer interview questions.

ACTIVITY 16-6 EMPLOYMENT APPLICATION

Complete an employment application such as the one pictured in Figure 16-1, or use an application from a local health care facility. Follow the guidelines given in Procedure 16-3.

DISCUSSION

The following topics can be used for class discussion or for individual student essay.

DISCUSSION 16-1

Define professionalism, and give examples of professional behavior.

DISCUSSION 16-2

Review your personal strengths and weaknesses. How would you discuss them with a potential employer?

DISCUSSION 16-3

Identify examples of how you could locate employment opportunities in your community using each of the following resources:

Networking
Academic placement services
Professional employment services
Classified ads
Internet job search
Professional associations
Cold calls
Internship opportunities

Bibliography

U.S. Office of Personnel Management: Federal Employees Health Benefits. U.S. Department of Labor. http://www.opm.gov.

U.S. Bureau of Labor and Statistics. http://www.bls.gov.

APPENDIX I Answers to Checkpoint Questions

Chapter 1

Explain why education as a medical administrative assistant would be beneficial for employment in a dental office.

Students of medical administrative assistant programs take courses in medical office procedures, anatomy and physiology, medical terminology, and computer technology; the skills and knowledge acquired in such a program would be used frequently in a dental office setting.

Chapter 2

Explain why a group practice may want to employ more primary care physicians than specialists.

Primary care physicians provide comprehensive general health care for patients. Because of their training, primary care physicians are able to treat patients with a huge variety of medical conditions. This training can improve access to medical care for patients. In addition, the primary care physician is usually the first physician a patient with a health concern would consult, and patients often are required to obtain a referral from a primary care physician before seeing a specialist.

What advantage(s) would a health care facility gain by hiring health care providers other than physicians?

If there is a shortage of physicians in a particular area, a health care provider such as a nurse practitioner or a physician' assistant can help fulfill the need for additional health care providers. Nurse practitioners and physician assistants can provide general health care services or can specialize in areas such as women's health, orthopedics, or neurology, for example. With regard to the financial aspect of using other health care providers, the salary for a nurse practitioner or a physician' assistant is lower than that required for a physician.

Nursing homes are required to have a certain number of registered nurses (RNs) on duty at all times. A clinic may choose to hire licensed practical nurses (LPNs) to work with patients and may or may not have an RN present in the facility. Given what you know about the makeup of those facilities, explain why a clinic may not be required to hire RNs.

Because a physician does not continually work in a nursing home, a higher level of health care is required for the care of nursing home residents. The level of nursing care required in a clinic may not be as great as that required in a nursing home.

Chapter 3

Identify whether the following situations could indicate malpractice on the part of a health care professional:

1. A nurse gives the wrong dosage of a drug, and that dosage causes harm to the patient.
2. A patient calls the clinic with chest pain, and the nurse fails to inform the physician of the phone call. Later in the day, the patient suffers a massive heart attack while at home and dies.
3. A physician fails to notify a patient of normal laboratory results.
4. A physician fails to inform the patient of suspicious Pap smear results. The patient is not informed of the need for follow-up care, and 1 year later, the patient is diagnosed as having cervical cancer.

Referring to the information in the chapter regarding proving negligence in a malpractice suit, all cases except number 3 probably would be considered negligence because the patient would be harmed. The patient in case number 3 probably would not be able to prove harm.

Could a patient with Alzheimer disease enter into a contract?

No. If a patient has been given the diagnosis of Alzheimer disease, the patient may no longer be of sound mind, and enforcing a contract signed by the patient (while suffering from the disease) would be difficult. Contracts made before the diagnosis may be valid but may be challenged if the contract was made close to the time of diagnosis.

Chapter 4

Physicians often provide treatment at no cost to their fellow physicians and their families. Is this in keeping with the Hippocratic Oath?

The Oath declares that a physician should "consider dear to me as my parents him who taught me this art; to live in common with him and if necessary to share my goods with him." This might be interpreted to support the practice of professional courtesy.

Professional courtesy is mentioned in the Current Opinions of the AMA, Opinion E-6.13, which identifies professional courtesy as "a long-standing tradition in the medical profession." However, professional courtesy is not required of physicians, and physicians must be careful not to forgive copayments or deductibles from patients and then or accept insurance only for payment of a patient's account. Such action may be unethical.

Examine the following examples of conduct, decide whether the conduct is in keeping with the information given about the AMA Principles of Medical Ethics, and state the reason for your answer.

1. Dr. Gonzalez is an obstetrician practicing in a large metropolitan city. Dr. Gonzalez has decided that she will not accept any new obstetrics patients in her practice. *This practice is ethical because physicians are allowed to choose whom they will accept as patients (with the exception of emergency cases) (Principle VI). See also Current Opinion E-10.05.*
2. Dr. Smith is an internist practicing in a state that has a law against physician-assisted suicide. Dr. Smith believes that patients should have the right to choose physician-assisted suicide if they are terminally ill, so he helps a patient commit suicide. *Euthanasia is not supported by the AMA as ethical behavior (Opinion 2.21). Physicians are dedicated to protecting life. A physician who commits such an act would be practicing unethically and would likely face criminal charges if such an act was illegal (Principle III).*
3. Dr. Anderson is aware of a physician in his health care facility who often bills Medicare for services that have not been performed. She does not report the physician's activity to the board of directors or to Medicare officials. *Physicians should report fraudulent activity of other physicians. If a physician has proof that fraudulent activity is occurring, the physician has an obligation to protect patients and the public (Principle II).*
4. Dr. Kowalski has developed a new technique for suturing operative wounds. He demonstrates this new technique to colleagues at the AMA National Convention. *Physicians are encouraged to develop new procedures and to willingly share their discoveries with their colleagues (Principle IV).*

A medical administrative assistant is confronted daily with situations to which she or he must decide how to respond. The Code of Medical Ethics of the AMA provides a framework from which the assistant can determine appropriate behavior. Consider the following instances, and determine whether or not the assistant's behavior is in keeping with the code of ethics:

1. An assistant volunteers for a local nonprofit health care organization. *Yes. Participation in service activities is encouraged.*
2. An assistant attends additional training to upgrade job skills. *Yes. An assistant should continually seek to improve skills and knowledge.*
3. An assistant unnecessarily discusses a patient's medical condition with a fellow employee. *No. Such activity is a breach of confidentiality.*

Consider the following case and determine the appropriate action that you as a medical administrative assistant should take:

Sue Adams, an unmarried pregnant patient of the office, cannot decide whether or not she should have an abortion. Sue asks Dr. Johnson what she thinks should be done. How would Dr. Johnson reply?
Dr. Johnson probably has a personal opinion about abortion, but she would likely present the facts (e.g., risks, alternatives) to the patient and leave it up to the patient to decide. Sue is the one who will have to live with her decision, not Dr. Johnson.

Is euthanasia a procedure that is consistent with the Hippocratic Oath? Why?
Not likely. The Hippocratic Oath, as given in the chapter, states, "to please no one will I prescribe a deadly drug, nor give advice which may cause his death."

Chapter 5

A physician who specializes in family practice often sees patients who bring their young children to the office. Explain how and why the office staff might be expected to assist with the children in the office.
Although it is not the office staff's responsibility to take care of every child who accompanies a patient to the office, once in a while a child will not be able to be present in an examination room during an examination or procedure. At that time, an assistant should keep a watchful eye on the child until the procedure or examination is completed and the child can rejoin the parent.

Chapter 6

A few people in the office like to gossip about other staff members. How could this affect the medical office environment?
The more people who work in a medical office, the more likely it is that there may be problems among some of the staff members. Office gossip can divide an office staff and create an unpleasant atmosphere in which to work. Gossip is negative and detrimental to the medical office environment and should not be tolerated.

Explain why training in proper telephone technique is important for every staff member of the medical office.
Although the front desk staff may be chiefly responsible for answering the telephone, other staff members frequently use the telephone to talk with patients or other staff members. Everyone may be needed to answer a call, whether the call is coming from outside the office or is being transferred. Training in proper telephone technique will help all personnel use the telephone more efficiently and effectively.

Explain the importance of deleting patient references from sample letters even though the letters remain in the office.
Although it is acceptable to keep samples of letters in an office, anything that could potentially identify a patient must be obliterated from them. Names, chart numbers, addresses, account numbers—anything that could possibly be linked to a particular patient should be blacked out from a copy. Samples usually are kept near a transcriptionist's workstation and are not part of the medical records; thus, samples may not have the confidentiality protection (i.e., locked cabinets or rooms) that a medical record would

have. All sample letters must be de-identified so as to comply with HIPAA regulations.

Chapter 7

The medical office where you are employed is evaluating two pieces of appointment scheduling software for implementation in the office. Software A is cheaper but allows only one user at a time to access the appointment system. Software B is twice as expensive but allows an unlimited number of users to access the appointment system at one time. Three physicians, a nurse practitioner, three nurses, and three medical office assistants are employed at the clinic. It is your job to recommend to the providers the appropriate software package for purchase. Which software package would you recommend? Defend your answer.
Of course, costs will be a factor, but if the office has sufficient funds to purchase software B, that should be the choice. Three assistants will be expected to schedule appointments for four health care providers. Software B allows more than one user at a time, so it is the better choice because assistants will have to schedule appointments and providers may need to access the system at the same time. Software B will enable the office staff to provide better service for patients.

Which of the following appointments could be scheduled as a double-booked appointment? (There may be more than one possible answer.)

Wart treatment	Headache	Depression
Lump	Sinus pain	Cough
Ear infection	Hearing check	Burn

Given the selections in the table, the following appointments could be double-booked: ear infection, sinus pain, and cough. Double-booked appointments are usually appointments of an urgent care nature. The three appointments identified are conditions that if left untreated could potentially become something more serious. Although the wart treatment is identified as a 15-minute appointment, wart treatment is usually not of an urgent nature. In addition, a physician may also approve a double-booked appointment for a patient with a headache if it is acute and the patient needs urgent pain control.

Why is it convenient for a patient to have a series of appointments established for a medical condition that needs regular attention?
If a patient needs to be seen on a regular basis by the physician, a series of appointments scheduled for the same day and time will help the patient remember when appointments are scheduled. For example, if a patient needs physical therapy twice a week for 6 weeks, if the appointments are always scheduled on the same days and times, the patient will be less likely to forget an appointment.

Why is it important for the medical office assistant to have an excellent understanding of anatomy, physiology, and disease processes before appropriately scheduling appointments in the medical office?
A basic understanding of the human body and conditions that affect a patient is absolutely essential for a medical administrative assistant. Although an assistant should never diagnose a patient, knowledge of the human body will enable an assistant to understand how extensive some health concerns could be. Also, it is usually an assistant who takes a patient's telephone call, screens the call, and decides how the call is handled (i.e., takes a message, makes an appointment, or transfers the call to a nurse or physician).

Chapter 8

An assistant who is new to the office likes to help make new patients feel more welcomed to the practice by sitting next to the patient in the lobby to answer any questions the patient may have while completing the paperwork for registration. Is this a good idea?
No, this is not a good idea. Oftentimes on patient registration and history forms, personal questions may be listed, and the patient's confidentiality may be in jeopardy if questions are asked while the patient is seated in the lobby.

Explain why music or television or both can be an important addition to a reception area.
Some type of entertainment that is appropriate for all ages will create a pleasant atmosphere and will help pass the time while patients and family members wait for appointments.

Explain why CPR training is a good idea for all medical office staff.
Whether an office is large or small, staff members never know whether they will be the first to encounter a patient who needs help. A staff member who is walking down a hallway or entering a restroom may be the first to encounter a patient who may need immediate attention.

Chapter 9

A medical office is using a terminal digit filing system in its records room. All chart numbers are composed of at least six digits. Charts will be marked with labels that correspond to the first unit used for filing. Should the medical office use colored chart folders, in addition to the colored labels, or will manila folders suffice?
Colored folders could provide another check when charts are filed. If a 10-color filing system such as the one pictured in Table 9-2 were implemented, the first digit in the secondary unit could signify the color. For example, the chart number 126342 would have labels identifying the 42, and the chart would have a green folder. Other charts—such as 126042, 126542, and 126842—would be filed near 126342, and would all be of the same color. If someone accidentally tried to file the chart numbered 123642 near those numbers, it would be recognized as a mistake because 123642 would be a white chart.

The credit department of the medical office has asked that an assistant place a colored label on the front of a patient's

chart if the patient's account has a large balance that is grossly overdue. Is this a good idea? Why?
No, this is not a good idea. A patient's or guarantor's financial status or information regarding the balance of a patient's or guarantor's account should not be included with the patient's medical record. A medical office would never want a patient to infer that treatment was not given because a large balance was owed on an account. Such activity might be an invitation to litigation.

Chapter 10

The office manager decides to not purchase a new edition of the CPT because there were not a lot of changes from the previous year. What impact, if any, would the office manager's decision have?
The decision to not purchase a new edition could have significant financial consequences, even if only one code (that the office uses) is updated or changed. Failure to use current codes could cause a delay in payment from an insurance company or a decrease in revenue if a new code is more appropriate for a claim.

Chapter 11

A patient telephones the office to report that she has not yet received a bill for services performed a month ago. What do you do?
Take the patient's name and number, and say that you will need to check the status of the bill. You may tell the patient that depending on the services that were rendered, it sometimes takes a short time for charges to be posted to an account. You would then need to trace the bill to determine why it has not appeared on the patient's account. After you find out the status of the bill, telephone the patient with the answer.

A minor calls the office and wishes to see a physician for information on birth control. The minor does not want her parents to know about the visit. Based on what you learned in Chapter 3 and in this chapter, what might your answer be?
It is likely that the physician will see the patient without the parents' consent. Before scheduling any type of appointment, confirm with the physician that the physician will see the patient for such a visit.

Chapter 12

Which coverage could potentially be more costly for an insurance company to provide: a fee-for-service plan or a managed care plan?
A fee-for-service plan is usually more costly because a patient usually is not required to get approval to see a specialist. Under a managed care plan, patients are required to see a primary care physician in order to get approval to see a specialist. Often, the primary care physician will be able to treat the patient's condition, and the cost of a specialist will be avoided. With a fee-for-service plan, an insurance company will have to pay for every visit covered by the policy.

Chapter 13

A medical office employee trips and falls over some boxes in the medical records room. One of the staff physicians examines the employee, obtains radiographs of the employee's wrist, and determines that the radiographs are negative and that the employee has sustained only a wrist sprain. Because the worker is already employed by the clinic, these services are performed at no charge. Should anything else be done by the employee?
The employee must file a first report of injury form to document the case for Workers' Compensation reasons. In addition, the employee should make sure that the visit is documented in the employee's medical record. Regardless of whether or not anyone is billed, both the Workers' Compensation and the medical record documentation must be done.

Chapter 14

At the end of many workdays, your coworkers comment that there is "too much to be done" to get ready for patients the next day, and that the receipts of the day should be handled when the office atmosphere is less hectic—maybe at the end of the week or the next week. What is your response?
If assistants are having trouble meeting all responsibilities of a position because of their workload, something must be done. Receipts should not sit until they can be processed; lack of deposits will affect cash flow, and this, in turn, will have an impact on the ability of the office to pay accounts payable. Letting receipts pile up also increases the chance that some payments will be lost or misplaced. Receipts must be handled on a timely basis. In this particular situation, employees may need to work overtime, additional office help may need to be hired, or office duties may need to be reassigned.

One of the assistants in the office proposes that receipts should no longer be written for payments received in person in the office, citing that patients who send checks in the mail do not get a receipt. What is your response?
Payments made in person in the office (e.g., small copayments may be required by insurance companies) occasionally may be made in cash. Without a receipt, persons who are paying cash will have no record of payment. In addition, receipts provide an excellent tracking device for recording information regarding a payment. It is likely that checks received in the mail will be returned with a portion of the patient's statement, which will allow an assistant to identify which account should be credited with the payment. The receipt that accompanies a payment also identifies which account should be credited with the payment.

Chapter 15

You are responsible for hiring an additional medical assistant to work in the office. A physician in the practice has asked you to find an older woman whose children are grown so that she will be able to stay late if necessary. How do you reply?
Such a question should never be asked. The question that could be asked of an applicant is whether the applicant would be able

to stay late if necessary, and the question should be asked of all applicants.

You are working for a pediatric practice. When hiring, the pediatricians have asked you to screen for an assistant who likes children. Would this be acceptable in an interview?
Most likely, this is an acceptable question. The question must be asked of all applicants, but because working with children is an essential part of the job, such a quality would be critical in an applicant.

Chapter 16

You want to work in a large well-known facility that is located about 700 miles from your current home. What are some good strategies for locating and applying for a position there?

The Internet is a good place to start. Because the facility is large and well known, chances are that information will be available from a website. In addition, you may decide to phone the human resources department of the facility in order to inquire about any current openings or to ask questions about applying for an open position.

APPENDIX II Competency Assessment Checklist

PROCEDURE 6-1

Demonstrate Telephone Techniques

Student Name ______________________ **Date** ______________________

Learning Outcome: Demonstrate telephone techniques.

Performance Standards: Time allowed ____________ min
Accuracy____________ %

Conditions: The student will follow the procedure outlined below to demonstrate telephone techniques within the standards identified using the following materials:

- Telephone setup with two separate lines
- Pen or pencil

EVALUATION CRITERIA

Symbol	Category	Point value
•	crucial step	______
■	essential step	______
▲	theory	______

Evaluation Criterion	Performance Evaluation Checklist	Points Possible	STUDENT'S SCORE	
			1st	2nd
	1. Answer the telephone within three rings.			
■	2. Answer the telephone using a proper greeting: • Welcome • Identification of facility • Identification of operator • Offer to help			
•	3. Determine the reason for the call.			
■	4. Identify the caller.			
▲	5. Determine the appropriate action based on the reason for the call.			
•	6. Confirm the call			
■	7. Close the call.			
	Optional			
▲	8. Demonstrate holding.			
▲	9. Demonstrate transferring a call.			
	Total Points			

Minimum total points required for satisfactory score ______

Evaluator's Comments:

Evaluator's Name ______________________ Date ______________________

- Denotes crucial step in procedure. Student must complete this step satisfactorily in order to complete the procedure.

National curriculum competencies achieved:

- Demonstrate telephone techniques.
- Recognize and respond to verbal and nonverbal communication.
- Use proper telephone techniques.

PROCEDURE 6-2

Demonstrate Taking Telephone Messages

Student Name ______________________ **Date** ______________________

Learning Outcome: Demonstrate taking telephone messages.

Performance Standards: Time allowed ____________ min
Accuracy____________ %

Conditions: The student will follow the procedure outlined below to demonstrate taking telephone messages within the standards identified using the following materials:

- Telephone setup with two separate lines
- Message blanks
- Pen or pencil

EVALUATION CRITERIA

Symbol	Category	Point value
•	crucial step	________
▪	essential step	________
▴	theory	________

Evaluation Criterion	Performance Evaluation Checklist	Points Possible	STUDENT'S SCORE	
			1st	2nd
▴	1. Demonstrate that a message is needed for an incoming telephone call and obtain a message blank to record the message.			
▪	2. Record date and time on message blank.			
▪	3. Record caller's name on message blank.			
•	4. Record patient's name on message blank.			
▪	5. Obtain patient's chart number. If chart number is not available, obtain patient's date of birth to help locate the chart number.			
▪	6. Record name of individual to whom the call is directed– physician or another individual.			
▪	7. Record message narrative, including action requested, on message blank.			
▪	8. Record telephone number for return call.			
	Total Points			

Minimum total points required for satisfactory score ______

Evaluator's Comments:

Evaluator's Name ______________________ Date ______________________

• Denotes crucial step in procedure. Student must complete this step satisfactorily in order to complete the procedure.

National curriculum competencies achieved:

- Demonstrate telephone techniques.
- Recognize and respond to verbal and nonverbal communication.
- Use proper telephone techniques.

PROCEDURE 6-3

Prepare a Patient Letter

Student Name ______________________ **Date** ______________________________

Learning Outcome: Prepare a patient letter.

Performance Standards: Time allowed ____________ min
Accuracy____________ %

Conditions: The student will follow the procedure outlined below to prepare a patient letter within standards identified using the following materials:

- Computer with word processing software
- Printer
- Letterhead stationery
- #10 business envelope
- Reference materials as necessary (dictionary, grammar reference)

EVALUATION CRITERIA

Symbol	Category	Point value
•	crucial step	________
▪	essential step	________
▲	theory	________

Evaluation Criterion	Performance Evaluation Checklist	Points Possible	STUDENT'S SCORE 1st	STUDENT'S SCORE 2nd
▪	1. Prepare a letter to a patient using the proper format illustrated in Figures 6-9, 6-10, and 6-11. a. Margins b. Date c. Inside Address d. Salutation e. Subject line f. Body g. Closing h. Notations i. Reference initials ii. Computer file name iii. Enclosure notation iv. Copy notation			
•	2. Proofread the letter for proper grammar and punctuation.			
▪	3. Print enough copies of the letter.			
▪	4. Address a business envelope using proper format for an OCR as shown in Figure 6-12. a. Addressee b. Street address c. City ST ZIP			
▪	5. Fold and insert letter in an envelope as shown in Figure 6-13.			
	Total Points			

Minimum total points required for satisfactory score ______

Evaluator's Comments:

Evaluator's Name ______________________ Date ______________________

- Denotes crucial step in procedure. Student must complete this step satisfactorily in order to complete the procedure.

National curriculum competencies achieved:

- Compose professional/business letters.
- Use correct grammar, spelling, and formatting techniques in written works.
- Apply computer concepts for office procedures.
- Perform basic secretarial skills.
- Perform basic keyboarding skills including typing medical correspondence and basic reports.

PROCEDURE 6-4

Prepare an Interoffice Memo

Student Name ______________________ **Date** ______________________

Learning Outcome: Prepare an interoffice memo.

Performance Standards: Time allowed ____________ min
Accuracy____________ %

Conditions: The student will follow the procedure outlined below to prepare an interoffice memo within the standards identified using the following materials:

- Computer with word processing software
- Printer
- Reference materials as necessary (dictionary, grammar reference)

EVALUATION CRITERIA

Symbol	Category	Point value
•	crucial step	________
▪	essential step	________
▴	theory	________

Evaluation Criterion	Performance Evaluation Checklist	Points Possible	STUDENT'S SCORE 1st	STUDENT'S SCORE 2nd
▪	1. Prepare an interoffice memo using the proper format, as illustrated in Figure 6-14. a. Margins b. To c. From d. Date e. Subject f. Body g. Reference initials h. Computer file name			
•	2. Proofread the memo for proper grammar and punctuation.			
▪	3. Print enough copies of the memo for distribution.			
	Total Points			

Minimum total points required for satisfactory score ______

Evaluator's Comments:

Evaluator's Name ______________________ Date ______________________

• Denotes crucial step in procedure. Student must complete this step satisfactorily in order to complete the procedure.

National curriculum competencies achieved:

- Use correct grammar, spelling, and formatting techniques in written works.
- Apply computer concepts for office procedures.
- Perform basic secretarial skills.

PROCEDURE 7-1

Prepare an Appointment Schedule for a Medical Office

Student Name ______________________ **Date** ______________________

Learning Outcome: Prepare an appointment schedule for a medical office.

Performance Standards: Time allowed __________ min
Accuracy__________ %

Conditions: The student will follow the procedure outlined below to prepare an appointment schedule for a medical office within the standards identified using the following materials:

- Appointment scheduling software on a computer system

EVALUATION CRITERIA

Symbol	Category	Point value
•	crucial step	________
■	essential step	________
▲	theory	________

Evaluation Criterion	Performance Evaluation Checklist	Points Possible	STUDENT'S SCORE 1st	STUDENT'S SCORE 2nd
■	1. Identify and mark off days the office is closed (weekends, holidays, whatever applies).			
■	2. Identify and mark off time of each day that the office is closed.			
■	3. Identify and mark off time of each day that the physician is unavailable.			
	Total Points			

Minimum total points required for satisfactory score ______

Evaluator's Comments:

Evaluator's Name ______________________ Date ______________________

- Denotes crucial step in procedure. Student must complete this step satisfactorily in order to complete the procedure.

National curriculum competencies achieved:

- Manage appointment schedule, using established priorities.
- Use office hardware and software to maintain office systems.
- Schedule and manage appointments.
- Identify and properly utilize office machines, computerized systems and medical software such as:
  - Apply computer application skills using variety of different electronic programs including both practice management software and EMR software.

PROCEDURE 7-2

Schedule Appointments

Student Name ______________________ **Date** ______________________

Learning Outcome: Schedule appointments.

Performance Standards: Time allowed ____________ min
Accuracy____________ %

Conditions: The student will follow the procedure outlined below to schedule appointments within the standards identified using the following materials:

- List of appointments and scheduling guidelines.
- Appointment scheduling software on a computer system
  or
- Appointment book and pencil

EVALUATION CRITERIA

Symbol	Category	Point value
•	crucial step	______
▪	essential step	______
▴	theory	______

Evaluation Criterion	Performance Evaluation Checklist	Points Possible	STUDENT'S SCORE 1st	2nd
•	1. Determine the reason for the appointment.			
▴	2. Using scheduling guidelines, determine the length of the appointment.			
▪	3. Identify the patient's name.			
▪	4. Determine the patient's preferences for desired appointment time.			
▪	5. Identify date and time for appointment and obtain approval for date and time with patient (or patient's representative).			
▪	6. Enter appointment on the schedule.			
•	7. Confirm appointment with patient (or patient's representative).			
▪	***Optional*** 8. If patient is in the office, give patient a written reminder for the appointment.			
	Total Points			

Minimum total points required for satisfactory score ______

Evaluator's Comments:

Evaluator's Name ______________________ Date ______________________

• Denotes crucial step in procedure. Student must complete this step satisfactorily in order to complete the procedure.

National curriculum competencies achieved:

- Manage appointment schedule, using established priorities.
- Use office hardware and software to maintain office systems.
- Schedule and monitor appointments.
- Apply computer concepts for office procedures.

PROCEDURE 7-3

Document Appointment Changes

Student Name ______________________ **Date** ________________________________

Learning Outcome: Document appointment changes.

Performance Standards: Time allowed ____________ min
Accuracy____________ %

Conditions: The student will follow the procedure outlined below to document appointment changes within standards identified using the following materials:

- Patient's medical record.
- Black ink pen (if paper record is used)

EVALUATION CRITERIA

Symbol	Category	Point value
•	crucial step	______
▪	essential step	______
▲	theory	______

Evaluation Criterion	Performance Evaluation Checklist	Points Possible	STUDENT'S SCORE	
			1st	2nd
▪	1. Identify appoint change (no-show, cancellation, reschedule, etc.)			
•	2. Locate patient's medical record.			
•	3. In appropriate location in the patient's record, enter the date and document the appointment change.			
•	4. Sign the record entry.			
	Total Points			

Minimum total points required for satisfactory score _______

Evaluator's Comments:

Evaluator's Name ________________________ Date ____________________________

• Denotes crucial step in procedure. Student must complete this step satisfactorily in order to complete the procedure.

National curriculum competencies achieved:

- Manage appointment schedule, using established priorities.
- Use office hardware and software to maintain office systems.
- Schedule and manage appointments.
- Identify and properly utilize office machines, computerized systems and medical software such as:
  - Apply computer application skills using variety of different electronic programs including both practice management software and EMR software.

PROCEDURE 7-4

Reschedule Appointments

Student Name ______________________ **Date** ______________________________

Learning Outcome: Reschedule appointments.

Performance Standards: Time allowed ____________ min
Accuracy____________ %

Conditions: The student will follow the procedure outlined below to reschedule appointments within standards identified using the following materials:

- Appointment scheduling software on a computer system

EVALUATION CRITERIA

Symbol	Category	Point value
•	crucial step	________
▪	essential step	________
▴	theory	________

Evaluation Criterion	Performance Evaluation Checklist	Points Possible	STUDENT'S SCORE 1st	STUDENT'S SCORE 2nd
•	1. Obtain the patient's name.			
•	2. Locate the original appointment.			
▴	3. Verify the reason for the appointment. Using scheduling guidelines, determine whether the length of the appointment is correct.			
▪	4. Determine preferences for desired appointment time.			
▪	5. Identify date and time for appointment and obtain approval for date and time with patient (or patient's representative).			
▪	6. Enter new appointment on the schedule.			
•	7. Confirm new appointment with patient (or patient's representative).			
▪	8. Delete original appointment.			
	Optional			
▪	9. If patient is in the office, give patient a written reminder for the new appointment.			
	Total Points			

Minimum total points required for satisfactory score ______

Evaluator's Comments:

Evaluator's Name ________________________ Date ____________________________

- Denotes crucial step in procedure. Student must complete this step satisfactorily in order to complete the procedure.

National curriculum competencies achieved:

- Manage appointment schedule, using established priorities.
- Use office hardware and software to maintain office systems.
- Schedule and manage appointments.
- Identify and properly utilize office machines, computerized systems and medical software such as:
  - Apply computer application skills using variety of different electronic programs including both practice management software and EMR software.

PROCEDURE 8-1

Update Existing Patient Registration Information

Student Name ____________________ **Date** ____________________

Learning Outcome: Update existing patient registration information.

Performance Standards: Time allowed ____________ min
Accuracy____________ %

Conditions: The student will follow the procedure outlined below to update existing patient registration information within standards identified using the following materials:

- Patient information.
- Computer software for a medical office.

EVALUATION CRITERIA

Symbol	Category	Point value
•	crucial step	________
▪	essential step	________
▲	theory	________

Evaluation Criterion	Performance Evaluation Checklist	Points Possible	STUDENT'S SCORE 1st	STUDENT'S SCORE 2nd
•	1. Ask patient for full legal name and locate patient information in patient database. Verify patient's date of birth to ensure that correct record is updated.			
▪	2. Verify that the following information for the patient is current: • address • telephone number • employer • insurance company name, address, policy number, and group number (copy insurance card if necessary) Record any changes given by patient.			
▪	3. Thank the patient for information and tell the patient to be seated in the reception area.			
▪	4. Record any changes in registration information in the patient's medical record (as applicable).			
	Total Points			

Minimum total points required for satisfactory score ______

Evaluator's Comments:

Evaluator's Name ____________________ Date ____________________

- Denotes crucial step in procedure. Student must complete this step satisfactorily in order to complete the procedure.

National curriculum competencies achieved:

- Use office hardware and software to maintain office systems.
- Execute data management using electronic healthcare records such as the EMR.
- Identify and properly utilize office machines, computerized systems and medical software such as:
  - Apply computer application skills using variety of different electronic programs including both practice management software and EMR software.
- Prepare and maintain medical records.
- Apply electronic technology.

PROCEDURE 8-2

Obtain New Patient Registration Information

Student Name ______________________ **Date** ______________________

Learning Outcome: Obtain new patient registration information.

Performance Standards: Time allowed ____________ min
Accuracy____________ %

Conditions: The student will follow the procedure outlined below to obtain registration information from a new patient within standards identified using the following materials:

- New patient registration form
- Patient medical history form
- Clipboard and pen or pencil
- Photocopier

EVALUATION CRITERIA

Symbol	Category	Point value
•	crucial step	________
▪	essential step	________
▴	theory	________

Evaluation Criterion	Performance Evaluation Checklist	Points Possible	STUDENT'S SCORE 1st	2nd
•	1. Ask patient for full legal name and check patient database to determine whether patient is new to the medical office.			
▪	2. Attach a registration form and a patient history form to the clipboard and give to the patient, asking the patient to complete the forms and return them to you when completed.			
▪	3. After patient returns forms, review each form to determine whether forms are complete. Ask patient for information if forms are incomplete.			
▪	4. Ask patient for insurance card. Copy insurance card.			
▪	5. Thank the patient for information and tell the patient to be seated in the lobby.			
	Total Points			

Minimum total points required for satisfactory score ______

Evaluator's Comments:

Evaluator's Name ______________________ Date ______________________

- Denotes crucial step in procedure. Student must complete this step satisfactorily in order to complete the procedure.

National curriculum competencies achieved:

- Use office hardware and software to maintain office systems.
- Execute data management using electronic healthcare records such as the EMR.
- Identify and properly utilize office machines, computerized systems and medical software such as:
  - Apply computer application skills using a variety of different electronic programs including both practice management software and EMR software.
- Prepare and maintain medical records.
- Apply electronic technology.

PROCEDURE 8-3

Record New Patient Registration Information

Student Name ______________________ **Date** ______________________________

Learning Outcome: Record new patient registration.

Performance Standards: Time allowed ____________ min
Accuracy____________ %

Conditions: The student will follow the procedure outlined below to record new patient registration within standards identified using the following materials:

- Computer software for a medical office
- Completed new patient registration form

EVALUATION CRITERIA

Symbol	Category	Point value
•	crucial step	______
▪	essential step	______
▴	theory	______

Evaluation Criterion	Performance Evaluation Checklist	Points Possible	STUDENT'S SCORE 1st	STUDENT'S SCORE 2nd
•	1. Check computer database to determine whether a previous record exists for the new patient.			
▪	2. Once the patient has been verified as a new patient to the medical office, assign a medical record number to the patient.			
▪	3. Enter all pertinent data for the patient.			
▪	4. Save the new record.			
	Total Points			

Minimum total points required for satisfactory score ______

Evaluator's Comments:

Evaluator's Name ________________________ Date ___________________________

- Denotes crucial step in procedure. Student must complete this step satisfactorily in order to complete the procedure.

National curriculum competencies achieved:

- Use office hardware and software to maintain office systems.
- Execute data management using electronic healthcare records such as the EMR.
- Identify and properly utilize office machines, computerized systems and medical software such as:
    - Apply computer application skills using a variety of different electronic programs including both practice management software and EMR software.
- Prepare and maintain medical records.
- Apply electronic technology.

PROCEDURE 9-1

Document an Event in a Patient's Chart

Student Name ____________________ **Date** ____________________

Learning Outcome: Document an event in a patient's chart.

Performance Standards: Time allowed ____________ min
Accuracy____________ %

Conditions: The student will follow the procedure outlined below to document an event in a patient's chart within standards identified using the following materials:

- Patient's medical record
- Black ink pen

EVALUATION CRITERIA

Symbol	Category	Point value
•	crucial step	________
▪	essential step	________
▴	theory	________

Evaluation Criterion	Performance Evaluation Checklist	Points Possible	STUDENT'S SCORE 1st	STUDENT'S SCORE 2nd
•	1. Obtain patient's medical record. Locate next available place for documentation in the progress notes (continuation sheet).			
▪	2. Determine information to be written in patient's chart. Be sure you are authorized to enter such information.			
•	3. With black ink pen, record date and information regarding the patient.			
•	4. Sign the chart entry.			
	Total Points			

Minimum total points required for satisfactory score ______

Evaluator's Comments:

Evaluator's Name ____________________ Date ____________________

• Denotes crucial step in procedure. Student must complete this step satisfactorily in order to complete the procedure.

National curriculum competencies achieved:

- Describe various types of content maintained in a patient's medical record.
- Prepare and maintain medical records.

PROCEDURE 9-2

Transcribe a Medical Report

Student Name ______________________ **Date** ______________________________

Learning Outcome: Transcribe a medical report.

Performance Standards: Time allowed ____________ min
Accuracy____________ %

Conditions: The student will follow the procedure outlined below to transcribe a medical report within standards identified using the following materials:

- Dictated medical report
- Equipment to play report (digital or tape transcriber)
- Computer with word processing software
- Printer

EVALUATION CRITERIA

Symbol	Category	Point value
•	crucial step	______
▪	essential step	______
▴	theory	______

Evaluation Criterion	Performance Evaluation Checklist	Points Possible	STUDENT'S SCORE 1st	2nd
▪	1. Locate beginning of report dictation.			
▪	2. Adjust volume and speed of the dictation as necessary.			
▴	3. Choose appropriate report format.			
▪	4. Type dictated report.			
•	5. Proofread report and make any necessary corrections.			
▪	6. Print report for physician signature and insertion in patient's medical record.			
	Total Points			

Minimum total points required for satisfactory score _______

Evaluator's Comments:

Evaluator's Name ___________________________ Date ______________________________

- Denotes crucial step in procedure. Student must complete this step satisfactorily in order to complete the procedure.

National curriculum competencies achieved:

- Describe various types of content maintained in the patient's medical record.
- Use office hardware and software to maintain office systems.
- Prepare and maintain medical records.
- Apply computer concepts for office procedures.

PROCEDURE 9-3

Organize a Patient's Medical Record

Student Name ______________________ **Date** ______________________

Learning Outcome: Organize a patient's medical record.

Performance Standards: Time allowed ____________ min
Accuracy____________ %

Conditions: The student will follow the procedure outlined below to organize a patient's medical record within standards identified using the following materials:

- Patient's medical record
- Medical reports

EVALUATION CRITERIA

Symbol	Category	Point value
•	crucial step	________
▪	essential step	________
▴	theory	________

Evaluation Criterion	Performance Evaluation Checklist	Points Possible	STUDENT'S SCORE	
			1st	2nd
•	1. Verify patient's name on reports and on the medical record.			
▪	2. Determine where the reports should be inserted in the medical record.			
▪	3. Open fasteners that hold together chart documents.			
▪	4. Insert the reports in the appropriate location in the patient's medical record.			
▪	5. Close fasteners to secure chart documents.			
	Total Points			

Minimum total points required for satisfactory score _______

Evaluator's Comments:

Evaluator's Name ______________________ Date ______________________

• Denotes crucial step in procedure. Student must complete this step satisfactorily in order to complete the procedure.

National curriculum competencies achieved:

- Describe various types of content maintained in a patient's medical record.
- Organize a patient's medical record.
- Maintain organization by filing.
- Prepare and maintain medical records.

PROCEDURE 9-4

Index and File Medical Records

Student Name ______________________ **Date** ______________________

Learning Outcome: Index and file medical records.

Performance Standards: Time allowed ____________ min
Accuracy____________ %

Conditions: The student will follow the procedure outlined below to index and file medical records within standards identified using the following materials:

- Medical records

EVALUATION CRITERIA

Symbol	Category	Point value
•	crucial step	________
▪	essential step	________
▲	theory	________

Evaluation Criterion	Performance Evaluation Checklist	Points Possible	STUDENT'S SCORE 1st	STUDENT'S SCORE 2nd
▪	1. Place medical records in indexing order following the guidelines for the filing system adopted by the medical office.			
•	2. Determine where the record will be filed.			
▪	3. Verify that the filing location is correct by checking the record in front and the record in back of the record to be filed.			
▪	4. Complete filing of each record by repeating steps 2 and 3 for each record.			
	Total Points			

Minimum total points required for satisfactory score ______

Evaluator's Comments:

Evaluator's Name ______________________ Date ______________________

- Denotes crucial step in procedure. Student must complete this step satisfactorily in order to complete the procedure.

National curriculum competencies achieved:

- Describe indexing rules.
- Maintain organization by filing.
- File medical records.
- Prepare and maintain medical records.

PROCEDURE 9-5

Color Code Medical Records

Student Name ____________________ **Date** ______________________________

Learning Outcome: Color code medical records.

Performance Standards: Time allowed ___________ min
Accuracy___________ %

Conditions: The student will follow the procedure outlined below to color code medical records within standards identified using the following materials:

- Medical records
- Color-coding scheme
- Labels compatible with color-coding scheme

EVALUATION CRITERIA

Symbol	Category	Point value
•	crucial step	________
▪	essential step	________
▲	theory	________

Evaluation Criterion	Performance Evaluation Checklist	Points Possible	STUDENT'S SCORE 1st	2nd
▪	1. Obtain scheme for color coding medical records.			
•	2. Affix appropriate label to each medical record that corresponds to the filing system and associate color scheme. Alphabetical filing – use label corresponding to first letter of patient's last name. Consecutive number filing – use label corresponding to thousandth digit of chart number Terminal digit filing – use labels corresponding to the two digits in the primary indexing unit.			
▪	3. Verify that color coding is correct by placing the records in order for filing. Colors will appear together.			
	Total Points			

Minimum total points required for satisfactory score _______

Evaluator's Comments:

Evaluator's Name ______________________ Date ______________________

• Denotes crucial step in procedure. Student must complete this step satisfactorily in order to complete the procedure.

National curriculum competencies achieved:

- Discuss pros and cons of various filing methods.
- Identify both equipment and supplies needed for filing medical records.
- Describe indexing rules.
- Discuss filing procedures.
- Prepare and maintain medical records.

PROCEDURE 9-6

Create Electronic Tickler File

Student Name ______________________ **Date** ________________________________

Learning Outcome: Create electronic tickler file.

Performance Standards: Time allowed ____________ min
Accuracy____________ %

Conditions: The student will follow the procedure outlined below to create electronic tickler file within standards identified using the following materials:

- Computer and scheduling software
- Lists of tasks to be scheduled

EVALUATION CRITERIA

Symbol	Category	Point value
•	crucial step	____________
▪	essential step	____________
▲	theory	____________

Evaluation Criterion	Performance Evaluation Checklist	Points Possible	STUDENT'S SCORE	
			1st	2nd
▪	1. Open the computer scheduling software.			
▲	2. Identify task to be scheduled.			
▪	3. Identify due date of task.			
▪	4. Identify task priority.			
•	5. Save all changes to task list.			
	Total Points			

Minimum total points required for satisfactory score ______

Evaluator's Comments:

Evaluator's Name _________________________ Date ____________________________

- Denotes crucial step in procedure. Student must complete this step satisfactorily in order to complete the procedure.

National curriculum competencies achieved:

- Use office hardware and software to maintain office systems.
- Implement time management principles to maintain effective office function.
- Apply electronic technology.

PROCEDURE 9-7

Process a Request to Release Medical Information

Student Name ______________________ **Date** ______________________________

Learning Outcome: Process a request to release medical information from the medical office.

Performance Standards: Time allowed ____________ min
Accuracy____________ %

Conditions: The student will follow the procedure outlined below to process a request to release medical information from the medical office within standards identified using the following materials:

- Release of information form
- Black ink pen
- Patient's medical record (paper or electronic)

EVALUATION CRITERIA

Symbol	Category	Point value
•	crucial step	______
▪	essential step	______
▴	theory	______

Evaluation Criterion	Performance Evaluation Checklist	Points Possible	STUDENT'S SCORE	
			1st	2nd
▪	1. If needed, help patient complete release request.			
▴	2. Verify that all necessary information is included on the release.			
•	3. Obtain patient's medical record and verify patient's name on release with name on medical record.			
▪	4. Photocopy or print requested information to be released.			
▪	5. Arrange information in logical order.			
▪	6. Attach copy of release of information request on top of information to be released.			
▪	7. Place original release request in correct section of patient's medical record.			
•	8. Send information to the medical facility identified on the release.			
•	9. In a chart entry, document that the release was processed.			
	Total Points			

Minimum total points required for satisfactory score ______

Evaluator's Comments:

Evaluator's Name ______________________ Date ______________________

• Denotes crucial step in procedure. Student must complete this step satisfactorily in order to complete the procedure.

National curriculum competencies achieved:

- Apply HIPAA rules in regard to privacy/release of information.
- Document accurately in patient record.
- Prepare and maintain medical records.

PROCEDURE 10-1

Assign Procedure Codes for a Patient's Encounter

Student Name ______________________ **Date** ______________________

Learning Outcome: Assign procedure codes for a patient's encounter.

Performance Standards: Time allowed __________ min
Accuracy__________ %

Conditions: The student will follow the procedure outlined below to assign procedure codes for a patient's encounter within standards identified using the following materials:
- Medical records
- CPT manual, current year's edition

EVALUATION CRITERIA

Symbol	Category	Point value
•	crucial step	______
▪	essential step	______
▴	theory	______

Evaluation Criterion	Performance Evaluation Checklist	Points Possible	STUDENT'S SCORE 1st	STUDENT'S SCORE 2nd
▪	1. From the patient's record, identify all procedures performed during a patient's encounter.			
▪	2. Locate the main term for each procedure in the index by identifying the condition, the anatomic site procedure, or the service provided.			
▪	3. Look beneath in the main term for any additional modifiers. Identify all codes that may fit the procedure.			
▪	4. Locate each of the codes from #3 in the appropriate section of CPT.			
•	5. Read the description for each code and choose the appropriate code for each procedure identified.			
	Total Points			

Minimum total points required for satisfactory score ______

Evaluator's Comments:

Evaluator's Name ______________________ Date ______________________

• Denotes crucial step in procedure. Student must complete this step satisfactorily in order to complete the procedure.

National curriculum competencies achieved:
- Perform accounts receivable procedures, including:
  - Perform billing procedures.
- Describe how to use the most current procedural coding system.
- Perform procedural coding.
- Perform billing and collection procedures.
- Perform diagnostic and procedural coding.

PROCEDURE 10-2

Assign Diagnosis Codes for a Patient's Encounter

Student Name ______________________ **Date** ______________________

Learning Outcome: Assign diagnosis codes for a patient's encounter.

Performance Standards: Time allowed ____________ min
Accuracy____________ %

Conditions: The student will follow the procedure outlined below to assign diagnosis codes for a patient's encounter within standards identified using the following materials:

- Medical records
- ICD-9-CM manual (current year)

EVALUATION CRITERIA

Symbol	Category	Point value
•	crucial step	____________
▪	essential step	____________
▲	theory	____________

Evaluation Criterion	Performance Evaluation Checklist	Points Possible	STUDENT'S SCORE 1st	STUDENT'S SCORE 2nd
▲	1. Identify all diagnoses treated during a patient's encounter.			
▲	2. Determine the primary reason for the patient's office visit.			
▪	3. Locate the main term for the diagnosis in the index (Volume II)			
▪	4. Locate any modifiers beneath the main term.			
▪	5. Identify the numerical code reference in Volume II.			
▪	6. Locate the code from Volume II in the tabular (numerical) listing (Volume I) in the manual.			
•	7. Read the description of the code. Determine whether the code fits the diagnosis given for the patient.			
▪	8. Code any additional diagnoses listed in the patient's encounter by repeating steps 3 through 7.			
	Total Points			

Minimum total points required for satisfactory score ______

Evaluator's Comments:

Evaluator's Name ______________________ Date ______________________

• Denotes crucial step in procedure. Student must complete this step satisfactorily in order to complete the procedure.

National curriculum competencies achieved:

- Perform accounts receivable procedures, including:
  - Perform billing procedures.
- Describe how to use the most current diagnostic coding system.
- Perform diagnostic coding.
- Perform billing and collection procedures.
- Perform diagnostic and procedural coding.

PROCEDURE 11-1

Enter Patients' Charges Into a Billing System

Student Name ______________________ **Date** ______________________

Learning Outcome: Enter patients' charges into a billing system.

Performance Standards: Time allowed ____________ min
Accuracy____________ %

Conditions: The student will follow the procedure outlined below to enter patients' charges into a billing system within standards identified using the following materials:

- Computer billing system or pegboard system
- Superbills from patients' encounters

EVALUATION CRITERIA

Symbol	Category	Point value
•	crucial step	____________
▪	essential step	____________
▲	theory	____________

Evaluation Criterion	Performance Evaluation Checklist	Points Possible	STUDENT'S SCORE 1st	STUDENT'S SCORE 2nd
▲	1. Gather superbills to be recorded.			
•	2. Assign correct procedure codes for each encounter.			
•	3. Assign correct diagnosis codes for each encounter.			
•	4. Record encounters in billing system. Enter correct information in each billing category.			
	Total Points			

Minimum total points required for satisfactory score ______

Evaluator's Comments:

Evaluator's Name ______________________ Date ______________________

- Denotes crucial step in procedure. Student must complete this step satisfactorily in order to complete the procedure.

National curriculum competencies achieved:

- Perform accounts receivable procedures including:
  - Perform billing procedures
- Utilize computerized office billing systems.
- Perform billing and collection procedures.
- Perform accounts receivable procedures.
- Use manual or computerized bookkeeping systems.

PROCEDURE 11-2

Produce Monthly Statements for Patient Accounts

Student Name ______________________ **Date** ______________________________

Learning Outcome: Produce monthly statements for patient accounts.

Performance Standards: Time allowed ____________ min
Accuracy____________ %

Conditions: The student will follow the procedure outlined below to produce monthly statements for patients' accounts within standards identified using the following materials:

- Patients' account (billing) information
- Outstanding charges and payments

EVALUATION CRITERIA

Symbol	Category	Point value
•	crucial step	________
▪	essential step	________
▲	theory	________

Evaluation Criterion	Performance Evaluation Checklist	Points Possible	STUDENT'S SCORE 1st	STUDENT'S SCORE 2nd
▲	1. Establish statement date.			
▲	2. Determine which accounts should have a statement generated. If a cycle billing system is used, only certain statements may have to be generated.			
▪	3. Post any outstanding charges to patients' accounts.			
▪	4. Post any outstanding payments to patients' accounts.			
•	5. Print statements.			
	Total Points			

Minimum total points required for satisfactory score ______

Evaluator's Comments:

Evaluator's Name ________________________ Date ____________________________

- Denotes crucial step in procedure. Student must complete this step satisfactorily in order to complete the procedure.

National curriculum competencies achieved:

- Perform accounts receivable procedures including:
  - Perform billing procedures
- Utilize computerized office billing systems.
- Perform billing and collection procedures.
- Perform accounts receivable procedures.
- Use manual or computerized bookkeeping systems.

PROCEDURE 12-1

Complete an Insurance Claim Using the CMS-1500

Student Name ______________________ **Date** ______________________

Learning Outcome: Complete an insurance claim using the CMS-1500.

Performance Standards: Time allowed ____________ min
Accuracy____________ %

Conditions: The student will follow the procedure outlined below to complete an insurance claim using the CMS-1500 within standards identified using the following materials:

- Billing and insurance information for a patient
- Computer software or typewriter to complete form
- CMS-1500 claim form

EVALUATION CRITERIA

Symbol	Category	Point value
•	crucial step	________
▪	essential step	________
▲	theory	________

Evaluation Criterion	Performance Evaluation Checklist	Points Possible	STUDENT'S SCORE 1st	STUDENT'S SCORE 2nd
▲	1. Obtain billing information for the claim.			
•	2. Code procedures and diagnoses for the claim.			
•	3. Obtain patient's insurance information for the claim.			
•	4. Complete CMS-1500 claim form following guidelines established by the insurance plan.			
	Total Points			

Minimum total points required for satisfactory score _______

Evaluator's Comments:

Evaluator's Name ______________________ Date ______________________

• Denotes crucial step in procedure. Student must complete this step satisfactorily in order to complete the procedure.

National curriculum competencies achieved:

- Complete insurance claim forms.
- Apply third-party guidelines.
- Utilize computerized office billing systems.
- Prepare and submit insurance claims.
- Use manual or computerized bookkeeping systems.

PROCEDURE 13-1

Prepare a Meeting Agenda

Student Name ______________________ **Date** ______________________

Learning Outcome: Prepare a meeting agenda.

Performance Standards: Time allowed ____________ min
Accuracy____________ %

Conditions: The student will follow the procedure outlined below to prepare a meeting agenda within standards identified using the following materials:

- Information about meeting
- Computer
- Printer

EVALUATION CRITERIA

Symbol	Category	Point value
•	crucial step	______
▪	essential step	______
▲	theory	______

Evaluation Criterion	Performance Evaluation Checklist	Points Possible	STUDENT'S SCORE 1st	STUDENT'S SCORE 2nd
▪	1. Identify meeting date, time, and place.			
▪	2. Identify agenda items to be discussed and order of discussion.			
▪	3. List agenda items in order of discussion.			
▪	4. Proofread the agenda for typos and grammatical errors.			
•	5. Print a copy of the agenda.			
▪	6. Make a required number of copies of agenda and distribute to designated individuals.			
	Total Points			

Minimum total points required for satisfactory score ______

Evaluator's Comments:

Evaluator's Name ______________________ Date ______________________

- Denotes crucial step in procedure. Student must complete this step satisfactorily in order to complete the procedure.

National curriculum competencies achieved:

- Use office hardware and software to maintain office systems.
- Perform basic clerical functions.
- Apply electronic technology.

PROCEDURE 13-2

Prepare Minutes of a Meeting

Student Name ______________________ **Date** ______________________

Learning Outcome: Prepare minutes of a meeting.

Performance Standards: Time allowed ____________ min
Accuracy____________ %

Conditions: The student will follow the procedure outlined below to prepare a travel itinerary within standards identified using the following materials:

- Meeting agenda
- Attendance at a meeting
- Computer and/or paper and pencil
- Printer

EVALUATION CRITERIA

Symbol	Category	Point value
•	crucial step	________
▪	essential step	________
▲	theory	________

Evaluation Criterion	Performance Evaluation Checklist	Points Possible	STUDENT'S SCORE 1st	STUDENT'S SCORE 2nd
▪	1. Identify meeting date, time, and place.			
▪	2. Obtain copy of agenda.			
▪	3. Attend meeting and list those present at the meeting.			
▪	4. During the meeting, take notes regarding meeting discussion.			
▪	Record the minutes in chronological order.			
▪	5. Prepare minutes using the format provided in Chapter 12.			
•	6. Proofread the minutes for typos and grammatical errors.			
▪	7. Print a copy of the minutes.			
▪	8. Make required number of copies of minutes and distribute to designated individuals.			
	Total Points			

Minimum total points required for satisfactory score ______

Evaluator's Comments:

Evaluator's Name ______________________ Date ______________________

- Denotes crucial step in procedure. Student must complete this step satisfactorily in order to complete the procedure.

National curriculum competencies achieved:

- Use office hardware and software to maintain office systems.
- Perform basic clerical functions.
- Apply electronic technology.

PROCEDURE 13-3

Prepare a Travel Itinerary

Student Name _______________ **Date** _______________

Learning Outcome: Prepare a travel itinerary.

Performance Standards: Time allowed __________ min
Accuracy__________ %

Conditions: The student will follow the procedure outlined below to prepare a travel itinerary within standards identified using the following materials:

- Information regarding travel plans
- Computer
- Printer

EVALUATION CRITERIA

Symbol	Category	Point value
•	crucial step	______
▪	essential step	______
▴	theory	______

Evaluation Criterion	Performance Evaluation Checklist	Points Possible	STUDENT'S SCORE 1st	STUDENT'S SCORE 2nd
▪	1. Obtain information on air or ground transportation. Identify name of transportation provider, departure and arrival locations, and travel confirmation numbers			
▪	2. Obtain information on hotel accommodations. Identify name, address, phone number, and confirmation numbers			
▪	3. Obtain information on any meetings, conferences, or other activities that will be attended. Identify name, address, and phone numbers where possible.			
•	4. Prepare itinerary listing in chronological order all information obtained above. Print if necessary.			
▪	5. Distribute two copies of the itinerary to the traveler (one for traveler, one for traveler's family) and retain one copy for the office.			
	Total Points			

Minimum total points required for satisfactory score ______

Evaluator's Comments:

Evaluator's Name _______________ Date _______________

• Denotes crucial step in procedure. Student must complete this step satisfactorily in order to complete the procedure.

National curriculum competencies achieved:

- Use office hardware and software to maintain office systems.
- Perform basic clerical functions.
- Apply electronic technology.

PROCEDURE 14-1

Prepare a Receipt for a Payment Received

Student Name ______________________ **Date** ______________________________

Learning Outcome: Prepare a receipt for a payment received.

Performance Standards: Time allowed ____________ min
Accuracy____________ %

Conditions: The student will follow the procedure outlined below to prepare a receipt for a payment received within standards identified using the following materials:

- Receipts
- Payments received
- Pen

EVALUATION CRITERIA

Symbol	Category	Point value
•	crucial step	________
▪	essential step	________
▲	theory	________

Evaluation Criterion	Performance Evaluation Checklist	Points Possible	STUDENT'S SCORE 1st	STUDENT'S SCORE 2nd
▪	1. Using the receipts in number order, enter the date the payment is received.			
▪	2. Enter the name of the payee.			
▪	3. Specify the method of payment (check or cash).			
•	4. Enter the amount of payment numerically and in words in the spaces provided.			
•	5. Identify the account to which the payment should be applied			
▪	6. Enter the account balances if known.			
•	7. Sign the receipt.			
	Total Points			

Minimum total points required for satisfactory score _______

Evaluator's Comments:

Evaluator's Name ________________________ Date ________________________

• Denotes crucial step in procedure. Student must complete this step satisfactorily in order to complete the procedure.

National curriculum competencies achieved:

- Perform accounts receivable procedures.
- Perform billing and collection procedures.

PROCEDURE 14-2

Prepare a Bank Deposit

Student Name ______________________ **Date** ______________________________

Learning Outcome: Prepare a bank deposit.

Performance Standards: Time allowed ___________ min
Accuracy___________ %

Conditions: The student will follow the procedure outlined below to prepare a bank deposit within standards identified using the following materials:

- Checks and currency deposited
- Deposit slip
- Pen

EVALUATION CRITERIA

Symbol	Category	Point value
•	crucial step	___________
▪	essential step	___________
▴	theory	___________

Evaluation Criterion	Performance Evaluation Checklist	Points Possible	STUDENT'S SCORE 1st	STUDENT'S SCORE 2nd
▪	1. Enter date of deposit on deposit slip.			
▪	2. Count currency to be deposited. Enter amount after currency on the deposit slip.			
▪	3. Count currency to be deposited. Enter amount after currency on the deposit slip.			
▪	4. Individually write the amount of each check to be deposited in the checks portion of the deposit slip.			
▪	5. Calculate total of currency, coin, and checks to be deposited and enter amount under total.			
•	6. Verify that deposit is correct by adding currency, coin, and the amount of each check.			
▪	7. Record deposit in check register.			
	Total Points			

Minimum total points required for satisfactory score ______

Evaluator's Comments:

Evaluator's Name ______________________ Date ___________________________

- Denotes crucial step in procedure. Student must complete this step satisfactorily in order to complete the procedure.

National curriculum competencies achieved:

- Prepare a bank deposit.
- Prepare and reconcile a bank statement and deposit record.

PROCEDURE 14-3

Maintain a Petty Cash Fund

Student Name ______________________ **Date** ______________________

Learning Outcome: Maintain a petty cash fund.

Performance Standards: Time allowed ____________ min
Accuracy____________ %

Conditions: The student will follow the procedure outlined below to maintain a petty cash fund within standards identified using the following materials:

- Petty cash record
- Receipts for expenditures
- Pen/pencil

EVALUATION CRITERIA

Symbol	Category	Point value
•	crucial step	________
▪	essential step	________
▴	theory	________

Evaluation Criterion	Performance Evaluation Checklist	Points Possible	STUDENT'S SCORE 1st	2nd
▪	1. A cash fund of a predetermined amount, possibly $100, is put in a secure location in a locked, zippered bank bag.			
▪	2. When an approved purchase must be made, cash is removed from the bag that will cover the purchase and an employee makes the purchase.			
▪	3. When the employee returns, a receipt for the item and change (if any) are placed in the bag. *The receipt and the change should total the amount that was removed to make the purchase.*			
•	4. The item purchased is written in a petty cash log (see Fig. 14-5).			
▪	5. When the fund becomes depleted, the expenses from the petty cash log are totaled and the log and receipts are kept as proof of expenses. A check then is written to Petty Cash for the amount of the expenses.			
▪	6. The check is cashed by the employee responsible for the fund and the fund is replenished by placing the check proceeds in the bank bag. A new log sheet is started.			
•	7. After the fund is replenished, the cash in the bank bag should equal the original amount of the petty cash fund.			
	Total Points			

Minimum total points required for satisfactory score ______

Evaluator's Comments:

Evaluator's Name ______________________ Date ______________________

• Denotes crucial step in procedure. Student must complete this step satisfactorily in order to complete the procedure.

National curriculum competencies achieved:

- Establish and maintain a petty cash fund.

PROCEDURE 14-4

Write a Check for Payment of an Invoice

Student Name ______________________ **Date** ______________________

Learning Outcome: Write a check for payment of an invoice.

Performance Standards: Time allowed ____________ min
Accuracy____________ %

Conditions: The student will follow the procedure outlined below to write a check for payment of an invoice within standards identified using the following materials:

- Check register with checks
- Invoices to be paid
- Pen

EVALUATION CRITERIA

Symbol	Category	Point value
•	crucial step	________
▪	essential step	________
▲	theory	________

Evaluation Criterion	Performance Evaluation Checklist	Points Possible	STUDENT'S SCORE 1st	STUDENT'S SCORE 2nd
▪	1. Complete the check stub, subtracting the amount of the check from the current balance of the account.			
•	2. Complete check using a pen. Use checks in numerical order.			
▪	3. Enter current date on check.			
•	4. On the PAY TO THE ORDER OF line, enter the payee's name.			
•	5. Enter the amount of the check numerically in the blank provided after the $ sign. Begin to enter the amount immediately after the $ sign to prevent anything from being added to the check amount.			
•	6. Enter the amount of the check in words on the line below the PAY TO THE ORDER OF line. If the entire line is not used, use dashes or a solid line to cross out the remainder of the line.			
•	7. The check then is signed by an individual who has been authorized to sign checks for the account. The check then can be placed in a window envelope for mailing to the payee if necessary.			
	Total Points			

Minimum total points required for satisfactory score ______

Evaluator's Comments:

Evaluator's Name ______________________ Date ______________________

• Denotes crucial step in procedure. Student must complete this step satisfactorily in order to complete the procedure.

National curriculum competencies achieved:

- Describe banking procedures.
- Perform accounts payable procedures.

PROCEDURE 14-5

Reconcile a Bank Statement

Student Name ____________________ **Date** ____________________

Learning Outcome: Reconcile a bank statement.

Performance Standards: Time allowed __________ min
Accuracy__________ %

Conditions: The student will follow the procedure outlined below to reconcile a bank statement within standards identified using the following materials:

- Current month's bank statement
- Record of checks drawn or check register
- Calculator
- Pen or pencil

EVALUATION CRITERIA

Symbol	Category	Point value
•	crucial step	______
▪	essential step	______
▴	theory	______

Evaluation Criterion	Performance Evaluation Checklist	Points Possible	STUDENT'S SCORE 1st	2nd
▪	1. All checks that have been paid by the bank should be checked on the record of checks drawn or the check register.			
▪	2. Any charges applied to the account by the bank should be listed on the record/register and subtracted from the balance.			
▪	3. Any interest deposits from the bank should be listed on the record/register and added to the balance.			
•	4. Take the ending monthly balance on the account and do the following. Add any deposits made by the practice that are not included on the statement. Subtract any checks written by the practice that have not been paid by the bank. The total should then equal the ending balance in the record. If the total does not equal the balance in the record, you should look for errors in addition and subtraction when figuring the ending balance, as well as any other errors that may be present in the record/register.			
	Total Points			

Minimum total points required for satisfactory score ______

Evaluator's Comments:

Evaluator's Name ____________________ Date ____________________

• Denotes crucial step in procedure. Student must complete this step satisfactorily in order to complete the procedure.

National curriculum competencies achieved:

- Describe banking procedures.
- Prepare and reconcile a bank statement and deposit record.

PROCEDURE 15-1

Select Candidates for Interviewing

Student Name ______________________ **Date** ______________________

Learning Outcome: Select candidates for interviewing.

Performance Standards: Time allowed ____________ min
Accuracy____________ %

Conditions: The student will follow the procedure outlined below to select candidates for interviewing within standards identified using the following materials:

- Résumés or job applications
- Selection criteria
- Pen or pencil

EVALUATION CRITERIA

Symbol	Category	Point value
•	crucial step	________
▪	essential step	________
▲	theory	________

Evaluation Criterion	Performance Evaluation Checklist	Points Possible	STUDENT'S SCORE	
			1st	2nd
▪	1. If at all possible, form a committee that will be involved in all aspects of the selection process. Using the committee selection process helps to eliminate potential biases and future conflicts. (Sometimes this is not possible and the applicants will be interviewed by only one individual.) There should always be more than one interview. A second interview ensures proper selection of the most qualified candidate.			
▪	2. The committee or interviewer should establish a list of criteria necessary for the position and should assign points to each of those criteria.			
▪	3. After all résumés are received, give copies of each résumé to each member on the committee.			
•	4. Résumés are evaluated by each member and points are assigned for each candidate's qualifications.			
▪	5. Point assignments are totaled and reviewed by the committee. Candidates with the greatest number of points are invited for an interview.			
	Total Points			

Minimum total points required for satisfactory score ______

Evaluator's Comments:

Evaluator's Name ______________________ Date ______________________

• Denotes crucial step in procedure. Student must complete this step satisfactorily in order to complete the procedure.

PROCEDURE 15-2

Prepare Payroll

Student Name ______________________ **Date** ______________________________

Learning Outcome: Prepare payroll.

Performance Standards: Time allowed ____________ min
Accuracy____________ %

Conditions: The student will follow the procedure outlined below to prepare payroll within standards identified using the following materials:

- Timecards and records (as in Figure 15-6 or a similar form)
- Tax tables or percentages
- Calculator

EVALUATION CRITERIA

Symbol	Category	Point value
•	crucial step	______________
▪	essential step	______________
▴	theory	______________

Evaluation Criterion	Performance Evaluation Checklist	Points Possible	STUDENT'S SCORE 1st	STUDENT'S SCORE 2nd
•	1. Calculate wages earned by multiplying hours worked by hourly rate. If the employee has worked overtime, the overtime hours worked will be multiplied by 1½ times the employee's hourly rate.			
•	2. Enter the total wages earned for the period in the gross (earnings) column.			
•	3. Enter FICA (social security and Medicare) tax in FICA column.			
•	4. Using amount of employee's wages and withholding allowances, determine the amount of tax to be withheld. Refer to employee's Form W-4 to obtain marital status and withholding allowances. Note any additional amount the employee wishes withheld. Enter federal income tax in FWT column.			
•	5. Determine the amount of state tax to be withheld by referring to the employee's wages and withholding allowances amounts. Enter state tax in SWT column.			
•	6. Enter any other deductions on the payroll record.			
•	7. To figure employee's net salary, subtract total deductions from gross earnings.			
•	8. Prepare payroll checks by listing all payroll amounts in the check summary.			
	Total Points			

Minimum total points required for satisfactory score ______

Evaluator's Comments:

Evaluator's Name ________________________ Date ______________________________

- Denotes crucial step in procedure. Student must complete this step satisfactorily in order to complete the procedure.

National curriculum competencies achieved:

- Process employee payroll.

PROCEDURE 16-1

Prepare a Résumé

Student Name ______________________ **Date** ______________________

Learning Outcome: Prepare a Résumé.

Performance Standards: Time allowed ____________ min
Accuracy____________ %

Conditions: The student will follow the procedure outlined below to prepare a résumé within standards identified using the following materials:

- Professional résumé paper (white or off-white) and matching envelope
- Computer with word processing software
- Education, work experience, and student portfolio information

EVALUATION CRITERIA

Symbol	Category	Point value
•	crucial step	________
▪	essential step	________
▲	theory	________

Evaluation Criterion	Performance Evaluation Checklist	Points Possible	STUDENT'S SCORE 1st	STUDENT'S SCORE 2nd
▪	1. Choose format for résumé. A résumé computer program or a résumé template from a word processing program may be used.			
▪	2. List full name, address, telephone number, and email address at the top of the résumé.			
▪	3. Write career objective specific to position desired.			
▪	4. List education with most recent first.			
▪	5. List work experience with most recent first. Any volunteer experience or student internship experience can be listed under work experience.			
▪	6. List personal achievements, awards, interests, and/or skills.			
▪	7. List personal references. Instructors and work supervisors are good choices. Friends and relatives should not be listed as personal references. Be sure to ask each individual for permission before listing him or her as a reference.			
•	8. Proofread résumé for typos or grammatical errors. If possible, have another person read the résumé for the same.			
▪	9. Review résumé to ensure that the format is easy to read. Make any adjustments necessary.			
▪	10. Print a copy of the résumé and retain a copy for yourself.			
	Optional			
▪	11. If mailing the résumé, print an envelope.			
	Total Points			

Minimum total points required for satisfactory score ______

Evaluator's Comments:

Evaluator's Name ______________________ Date ______________________

• Denotes crucial step in procedure. Student must complete this step satisfactorily in order to complete the procedure.

PROCEDURE 16-2

Prepare a Cover Letter

Student Name ______________________ **Date** ______________________

Learning Outcome: Prepare a cover letter.

Performance Standards: Time allowed ____________ min
Accuracy____________ %

Conditions: The student will follow the procedure outlined below to prepare a cover letter within standards identified using the following materials:

- Professional résumé paper (white or off-white) and matching envelope
- Computer with word processing software
- Completed résumé

EVALUATION CRITERIA

Symbol	Category	Point value
•	crucial step	________
■	essential step	________
▲	theory	________

Evaluation Criterion	Performance Evaluation Checklist	Points Possible	STUDENT'S SCORE 1st	2nd
▲	1. Use proper format for the letter. (Formats are located in Chapter 6.)			
■	2. Address the letter to the individual designated to receive applications.			
■	3. Write a letter to express your interest in a position and to identify some of your qualifications and strengths.			
▲	4. Close the letter with an appropriate salutation and your full name.			
•	5. Proofread the letter for typos and grammatical errors. If possible, have another person also proof the letter.			
■	6. Print a copy of the letter and retain a copy for yourself.			
•	7. Sign the letter that will go with your résumé.			
	Optional			
■	8. If mailing the résumé, print an envelope. Place the letter appropriately in a business envelope along with the résumé (see Fig. 16-3).			
	Total Points			

Minimum total points required for satisfactory score ______

Evaluator's Comments:

Evaluator's Name ______________________ Date ______________________

- Denotes crucial step in procedure. Student must complete this step satisfactorily in order to complete the procedure.

PROCEDURE 16-3

Complete an Employment Application

Student Name ______________________ **Date** ______________________________

Learning Outcome: Complete an employment application.

Performance Standards: Time allowed ____________ min
Accuracy____________ %

Conditions: The student will follow the procedure outlined below to complete an employment application within standards identified using the following materials:

- Employment application (Lately, many employment applications have been made available over the Internet. The same steps would be followed, only the information would be entered electronically.)
- Pen

EVALUATION CRITERIA

Symbol	Category	Point value
•	crucial step	____________
▪	essential step	____________
▴	theory	____________

Evaluation Criterion	Performance Evaluation Checklist	Points Possible	STUDENT'S SCORE 1st	STUDENT'S SCORE 2nd
▪	1. Read instructions on the form and follow them carefully. Provide the information requested below in addition to any other information requested on the application.			
▪	2. Identify personal information.			
▪	3. List educational history.			
▪	4. List employment history.			
▪	5. List medical office-related skills.			
▪	6. List personal references.			
•	7. Review the application to make sure it is complete.			
•	8. Sign and date the application.			
▪	9. Submit the application to the individual designated.			
	Total Points			

Minimum total points required for satisfactory score ______

Evaluator's Comments:

Evaluator's Name ______________________ Date ______________________

- Denotes crucial step in procedure. Student must complete this step satisfactorily in order to complete the procedure.

APPENDIX III Using Medisoft v18

Medisoft Version 18 software on the CD-ROM may be bundled with *Medical Office Administration* or may be purchased separately. Medisoft is a Windows-based medical practice management program. Students are encouraged to install and use this program to perform many administrative tasks of the medical office, such as

- Recording demographic and insurance information for patients
- Scheduling appointments
- Entering patient charges
- Entering payments
- Creating receipts, bills, and insurance billing
- Submitting electronic claims
- Creating reports such as day sheets and account aging reports

Installation and Setup

Medisoft is installed on the hard drive of the computer. To install Medisoft Version 18, complete the installation instructions on the Evolve site associated with the textbook. Be sure to follow the instructions exactly to ensure that the software will work properly. Once the software is installed, the CD will not have to be used.

The practice that will be used for exercises within this text is the Medisoft Tutorial practice entitled "Happy Valley Medical Clinic." The words "Medical Group (Tutorial Data)" will appear on the Medisoft title bar when the Happy Valley Medical Clinic practice is open. Be sure to consult Evolve for tips and updates on using Medisoft.

Starting Medisoft

All activities within Medisoft will be done within the Medisoft tutorial for the practice named Happy Valley Medical Clinic (or Happy Valley Medical Group). After the software has been installed, perform the following to begin working in the practice:

1. Open Medisoft using one of the following options:
   a. On the computer desktop, double-click the icon labeled **Medisoft Advanced Demo** or click **Programs>Medisoft>Medisoft Advanced Demo.**
2. Verify that the practice entitled **Medical Group (Tutorial Data)** is open. The practice name appears after Medisoft Advanced at the top of the Medisoft window. If no practice name appears, click **File>Open Practice>Medical Group,** then click **OK.** (If the tutorial is not on the list, click **Add tutorial** on the right side of the practice window and after the tutorial has installed, open the practice as previously instructed.

Using the Help Feature in Medisoft

For a quick overview of the features associated with Medisoft, click *Help>MedisoftHelp>Contents> Getting Started with Medisoft.* Expand the *Getting Started with Medisoft* option to become acquainted with Medisoft features.

The *content* tab of the help feature allows you to locate information by clicking on the subject area. The *index* and *search* tabs allow you to enter keywords for which you may need some information. The index and search features provide quick access to information on your keyword. When looking for information through the help feature, type a keyword under the index feature first. If no information is found, proceed to the search feature. The search feature provides a more comprehensive search of Medisoft information. If you have questions when using Medisoft, the help feature provides a myriad of information about the program's operation.

Patient Registration

To locate patient registration data, complete the following:

1. Click Lists>Patient/Guarantors and Cases.
2. From the Patient/Guarantors and Cases window, it is possible to search for patients or cases that are related to patients. Radio buttons on the upper right portion of the window allow the search to be specified for a patient or case. Click the Patient button.
3. In the Search for box, begin to type the patient's last name. The patient list will display only those patients' names that match your entry.
4. Double-click the patient's name in the patient list. The patient window will open.

Patient Tabs

Any one of the four tabs at the top of the window can be clicked to display information fields for a patient.

Name/Address tab— Basic demographic information that identifies the patient is located under this tab.

Chart number— This field will be filled in automatically if left blank. Once a chart number is assigned, it cannot be changed. If a chart number must be changed, the patient will need to be inactive or deleted and a new patient created.

Inactive– When selected, *Inactive* will deactivate a patient's record.

Last Name - Enter patient's last name. If the patient's last name contains punctuation, omit the punctuation and omit the space where the punctuation was located.

First Name – Enter the patient's legal name. Do not enter a nickname.

Street - Two lines exist for the address. If there is only one line for a patient's address, use the first line. If there are two lines for the patient's address, the second line should be used for the street address and the first line should be used for an appointment number, building location or name of a company.

When the tab is used to enter the address, the program will skip the City and State and will move to the ZIP code field. If the ZIP code has been saved to the database previously, the City and State fields will be completed automatically.

City – Enter the patient's city.

State – Enter the patient's state.

ZIP – Enter the patient's ZIP if necessary.

Email – Enter the patient's email address.

Home - Enter the patient's home phone number.

Work – Enter the patient's work phone number. Enter the number where the patient can be reached at work, NOT the employer's main number.

Cell – Enter the patient's cell number.

Other – Enter any other phone number.

Birth date— Patient's date of birth should be entered as follows: MMDDYYYY, to avoid any confusion with the century.

Sex – Identify the patient's gender.

Birth weight/units— Leave blank. This field is completed only for newborn records. *Units* refers to the type of measurement used (grams or pounds).

Social Security Number— Enter the patient's Social Security Number if available. Information should be entered as nine digits with no hyphens because hyphens are automatically inserted by the program.

Entity type— This field identifies whether the patient record pertains to a person or a nonperson. An example of a nonperson is a corporation.

Race – Enter if known. Enter this information ONLY if provided by the patient. Do not guess as to what this information might be.

Ethnicity – Enter if known. Enter this information ONLY if provided by the patient. Do not guess as to what this information might be.

Language – Enter if known. Enter this information ONLY if provided by the patient. Do not guess as to what this information might be.

Death Date: If the patient is deceased, enter the date of death.

Other Information Tab

Type—This field identifies whether the record is for a patient or a guarantor. If the patient is a patient, choose **Patient** from the drop-down list. If the individual is a guarantor for a patient's bill and not a patient at the clinic, choose **Guarantor.**

Assigned provider— If known, identify the patient's primary provider.

Patient ID #2— If patient has a maiden name or previous name, enter the name in this blank.

Patient billing code— This option can be used to identify a billing code that might be used to sort patients. For example, cycle billing identification could be set up in this field.

Patient indicator— Leave blank. This option provides an additional method by which to sort patients.

Flag— Patient records can be color coded to identify certain situations related to the patient, such as minor, past due on account or an auto accident patient. Only one flag can be used at a time, and no flags are required.

Health care ID— Leave blank. This field can be used as a unique identifier for the patient.

Signature on file/date— This field identifies whether the patient has signed an authorization to have information sent to his/her insurance carrier for processing claims. If an authorization has been signed, check the box, then identify the date the signature was obtained.

Emergency contact— Enter the name and phone number(s) of the patient's emergency contact.

Employment Information— Enter the patient's employer information if known. If there are two employer phone numbers, enter the work phone for the employer in this blank, not the patient's work phone.

Retirement date— Leave blank.

Payment Plan Tab

Payment code— If the patient has established a payment plan with the office, click the drop-down arrow to select the type of plan. When this feature is used, the account will be monitored to ensure that payments are received as required.

Custom Tab – Medisoft can customize this tab to accommodate information that a practice may wish to retain regarding a patient.

Entering Data for a New or Established Patient

Every patient of the practice will require a Medisoft patient record.

To update an established patient's record, do the following:

1. Click Lists>Patients/Guarantors and Cases.
2. Locate the patient by entering the patient's last name in the Search for box.
3. Double-click the patient's name, and the patient's record will open.
4. Update any information as necessary under the Name, Address, Other Information, and Payment Plan tabs.
5. Click Save to save updates to the patient's record.

To create a new patient record, follow these steps:

1. Click Lists>Patients/Guarantors and Cases.
2. Enter the patient's last name in the Search for box. If the patient is new to the practice, no record will be found in the patient list.
3. Click New on the bottom of the Patients window.
4. Complete any information as necessary under the Name, Address, Other Information, and Payment Plan tabs. (The fields within those tabs are described previously under Locating a Patient.)
5. Click Save to save information to the patient's record.

Appointments

All appointments are recorded in a separate part of the Medisoft software entitled **Office Hours Professional**. The **Office Hours Professional** window will open on the current day.

Establish Appointment Parameters for the Appointment System

To establish appointment parameters (appointment matrix), complete the following:

1. In the **Office Hours Professional** window, click **File>Program Options**. Make sure the **Options tab** is open. Note that the following choices will be established as a default and will be applied to the entire calendar:
   a. **Start time** and **End time**: The starting and ending times for the appointment book can be set. Set the **Start time** and the **End time.**
   b. **Interval**: Appointment lengths can be set to accommodate the type of medical practice. Family practice might prefer 10-minute appointments; neurosurgery might prefer 30-minute appointments.
   c. **Default colors**: This identifies the colors used for appointment display.
   d. Leave **Multi Views** tab and **Appointment Display** tab as is.

Establish Time Off or Breaks for Each Physician

To schedule physicians' time out of the office, complete the following:

1. In the **Office Hours Professional** window, click **Lists>Break Lists.** A separate break will have to be created for each **different** type of break.
2. Click **New.** Name the break or identify the type of break.
3. Use current date for the break to start from today forward.
4. Insert beginning **time** and **length** of the break.
5. Click **Change.** The **Repeat Change** window will open. Specify how oftenthe break should be repeated. The **End on** box should be completed to avoid too many breaks from filling up the demonstration version of the program. Click **OK** to close the **Repeat Change** window.
6. If the break does not apply to all providers, click **Some.** Click **Save.**
7. The **Provider Selection** window will appear. Select the name of the provider(s) for whom the break applies. Click **OK.**
8. When all breaks have been entered, click **Close.**

Establish Reasons for Appointments

Medisoft has the capability to link the reason for an appointment with the length of time needed for the appointment. To create reasons for appointments, complete the following:

1. On the Office Hours Professional menu, click Lists>Reason List.
2. Click New. The Appointment Reason Entry window will open.
3. In the Code box, enter the appointment abbreviation.
4. In the Description box, enter the complete description associated with the abbreviation.
5. Identify the appointment length associated with the appointment in the Default Appointment Length box. The Default Appointment Color should remain the same unless otherwise specified. Click Save.

Scheduling an Appointment

1. On the **Office Hours Professional** menu, click the drop-down arrow in the **Provider** box on the upper right side of the Office Hours window. Click on the provider's name. Once selected, the provider's name will appear in the provider box. **(Note: For training purposes, Medisoft has included several sample appointments in J.D. Mallard's schedule that appear on each day within the *Office Hours* program.)**
2. Select the appointment date by clicking on the correct date on the calendar displayed on the left side of the **Office Hours Professional** window. The appointment date should be highlighted.
3. Verify that the appointment time is available in Column 1. To schedule an appointment, double-click the box next to the desired time slot. The **New Appointment Entry** window will open. Be sure to double-check the name of the provider in the lower portion of the **New Appointment Entry** window.
4. In the **New Appointment Entry** window, click the magnifying glass on the right of the **Chart** box. The **Patient Search Window** will open. Patient information can be located a number of ways: by chart number, last name, social security number, etc. In the **Field** box, specify that the patient search should be **Last Name, First Name.** Locate the patient's information by typing the patient's last name in the **Search for** box, or by using the scroll bar on the patient list. If the practice has a large number of patients, the most expedient way to locate a patient would be to input the first three to four letters of the patient's last name in the **Search for** box. (The drop-down arrow on the text box will reveal the list of patients in chart number order.)
5. Select the correct patient by double-clicking on the patient's name. The patient's name then will appear in a **New Appointment Entry** window. Note that the information for the patient now appears in the window.
6. Use the **Tab** key to move to the **Reason** box. Select the reason for the appointment from the reason list. The length of the appointment will be automatically adjusted based on the reason for the appointment. (If the patient has repeating appointments at the same date and time, click **Change** to insert multiple appointments.) If the reason does not appear on the list, choose **Existing Patient** and specify the time needed for the appointment.
7. Any special comments about the patient's appointment may be entered in the **Note** box.
8. Click **Save.** The patient's appointment should appear on the physician's schedule with time slots color coded for the required time for the appointment.

Locating Appointments

Appointments can be located quickly by completing the following:

1. In **Office Hours Professional** click *Lists>Patients/Guarantors and Cases.*
2. Determine which patient's appointments you wish to locate and open the patient's file. In the **Name, Address** tab, click the **Appointments** button on the right.
3. The patient's appointments will appear in a new window. If needed, click **Print,** then **Preview>Print**, or **Export** to save a list of the patient's appointments. Then click **Close** to close the appointment list window, **Cancel** to close the patient information and **Close** to close the patient list.

Rescheduling Appointments

To reschedule appointments, do the following:

1. Locate the patient's appointment on the provider's schedule. Right-click the patient's appointment and click **Cut.**
2. Locate a new time slot for the appointment. Make sure that enough time is available to reschedule the original appointment. Right-click on the new appointment slot and click **Paste.**

Printing Appointment Schedules

1. Open Office Hours Professional. Click Reports> Appointment List. Select Preview report on screen. Click Start.
2. In the Data Selection window, enter first date to be printed and last date to be printed. In the provider fields, identify the first provider and last provider to be printed. (If no selection is made in the provider window, all providers will be printed.) Click OK.
3. Click the arrows on the toolbar to advance through the report. If the report is correct, click Print Report on the toolbar.

Saving an Appointment Schedule File

1. Click Reports>Appointment List.
2. Click Export the report to a file. Click Start. Specify which dates and providers should be printed. Name the file and save it to a location on your hard drive or on an external storage device. The file will be saved as a text file.

Patient Check-In

1. Open **Office Hours Professional.** Locate the appointment for the patient who is checking in and double-click the appointment to open the appointment.
2. On the right side of the **Edit Appointment** window, click the option for **Checked In.**
3. Right-click in the **Chart** box and select **Edit Patient.** Enter the information in the **Name, Address** tab and the **Other Information** tab. Each patient has signed an authorization for filing insurance claims for their visits. Select **Signature on File** for each patient and enter the **Signature date** as the date of their visit.
4. In the Chart box, **Case box** and select **New Case.** The tabs within the case window allow you to assign specific information to the patient's encounter.
   a. Under the **Personal tab**, enter the **Case Description** and **Guarantor** information. (The case description will consist of the type of insurance and date of service. Cases can be named in any way that the clinic chooses.)
   b. Under the **Account** tab, enter the assigned provider information.
   c. Under the **Policy 1** tab, enter the insurance information.
   d. Click **Save.**

1. Verify that the Case number appears in the Case box and the description is next to the case number box. Verify that you have marked "checked in" for the appointment.
2. Click Save. Note that a checkmark is placed next to the patient's name on the schedule.

Charges and Payments

Entering Charges

1. On the main menu, click **Activities>Enter Transactions.** The **Transaction Entry** window will open.
2. Begin to enter billing information as follows. (To move from field to field within this window, simply press the **Enter** or **Tab** key.)
   a. Chart– Click the drop-down arrow on the chart field. Double-click the name of the patient to be billed.
   b. **Case**– Click the drop-down arrow on the case field. Double-click the name of the case that was assigned for the billing. The case name used in this text is the date of service (MMDDYY).
   c. Date– Click the drop-down arrow, and click the date of the patient's encounter.
   d. **Procedure**– Type the procedure code in the box or click the drop-down arrow to select the procedure code for the patient's encounter. If a new code needs to be added to the procedure code list, it can be added by right-clicking on the **procedure** box.
   e. **Units** – This field indicates the number of times the procedure was performed. Usually this field has a value of 1. Leave the units as is unless instructed otherwise.
   f. Amount– The procedure amount will be entered automatically from the database information in Medisoft. This information also can be overwritten if a provider modifies a charge.
   g. Diagnosis **1, 2, 3, 4**– type the diagnosis code in the first box or click the drop-down arrow to select the diagnosis code for the patient's encounter. Enter the first-listed diagnosis and subsequent diagnoses in the order given by the provider. Use the type of diagnosis code that is currently required for processing claims: either an I-9 or I-10 code. DO NOT use both codes. If a new diagnosis code needs to be added to the diagnosis code list, it can be added by right-clicking on the **Diag 1** box.
   h. **1, 2, 3, 4**– If more than one diagnosis is listed for an encounter, place a checkmark under the diagnosis(es) that apply to each specific procedure code.

i. Provider– Medisoft defaults to the provider that is listed in the case information for the encounter being billed. Be sure that the provider who saw the patient gets credit for the charges for that encounter. If the provider needs to be changed, click the drop-down arrow to choose the provider who performed the service for the patient.

j. **POS (place of service)**– To set a default place of service code, click **File>Program Options>Data Entry.** The usual place of service for Happy Valley Medical Group is 11 – Office. Click **Save** when the default has been entered. (If a service is provided in another location, the correct code may be entered in the POS field.)

k. **Additional Charges**– If another line is needed to enter another procedure code for an additional charge, click the **New** button until a new line appears.

l. **Completed Charges**– If the charges are complete, click **Save Transactions.**

To begin to enter information for a new patient, click the drop-down arrow on the *Chart* field to select a new patient.

When all bills have been entered, click *Close* at the bottom of the window.

If a mistake is made after a transaction has been saved, select the patient's name and open the case that contains the billing error. Charges can be deleted by highlighting the line with the error and clicking **Delete**. New information can then be entered by clicking **New**.

Printing Patient Statements

Patient statements usually are printed monthly for each account of a practice.

To begin to print account statements for patient accounts, complete the following:

1. On the Medisoft main menu, click Reports>Patient Statements. Click Patient Statements (30, 60, 90). Click OK.
2. Specify Export the report to a file. Click Start.
3. Name the file your last name statements, save it as a text file and Save the file to a location you can remember.
4. In the Patient Statements Data Selection window, leave all entries blank. Click OK.
5. Statements for all patients who have had charges or who have a balance will be displayed on the screen. (Patients with balances previously in the software also will print.) Use the right and left arrows to scroll through the statements to ensure that the correct ones are displayed. If statements are correct, click the printer icon on the toolbar to print the statements.

Entering Payments

To record payments on the account, complete the following:

1. Open Medisoft. At the main menu, click **Activities>Enter Deposits/Payments.**
2. In the **Deposit List** window, list the deposit date as the date on which the deposits were made.
3. Click **New.**
4. Enter the following information into the identified fields in the **Deposits: New** window.
   a. **Payor type**: Identify whether the payment is from a patient or an insurance company.
   b. **Method**: identify the form of payment (check, cash, credit card, electronic). If a check, enter the check number field.
   c. **Payment Amount**: Enter total amount of payment.
   d. **Chart # or Insurance**: Identify who or what company made the payment.
   e. Leave other fields as is.
   f. Click **Save.**
   g. Highlight the deposit you just entered on the **Deposit List.** Click **Apply.**
   h. Uncheck the box **Show Remainder Only.**
   i. Enter the amount paid by the patient or insurance company in the **payment** field. Press **tab.** The payment will show as a negative number.
   j. Click **Save Payments/Adjustments.**
   k. In the **Create Statements** window, click **Cancel.** When asked **Do you want to print the last created statement for this patient,** click **No.**
   l. Click **Close.**
5. Enter the next deposit following the instructions in #4. When done entering and applying payments, click **Close.**

NOTE: At any time during this process, lines can be deleted to wipe out any mistakes.

Printing Insurance Claims

To prepare insurance claims, complete the following:

1. Open Medisoft. At the main menu, click **Activities>Claim Management.**
2. Click **Create Claims.** Specify the following: **Range of Transaction Dates**: First date: MM-DD-YYYY. Last date: MM-DD-YYYY.
3. Click **Create.** Claims will be added to the **Claims Management** window.
4. Click **Print/Send** in the claim management window. Specify **Paper Claim>OK.** Click **Laser CMS (Primary) W/Form.** Click **OK.**
5. Click **Export the report to a file>Start.**
6. Name the file **yourlastname claims.** Save as a **text document.** Click **Save.**
7. In the **Date Created Range** enter **today's date** if you created the claims today. Enter today's date in both date boxes. If you did not create the claims today, check the **Date Created Column** in the **Claim Management** window. The claims you created will be in the last group of claims on the list. Use the date in the **Date Created Column.**
8. Click **OK.**

If you wish to reprint claims after you complete this exercise, you must highlight the claims you wish to print and then choose the **Reprint Claims** option near the bottom of the Claim Management window.

Reports

A variety of report options are available under *Reports* on the Medisoft menu. It is a good idea when printing reports to click the *Preview* button before printing the reports to make sure that the information requested is included in the report.

Following is a list of instructions for some common reports.

Practice Analysis

1. Open Medisoft. At the main menu, click **Reports>Analysis Reports>Practice Analysis.**
2. Click *Print*>**Start or Preview>Start.** In the **Search** window, all options should have **Show All Values** checked.
3. After reviewing the report, explain how the report could be used in financial planning in the office.

Patient Aging

1. Open Medisoft. At the main menu, click *Reports>Aging Reports>Patient Aging.*
2. Click *Print*>**Start or Preview>Start.** In the **Search** window, all options should have **Show All Values** checked.
3. After reviewing the report, explain how the report could be used in financial planning in the office.

Patient Ledger

1. Open Medisoft. At the main menu, click *Reports>Patient Ledger.*
2. Click *Print*>**Start or Preview>Start.** In the **Search** window, all options should have **Show All Values** checked.
3. After reviewing the report, explain how the report could be used in financial planning in the office.

Patients by Diagnosis

1. Open Medisoft. At the main menu, click Reports>Standard Patient Lists>Patients by Diagnosis.
2. Click Print>**Start or Preview>Start.** In the **Search** window, all options should have **Show All Values** checked.
3. After reviewing the report, explain how the report could be used in financial planning in the office.

APPENDIX IV Abbreviations Commonly Used in the Medical Office

a.c.	*ante cibum* or before meals
AAMA	American Association of Medical Assistants
ABN	Advance Beneficiary Notice
AD	right ear
ADA	Americans With Disabilities Act
AHDI	Association for Healthcare Documentation Integrity
AHIMA	American Health Information Management Association
AIDS	acquired immune deficiency syndrome
AMA	American Medical Association
AMT	American Medical Technologists
AOA	American Osteopathic Association
ARRT	American Registry of Radiologic Technologists
AS	left ear
ASA	aspirin
AU	both ears
b.i.d.	twice per day
BC/BS	Blue Cross/Blue Shield
BCP	birth control pill
BM	bowel movement
BP	blood pressure
BSN	bachelors of science–nursing
BUN	blood urea nitrogen
Bx	biopsy
c̄	with
C#	C followed by a number from 1–7 identifies a particular cervical vertebra (C1–C7)
C&S	culture and sensitivity
Ca	cancer
CABG	coronary artery bypass graft
cap	capsule
CAP	Certified Administrative Professional
CBC	complete blood count
CC	chief complaint
cc	cubic centimeter
CCS	Certified Coding Specialist
CCS-P	Certified Coding Specialist–Physician-Based
CCU	Coronary Care Unit
CDC	Centers for Disease Control and Prevention
CEJA	(AMA) Council on Ethical and Judicial Affairs
CEU	continuing education unit
CHAMPVA	Civilian Health and Medical Program of the Department of Veterans Affairs
CHF	congestive heart failure
CHIP	Children's Health Insurance Program
chol	cholesterol
CLIA	Clinical Laboratory Improvement Amendments
cm	centimeter
CMA	Certified Medical Assistant
CMAS	Certified Medical Administrative Specialist
CMS	Centers for Medicaid and Medicare Services

CMT	Certified Medical Transcriptionist
CNA	certified nursing assistant
CNM	Certified Nurse Midwife
CNP	Certified Nurse Practitioner
COB	coordination of benefits
COBRA	Consolidated Omnibus Budget Reconciliation Act
COMLEX	Comprehensive Osteopathic Medical Licensing Examination
COPD	chronic obstructive pulmonary disease
COTA	Certified Occupational Therapy Assistant
CPC	Certified Professional Coder
CPC-H	Certified Professional Coder–Hospital
CPC-P	Certified Professional Coder–Payer
CPR	cardiopulmonary resuscitation; computerized patient record
CPT	Current Procedural Terminology
CRTT	Certified Respiratory Therapist Technician
CS	cesarean section
CSA	Controlled Substances Act
CT	computerized tomography (scanning)
CTR	certified tumor registrar
CTS	carpal tunnel syndrome
D&C	dilatation and curettage
D/C	discontinued
DC	Doctor of Chiropractic
DEA	Drug Enforcement Agency
DEERS	Defense Enrollment Eligibility Reporting System
DJD	degenerative joint disease
DM	diabetes mellitus
DNR	Do Not Resuscitate (Order)
DO	Doctor of Osteopathy
DOB	date of birth
DPM	Doctor of Podiatric Medicine
DTR	deep tendon reflex
DVT	deep vein thrombosis
Dx	diagnosis
E&M	evaluation and management
ECG, EKG	electrocardiogram
ECOA	Equal Credit Opportunity Act
ED	emergency department
EDC	estimated date of confinement (due date of a pregnancy)
EEG	electroencephalogram
EENT	eyes, ears, nose, and throat
EHR	electronic health record
EIN	employer identification number
ELL	English as a learned language
EMG	electromyogram
EMR	electronic medical record
ENT	ears, nose, and throat
EOB	explanation of benefits
EPA	Environmental Protection Agency
EPR	electronic patient record
EPSDT	early periodic screening, diagnosis, and treatment
ER	emergency room
ESA	Employment Standards Administration
ESL	English as a second language
ESR	erythrocyte sedimentation rate
FB	foreign body
FBS	fasting blood sugar

FH	family history
FICA	Federal Insurance Contributions Act
FLEX	Federation Licensing Examination
flex	proctosigmoidoscopy
FLSA	Fair Labor Standards Act
FMLA	Family and Medical Leave Act
FUTA	Federal Unemployment Tax
fx	fracture
GI	gastrointestinal
GP	general practitioner
gr	grain
GTT	glucose tolerance test
gtt.	drops
GU	genitourinary
gyn	gynecology
H&H	hemoglobin and hematocrit
H&P	history and physical
h.s.	at hour of sleep; bedtime
HA	headache
Hb, Hgb	hemoglobin
HBV	hepatitis B virus
HCFA	Health Care Financing Administration
HCPCS	Healthcare Common Procedure Coding System
HCT, Hct	hematocrit
HEENT	head, eyes, ears, nose, and throat
HHS	(Department of) Health and Human Services
HIPAA	Health Insurance Portability and Accountability Act
HIV	human immunodeficiency virus
HMO	health maintenance organization
HOH	hard of hearing
HTN	hypertension
hx	history
I&D	incision and drainage
ICD-9	International Classification of Disease, 9th revision
ICU	Intensive Care Unit
IDDM	insulin-dependent diabetes mellitus
IM	intramuscular
Inj	injection
IPA	independent practice association
IUD	intrauterine device
IV	intravenous
IVP	intravenous pyelogram
JCAHO	Joint Commission on Accreditation of Health Care Organizations
L	left, liter
L#	L followed by a number from 1–5 identifies a particular lumbar vertebra (L1–L5)
lat	lateral
lb	pound
LBP	low back pain
LLQ	left lower quadrant
LMCC	Licentiate of the Medical Council of Canada
LMP	last menstrual period
LOC	loss of consciousness
LPN	licensed practical nurse
LUQ	left upper quadrant
LVN	licensed vocational nurse
MAC	Medicare Administrative Contractor
mcg	microgram

MD	Doctor of Medicine
MI	myocardial infarction
min	minute
mL	milliliter
MRI	magnetic resonance imaging
MS	multiple sclerosis
MSD	musculoskeletal disorder
MSDS	material safety data sheet
MSN	Medicare Summary Notice
Na	sodium
NAD	no acute distress
NBOME	National Board of Osteopathic Medical Examiners
NBME	National Board of Medical Examiners
neg	negative
NIDDM	non–insulin-dependent diabetes mellitus
NKA	no known allergies
NP	nurse practitioner
NPO	nothing by mouth
NPP	Non-physician providers
NSAID	nonsteroidal anti-inflammatory drug
NSF	nonsufficient funds
OB	obstetrics
OB-GYN	obstetrics and gynecology
OCR	Optical Character Reader
OD	Doctor of Optometry; right eye
ORIF	open reduction internal fixation
OS	left eye
OSHA	Occupational Safety and Health Administration
OT	occupational therapy, occupational therapist
OTA	Occupational Therapy Assistant
OTC	over-the-counter
OU	both eyes
$\bar{p}$	after
p.c.	post cibum; after meals
p.o.	by mouth
p.r.n.	as needed
PA	Physician Assistant
PAR	participating provider
PE	physical examination
PH	past history
Ph.D.	Doctor of Philosophy
Pharm.D.	Doctor of Pharmacy
PHI	protected health information
PMH	past medical history
PMS	premenstrual syndrome
PO	purchase order
POMR	problem-oriented medical record
PPO	preferred provider organization
PRO	peer review organization
procto	proctosigmoidoscopy
Psy.D.	Doctor of Psychology
pt	patient
PT	physical therapy, physical therapist, prothrombin time
PTA	physical therapy assistant
PTT	partial thromboplastin time
px	physical examination
q	every

q.h.	every hour
q.i.d.	four times per day
R	right
R/O	rule out
RA	rheumatoid arthritis
RBC	red blood (cell) count
rbc	red blood cell
RHIA	Registered Health Information Administrator
RHIT	Registered Health Information Technician
RLQ	right lower quadrant
RMA	Registered Medical Assistant
RMT	Registered Medical Transcriptionist
RN	registered nurse
ROI	Release of information
ROM	range of motion
ROS	review of systems
RRT	Registered Respiratory Therapist
RUQ	right upper quadrant
Rx	prescription, treatment, therapy
$\bar{s}$	without
S#	S followed by a number from 1–5 identifies a particular sacral vertebra
s/p	status post
sed rate	erythrocyte sedimentation rate
SOAP	subjective, objective, assessment, plan
SOB	shortness of breath
SOMR	source-oriented medical record
SSI	supplemental security income
SSN	Social Security number
stat	immediately
STD	sexually transmitted disease
Sx	symptoms
T#	T followed by a number from 1–12 identifies a particular thoracic vertebra
T&A	tonsillectomy and adenoidectomy
t.i.d.	three times per day
TAHBSO	total abdominal hysterectomy bilateral salpingo-oophorectomy
TB	tuberculosis
TEMP	temperature
tx	treatment
UA	urinalysis
UCR	usual, customary, reasonable
URI	upper respiratory infection
USMLE	United States Medical Licensing Examination
UTI	urinary tract infection
WBC	white blood (cell) count
wbc	white blood cell
WNL	within normal limits
×	times

Glossary

Abandonment Occurs when a physician neglects to provide care for a patient when the physician is obligated to provide care.

Abortion Termination of a pregnancy before the fetus is viable.

Accession ledger Used to keep track of chart numbers assigned to patients.

Accounting Development and analysis of financial reports derived from a practice's financial transactions.

Accounts payable Liabilities of a practice; expenses that are owed by a practice.

Accounts receivable Payment owed to the practice by patients, etc.

Active record Medical record of a patient who is currently undergoing or has recently undergone treatment.

Administrative law Regulations, or laws, established by government agencies to regulate activities within that agency's control.

Advance Beneficiary Notice (ABN) Medicare document which states that Medicare may not provide coverage for certain services.

Advance directive Legal document that establishes a patient's wishes for medical care when the patient is no longer able to make those decisions.

Agenda Summary of items to be discussed at a meeting.

Alphanumeric Combination of letters and numbers are used to identify a patient's record.

Ambulatory care Medical care provided for patients on an outpatient basis.

American Academy of Professional Coders (AAPC) Largest coding certification organization in the United States.

Ancillary appointments Appointments that are made with departments such as laboratory or x-ray to run special diagnostic tests.

Arrival Term used to describe a patient who has appeared for his/her appointment.

Assessment Part of the chart note in which a physician considers the subjective and the objective information gathered about the patient and comes to a conclusion, diagnosis, or impression.

Assets Items of value such as bank accounts, furniture, and equipment.

Assignment Health care provider agrees to accept the Medicare (or other insurance program's) approved amount as payment in full.

Assignment of benefits Patient's insurance claim benefits are sent directly from the insurance company to the physician's office.

Assisted living facility Health care facility in which residents live in an apartment-type setting with services such as medication administration and meal preparation available.

Authorization Insurance plan's approval for a health care provider to provide a health care service to a patient.

Balance sheet Financial report showing the financial condition of a business. A balance sheet lists the amount of assets, liabilities, and capital.

Beneficiary Any individual who qualifies for benefits under an insurance policy.

Birthday rule Dependents are covered by the policy of the parent that has a birthday closest to the beginning of the year.

Block style Letter formatting style in which all letter components are flush with the left margin; also known as *full-block style*.

Board certified Physician who has passed an examination in a specific specialty; once a physician successfully completes the examination, the physician is known as a "diplomate" and is *board certified*.

Body Portion of a letter that contains the message to be conveyed to the addressee.

Bookkeeping Recording the financial transactions of a business.

Breach of confidentiality Release of medical information that should not be released.

Capital Investments to a business made by the owners of a business.

Capitation Prepaid plan (HMO) that provides all the care a patient needs for a flat fee or premium.

Caring response Realization that the focus of all patient care is the patient

Case law Common law; law established by the judicial system.

Cash flow statement Financial report summarizing the cash transactions of a business.

Centers for Medicaid and Medicare Services (CMS) Agency of the federal government responsible for administering Medicaid, Medicare and the State Children's Health Insurance Program.

Certified Administrative Professional (CAP) Certification awarded by the International Association of Administrative Professionals.

Certified Coding Specialist (CCS) Coding certification awarded by the American Health Information Management Association.

Certified Coding Specialist-Physician based (CCS-P) Coding certification awarded by the American Health Information Management Association.

Certified Medical Administrative Specialist (CMAS) Certification awarded by American Medical Technologists.

Certified Medical Assistant (CMA) Certification awarded by the American Association of Medical Assistants.

Certified Healthcare Documentation Specialist (CHDS) The AHDI has established guidelines for the Certified Healthcare Documentation Specialist (CHDS) examination. This examination is given to transcriptionists who have 2 or more years' experience in an acute care health care setting.

Certified Professional Coder (CPC) Coding certification awarded by the American Academy of Professional Coders.

Certified Professional Coder–Hospital (CPC-H) Coding certification awarded by the American Academy of Professional Coders.

Certified Professional Coder–Payer (CPC-P) Coding certification awarded by the American Academy of Professional Coders.

Change fund Cash on hand that is used for making change for cash transactions.

Charge slip Documentation of a patient's office visit listing the charges incurred and the patient's diagnosis; an invoice for a physician's services. Also called a *superbill, fee slip, service record,* or *encounter form.*

Chart entries or Chart notes Entries or notes made in a patient's chart regarding the patient's visit to the doctor.

Chief complaint Primary reason a patient visits the doctor; this is noted in the subjective portion of the chart note.

Children's Health Insurance Program (CHIP) A federal program designed to provide health care benefits to children who do not qualify for Medicaid because their families earn too much money.

Civilian Health and Medical Program of the Department of Veterans Affairs (CHAMPVA) A federal program providing health care coverage for dependents of veterans who have a total, permanent service-connected disability, survivors of veterans who died because of a service-connected disability or who at the time of death were totally disabled from a service-connected condition, and survivors of persons who died in the line of duty.

Civil law Type of law that involves a relationship between individuals or groups (as opposed to criminal law).

Claim Any request to the insurance company or government insurance program to receive benefits on the behalf of the insured.

Clinic Facility in which a group of health care providers render medical treatment. A variety of medical specialties may be represented, or a clinic may consist of providers in one medical specialty, such as a family practice or pediatric clinic.

Clinical Process in which a student works under the supervision of a medical office employee and receives on-the-job experience; also known as an *externship, internship,* or *practicum.*

Closed record Medical record of a patient who has died, moved away, or will not likely return for treatment.

Closing Complimentary closing of a letter is a phrase such as "Sincerely," or "Cordially"; appears after the body of the letter and before the signature.

Consolidated Omnibus Budget Reconciliation Act (COBRA) Federal law that requires that an employee be allowed to continue health insurance coverage if the employee is laid off or if the employee leaves the job.

Code team Specific people within a medical facility who respond immediately to emergency medical situations within the facility.

Coding Practice of assigning a numerical or alphanumerical code to identify a procedure that has been performed or a condition that has been treated.

Coinsurance Percentage of a claim required to be paid by the patient.

Color coding Involves assigning colors to represent letters and numbers to aid in record filing and retrieval.

Common law Law established as precedence by the judicial branch or court system; also known as case law.

Communication Conveying information from one person to another.

Compassion Genuine caring and concern for people.

Compensatory damages Monetary awards to compensate a plaintiff for damages such as physical injury, lost wages, emotional suffering, and loss of companionship.

Compliance Practice of ensuring that federal, state, and local requirements pertaining to health insurance or benefits are being followed.

Computer file name notation Notation at the end of the letter that identifies the computer file name given to the letter.

Computerized Patient Record (CPR) Another name for an electronic health record; an individual's health information kept in a computer system.

Confidentiality Keeping secret everything that is seen, heard, or performed in the medical office.

Consecutive number filing Method of filing medical charts in the order of lowest to highest number.

Consent To give approval.

Consideration Something of value that is exchanged between two parties; consideration is required as part of a contract.

Consultation When a patient is referred by a primary physician to a specialist, the encounter between the patient and the specialist is a *consultation.*

Continuation sheets Document used to record information regarding a patient's visits to the doctor; may also be known as *progress notes.*

Contract Legal agreement between two parties that creates an obligation.

Contrast medium Substance that can be traced in a radiologic study.

Conventions Symbol such as a set of parentheses or an abbreviation that alerts an assistant to any special notations or conditions of selecting a certain diagnosis code.

Coordination of Benefits (COB) Process used to determine benefits for a patient who is covered by more than one insurance plan; the process ensures that a health care expense is not paid for more than once.

Copayment Set amount that must be paid by a patient or policy holder for each office visit regardless of the cost of the visit.

Copy notation Notation at the end of a letter that identifies who will receive a copy of the letter.

Corporation Recognized separate entity operating independently of its employees and stockholders.

Criminal law Type of law that involves a relationship between an individual and the government.

Cross-reference Filing method that allows a patient's medical record to be easily located in the case of a name change. A patient with a name change would be referenced under the old name and the new name in the master patient index.

Culture Beliefs, behaviors, and attitudes shared by a particular group of people, passed from generation to generation.

Culture care diversity and universality Theory developed by Madeline Leininger stating that a patient's culture should be taken into consideration when providing nursing services to the patient.

Current Procedural Terminology (CPT) Numerical codes representing procedures for which a physician charges fees. The CPT manual contains a listing of codes assigned to medical procedures performed by physicians.

Cycle billing Billing method in which patients are billed at designated intervals throughout the month.

Damages Monetary amounts requested by a plaintiff in consideration for injuries the plaintiff alleges to have received.

Database Computer-based information storage system containing health information about patients, their appointments, diagnoses, and procedures that will appear on insurance claims; results of diagnostic studies, laboratory tests, and x-rays can also be entered.

Day surgery Patients have surgery and go home all within the same day.

Deductible Set amount of money that an insured person must pay each year before insurance benefits will be paid.

Defendant Party or parties accused of wrongdoing.

Deposition Sworn testimony given outside the courtroom.

Diagnosis Physician's determination of a patient's illness or reason for the office visit.

Dictation Voice recording by a health care provider of health information for a patient's medical report.

Digital sender Equipment that can scan many pages quickly and convert the pages into a pdf document; then send the pdf file to any email address.

Discharge summary Synopsis of a patient's hospital treatment.

Double booking Occurrence of overbooking a physician's appointment schedule.

Double-entry bookkeeping Type of bookkeeping system in which entries of equal amounts are made as debits and credits to accounts.

Dual-eligibles Patients who are covered under both Medicare and Medicaid.

Dun Repetitive action to collect payment.

Dunning message Any type of message that makes a request for payment on an account.

Durable power of attorney for health care Legal document giving authority to one person to make health care decisions for another person who is not able to make health care decisions.

Edits Insurance claim review to evaluate compliance with Health Insurance Portability and Accountability Act (HIPAA) standards and the accuracy of the claims

Electronic Data Interchange (EDI) Way of submitting insurance claims electronically between a health care provider and an insurance company.

Electronic Health Record (EHR) Individual's health information kept in a computer system.

Electronic mail (email) Written message sent electronically by computer through a connection to the Internet.

Electronic Medical Record (EMR) Another name for an electronic health record; an individual's health information kept in a computer system.

Electronic Patient Record (EPR) Another name for an electronic health record; an individual's health information kept in a computer system.

Emancipated minor Minor declared by the court to be capable of making adult decisions.

Emergency Department or Emergency Room (ED, ER) Location in a hospital that receives patients who are acutely, seriously, or critically ill or injured.

Emoticon Use of symbols in email to convey feeling.

Empathy Understanding of another person's feelings regarding his or her experiences.

Employee compensation record Payroll data for each individual employee; includes amounts paid and deducted from each check. This information is used at the end of the year to produce W-2 forms.

Employer Identification Number (EIN) Unique number assigned to each employer to use when reporting employment taxes or when giving tax statements to employees. This number identifies the tax account of the employer.

Empower, empowerment To give employees some degree of responsibility (within their expertise) in achieving the mission of an organization.

Enclosure notation Notation at the end of a letter that identifies if additional documents or items are included with the letter.

Encounter form Documentation of a patient's office visit listing the charges incurred and the patient's diagnosis; an invoice for a physician's services; also called a *superbill, fee slip, service record,* or *charge ticket*.

Equal Credit Opportunity Act (ECOA) Enacted in 1975; requires that once credit is extended to one individual, it must be extended to all others. Individuals cannot be denied credit on the basis of race, color, religion, national origin, sex, marital status, or age. Credit can be refused based only on the individual's inability to pay.

Ergonomics Designing work to fit the worker's physical capabilities.

Ethics Rules or principles of right conduct.

Euthanasia Aggressive action intended to hasten a patient's death.

Executive branch Branch of government at both the state and federal level that is responsible for ensuring that laws within its jurisdiction are observed.

Exemplary Damages Monetary awards designed to punish a defendant for wrongdoing. Exemplary damages are also known as punitive damages.

Explanation of Benefits (EOB) Explanation of insurance benefits paid and what, if any, subtractions have been made from a claim. If the claim is rejected, the reason for the rejection is on the EOB.

Express mail Fastest type of delivery offered by the U.S. Postal Service.

Expressed consent Statement from a patient that a physician should provide medical treatment for the patient.

Externship Process in which a student works under the supervision of a medical office employee and receives on-the-job experience; also known as an *internship, clinical,* or *practicum.*

Face sheet Usually the first sheet in a patient's medical record; it includes patient's name, address, phone number, employer and insurance information; also known as a *summary sheet* or *identification sheet.*

Fair Debt Collection Practices Act Legislation that protects debtors against debt collectors who use unfair practices when collecting a debt. Collectors cannot misrepresent themselves, or use threats of violence or offensive language.

Fee-for-service Insurance plan that pays a physician a fee for every patient encounter.

Fee schedule Listing of every procedure done by a practice's physicians and the charge for each procedure.

Fee slip A documentation of a patient's office visit listing the charges incurred and patient's diagnosis; an invoice for a physician's services; also called a *superbill, encounter form, service record,* or *charge ticket.*

Fee splitting Unethical practice of one physician paying another for the referral of a patient.

Feedback Information about a message that a receiver gives to the message's sender.

First-listed diagnosis Chief reason for a patient's outpatient encounter with a physician; also known as *primary diagnosis.*

Fiscal intermediary An insurance company that has been contracted to process claims for Medicare.

Five stages of loss Theory developed by Elizabeth Kübler-Ross that identifies five stages in the grief process. Stages are denial, anger, bargaining, depression, and acceptance.

Fraud Knowingly and willingly billing an insurance company or individual for something that did not occur.

Full-block style Letter formatting style in which all letter components are flush with the left margin; also known as *block style.*

Group insurance Group of people (usually with the same employer) who have the same insurance policy and related benefits.

Group number Number used to identify a group of people who have the same insurance policy and related benefits.

Group (block) scheduling Practice of scheduling more than one patient at the same time, with the idea that those patients will be served by different areas of the clinic.

Guarantor Party responsible for payment of account.

Healthcare Common Procedure Coding System (HCPCS) Coding system established by the federal government; consists of three levels of coding: level I codes are for physician procedures and level II codes are for nonphysician services, supplies, and procedures. Level III codes are no longer used.

Health information management Directing and organizing all activities related to keeping and caring for information concerning health care provided for patients.

Health Maintenance Organization (HMO) Prepaid plan that provides all the care a patient may need in exchange for a flat monthly fee or premium.

Highly confidential information The following health information is identified by HIPAA as highly confidential: mental illness or developmental disability, HIV/AIDS treatment, communicable or venereal diseases, substance abuse, physical abuse, and genetic testing.

History and Physical (H&P) Documents the patient's condition on admission to the hospital.

Home health Care given to a patient in his or her own home.

Hospice care Care provided for terminally ill persons who have a life expectancy of less than 6 months.

Hospital Facility that provides inpatient care—health care that necessitates the patient staying overnight (usually more than a 24-hour period) and having the constant attention of the nursing staff.

Human resources Department of a health care organization that provides services for the people who work for the organization.

ICD-9-CM Diagnosis coding system of numerical codes; the *International Classification of Diseases, 9th Revision, Clinical Modification.* Coding consists of three parts: Volume 1, Tabular List of Diseases (in numerical order); Volume 2, Index of Diseases (in alphabetical order); Volume 3, Index and Tabular List of Procedures.

ICD-10-CM Diagnosis coding system of numerical codes; the *International Classification of Diseases, 10th revision, Clinical Modification.*

Identification sheet Sheet in a patient's chart that identifies the patient and contains pertinent information, such as name, address, telephone number, and insurance.

Identity theft Stealing a person's identification; usually for personal gain.

Implied consent Consent evidenced by a patient's actions; the very act of arriving at an appointment made with a physician may be interpreted as implied consent.

Impression Diagnosis or assessment.

Inactive record Medical record of a patient who has not received treatment within a specified period of time.

Income statement Financial report detailing the profit earned during a specific period of time; also called a profit and loss statement.

Independent Practice Association An independent group of providers which provides coverage under an HMO plan.

Informed consent Patient is given information about his/her medical condition, the treatment alternatives and why treatment is recommended.

Inpatient Patient care given within a hospital setting, usually involving an overnight stay.

Inside address Complete name and address of the person to whom a letter is sent.

Insurance contract or policy Specifies what types of health treatments are covered as well as the amount for which the treatments are covered.

Insured Refers to the individual who holds an insurance policy; also called a *subscriber* or *policyholder*.

Insurer Insurance company.

Internship Process whereby a student works under supervision of a medical office employee and receives on-the-job experience; also known as an *externship*, *clinical*, or *practicum*.

Interrogatories Set of written questions asked of both the defendant and the plaintiff involved in a lawsuit.

Job description Identifies what a person employed in a particular position will be required to do.

Judicial branch Branch of government that establishes case (common) law.

Laboratory report Report documenting results from a laboratory test (e.g., results of urinalysis, complete blood cell count).

Laterality The function of the ICD-10-CM system which allows for a location, such as right or left side, to be identified with a unique diagnosis code.

Law Written rule established by society.

Legal capacity Person's ability to enter into a contract.

Legislative branch Branch of government that consists of senators and representatives elected by the people.

Liabilities Debts of a business.

Limiting charge Maximum amount that a nonparticipating Medicare provider can charge a patient.

Litigation Legal action.

Living will Legal document that communicates a patient's wishes with regard to life-sustaining treatment.

Malpractice Professional misconduct, illegal or immoral, involving an unreasonable lack of skill or fidelity in the performance of professional duties.

Managed care Type of insurance plan that often requires an insured to see a primary care physician initially for treatment. The primary care physician refers the patient to a specialist only if necessary. Managed care plans often require patients to obtain authorizations before beginning certain types of medical treatment.

Master patient index Alphabetical system of filing medical records.

Material Safety Data Sheet (MSDS) All facilities with hazardous substances on site are required to have an MSDS on file for every hazardous substance. The MSDS details the ingredients of the product as well as first aid measures to take in case of wrongful exposure.

Mature minor Minor recognized by some states as capable of making medical decisions without parental consent.

Medical administrative assistant Multiskilled individual who performs administrative support services for the efficient operation of a medical office.

Medical assistant Individual who is qualified to perform both administrative and clinical duties in a medical office.

Medical ethics Values and guidelines governing decisions in medical practice.

Medical history Questionnaire detailing a patient's past illnesses and treatment.

Medical transcription Production of a typewritten medical report from a physician dictation for placement in a patient's file.

Medical transcriptionist Person preparing medical reports from dictation.

Medicaid Federal government health benefits program for low-income or medically needy individuals.

Medicare Federal government health benefits program for persons over 65 or other individuals who meet other conditions.

Medicare Administrative Contractor (MAC) A company that has contracted with Medicare to process claims for Medicare.

Memo Written document used internally in a business to inform employees of routine information.

Mid-level provider Nonphysician provider such as a nurse practitioner or physician assistant.

Minutes Summary of information and discussion that occurred during a meeting.

Modified-block style Letter formatting style in which the date, complimentary closing and signature begin at the center of the page and the remainder of the letter components is flush with the left margin.

Modified-block style with indented paragraphs Letter style in which the date, complimentary closing, and signature begin at the center of the page; paragraphs are indented; and the remainder of the letter components are flush with the left margin. Also known as *semiblock style*.

Modifier Code used to communicate something different about a procedure or service (when coding); used in addition to a procedure code.

Musculoskeletal Disorders (MSDs) Injury or disorder of the muscles, nerves, tendons, ligaments and/or joints brought on by repetitive motion.

Non-Physician Provider practitioner (NPP) Health care provider who is not a physician, such as a nurse practitioner or physician's assistant.

Nonsufficient Funds (NSF) check Check returned by the bank because there are not enough funds in the payer's account to pay the check.

No-show Appointment for which the patient has failed to arrive.

Notation Information written at the end of a letter and intended for use by the practice.

Notice of Privacy Practices Document required by HIPAA that is given to each patient and identifies how the patient's demographic and medical information will be used.

Nursing home Facility providing round-the-clock medical care for residents. Residents are often too ill to be cared for at home, but they are not sick enough to be hospitalized.

Objective Portion of a chart note in which the results of the patient's physical examination are documented.

Occupational Safety and Health Administration (OSHA) Agency of the federal government that establishes and enforces safe work practices.

Offer and acceptance Initial step in establishing a contract—an offer is made by one individual, and the other accepts the offer.

Operative report Detailed account of a patient's surgical procedure.

Optical Character Reader (OCR) Device that allows envelopes to be read by machine to enable speedy processing of mail within the U.S. Postal Service.

Outguide Plastic envelope with pockets; used to mark the place from which a medical record was removed.

Outpatient Medical care provided for patients outside a hospital setting.

Outpatient surgery center Health care facility that provides same day surgery services. Patients check in, receive surgery, and are sent home within the same day.

Participating Provider (PAR) Providers who accept assignment.

Participatory management Management style in which empowerment is present.

Partnership Two or more physicians who do not wish to incorporate can form a *partnership*. Partner physicians share all income and expenses of the practice.

Pathology report Analysis of diseased body tissue that has been sent for testing.

Performance review Review of an employee's performance over a period of one year; it is usually used to determine employee raises.

Physician extender Nonphysician health care provider.

Plaintiff Initiator of a lawsuit.

Plan Portion of a medical report describing what treatment is recommended for the patient.

Policy Agreement between an insurance company (otherwise known as an insurer) and an individual or group of individuals.

Policyholder Individual who holds an insurance policy; also called the *subscriber* or the *insured*.

Policy manual Office publication that details job descriptions and the practice's policies on various human resource–related topics.

Practicum Process in which a student works under the supervision of a medical office employee and receives on-the-job experience; also known as an *externship, internship,* or *clinical*.

Preauthorization Insurance plan's approval for a health care provider to provide a health care service to a patient.

Precertification Insurance plan's approval for a health care provider to provide a health care service to a patient.

Preferred Provider Organization (PPO) Network of health care providers who agree to provide services at a discount for members of the PPO. A PPO may require patients to choose a primary care physician or a primary care clinic.

Premium Payment required for insurance coverage.

Primary care Health services focused on providing care for routine injury and illness. Common providers of primary care are family practice and internal medicine physicians, pediatricians, nurse practitioners, and physician assistants.

Primary care physician Physician designated by a patient to provide initial care for a medical condition.

Principal diagnosis ICD-9 term used to describe a patient's chief reason for admission to a hospital.

Private practice Physician providing outpatient care from a private office in which the physician is the only provider.

Probationary period Specific amount of time, such as 90 days, when an employee is working under a temporary employment arrangement.

Problem-Oriented Medical Record (POMR) Method of organizing a medical record in which all information pertaining to one specific problem is grouped together.

Procedure Service provided for a patient in the course of medical treatment.

Procedure manual Book or booklet that gives instructions for procedures, guidelines, and protocols in a medical office.

Progress notes Information regarding a patient's visits to the doctor.

Protocol Instructions given to use in response to an event.

Provider Individuals who are chiefly responsible for coordinating and delivering health care services; such as physicians, nurses, and nurse practitioners.

Public health agency Agency that provides health care at little or no cost to lower-income individuals. These agencies often educate the community about healthy living, work to prevent or control epidemics, and track and report infectious and communicable diseases to state health departments.

Punitive damages Monetary awards designed to punish a defendant for wrongdoing. Punitive damages are also known as exemplary damages.

Purchase Order (PO) Request to purchase merchandise from an identified supplier.

Quantitative analysis Process in which a patient's record is reviewed to make sure that all necessary components are included in the chart; usually performed after the patient record has been returned to the record room.

Radiology report Results of a patient's radiologic study.

Reciprocity Agreement between states that allow an individual who has met the requirements in one state to meet requirements in another state; applies in the case of licensure of many medical professionals.

Reconciling Making sure that the bank statement and the bank balance are in agreement.

Redacted Removed. If a record is being used for the purpose of research or medical education, all identifying information in the record is redacted.

Reference initials Notation at the end of a letter identifying the author and typist/transcriptionist of a letter.

Referral Approval by the primary care physician for a patient to receive the services of a specialist.

Registered Medical Assistant (RMA) Award given by American Medical Technologists.

Registered Healthcare Documentation Specialist (RHDS) The AHDI has established guidelines for the Registered Healthcare Documentation Specialist (RHDS) examination. This examination is intended for the transcriptionist who is not eligible to complete the CHDS examination. Recent graduates of medical transcription programs are eligible to complete the RHDS.

Referral appointments Appointment made for a patient to see a specialist.

Release Of Information (ROI) Document that specifies what medical information regarding the patient is to be released. The release must be signed by the patient.

Res ipsa loquitur Latin term meaning "the thing speaks for itself." In legal cases involving medical practice, *res ipsa loquitur* means that physical evidence of wrongdoing is proof enough to demonstrate negligence.

Residency Period of time in which a physician is educated in the specialty of his or her choice; the physician is known as a *resident*.

Resident 1. Medical school graduate studying in a medical specialty. 2. Person residing in a nursing home.

Resources Supply of goods or people used to complete necessary tasks.

Respondeat superior Latin term meaning "let the master answer." *Respondeat superior* means that the employer is responsible for the actions of the employee; the employee is deemed to have acted for the employer.

Résumé Document outlining an individual's qualifications for a position; allows the individual give detailed information about his/her education, work experience, personal achievements, strengths, and qualities.

Restrictive endorsement Instructions allowing a check to be deposited only in the account of a particular business, practice, or physician. A check with a *restrictive endorsement* cannot be cashed if lost.

Risk management Means of minimizing the potential for legal action being taken against a practice.

Rotation Third- and fourth-year medical students' experience in different medical specialties.

Salutation Greeting at the beginning of a letter; usually "Dear."

Semiblock style Letter formatting style in which the date, complimentary closing, and signature begin at the center of the page, paragraphs are indented, and the remainder of the letter components are flush with the left margin; also known as *modified-block style* with indented paragraphs.

Service record Documentation of a patient's office visit listing the charges incurred and patient's diagnosis; an invoice for a physician's services. Also called a *superbill, fee slip, encounter form,* or *charge ticket*.

Sexual harassment Unwelcome sexual behavior or innuendo.

Shingling Placing the oldest laboratory report near the back of the chart and laying new reports slightly above and overlapping the top of the previously placed report. This method is used to save space in a patient's chart.

SOAP method Method of documenting patient visits in a chart note. Each letter stands for the type of information in that section of the note: for example, S = Subjective, O = Objective, A = Assessment, P = Plan.

Sole proprietorship Business arrangement that assumes all the liabilities for a practice and receives all income generated by the practice.

Sponsor Veteran on whom CHAMPVA eligibility is based.

Source-Oriented Medical Record (SOMR) Related information grouped together in a patient's medical record.

SSN Social Security number.

Standards of care Level of acceptable care a health care provider is expected to give, usually reasonable and prudent.

Standard precautions Protocol that treats all human blood and bodily fluids as potentially infectious for pathogens, such as the human immunodeficiency virus and hepatitis.

Statute Law established by legislative branch of government.

Statute of limitations Time period in which a patient must file suit for medical malpractice.

Statutory adults Minors who may consent to medical treatment at 14 years of age.

Statutory law Law established by the legislative branch of government; also know as legislative law.

Student portfolio Folder in which students have collected samples of projects and course work they have completed. Students should also keep track of accomplishments and special activities they participated in to present to prospective employers.

Subjective Portion of the chart notes that documents information received from the patient.

Subpoena Order to appear in court.

Subpoena duces tecum Order to produce medical records for trial.

Subscriber Individual who holds the insurance policy; *policyholder*.

Summary sheet Top sheet in a medical file containing a patient's demographic information, including address, telephone, employer, date of birth, insurance information, and next of kin. May also include a brief summary of significant diagnoses, release information, and other necessary information.

Superbill Documentation of a patient's office visit listing the charges incurred and patient's diagnosis; an invoice for a physician's services; also called an *encounter form, fee slip, service record,* or *charge ticket*.

Terminal digit filing Filing method that involves breaking a chart number into a series of groups and filing within each group.

Tickler file System that reminds an assistant to perform a certain activity at a certain time.

Transposition Reversing the order of digits within a number.

Triage Process of determining which patient will receive care first.

TRICARE U.S. military health care benefit program for active-duty service members and other military personnel.

Unbundling Illegal billing practice involving charging individually for items that should be billed together as a package.

Universal precautions Treatment of all human blood and certain bodily fluids as potentially infectious.

Upcoding Illegal billing practice involving coding a higher level of service than was administered to the patient.

Urgent care Providing quick attention to a patient's health problem with immediate access to health care; urgent care centers usually operate on a walk-in basis.

Usual, Customary, and Reasonable (UCR) fee Average amount charged by local physicians for services rendered. Insurers may not pay the portion of a fee that is higher than the UCR fee.

Vendor Business or supplier from which merchandise is being purchased.

Voice mail Telephone system that works like an answering machine: a message is recorded for the caller and the caller can leave a message.

Walk-in Patient who enters a clinic or outpatient facility without an appointment.

Workers' Compensation Insurance coverage for employees who suffer from work-related injuries, diseases, illnesses, or even death.

Index

Page numbers followed by f indicate figures; t, tables; b, boxes.

D

N

O

P